THE SCIENCE
OF SUBJECTIVE WELL-BEING

The
Science of
Subjective
Well-Being

EDITED BY
MICHAEL EID
RANDY J. LARSEN

THE GUILFORD PRESS
New York   London

© 2008 The Guilford Press
A Division of Guilford Publications, Inc.
72 Spring Street, New York, NY 10012
www.guilford.com

Printed in the United States of America

This book is printed on acid-free paper.

Last digit is print number: 9 8 7 6 5 4 3 2 1

Library of Congress Cataloging-in-Publication Data

The science of subjective well-being / edited by Michael Eid and Randy J. Larsen.
   p. cm.
  Includes bibliographical references and index.
  ISBN-13: 978-1-59385-581-9 (hardcover : alk. paper)
  ISBN-10: 1-59385-581-8 (hardcover : alk. paper)
  1. Happiness. 2. Well-being. I. Eid, Michael. II. Larsen, Randy J.
  BF575.H27S39 2008
  158—dc22

                                            2007027502

About the Editors

Michael Eid, DSc, is Professor of Psychology at the Free University of Berlin, Germany. Dr. Eid is currently Editor of *Methodology—European Journal of Research Methods for the Behavioral and Social Sciences* and Associate Editor of the *Journal of Positive Psychology*. His main research interests are subjective well-being, mood regulation, multimethod measurement, and longitudinal data analysis.

Randy J. Larsen, PhD, is the William R. Stuckenberg Professor of Human Values and Moral Development and Chair of the Psychology Department at Washington University in St. Louis. He conducts research on emotion, primarily in terms of differences between people, and studies such topics as subjective well-being, mood variability, jealousy, attraction, depression, and strategies for the self-management of self-esteem and emotion. Dr. Larsen is an elected member of the Society of Multivariate Experimental Psychology and is listed as one of the highly cited psychologists by the Institute for Scientific Information.

Contributors

Robert M. Biswas-Diener, MS, Department of Psychology, Portland State University, Portland, Oregon

David M. Buss, PhD, Department of Psychology, University of Texas at Austin, Austin, Texas

John T. Cacioppo, PhD, Department of Psychology, University of Chicago, Chicago, Illinois

Rebecca J. Compton, PhD, Department of Psychology, Haverford College, Haverford, Pennsylvania

Carol Diener, PhD, JD, Department of Psychology, University of Illinois at Urbana–Champaign, Champaign, Illinois

Ed Diener, PhD, Department of Psychology, University of Illinois at Urbana–Champaign, Champaign, Illinois

Marissa L. Diener, PhD, Department of Family and Consumer Studies, University of Utah, Salt Lake City, Utah

Mary Beth Diener McGavran, PhD, Department of Psychology, University of Kentucky, Lexington, Kentucky

Michael Eid, DSc, Department of Psychology, Free University of Berlin, Berlin, Germany

Robert A. Emmons, PhD, Department of Psychology, University of California at Davis, Davis, California

Barbara L. Fredrickson, PhD, Department of Psychology, University of North Carolina at Chapel Hill, Chapel Hill, North Carolina

Frank Fujita, PhD, Department of Psychology, Indiana University South Bend, South Bend, Indiana

Louise C. Hawkley, PhD, Department of Psychology, University of Chicago, Chicago, Illinois

Daniel M. Haybron, PhD, Department of Philosophy, Saint Louis University, St. Louis, Missouri

E. Scott Huebner, PhD, Department of Psychology, University of South Carolina at Columbia, Columbia, South Carolina

M. E. Hughes, PhD, Center for the Study of Aging and Human Development, Duke University Medical Center, Durham, North Carolina

Sarah E. Hill, PhD, Department of Psychology, California State University– Fullerton, Fullerton, California

Timothy A. Judge, PhD, Department of Management, University of Florida, Gainesville, Florida

Ariel Kalil, PhD, Harris School of Public Policy Studies, University of Chicago, Chicago, Illinois

Laura A. King, PhD, Department of Psychological Sciences, University of Missouri, Columbia, Missouri

Ryan Klinger, MSM, Department of Management, University of Florida, Gainesville, Florida

Jayoung Koo, MA, Department of Psychology, Yonsei University, Seoul, South Korea

Minkyung Koo, MA, Department of Psychology, University of Virginia, Charlottesville, Virginia

Randy J. Larsen, PhD, Department of Psychology, Washington University in St. Louis, St. Louis, Missouri

Richard E. Lucas, PhD, Department of Psychology, Michigan State University, East Lansing, Michigan

Darrin M. McMahon, PhD, Department of History, Florida State University, Tallahassee, Florida

David G. Myers, PhD, Department of Psychology, Hope College, Holland, Michigan

Shigehiro Oishi, PhD, Department of Psychology, University of Virginia, Charlottesville, Virginia

William Pavot, PhD, Department of Social Science, Southwest Minnesota State University, Marshall, Minnesota

Zvjezdana Prizmic, PhD, Department of Psychology, Washington University in St. Louis, St. Louis, Missouri

Michael D. Robinson, PhD, Department of Psychology, North Dakota State University, Fargo, North Dakota

Ulrich Schimmack, PhD, Department of Psychology, University of Toronto at Mississauga, Mississauga, Ontario, Canada

Eunkook M. Suh, PhD, Department of Psychology, Yonsei University, Seoul, South Korea

Ronald A. Thisted, PhD, Departments of Health Studies and Statistics, University of Chicago, Chicago, Illinois

Ruut Veenhoven, PhD, Faculty of Social Science, Erasmus University of Rotterdam, Rotterdam, The Netherlands

Linda Waite, PhD, Department of Sociology, University of Chicago, Chicago, Illinois

Preface

What is happiness? Does happiness have distinct components, or is it a singular global state? How can it be measured? What causes happiness? What are the consequences of happiness? What predicts happiness? Are there national or cultural differences in happiness? How might people become happier, if they wanted to? Although answers to questions such as these are fundamental to our understanding of human functioning and flourishing, it has only been over the last 25 years that we have seen an increasing amount of empirical research in the social and behavioral sciences on the topic of happiness. This interest has crystallized in the foundation of a new discipline of psychology called "positive psychology." The development of positive psychology has its roots in the prescient and ground-breaking work of Ed Diener, who has devoted his scientific life over the last 25 years to the kinds of questions with which we began this paragraph. His scientific work has strongly influenced psychology and made him one of the most cited living psychologists. His work has also attracted many collaborators from all over the world, and his encouraging and warmhearted approach has strongly influenced many scientific careers. It was the desire of many of his former students, postdocs, and collaborators to take the occasion of his 60th birthday, and his approaching retirement, to honor Ed and to thank him for his scientific and personal inspiration, support, and friendship.

In publishing over 200 scientific articles and several books on subjective well-being, Ed Diener has been active in defining the field and training an entire new generation of scholars in this area. Many of these scholars have gone on to develop outstanding careers of their own in the field of positive psychology and related areas. Ed Diener and his former students and current colleagues form a large corps of researchers who are working at the cutting edge of the science of subjective well-being. Our intent in producing this book was to bring together this corps of researchers and scholars, along with others working in related disciplines, and have them each contribute a chapter to a volume that will be a definitive statement about the state of knowledge in the broad area of subjective well-being. Although the book takes its focus from topics connected to the work of Ed Diener, we have not asked the authors to address this connection in their chapters. Rather, authors were asked to contribute authoritative summaries of the key issues and current state of knowledge in regard to specific themes concerning subjective well-being.

We organized the book around five major themes. These include a broad overview of subjective well-being from multiple perspectives, including philosophy, history, sociology, and evolution. The second broad theme is measurement, which is of great importance to any discipline purporting to be a science. The third theme concerns aspects of life that are related to subjective well-being, including personality, social connectedness, social comparison, material wealth, religion, and emotion regulation. The fourth theme concerns different life domains wherein subjective well-being is manifest in important ways, including the family, institutions such as schools and the workplace, and in cultural contexts. The fifth theme focuses on interventions that may work to make people happier.

This handbook is the product of a common enterprise among many active researchers in the field of subjective well-being and happiness. It is not a festschrift in the usual sense but a handbook or upper-level textbook that gives an overview of the science of subjective well-being and covers contributions not only from psychology but from many other disciplines that deal with fundamental questions of subjective well-being. This book should assist readers from psychology as well as other disciplines in forming a deeper understanding of the many facets of subjective well-being—its definition and measurement, its predictors and consequences, and the ways it can be enhanced. It is suitable for self-study or as a foundation for a course or seminar on subjective well-being. We hope that readers enjoy the book and profit from the enthusiasm with which the many contributors have written their chapters, in honoring one of the leading scientists in this area of research.

Contents

III. THE HAPPY PERSON

IV. SUBJECTIVE WELL-BEING
IN THE INTERPERSONAL DOMAIN

V. MAKING PEOPLE HAPPIER

VI. CONCLUSIONS AND FUTURE DIRECTIONS

1

Ed Diener and the Science of Subjective Well-Being

RANDY J. LARSEN and MICHAEL EID

Although this book is not intended to be a festschrift, the opening chapter does highlight the contributions of one person: We show how the field of subjective well-being has been shaped and influenced by the efforts of Ed Diener. His impact has resulted not just from his own extensive body of empirical work, but also from his thoughtful and integrative review papers, his edited volumes, his wide-ranging collaborations with a large number of scientists around the world, his work with the popular press, and his success in training a substantial number of well-equipped PhD and postdoctoral students who have gone on to make their own contributions to the field of subjective well-being.

In tracing Ed Diener's contributions, we begin by noting that he had a successful research career before he turned to subjective well-being. In fact, prior to his work on positive characteristics, Ed Diener focused on some of the darker aspects of human nature. Before the 1980s he worked primarily on the topic of deindividuation (e.g., Diener, Fraser, Beaman, & Kelem, 1976), the notion that people in a group would sometimes behave in ways that were against the values and morals of the individuals in the group, such as is often the case with lynching, pillaging, gang rape, genocide and other autocracies committed by groups. The title of his dissertation, completed in 1975, was: "Prior destructive behavior, anonymity, and group presence as antecedents of deindividuation and aggression," so it is obvious that Ed Diener was a card-carrying member of the Dark Side before he helped define the field of positive psychology. By the time he achieved tenure at the University of Illinois, he was a leading authority on aggression and group violence, and had produced important papers on related topics such as gun ownership and crime, stealing, and television violence. He was a poster child for normative psychology at the time, which focused on negative aspects of human nature and behavior.

All this changed in the early 1980s, however. In 1980, Ed Diener took his first sabbatical. He went to the Virgin Islands for a year, with the explicit goal of changing the focus of his research career. He felt he had gone about as far as he wanted to go with the topic of deindividuation, and so went to the Virgin Islands to think long and hard about what to do next. He kept in touch with his graduate students back at Illinois, via letters, since the Internet and e-mail had not been invented yet. During that year he read through several distinct literatures, including political psychology and evolution, but reported to his graduate students that he found them unsatisfying for a number of reasons. When he finally got back to Illinois, no one knew what to expect. He called his research team together and made the announcement that he wanted to study what makes people happy. His graduate students were shocked, and most thought he had spent too much time on the beach during his sabbatical. Nevertheless, they went along with him, partly to humor him and partly because the topic was something that seemed new and interesting.

In 1980 most of the research that had been done on happiness and related constructs was survey research. Not much systematic work had been done in terms of defining and measuring this construct. And so Ed Diener and his research team set out to do some basic descriptive and measurement evaluation research, turning first to the experience sampling method to track people over time in terms of their day-to-day reports of subjective well-being. Diener also began a systematic review of the existing literature and taught a graduate seminar on subjective well-being in 1982.

Ed Diener's review of the literature culminated in 1984 when he published an article titled "Subjective Well-Being" in the *Psychological Bulletin*. This paper soon became a citation classic, and then a mega-citation classic, having been cited, as of this writing, over 1,265 times. Diener (1984) gave an overview of the field of subjective well-being that was, at the time, not the focus of psychological research. This paper was not only the cornerstone of a very fruitful and successful empirical research program of the Diener lab but also ignited many other laboratories, in the United States and around the world, to study the topic of subjective well-being. Starting in 1984 the number of papers published each year on subjective well-being doubled from the previous year, with this rapid acceleration in research output being sustained for almost a decade. Ed Diener himself has published over 200 papers since 1984, along with three books. His work has had a strong impact on the field. His work has been cited over 10,000 times, and he has 22 papers that are citation classics (over 100 citations each) and two papers that are mega-citation classics (over 1,000 citations each; one was the *Psychological Bulletin* paper mentioned above, and the other was the publication of his Satisfaction with Life Scale, the most widely used assessment instrument in subjective well-being research).

Ed Diener's contributions to the field are manifold and lasting. He is interested in the refinement of theoretical models of subjective well-being, the development and application of measurement instruments for assessing subjective well-being, and the conditions, consequences, and correlates of subjective well-being. He is fascinated by the possibilities that cross-cultural settings are opening for researching the universal causes of happiness, but also for detecting indigenous structures and correlates of subjective well-being. Most recently, his work concerns the many positive consequences that subjective well-being has for the single individual and also for society in general. The insights he has gained from all of his work have convinced him that it is necessary for policy makers to not only consider economic criteria for evaluating the state of a society and its members, but they must also include national indicators of subjective well-being as a basis for policy decision and improving the wealth and the well-being of a society. We now review a few selected aspects of his contributions in more detail.

The Structure of Subjective Well-Being

In the mid-1980s there was an active debate about the nature of, and relationship between, positive and negative affect. Diener and Emmons (1984) wrote an influential paper demonstrating that trait measures of positive affect (PA) and negative affect (NA) were essentially uncorrelated, meaning that how much of one affect a person tended to experience had no bearing on how much of the other he or she experienced. This finding led the way for conceptualizing the independent contributions of each to the hedonic component of overall subjective well-being. Today, many researchers view this hedonic component of subjective well-being as the ratio of PA to NA, over time, in a person's life (Larsen & Prizmic, Chapter 13, this volume) and view it as an important component in the overall structure of subjective well-being.

Diener and colleagues also investigated other dimensions of affective experience in relation to subjective well-being, including the characteristic intensity and frequency of affective experience (Diener, Larsen, Levine, & Emmons, 1985). It turns out that the typical intensity with which people experience their affective states, although an interesting dimension in its own right (e.g., Larsen & Diener, 1987), has no impact on overall subjective well-being (Larsen & Diener, 1985). Rather, what turns out to be the best predictor of global subjective well-being, in terms of affective experience, is the frequency of positive compared to negative states in a person's life over time (Larsen, Diener, & Emmons, 1985). Indeed, one of the best short measures of the affective component of subjective well-being is that developed by Fordyce (1988), which asks people to estimate the percent of time they feel happy, the percent of time they feel neutral, and the percent of time they feel unhappy over a given time period (e.g., the past year), such that it adds up to 100%. This measure correlates very highly with a wide variety of criterion measures of subjective well-being, including the long-term ratio of PA to NA assessed with experience sampling measures (Larsen et al., 1985).

Subjective well-being has another component in addition to the hedonic component; it includes a cognitive judgment about one's life, as a whole, as satisfying. Some researchers refer to this as life satisfaction, and most see it as an essential feature in the overall structure of subjective well-being. It is possible for judgments of life satisfaction to be at variance with the hedonic component (e.g., a starving artist who has a lot of negative affect and little positive affect in his or her life, but nevertheless judges his or her life to be satisfying and worthwhile). However, in most populations the life satisfaction component and the hedonic component of subjective well-being are at least moderately and sometimes highly correlated (Diener, Napa-Scollon, Oishi, Dzokoto, & Suh, 2000).

The Measurement of Subjective Well-Being

Can happiness be measured—and, if yes, in which way? An answer to this question is fundamental for an empirical science of subjective well-being. Ed Diener often tells the anecdote about his interest as a student, in the happiness of farm workers (because his parents owned a big farm) and that he wanted to conduct a study on this topic as a part of his school requirements. His professor refused this project for two reasons. First, he thought that happiness could not be measured, and second, he was convinced that farm workers could not be happy. This experience might have motivated Ed Diener's strong emphasis on measurement issues, particularly the development of measurement methods and their validation.

Because *subjective well-being* refers to affective experiences and cognitive judgments, self-report measures of subjective well-being are indispensable. With his collaborators Ed Diener developed the Satisfaction with Life Scale (Diener, Emmons, Larsen, & Griffin, 1985), which became the standard measure of life satisfaction in the field and has been translated into many languages. Moreover, he developed measurement procedures for the affective components of subjective well-being such as the intensity and frequency of emotion (Larsen & Diener,

1985; Schimmack & Diener, 1997), and was one of the early proponents of experience sampling methods using beepers and hand-held computers to assess affective states in people's natural lives. His main messages concerning the measurement of subjective well-being are (1) that subjective well-being can be assessed by self-report with substantial reliability and validity, (2) that each measurement method has advantages and pitfalls, and (3) that the more complete assessment of subjective well-being requires a multimethod assessment tool (e.g., Diener, 1994; Diener & Eid, 2006; Scollon, Kim-Prieto, & Diener, 2003). Psychology offers many methods that can be used to assess facets of subjective well-being, such as self-reports, peer reports, observational methods, physiological methods, emotion-sensitive tasks such as the speeded recall of happy experiences, and other cognitive tasks such as word-completion and word recognition tasks (Sandvik, Diener, & Seidlitz, 1993; Lucas, Diener, & Larsen, 2003). All these different methods do not perfectly converge, because they assess different facets of subjective well-being and can be affected by specific biases, but the differences between these methods often contain important information. Thomas and Diener (1990), for example, found that people overestimate their emotional intensity and underestimate the frequency of their positive affect when recalling emotional experiences. This finding shows that there is a bias in the recall of affective experiences that only can be detected by using several methods (in situ assessment vs. recall assessment). Both methods contain important information. Although the recall might be biased, it might strongly determine how people reconstruct their lives and might guide future behavior. In contrast, experience sampling methods measure affect in situ and might provide more information about subjective well-being in real time. Multimethod assessment procedures of emotions offer many important insights into the structure and processes of subjective well-being (Larsen & Prizmic-Larsen, 2006), and Ed Diener's ideas of measurement issues have strongly influenced the development of assessment methods (Pavot, Chapter 7, this issue) as well as the development and application of sophisticated statistical tools for analyzing subjective well-being data (Eid, Chapter 8, this issue).

The Determinants of Subjective Well-Being

Diener's research indicates that there is no sole determinant of subjective well-being. Some conditions seem to be necessary for high subjective well-being (e.g., mental health, positive social relationships), but they are not, in themselves, sufficient to cause happiness. His research has identified a number of conditions that appear to be necessary for happiness, or are correlated with happiness, though no single condition or characteristic is sufficient to bring about happiness in itself.

Research out of the Diener lab supports the idea of Costa and McCrae (1980) that personality factors, especially extraversion and neuroticism, are important contributors to subjective well-being. Extraversion most likely influences subjective well-being because it is related to feeling more positive emotions and having a lower threshold for activating positive affect. On the other hand, neuroticism is strongly related to feeling more negative emotions and a lower threshold for activating negative affect. The two personality traits thus work in reciprocal fashion to influence the hedonic component of subjective well-being.

Diener and Seligman (2002) examined the characteristics of the happiest 10% of a college student sample. They compared the upper 10% of consistently very happy people to average and very unhappy people. The very happy people were highly social, with strong romantic and other close social relationships, compared to less happy groups. They were more extraverted, more agreeable, less neurotic, and lower on several Minnesota Multiphasic Personality Inventory (MMPI) psychopathology scales. The happiest subjects did not exercise significantly more, participate in religious activities significantly more, or experience more objectively defined good events. Diener and Seligman (2002) concluded that good social relations were necessary for happiness. The happiest group experienced generally positive, but not ecstatic feelings, most of the time, though they also reported occasional negative moods. This finding suggests that even very happy people have a responsive emotion system that reacts appropriately to life events.

Some researchers have implicated genetic determinants of subjective well-being based on data from twin studies. Some of these studies, conducted at the University of Minnesota and reviewed by Lykken (1999), found that monozygotic twins reared apart are more similar in happiness levels than are dyzygotic twins who were reared together. The twin studies (and adoption studies as well) suggest that some portion of the variability in happiness is likely due to genetic contributions. Studies of specific gene influences suggest that genes linked with a propensity toward depression or extraversion and neuroticism might be responsible for the genetics of subjective well-being.

Some researchers, and many popular writers, have interpreted the genetic evidence to mean that happiness is determined by DNA endowment. This is not true for several reasons, as Diener has argued in several places. First, in most genetic studies, there is a fair amount of variability in happiness over time. Although the long-term or setpoint level of happiness a person reports across two or more time periods has a heritable component, people's moods and emotions and level of satisfaction—and hence their subjective well-being—moves up and down, over time, in reaction to life events. A second piece of evidence supporting environmental effects on subjective well-being also comes from the twin studies. Researchers typically find that early family environment (twins who grow up in the same home) has an influence on levels of positive affect that the twins experience as adults. In other words, something about the shared family environment in childhood predisposes individuals to later feeling less or more positive emotions, such as joy, enthusiasm, and engagement.

Diener's lab has also provided evidence for environmental effects on subjective well-being in terms of the large differences between nations in life satisfaction and other subjective well-being variables. The poorest and richest nations, for example, differ substantially in subjective well-being (Diener & Suh, 1999). Former Communist nations, which have recently gone through political transition, show much lower rates of subjective well-being than nearby non-Communist nations (Diener & Seligman, 2004). So the larger environment seems to influence happiness, and it would appear unlikely that these national differences are due to genetic differences (see Inglehart & Klingemann, 2000, for a fuller exposition of this argument).

Other results that also argue against the idea that subjective well-being is determined by genetic inheritance come from Diener and colleagues' longitudinal studies in Germany (Diener, Nickerson, Lucas, & Sandvik, 2002; Lucas, Clark, Georgellis, & Diener, 2004). They repeatedly find that people who become unemployed are less happy, and they remain so for many years, compared to people with steady employment. Diener and colleagues also report, similarly, that women who get married are, on average, somewhat happier than their unwed counterparts for several years (Lucas, Clark, Georgellis, & Diener, 2003).

A final piece of evidence for environmental effects comes from data on widows. Studies show that widows remain less happy for several years after their partner dies. That is, genetic predisposition notwithstanding, widows, on average, are made less happy by the tragedy that befalls them. In sum, many findings argue that happiness is not solely genetic—the environment matters too. Although genetic effects are undoubtedly important, cultural and situational factors also influence subjective well-being, sometimes strongly.

Furthermore, there is evidence that different conditions and outcomes make different people happy. For example, Diener and colleagues have shown that the correlates of happiness vary between young versus old people (Diener & Suh, 1998). Similarly, Diener, Suh, Smith, and Shao (1995) reported that there are different correlates of happiness in different cultures. Of course, at some basic level, Diener (e.g., Diener, Diener, & Diener, 1995) has argued that there are probably universals—for example, having close social relationships—but there are also specific conditions, characteristics, and activities that make some people more satisfied but that have little effect on others.

When it comes to considering the determinants of subjective well-being, Diener has made the analogy to a recipe rather than a single cause. Most good recipes call for several ingredients. Some ingredients are essential, others are merely helpful or add a particular flavor or texture to the outcome. But there is no single key ingredient that, by itself, produces the outcome; instead one needs to have multiple ingredients put together in the right way. A similar case holds for subjective well-being—one needs several important and necessary ingredients, but no single one of them, by itself, produces a happy person.

The Consequences of Subjective Well-Being

The pursuit of happiness is a right that every American possesses, according to the Declaration of Independence. The term *happiness* even appears in several drafts of the European Union constitution. To be happy is one of the major goals, if not the ultimate goal, of human beings. To be happy is a quality itself, and a lot of research has been devoted to identifying the conditions for, and the causes of, happiness. During the last few years the consequences and benefits of happiness have also come into the focus of research. Happiness might not only be a goal of life but also a means for reaching other goals and for facilitating desirable behaviors and outcomes. In a recent review Lyubomirsky, King, and Diener (2005) showed that happy people are successful in many life domains and that this success is at least partly due to their happiness (see Oishi & Koo, Chapter 14, this volume; King, Chapter 21, this volume). Happy people are more social, altruistic, active, like themselves and others more, have strong bodies and immune systems, and have better conflict resolution skills. Moreover, pleasant moods promote creative thinking. Many of these results have been found in cross-sectional and experimental studies, and it will be one of the most fascinating research questions of the future to analyze the consequences of subjective well-being in long-term studies over the lifespan and to see whether interventions to enhance subjective well-being (see Emmons, Chapter 23, this volume; King, Chapter 23, this volume) will have sustainable and long-lasting effects.

Cross-Cultural Research on Subjective Well-Being

Although the pursuit of happiness seems to be a general drive of life, there are strong inter- and intracultural differences in the way people appreciate happiness and in the routes to happiness (Suh & Koo, Chapter 20, this volume). Ed Diener's lab has contributed to our understanding of cultural differences in subjective well-being in many important ways (for an overview, see Diener & Suh, 2000). There are strong national differences in citizens' overall satisfaction with life. Although most people are happy, Diener, Diener, and Diener (1995) could show that international differences in subjective well-being are positively correlated with international differences in income, individualism, human rights, and societal equality. There are universal predictors of subjective well-being that have been found in several nations, such as extraversion (Diener, Oishi, & Lucas, 2003) and marriage (Lucas, Clark, Georgellis, & Diener, 2003), but there are also differences between nations. In individualistic nations judgments of subjective well-being are more strongly based on the emotions people experience and their self-esteem, whereas financial satisfaction was a stronger predictor in poorer countries. Life satisfaction is more strongly related to autonomy, feelings of meaning, and growth in Western cultures than in Eastern ones. However, in collectivistic cultures, those higher in autonomy are also higher in levels of problems such as suicide and divorce (Diener & Suh, 2003). Nations also differ in the norms for experiencing positive emotions, with Eastern nations devaluing some positive emotions such as pride and satisfaction (Eid & Diener, 2001). There are also strong differences between cultures in the stability and variability of affective experiences across situations, with Japanese and Hispanic Americans showing higher intraindividual variability in positive affect than European Americans, for example (Oishi, Diener, Scollon, & Biswas-Diener, 2004). These few results show that Ed Diener's work has formed the cornerstones of a cross-cultural psychology of subjective well-being that helps us to understand how to live a happy life all over the world.

National Indicators of Subjective Well-Being

People pursue happiness, and the happiness of citizens has many benefits for society. How can policy use the insights that research on subjective well-being has uncovered? Diener and Seligman (2004) argue that national indicators are needed to inform policy makers about the well-being of their citizens. In their article "Beyond Money: Toward an Economy of Well-Being" they discuss the shortcomings of economic measures and outline the profits society can gain from enhancing the well-being of its citizens. Citizens that are high in well-being might facilitate governance, they can increase the wealth of a nation by earning more money and creating more opportunities for others, they might be more productive and profitable, they might be healthier and live longer, they might be less prone to mental disabilities and create more satisfying social relationships. Diener and Seligman (2004) outline the requirements that a national indicator of subjective well-being has to fulfill and propose a large-scale research program to develop and refine such indicators. Although the development of national indicators is in its initial stage, it is likely that Ed Diener will promote this topic in his future research and that this idea will gain the attention from policy makers that it deserves.

Summary

Interest in subjective well-being and happiness has been an undercurrent in scholarly thinking for a long time. After all, Aristotle wrote an entire treatise—*The Nicomachean Ethics*—on happiness and the "good" life centuries ago. Even in psychology there has been a continuous line of scholars writing on optimal functioning, such as Maslow's work on self-actualization. So what is really "new" in Ed Diener's work and in the positive psychology movement that he helped create? What is new, and important, is that Diener and his colleagues have employed the empirical methods of scientific psychology to build up the knowledge base on subjective well-being, to create reliable and valid measures of subjective well-being, and to empirically test predictions derived from theories about subjective well-being. Previous scholars were more of the armchair variety, whereas Ed Diener and the new cohort of subjective well-being scientists represented in this volume are of a more empirical tradition. The application of the scientific method to various topics has proven amazingly powerful in the past two centuries in such areas as medicine, chemistry, and physics. It is now being applied to questions in psychology that have formerly been approached through such prescientific methods as introspection, narrative, or qualitative strategies.

The scientific method applied to questions of subjective well-being is yielding tremendous gains in our knowledge. We reviewed several areas of knowledge gain above that were mainly due to the work of Ed Diener, who is a relentless proponent of the scientific method. The scientific method is useful for several reasons. First, it is self-correcting. Scientists are methodologically skeptical, always searching for ways to put their best ideas in grave danger of being refuted. Science also awards higher credibility to findings that replicate, and the field encourages scientists to check each other's work. And finally, science is incremental; individual scientists build on the work of others, adding pieces to the knowledge base as a field progresses. In this chapter, we have highlighted several areas where Ed Diener has laid the foundational findings upon which others are now building. The strength of this scientific foundation will ensure that knowledge built on it will survive the test of time and achieve a degree of permanence and credibility lasting well into the future.

Another way Ed Diener's work is significant is his emphasis on how happiness is important, in and of itself. When people are asked, they say that subjective well-being is extremely important in their lives. For example, Diener has shown that college students the world over rated happiness and life satisfaction as very important or extremely important. In fact, in only one country did students rate money as more important than life satisfaction, and happiness was rated as more important than money in every single country examined. Attaining happiness in life appears to be an almost universal human goal.

Another way subjective well-being is important is that it appears to lead to many good outcomes in life. The work of Diener and colleagues has established that happy people are, among other things, more sociable and creative, they live longer and have stronger immune systems, they make more money, are better leaders, and are better "citizens" in their workplace. A host of good outcomes (e.g., marital satisfaction, job satisfaction, better coping) often follows from happiness. Thus, there are many reasons to suggest that high subjective well-being is extremely desirable at both individual and societal levels.

Given findings such as these, Diener has recently moved beyond science into the realm of social policy. He has shown that nations with higher mean subjective well-being (compared to low) have longer life expectancy, more job security, more political stability, lower divorce rates, better records of civil liberty, and more gender equality. He has argued that social policies need to be evaluated with respect to impact on national subjective well-being, not just economic or job-related outcomes. If the rights of citizens include the right to pursue happiness, then policies need to be established and evaluated with respect to fostering that right. In this way, the legacy of Ed Diener's work will extend beyond his outstanding scientific record and may actually have an impact on how governments and businesses develop and evaluate social policy.

References

Costa, P. T., & McCrae, R. R. (1980). Influence of extraversion and neuroticism on subjective well-being: Happy and unhappy people. *Journal of Personality and Social Psychology, 38,* 668–678.

Diener, E. (1984). Subjective well-being. *Psychological Bulletin, 95,* 542–575.

Diener, E. (1994). Assessing subjective well-being: Progress and opportunities. *Social Indicators Research, 31,* 103–157.

Diener, E., Diener, M., & Diener, C. (1995). Factors predicting the subjective well-being of nations. *Journal of Personality and Social Psychology, 69,* 851–864.

Diener, E., & Eid, M. (2006). The finale: Take-home messages from the editors. In M. Eid & E. Diener (Eds.), *Handbook of multimethod measurement in psychology* (pp. 457–463). Washington, DC: American Psychological Association.

Diener, E., & Emmons, R. A. (1985). The independence of positive and negative affect. *Journal of Personality and Social Psychology, 47,* 1105–1117.

Diener, E., Emmons, R. A., Larsen, R. J., & Griffin, S. (1985). The Satisfaction With Life Scale. *Journal of Personality Assessment, 49,* 71–75.

Diener, E., Fraser, S. C., Beaman, A. L., & Kelem, R. T. (1976). Effects of deindividuation variables on stealing among Halloween trick-or-treaters. *Journal of Personality and Social Psychology, 33,* 178–183.

Diener, E., Larsen, R. J., Levine, S., & Emmons, R. A. (1985). Frequency and intensity: Dimensions underlying positive and negative affect. *Journal of Personality and Social Psychology, 48,* 1253–1265.

Diener, E., Napa-Scollon, C. K., Oishi, S., Dzokoto, V., & Suh, E. M. (2000). Positivity and the construction of life satisfaction judgments: Global happiness is not the sum of its parts. *Journal of Happiness Studies, 1,* 159–176.

Diener, E., Nickerson, C., Lucas, R. E., & Sandvik, E. (2002). Dispositional affect and job outcomes. *Social Indicators Research, 59,* 229–259.

Diener, E., Oishi, S., & Lucas, R. E. (2003). Personality, culture, and subjective well-being: Emotional and cognitive evaluations of life. *Annual Review of Psychology, 54,* 403–425.

Diener, E., & Seligman, M. E. P. (2002). Very happy people. *Psychological Science, 13,* 81–84.

Diener, E., & Seligman, M. E. P. (2004). Beyond money: Toward an economy of well-being. *Psychological Science in the Public Interest, 5,* 1–31.

Diener, E., & Suh, E. M. (1998). Subjective well-being and age: An international analysis. In K. W. Schaie & M. P. Lawton (Eds.), *Annual review of gerontology and geriatrics, Vol. 17: Focus on emotion and adult development* (pp. 304–324). New York: Springer.

Diener, E., & Suh, E. M. (1999). National differences in subjective well-being. In D. Kahneman, E. Diener, & N. Schwarz (Eds.), *Well-being: The foundations of hedonic psychology* (pp. 434–450). New York: Sage.

Diener, E., & Suh, E. M. (2000). *Culture and subjective well-being.* Cambridge, MA: MIT Press.

Diener, E., Suh, E. M., Smith, H., & Shao, L. (1995). National differences in reported subjective well-being: Why do they occur? *Social Indicators Research Special Issue: Global Report on Student Well-Being, 34,* 7–32.

Eid, M., & Diener, E. (2001). Norms for experiencing emotions in different cultures: Inter- and intranational differences. *Journal of Personality and Social Psychology, 81,* 869–885.

Fordyce, M. W. (1988). A review of results on the happiness measures: A 60-second index of happiness and mental health. *Social Indicators Research, 20,* 355–381.

Inglehart, R., & Klingemann, H. D. (2000). Genes, culture, democracy, and happiness. In E. Diener & E. M. Suh (Eds.), *Culture and subjective well-being* (pp. 165–183). Cambridge, MA: MIT Press.

Larsen, R. J., & Diener, E. (1985). A multitrait–multimethod examination of affect structure: Hedonic level and emotional intensity. *Personality and Individual Differences, 6,* 631–636.

Larsen, R. J., & Diener, E. (1987). Affect intensity as an individual difference characteristic: A review. *Journal of Research in Personality, 21,* 1–39.

Larsen, R. J., Diener, E., & Emmons, R. A. (1985). An evaluation of subjective well-being measures. *Social Indicators Research, 17,* 1–18.

Larsen, R. J., & Prizmic-Larsen, Z. (2006). Measuring emotions: Implications of a multimethod perspective. In M. Eid & E. Diener (Eds.), *Handbook of multimethod measurement in psychology* (pp. 337–351). Washington, DC: American Psychological Association.

Lucas, R. E., Clark, A. E., Georgellis, Y., & Diener, E. (2003). Reexamining adaptation and the set point model of happiness: Reactions to changes in marital status. *Journal of Personality and Social Psychology, 84,* 527–539.

Lucas, R. E., Clark, A. E., Georgellis, Y., & Diener, E. (2004). Unemployment alters the set point for life satisfaction. *Psychological Science, 15*, 8–13.

Lucas, R. E., Diener, E., & Larsen, R. J. (2003). Measuring positive emotions. In S. J. Lopez & C. R. Snyder (Eds.), *Positive psychological assessment: A handbook of models and measures* (pp. 201–218). Washington, DC: American Psychological Association.

Lykken, D. (1999). *Happiness: What studies on twins show us about nature, nurture, and the happiness set-point.* New York: Golden Books.

Lyubomirsky, S., King, L., & Diener, E. (2005). The benefits of frequent positive affect: Does happiness lead to success? *Psychological Bulletin, 131*, 803–855.

Oishi, S., Diener, E., Scollon, N. C., & Biswas-Diener, R. (2004). Cross-situational consistency of affective experiences across cultures. *Journal of Personality and Social Psychology, 86*, 460–472.

Sandvik, E., Diener, E., & Seidlitz, L. (1993). Subjective well-being: The convergence and stability of self-report and non-self-report measures. *Journal of Personality, 61*, 317–342.

Schimmack, U., & Diener, E. (1997). Affect intensity: Separating intensity and frequency in repeatedly measured affect. *Journal of Personality and Social Psychology, 73*, 1313–1329.

Scollon, C. N., Kim-Prieto, C., & Diener, E. (2003). Experience sampling: Promises and pitfalls, strengths and weaknesses. *Journal of Happiness Studies, 4*, 5–34.

Thomas, D. L., & Diener, E. (1990). Memory accuracy in the recall of emotions. *Journal of Personality and Social Psychology, 59*, 291–297.

I

THE REALM OF SUBJECTIVE WELL-BEING

2

Philosophy and the Science of Subjective Well-Being

Daniel M. Haybron

The Renaissance of Prudential Psychology

Philosophical reflection on the good life in coming decades will likely owe a tremendous debt to the burgeoning science of subjective well-being and the pioneers, such as Ed Diener, who brought it to fruition. Although the psychological dimensions of human welfare now occupy a prominent position in the social sciences, they have gotten surprisingly little attention in the recent philosophical literature. The situation appears to be changing, however, as philosophers, inspired by the empirical research, begin to examine more seriously the psychology of human flourishing. This is not to say that the philosophers of any era have kept entirely silent about such matters. Although the term "subjective well-being" has yet to take a significant place in the philosophical lexicon, philosophers have always evinced some interest—and sometimes quite a lot—in the subjective or psychological dimensions of human welfare.

Philosophical work on the good life has traditionally been the province of *ethical theory*, which may be understood to include all aspects of value theory. Ethics in this broad sense is one of three main branches of philosophical inquiry, alongside metaphysics and epistemology. Philosophers sometimes use "ethics" more narrowly, as a synonym for "morality" or "moral theory." But ethical theorists frequently claim to be in the business of trying to answer Socrates' question: How ought one to live? And this question ranges well beyond matters of right and wrong, dealing also with matters of *well-being, flourishing, welfare, eudaimonia*, or *prudential value*. There is some dispute about the precise equivalence of these expressions, each of which carries differing connotations. But all seem to concern the same cluster of issues: what benefits a person, is in his or her interest, or makes life go best for him or her. Thus contemporary theories of "well-being" or "welfare" appear to be direct competitors to ancient theories of "eudaimonia." It can be useful, then, to employ these expressions interchangeably, whether or not they are strictly synonymous.

Some philosophers have maintained that well-being is entirely a psychological affair: The only ingredient necessary for well-being is, ultimately, pleasure or some other mental state. Most, however, have tended toward the view that mental states comprise only a *part* of well-being. Nozick's (1974) "experience machine" case, for example, is widely taken to show that welfare cannot depend solely on mental states, or at least experiential states, because most people recoil at the thought of permanently plugging into a virtual reality machine, à la *The Matrix*, that offers a simulated life containing whatever experiences its occupant—who would think they were real—might want. Such a life strikes many as pathetic, not enviable. Examples of this sort suggest that well-being depends on what our lives are actually like, and not just how they seem to us. If this suggestion is right, then well-being is not purely a psychological matter.

Judging by the dearth of recent philosophical work on the psychological dimensions of well-being, one might wonder whether philosophers have concluded that such matters aren't terribly important or interesting. When happiness gets discussed at all, for instance, it is often only to be dismissed as a superficial state of cheerfulness. But perhaps the superficiality lies in the way people tend to *think* about happiness and related states, and not in the idea that such matters are of central importance in a good life. This, probably, would have been the view of most ancient philosophers, for whom the psychology of well-being was a major preoccupation. (For an excellent survey of Hellenistic ethics, see Annas, 1993.) Such thinkers took Socrates' question quite seriously and tried to articulate ideals of the good life that intelligent persons would, on reflection, find compelling. None of the major schools of ancient ethical thought failed to maintain that the good life was a pleasant one, and most took great pains to show how this was so, often developing sophisticated doctrines about the mental aspects of flourishing. Whereas the Cyrenaics espoused a simple form of hedonism centering on the pleasures of the moment, more discerning hedonists such as the Epicureans, and perhaps Democritus, held subtler views about the pleasures worth seeking: in the Epicurean case, the "static" pleasures of tranquility or *ataraxia*, and in the Democritean case, *euthymia*, which is often translated as "cheerfulness" but may have centered more on tranquility than this translation suggests. (The ideal of *ataraxia* also figured prominently in the work of the Skeptics.) The Epicureans had a lot to say, not just about pleasure but also about the varieties of desire and how to cultivate the proper desires. By contrast the Stoics, who posited virtue as the sole good and believed pleasure and pain to be "indifferents," might be expected to have been more reticent about such matters. But a highly developed psychology of well-being occupied the center of their ethics, partly because virtue for them involved getting one's inner life, particularly one's emotions, in proper order. And despite its freedom from the passions or *apatheia*, the virtuous life was clearly envisaged as a pleasant one involving *ataraxia* and various "good affects," or *eupatheiai*, including a kind of joy (*chara*). It was not a grueling or affectless "eat your vegetables" affair. They did, admittedly, maintain that one could be *eudaimon* on the rack, so perhaps the sage's life is only normally pleasant. But even persons on the rack could only flourish provided that they not let the rack disturb their tranquility.

In the *Republic* Plato tries hard to defend a similar view of well-being, arguing at great length that the unvirtuous must be plagued by psychic disharmony, so that only the virtuous life is truly pleasant. Aristotle moderates such views by identifying well-being with virtuous *activity* and counting goods of fortune in the assessment of well-being. He too discussed the psychological aspects of human flourishing at length, developing an influential view about the role of the emotions in a virtuous life, but also saying much about the character of pleasure and arguing that the life of virtue is the most pleasant.

It is doubtful that many ancients would have failed to grasp the significance of empirical research on subjective well-being. If, for instance, studies indicate that certain ways of life are surprisingly unfulfilling or downright unpleasant, this finding would likely qualify as important according to any of the doctrines noted above. To be sure, qualifications would need to be made regarding the value of such states for the ancients. For example, people can enjoy themselves in questionable ways, say, in leading lives of passive consumption that Aristotle deemed fit only for "grazing cattle." Hence most ancients would not have considered high levels of subjective well-being to be sufficient for well-being (though perhaps the highest reaches of subjective well-being are possible only for those leading the best sort of life—recall Aristotle's claim that the virtuous life is also the most pleasant). Second, some of the states we associate with being happy, such as giddy elation, would have been thought undesirable by many ancient theorists—in some cases, as among the Stoics, intrinsically bad. Third, many ancients—Stoics and Aristotelians, for instance—rejected the idea that happiness, or any part of it, should be our goal. It is, for them, just a by-product of virtue—an agreeable accompaniment to the life well lived. Finally, those same thinkers rejected the notion that happiness could be good in itself, apart from the activities and circumstances associated with it. It was essential that these mental states come about in the right way, at the right time. But such points hardly show subjective

complete latitude in defining their own subspecialties and theoretical approaches to the subject. It is not meant to supplant terms such as "positive psychology" but to place various fields in a broader context that highlights their common interests and significance. It is possible for intelligent people to disagree about the promise of, say, hedonic versus eudaimonic psychology. But there can be little dispute about the importance of prudential psychology.

The Philosophy of Well-Being and Happiness

Theories of Well-Being

To put subjective well-being research in historical and philosophical context, we need to understand how philosophers think about the more fundamental notion of *well-being*. The best-known philosophical taxonomy, offered by Parfit (1984), divides theories of well-being into three types: hedonistic, desire, and objective list. But an important new approach has entered the scene, and an ancient family of theories has gained substantially in prominence. Here I distinguish five basic approaches:

1. Hedonistic theories
2. Desire theories
3. Authentic happiness theories
4. Eudaimonistic (or "nature-fulfillment") theories
5. List theories

Hedonistic Theories

Crudely, hedonism identifies well-being with pleasure. A bit more precisely, well-being consists in a subject's balance of pleasant over unpleasant experience. Hedonism about well-being should not be confused with other forms of hedonism, notably hedonism about happiness. Historical hedonists include, among others, Epicureans and classical Utilitarians. (Recent defenses of welfare hedonism include Crisp, in press; Feldman, 2004; Sprigge, 1987.) Hedonists vary on the exact specification of the theory, some preferring to focus on enjoyment and suffering, others pleasure and pain, and so forth. (For a good discussion of philosophical views of pleasure, see Sumner, 1996.) But the central idea is that what ultimately matters for welfare is the hedonic quality of individuals' experience, and nothing more.

The chief attraction of this view is that it accommodates the plausible thought that, if anything matters for welfare, it is the pleasantness of our experience of life. Whereas it is far less obvious that something can benefit or harm us if it does not enter our experience; moreover, nothing else seems to matter in just the way that pleasure and suffering do. Despite its attractions, most philosophers have rejected hedonism, either because of experience machine-type worries or "philosophy of swine" objections such as those that led Mill (1979) to distinguish higher- and lower-quality pleasures. Crisp's (1997) example of Haydn and the oyster illustrates the latter worry: Supposing an oyster can have pleasant experiences—of low level and quality—then one could apparently be better off with an extremely long oyster life versus the normal-length life of Haydn, however fulfilling his life may have been. For given enough time the oyster will accumulate a greater quantity of pleasure than any human could achieve (Crisp, 1997). Many find it implausible that an oyster could be better off than Haydn, and few have endorsed Mill's attempt to remedy such concerns.

Desire Theories

Currently, the theory to beat is the desire theory of well-being, also called the desire or preference satisfaction or fulfillment account. The dominant account among economists and philosophers over the last century or so, the desire theory identifies well-being with the (actual) satisfaction of the individual's desires. Experience machines don't trouble such views, because many of our desires will go unfulfilled in an experience machine. Desire theories come in many varieties, the most important type being informed-desire theories, which restrict the desires that count to the ones we would have given full information (rationality, reflection, etc.). (Such theories include those of Brandt, 1979; Hare, 1981; Harsanyi, 1982; Rawls, 1971; and Sidgwick, 1966. For related views, see Carson, 2000; Darwall, 1983; Griffin, 1986, 2000; Railton, 1986a, 1986b.) These variants predominate, because many find it intuitively obvious that we don't gain from the satisfaction of desires that are grounded in ignorance or irrationality. Desire theories have a number of attractions, one being that they forge an obvious link between agents' welfare and their motives. Moreover, they are extremely flexible, able to accommodate the full range of goods that people seek in their lives. But most importantly, they seem to comport with the liberal sensibilities of modernity: What's best for me depends on what I care about, and on such matters I am sovereign. This position seems appealingly nonpaternalistic.

Yet desire theories have come in for withering criticism in recent decades on a variety of counts, and may be on the decline. One difficulty is that people's desires can be self-sacrificial or hostile to their own interests, or simply concerned with distant affairs having no bearing on their own lives. People can desire anything, including things that seem irrelevant or detrimental to their well-being (Darwall, 2002; Sumner, 1996). Another is how to devise an information or rationality constraint that gives sufficient critical power—recognizing that people do make mistakes—without departing so much from agents' actual perspectives that the theory loses the connection with individual sovereignty that drew people to it in the first place. (What do the priorities I would have if I were omniscient, perfectly rational, etc., have to do with *me*? See Loeb, 1995; Rosati, 1995.) Also influential have been "happy slave"-type worries concerning adaptation: Desires adapt to the possibilities people face, so that the aspirations of those with modest prospects tend likewise to be modest. Oppressed women, for instance, can content themselves with being treated like property. Merely getting what they want would, it seems, leave them with impoverished lives (Elster, 1983; Nussbaum, 2000b; Sen, 1987).

Authentic Happiness Theories

L. W. Sumner's authentic happiness view is meant to rectify the most serious difficulties with hedonistic and desire theories while retaining their emphasis on subjective experience and individual sovereignty (Sumner, 1996, 2000). His view identifies well-being with authentical happiness: being happy, wherein one's happiness is both *informed* about the conditions of one's life and *autonomous*, meaning that it reflects values that are truly one's own and not the result of manipulation or oppressive social conditioning. "Happiness" here is something like subjective well-being, involving both global attitudes of life satisfaction and positive affect, though Sumner calls his view a "life satisfaction" account. The root idea is that one's happiness should reflect a response *of* one's own, *to* a life that is one's own, ostensibly ruling out experience machine and happy-slave objections. Whereas desire theories face the problem of how irrelevant desires, or fulfillments that don't impact my experience, can affect my well-being, the authentic happiness view incorporates an experience requirement: Only what affects my happiness can benefit me. The response to Sumner's account is still taking shape (but see LeBar, 2004; Haybron, in press-b), but one concern is whether any subjectivist theory has the critical power to manage common intuitions about impoverished lives or when normal human goods are lacking. Why couldn't passive couch potatoes or even slaves be authentically happy, having reflected on their values and decided to affirm their life just as it is?

Eudaimonistic Theories

Aristotle's writings are so influential that commentators often use "eudaimonistic" or "eudaimonic" simply to denote Aristotelian theories of well-being or views that emphasize perfection or virtue. But Aristotelians formed only one of the schools of Hellenistic ethics that scholars denote, collectively, as eudaimonistic. Definitions vary, but (ethical) *eudaimonism* tends to refer to ancient theories that ground ethics in the notion of eudaimonia—the idea being that eudaimonia is our agreed-upon goal that properly structures our deliberations about how to live, and the theory's job is to determine the nature of this goal (see, e.g., Annas,

1993). Some ancient eudaimonists, for example, the Epicureans, denied that eudaimonia consists in perfection. If there was an important feature that eudaimonistic accounts of well-being shared in common, it was the teleological idea that well-being consists in *nature fulfillment*. Epicureans arguably agreed with Aristotle that well-being involves the fulfillment of our natures as human beings, but they believed that we fulfilled our natures by achieving pleasure.

Thus we might usefully distinguish *welfare eudaimonism* as a fourth approach to well-being, where we start with a conception of human nature—or, if we are specifically interested in *self*-fulfillment, the self—and take well-being to consist in the fulfillment of that nature. Aristotelian views form the best-known variety of eudaimonism. But this sort of approach is not limited to the ancients, and versions of it arguably inform Mill's (1991) discussion of individuality in *On Liberty*, eudaimonic approaches to the psychology of well-being, and the work of many other moderns. A eudaimonistic account incorporating a form of authentic happiness as a central element of self-fulfillment is sketched in Haybron, in press-b. (For a general discussion of the notion of self-fulfillment, see Gewirth, 1998; Feinberg, 1992. For a review of eudaimonic psychology, see Ryan & Deci, 2001.) It is even possible to base desire accounts and other subjectivisms on a eudaimonistic framework: Perhaps the self is defined by a person's desires, and thus we fulfill ourselves by fulfilling our desires. Eudaimonism merits classification as a distinct family of theories, however, because all share the same fundamental motivation: the idea that well-being consists in nature-fulfillment. Differences arise in their views of a person's nature, and of what it means to fulfill that nature. Subjectivists such as Sumner and most desire theorists, by contrast, start from very different foundations, such as the ideal of individual sovereignty.

Such concerns have given much impetus to Aristotelian accounts of well-being, which have stirred considerable interest since the revival of virtue ethics and the rise of the Sen–Nussbaum capabilities approach in political theory. Comprising the best-known variety of our fourth type of theory—to be explained shortly—Aristotelian views identify well-being with "well-functioning," which is to say, functioning or living well as a human being: the fulfillment of human nature. This fulfillment consists, in the first instance, of a life of excellent or virtuous activity, though this is sometimes put less astringently as a "fully" or "truly" human life. Aristotelian views and close relations appear in, for example, Darwall (2002), Foot (2001), Hurka (1993), Hursthouse (1999), Kraut (2002), LeBar (2004), Murphy (2001), Nussbaum (1988, 1992, 1993, 2000a, 2000b), Sher (1997), Toner (in press). (The Aristotelian literature has yet to be integrated fully with contemporary work on well-being, so it is often difficult to tell where an author stands on well-being. Hurka, e.g., rejects a "well-being" interpretation of his view.)

The idea behind such theories is that we flourish by fully exercising our human capacities. It is not simply a matter of being morally virtuous, although moral virtue is essential to well-being, as Aristotelians see it. Thus a ruthless corporate executive with little concern for others could not flourish, according to the Aristotelian, however successful he or she might be in relation to his or her own priorities. Such a life would be stripped bare of crucial elements of other-concern that give normal human lives much of their shape. Similarly, the couch potato's life of passive consumption would strike the Aristotelian as barely human, a sad waste of potential. Aristotelian theories address widespread intuitions about the importance of personal development and leading a "full life" replete with the essentials of a normal human life. (A disability that strips the individual of normal sexual capacities, say, seems to mark an irreplaceable loss for which no amount of happiness can compensate.) Yet these views face serious objections as well. First, they can seem to make well-being alien to the individual: How can what benefits *me* depend on what *human beings, in general,* are like? Species norms are not obviously relevant to questions of personal benefit. A second concern is that, although virtue does seem important for well-being in most cases, the connection might be weaker than Aristotelians think. Sometimes virtue seems not so beneficial, as in a talented philosopher whose excellence brings little satisfaction. And sometimes the unvirtuous really do seem to flourish. A related point is that Aristotelian accounts may seem to accord too marginal a role for pleasure and other aspects of subjective well-being. Although truly virtuous activity is indeed counted pleasant by Aristotelians, the pleasure apparently matters simply as a "completion" or by-product of excellence, a congenial bonus attending what really matters. This idea has some appeal when thinking about the way we plan our own lives, but less so from other perspectives, as when assessing our children's well-being: We do not think their happiness or suffering are mere by-products or concomitants of what really matters. They *are*, in great part, what really matters.

List Theories

Fifth, we have *list theories* of well-being, which identify well-being with some brute list of goods, such as knowledge, friendship, accomplishment, pleasure, etc. Likely examples of such accounts include Arneson (1999), Brink (1989), Gert (1998), Griffin (1986, 2000), and Scanlon (1993, 1999). (Finnis [1980] and Murphy [2001] offer lists grounded in a broadly Aristotelian natural law framework.) Their appeal derives from the fact that other approaches seem incapable of encompassing the full range of our intuitions about well-being. The elements on most proposed lists do strike many as intrinsically beneficial, so why adopt a theory that excludes them? On the other hand, with no principled basis for populating one's list of goods in a certain way, the whole enterprise can seem deeply ad hoc. Moreover, it does not illuminate the nature of well-being very much; what do all the items share, such that they all have the same kind of value? But even critics of list theories can grant their utility for laying out the appearances: If an item appears on most lists, then any account of well-being will likely need to make room for it, lest it seem implausibly counterintuitive.

When assessing theories of well-being, it is essential to distinguish well-being from the broader notion of the *good life*. Although we sometimes use "the good life" simply as a synonym for "well-being," it seems we usually mean a life that is desirable or choiceworthy: not just morally good, or good *for* the individual leading it, but good, *period*. Given that few would deny that it is desirable both to flourish and to be virtuous, most ethical doctrines maintain that the good life involves both virtue and well-being, and perhaps aesthetic or other values as well. Disagreements concern the relative importance of these values and the relation between them. The important point here is to see what happens when we don't carefully distinguish the notions of well-being and the good life: conflating this distinction can foster bad arguments for certain views of well-being. For instance, commentators often infer that well-being requires virtue because we wouldn't consider a life good without it: Bad people can't flourish because such lives do not strike us as good ones. But such contentions prove nothing: On the most natural reading of "good lives," virtually no one would dispute that the good life requires morality. For such a claim amounts to nothing more than the platitude that it is desirable to be moral, which is not a very interesting suggestion. What most contemporaries deny is that *well-being* is impossible absent moral goodness. This claim may well be true, but talking about the requirements of a good life won't help to establish it.

What Does "Happiness" Mean?

"Happiness" has many meanings, but most scholarly work centers on two of them. (For further discussion, see Haybron, 2000, 2003.) The first usage, more prominent in the philosophical literature than elsewhere, treats "happiness" as basically a synonym for "well-being." The uses of "happiness" to discuss premodern philosophy almost always take this meaning, as when it is used—controversially—to translate "eudaimonia." To ascribe happiness to people, in the well-being sense, is to say that their lives are going well for them. It is to make a value judgment about their lives. This usage is the most natural reading of talk about leading a happy *life*, as opposed simply to *being* happy. For whereas being happy seems to be a property of the person and can sensibly be regarded as a purely psychological matter, most people probably would not say as much about the idea of having a happy *life*, which plausibly involves nonmental states of affairs as well. Thus you might find it intuitive to say that Nozick's (1974) experience machine user could *be* happy, even if his or her *life* isn't a happy one at all. The abstract noun "happiness" often evokes the "well-being" reading as well, as in "life, liberty, and the pursuit of happiness."

hedonists do. (See, e.g., Brandt, 1979, 1989; Carson, 1978, 1981; Davis, 1981a, 1981b; Griffin, 1979, 1986; Kahneman, 1999; Mayerfeld, 1996, 1999; Sprigge, 1987, 1991.) The difference, of course, is that those who endorse hedonism about happiness need not accept the stronger doctrine of welfare hedonism; this emerges clearly in arguments against the classical utilitarian focus on happiness as the aim of social choice. Such arguments tend to grant the identification of happiness with pleasure, but challenge the idea that happiness should be our primary or sole social concern, and often as well the idea that happiness is all that matters for well-being.

Also common are life satisfaction theories, which identify happiness with having a favorable attitude toward one's life as a whole. This basic schema can be filled out in a variety of ways but typically involves some sort of global judgment, an endorsement or affirmation of one's life as a whole. This judgment may be more or less explicit, and may involve or accompany some form of affect. It may also involve or accompany some aggregate of judgments about particular items or domains within one's life. (Variants of the life satisfaction view appear to include Barrow, 1980, 1991; Benditt, 1974, 1978; Campbell, 1973; Montague, 1967; Nozick, 1989; Rescher, 1972, 1980; Sumner, 1996; Telfer, 1980; Veenhoven, 1984, 1997; Von Wright, 1963. Those making life satisfaction central or identical to well-being—often using the word "happiness" for it—appear to include Almeder, 2000; Kekes, 1982, 1988, 1992; McFall, 1989; Meynell, 1969; Tatarkiewicz, 1976; Thomas, 1968, among others.)

A third theory, the *emotional state* view, departs from hedonism in a different way: Instead of identifying happiness with pleasant experience, it identifies happiness with an agent's emotional condition as a whole (Haybron, 2005). This condition includes nonexperiential aspects of emotions and moods (or perhaps just moods) and excludes pleasures that don't directly involve the individual's emotional state. It might also include a person's *propensity* for experiencing various moods, which can vary over time. Happiness, on such a view, is more nearly the opposite of depression or anxiety, whereas hedonistic happiness is simply opposed to unpleasantness. One reason for taking such a view is intuitive: Psychologically superficial pleasures do not obviously make a difference in how happy one is—the typical pleasure of eating a cracker, say, or even the intense pleasure of an orgasm that nonetheless fails to move one, as can happen with meaningless sexual activity. The intuitive distinction seems akin to distinctions made by some ancient philosophers; consider, for instance, the following passage from Epictetus's (1925) *Discourses*: " 'I have a headache.' Well, do not say 'Alas!' 'I have an earache.' Do not say 'Alas!' And I am not saying that it is not permissible to groan, only *do not groan in the centre of your being*" (1.18.19, emphasis added). The Stoics did not expect us never to feel pain or unpleasant sensations, which would plainly be impossible; rather, the idea was not to let such things *get to us*, to impact our emotional conditions.

But why should we care to press such a distinction in characterizing happiness? The hedonic difference between happiness on an emotional state view versus a hedonistic view is probably minimal. But whereas little would be lost, what would be gained? For one, the more "central" affects involving our emotional conditions may bear a special relation to the person or the *self*, whereas more "peripheral" affects, such as the pleasantness of eating a cracker, might pertain to the subpersonal aspects of our psychologies. Because well-being is commonly linked to ideas of self-fulfillment, as we saw earlier, this sort of distinction might signal a difference in the importance of these states (Haybron, in press-b). Another reason to focus on emotional condition rather than experience alone is the greater psychological depth of the former: Its impact on our mental lives, physiology, and behavior is much deeper and more pervasive. This "depth" enhances the explanatory and predictive significance of happiness, but more importantly it captures the idea that happiness concerns the individual's psychological orientation or disposition: To be happy is not just to be subjected to a certain sequence of experiences; it is, instead, for one's very being to manifest a favorable orientation toward the conditions of one's life—a kind of psychic affirmation of one's life. This suggestion reflects a point of similarity with life satisfaction views of happiness: contra hedonism, both views take happiness to be substantially dispositional, involving some sort of favorable orientation toward one's life. Life satisfaction views tend to emphasize reflective or rational endorsement, whereas emotional state views emphasize the verdicts of our emotional natures.

A fourth family of views, *hybrid theories*, attempts an irenic solution to our diverse intuitions about happiness: Identify happiness with both life satisfaction and pleasure or emotional state, perhaps along with other states such as domain satisfactions. The most obvious candidate here is *subjective well-being*, which is typically defined as a compound of life satisfaction, domain satisfactions, and positive and negative affect. (Researchers often seem to identify happiness with subjective well-being, sometimes with life satisfaction, and perhaps most commonly with emotional or hedonic state.) The chief appeal of hybrid theories is their inclusiveness: All the components of subjective well-being seem important, and there is probably no component of subjective well-being that does not, at times, get included in happiness in ordinary usage.

Evaluating Theories of Happiness

How do we determine which theory is correct? Traditional philosophical methods of conceptual or linguistic analysis can give us some guidance, indicating that some accounts offer a better fit with the ordinary concept of happiness. Thus it has been argued that hedonism is false to the concept of happiness as we know it; the intuitions taken to support hedonism point instead to an emotional state view (Haybron, 2001, 2005). And some have argued that life satisfaction is compatible and may thus weaken the case for life satisfaction theories of happiness. It does not show that self-reports of life satisfaction aren't useful *measures* of well-being, in precisely the way we would expect: by giving information about how people's lives are going relative to their priorities. For even if such reports systematically deviate from well-being, possibly to the point that they are well nigh useless in the individual case, they can still tell us a lot about how *populations* of people are doing: Many discrepancies will wash out over large samples, and others may at most threaten claims about absolute levels of well-being, while leaving most correlational results intact. (Such points illustrate how philosophers' instincts can be misleading: we tend to worry about whether somewhere, in some possible world, there lives a strange person who constitutes an exception our theory. Thus many philosophers distrust self-report measures, given how easy it is to imagine someone getting it wrong. But science centers on generalizations, not individuals, and errors that seem epistemically fatal in the individual case may be benign for the study of populations.)

Given the limitations of narrower theories of happiness, a hybrid account may seem an attractive solution. But this strategy raises difficulties of its own. If we arrive at a hybrid theory by this route, it is liable to seem like either the marriage of two unpromising accounts, or of a promising account with an unpromising one. It is not obvious that such a union will yield wholesome results. And people have different intuitions about what counts as happiness, so that no theory can accommodate all of them—and any theory that tries to do so risks pleasing no one. A second concern is that the various components of any hybrid, such as subjective well-being, are liable to matter for quite different reasons. Although it is helpful to employ blanket concepts such as subjective well-being to encompass some broad domain in which we have an interest, most purposes may be better served by focusing on more specific psychological kinds, for instance, distinguishing life satisfaction from happiness, understood as a matter of hedonic or emotional state.

The Role of Intuitions in Value Inquiry

Some explanation of philosophical methodology is in order, because it can seem baffling or downright suspicious to researchers schooled in the scientific method. Here I focus on philosophical inquiry into matters of value. There is currently much dispute about the nature of philosophy and the methods appropriate to it, so anything I say will be contentious. But a glance through philosophy journals of recent decades, if not the history of philosophical reflection, suggests a considerable degree of consistency in approach, with disputes mainly concerning the relative weight of various considerations, or about theoretical issues with little bearing on philosophical practice. Perhaps the most common procedure is to reflect the way people think about matters of value, as we saw in connection with life satisfaction theories of happiness. Because philosophical reflection aims partly to clarify the concerns driving our responses to value, it may help us to understand the processes driving self-reports and hence to explain them and understand their significance (Haybron, 2007).

Virtue and Subjective Well-Being

A central concern of the positive psychology movement has been to research the strengths or virtues that contribute to human flourishing. Clearly, certain traits of character will tend more than others to foster subjective well-being; the question is what these traits are and how they promote subjective well-being. This sort of inquiry is interdisciplinary: Although it is an empirical question how a given trait impacts subjective well-being, philosophical inquiry is needed to establish which traits are virtues. (Tiberius is doing some important work along these lines, including a book in progress; see, e.g., Tiberius, 2002.) For example, perhaps some ways of being unrealistic amount to vices even while tending to promote subjective well-being. Empirical results can also be relevant to establishing the status of certain traits as virtues: If a trait tends to help its possessors lead more satisfying lives, this seems a point in favor of its being a virtue—at the very least, a prudential virtue. A further question is how far indicators of well-being should go beyond subjective well-being, perhaps tracking some of the virtues, such as optimism, that seem especially significant for a good life.

Challenges to Traditional Views in Ethics and Political Philosophy

Most ethical theories rest on some view of human nature and hence are susceptible to empirical challenge. Aristotelian ethics, for instance, gives our rational faculties a central role in the proper governance of human life. It is possible that the science of subjective well-being and associated disciplines will help to confirm or undermine this view, for instance, if it turns out that subrational processes play a larger role in the direction of human life than the Aristotelian account permits (see, e.g., Bargh & Chartrand, 1999). Also vulnerable may be views about the types of social arrangements that promote human well-being. Liberal modernity has it that people tend to fare best when given extremely broad scope to shape their lives as they see fit. Yet there is growing evidence that people are susceptible to a wide range of systematic errors in the pursuit of happiness. At least conceivably, we might find that people tend to fare better in certain social forms that offer individuals a narrower range of options in determining the shape of their lives than many affluent Westerners enjoy, or, perhaps, that paternalistic interventions aimed at correcting for certain errors will prove more effective than many would have guessed, so that governments may have a surprisingly large role to play in the promotion of happiness. Perhaps some interventions will be both effective at promoting well-being and Orwellian, threatening consequentialist arguments for liberal restrictions on paternalism—and thus threatening either consequentialism or liberalism itself. Political philosophers, among others, will probably be well advised to attend to developments in the science of happiness.

Acknowledgments

Thanks to Anna Alexandrova, Matthew Cashen, Monte Johnson, and Valerie Tiberius for helpful comments on material used in this chapter.

References

Almeder, R. (2000). *Human happiness and morality*. Buffalo, NY: Prometheus Press.

Annas, J. (1993). *The morality of happiness*. New York: Oxford University Press.

Aquinas, T. (1990). *A summa of the summa* (P. Kreeft, Ed.). San Francisco: Ignatius Press.

Arneson, R. J. (1999). Human flourishing versus desire satisfaction. In E. F. Paul, F. D. Miller, Jr., & J. Paul (Eds.), *Human flourishing* (pp. 113–142). New York: Cambridge University Press.

Bargh, J. A., & Chartrand, T. L. (1999). The unbearable automaticity of being. *American Psychologist, 54,* 462–479.

Barrow, R. (1980). *Happiness and schooling*. New York: St. Martin's Press.

Barrow, R. (1991). *Utilitarianism: A contemporary statement*. Brookfield, VT: Edward Elgar.

Benditt, T. M. (1974). Happiness. *Philosophical Studies, 25,* 1–20.

Benditt, T. M. (1978). Happiness and satisfaction: A rejoinder to Carson. *The Personalist, 59,* 108–109.

Block, N. (1995). On a confusion about a function of consciousness. *Behavioral and Brain Sciences, 18,* 227–247.

Brandt, R. B. (1979). *A theory of the good and the right*. New York: Oxford University Press.

Brandt, R. B. (1989). Fairness to happiness. *Social Theory and Practice, 15,* 33–58.

Brink, D. O. (1989). *Moral realism and the foundations of ethics*. New York: Cambridge University Press.

Campbell, R. (1973). The pursuit of happiness. *The Personalist, 54,* 325–337.

Carson, T. L. (1978). Happiness and the good life. *Southwestern Journal of Philosophy, 9,* 73–88.

Carson, T. L. (1981). Happiness, contentment, and the good life. *Pacific Philosophical Quarterly, 62,* 378–92.

Carson, T. L. (2000). *Value and the good life*. Notre Dame, IN: University of Notre Dame Press.

Crisp, R. (1997). *Mill on utilitarianism*. New York: Routledge.

Crisp, R. (in press). Hedonism reconsidered. *Philosophy and Phenomenological Research*.

Darwall, S. (1983). *Impartial reason*. Ithaca, NY: Cornell University Press.

Darwall, S. (2002). *Welfare and rational care*. Princeton, NJ: Princeton University Press.

Davis, W. (1981a). Pleasure and happiness. *Philosophical Studies, 39*, 305–318.

Davis, W. (1981b). A theory of happiness. *American Philosophical Quarterly, 18*, 111–120.

Diener, E., & Biswas-Diener, R. (2002). Will money increase subjective well-being? *Social Indicators Research, 57*, 119–169.

Diener, E., & Diener, C. (1996). Most people are happy. *Psychological Science, 7*, 181–185.

Diener, E., & Oishi, S. (2005). The nonobvious social psychology of happiness. *Psychological Inquiry, 16*, 162–167.

Diener, E., Sapyta, J. J., & Suh, E. (1998). Subjective well-being is essential to well-being. *Psychological Inquiry, 9*, 33–37.

Diener, E., & Scollon, C. N. (2003, October). *Subjective well-being is desirable, but not the summum bonum*. Paper presented at the Minnesota Interdisciplinary Workshop on Well-Being, Minneapolis.

Elster, J. (1983). *Sour grapes*. New York: Cambridge University Press.

Epictetus. (1925). *The discourses as reported by Arrian, the manual, and fragments* (W. A. Oldfather, Trans.). Cambridge, MA: Harvard University Press.

Epicurus. (1994). *The Epicurus reader* (B. Gerson & L. P. Gerson, Trans.). Indianapolis: Hackett.

Feinberg, J. (1992). Absurd self-fulfillment. In J. Feinberg (Ed.), *Freedom and fulfillment* (pp. 297–330). Princeton, NJ: Princeton University Press. (Original work published 1980)

Feldman, F. (2004). *Pleasure and the good life*. New York: Oxford University Press.

Finnis, J. (1980). *Natural law and natural rights*. New York: Oxford University Press.

Foot, P. (2001). *Natural goodness*. New York: Oxford University Press.

Gert, B. (1998). *Morality: Its nature and justification*. New York: Oxford University Press.

Gewirth, A. (1998). *Self-fulfillment*. Princeton, NJ: Princeton University Press.

Griffin, J. (1979). Is unhappiness morally more important than happiness? *Philosophical Quarterly, 29*, 47–55.

Griffin, J. (1986). *Well-being: Its meaning, measurement, and moral importance*. Oxford, UK: Clarendon Press.

Griffin, J. (2000). Replies. In R. Crisp & B. Hooker (Eds.), *Well-being and morality* (pp. 281–313). New York: Oxford University Press.

Griswold, C. (1996). Happiness, tranquillity, and philosophy. *Critical Review, 10*, 1–32.

Hare, R. M. (1981). *Moral thinking*. New York: Oxford University Press.

Harsanyi, J. (1982). Morality and the theory of rational behaviour. In A. Sen & B. Williams (Eds.), *Utilitarianism and beyond* (pp. 39–62). New York: Cambridge University Press.

Haybron, D. M. (2000). Two philosophical problems in the study of happiness. *Journal of Happiness Studies, 1*, 207–225.

Haybron, D. M. (2001). Happiness and pleasure. *Philosophy and Phenomenological Research, 62*, 501–528.

Haybron, D. M. (2003). What do we want from a theory of happiness? *Metaphilosophy, 34*, 305–329.

Haybron, D. M. (2005). On being happy or unhappy. *Philosophy and Phenomenological Research, 71*, 287–317.

Haybron, D. M. (in press-a). Do we know how happy we are? *Nous.*

Haybron, D. M. (in press-b). Happiness, the self, and human flourishing. *Utilitas.*

Haybron, D. M. (2007). Life satisfaction, ethical reflection and the science of happiness. *The Journal of Happiness Studies, 8,* 99–138.

Hurka, T. (1993). *Perfectionism.* New York: Oxford University Press.

Hursthouse, R. (1999). *On virtue ethics.* New York: Oxford University Press.

Kahneman, D. (1999). Objective happiness. In D. Kahneman, E. Diener, & N. Schwarz (Eds.), *Well-being: The foundations of hedonic psychology* (pp. 3–25). New York: Sage.

Kant, I. (1997). *Groundwork of the metaphysics of morals* (M. Gregor, Trans.), New York: Cambridge University Press. (Original work published 1785)

Kekes, J. (1982). Happiness. *Mind, 91,* 358–376.

Kekes, J. (1988). *The examined life.* Lewisburg, PA: Bucknell University Press.

Kekes, J. (1992). Happiness. In L. C. Becker & C. B. Becker (Eds.), *Encyclopedia of ethics* (pp. 430–435). New York: Garland.

Kraut, R. (1979). Two conceptions of happiness. *Philosophical Review, 138,* 167–197.

Kraut, R. (2002). *Aristotle: Political philosophy.* New York: Oxford University Press.

LeBar, M. (2004). Good for you. *Pacific Philosophical Quarterly, 85,* 195–217.

Loeb, D. (1995). Full-information theories of individual good. *Social Theory and Practice, 21,* 1–30.

Mayerfeld, J. (1996). The moral asymmetry of happiness and suffering. *Southern Journal of Philosophy, 34,* 317–338.

Mayerfeld, J. (1999). *Suffering and moral responsibility.* New York: Oxford University Press.

McFall, L. (1989). *Happiness.* New York: Lang.

Meynell, H. (1969). Human flourishing. *Religious Studies, 5,* 147–154.

Mill, J. S. (1979). *Utilitarianism.* Indianapolis: Hackett.

Mill, J. S. (1991). On liberty. In J. Gray (Ed.), *On liberty and other essays* (pp. 5–130). New York: Oxford University Press.

Montague, R. (1967). Happiness. *Proceedings of the Aristotelian Society, 67,* 87–102.

Murphy, M. C. (2001). *Natural law and practical rationality.* New York: Cambridge University Press.

Nozick, R. (1974). *Anarchy, state, and utopia.* New York: Basic Books.

Nozick, R. (1989). *The examined life.* New York: Simon & Schuster.

Nussbaum, M. (1988). Nature, function, and capability: Aristotle on political distribution. In J. Annas & R. H. Grimm (Eds.), *Oxford studies in ancient philosophy* (Suppl. Vol. I, pp. 145–184). New York: Oxford University Press.

Nussbaum, M. (1992). Human functioning and social justice: In defense of Aristotelian essentialism. *Political Theory, 20,* 202–246.

Nussbaum, M. (1993). Non-relative virtues: An Aristotelian approach. In M. Nussbaum & A. Sen (Eds.), *The quality of life* (pp. 242–269). New York: Oxford University Press.

Nussbaum, M. (2000a). Aristotle, politics, and human capabilities: A response to Antony, Arneson, Charlesworth, and Mulgan. *Ethics, 111,* 102–140.

Nussbaum, M. (2000b). *Women and human development: The capabilities approach.* New York: Cambridge University Press.

Parfit, D. (1984). *Reasons and persons.* New York: Oxford University Press.

Railton, P. (1986a). Facts and values. *Philosophical Topics, 14,* 5–31.

Railton, P. (1986b). Moral realism. *Philosophical Review, 95*, 163–207.

Rawls, J. (1971). *A theory of justice*. Cambridge, MA: Harvard University Press.

Rescher, N. (1972). *Welfare: The social issues in philosophical perspective*. Pittsburgh, PA: Pittsburgh University Press.

Rescher, N. (1980). *Unpopular essays on technological progress*. Pittsburgh, PA: University of Pittsburgh Press.

Rosati, C. (1995). Persons, perspectives, and full information accounts of the food. *Ethics, 105*, 296–325.

Ryan, R. M., & Deci, E. L. (2001). On happiness and human potentials: A review of research on hedonic and eudaimonic well-being. *Annual Review of Psychology, 52*, 141–166.

Scanlon, T. (1993). Value, desire, and quality of life. In A. Sen & M. Nussbaum (Eds.), *The Quality of Life* (pp. 185–200). New York: Oxford University Press.

Scanlon, T. (1999). *What we owe to each other*. Cambridge, MA: Harvard University Press.

Sen, A. (1987). *On ethics and economics*. Oxford, UK: Blackwell.

Sher, G. (1997). *Beyond neutrality: Perfectionism and politics*. New York: Cambridge University Press.

Sidgwick, H. (1966). *The methods of ethics*. New York: Dover.

Sprigge, T. L. S. (1987). *The rational foundations of ethics*. New York: Routledge & Kegan Paul.

Sprigge, T. L. S. (1991). The greatest happiness principle. *Utilitas, 3*, 37–51.

Sumner, L. W. (1996). *Welfare, happiness, and ethics*. New York: Oxford University Press.

Sumner, L. W. (2000). Something in between. In R. Crisp & B. Hooker (Eds.), *Well-being and morality* (pp. 1–19). New York: Oxford University Press.

Tatarkiewicz, W. (1976). *Analysis of happiness*. The Hague: Martinus Nijhoff.

Telfer, E. (1980). *Happiness*. New York: St. Martin's Press.

Thomas, D. A. L. (1968). Happiness. *Philosophical Quarterly, 18*, 97–113.

Tiberius, V. (2002). Perspective: A prudential virtue. *American Philosophical Quarterly, 39*, 305–324.

Toner, C. H. (2006). Aristotelian well-being: A response to L.W. Sumner's critique. *Utilitas, 18*, 218–231.

Veenhoven, R. (1984). *Conditions of happiness*. Dordrecht, The Netherlands: Reidel.

Veenhoven, R. (1997). Advances in understanding happiness. *Revue Québécoise de Psychologie, 18*, 29–79.

Von Wright, G. H. (1963). *The varieties of goodness*. London: Routledge & Kegan Paul.

Wilson, T. D., & Gilbert, D. T. (2003). Affective forecasting. In M. Zanna (Ed.), *Advances in experimental social psychology* (Vol. 35, pp. 345–411). New York: Elsevier.

3

Sociological Theories of Subjective Well-Being

RUUT VEENHOVEN

Subjective well-being is no great issue in sociology; the subject is not mentioned in sociological textbooks (a notable exception is Nolan & Lenski, 2004) and is rarely discussed in sociological journals. This absence has many reasons: pragmatic, ideological, and theoretical. To begin with *pragmatic reasons*: Sociologists are more interested in what people *do* than in how they *feel*. Their main objective is to explain social behavior, and subjective well-being is, at best, a variable in that context. A related point is that sociology is about collectivities, whereas subjective well-being is an individual-level concept. A further pragmatic reason is that sociologists earn their living dealing with social problems. So, if they look at well-being at all, they focus on "ill-being" in the first place. Next there are *ideological reasons*. Many sociologists are committed to notions of objective wellbeing, such as social equality and social cohesion. They are therefore not eager to investigate how people actually feel in such conditions and often ignore research results that contradict their favored views. When people appear to feel subjectively good in conditions deemed to be objectively bad, the discrepancy is easily disposed of as "desirability bias" or "false consciousness." Lastly, there are *theoretical reasons*. As we will see below, sociologists tend to think of subjective wellbeing as a mere idea that depends on social comparison with variable standards

44

and that is therefore a whimsical state of mind, not worth pursuing and hence not worth studying.

Nevertheless, the subject of subjective well-being is not entirely absent in sociology. Job satisfaction is a common topic in the sociology of work, marital satisfaction is a well-known variable in the sociology of family, and life satisfaction is a regular theme in the sociology of aging. Recently subjective well-being has also become a theme in comparative sociology and in social indicators research. I have reviewed this sociological literature elsewhere (Veenhoven, 2006a).

Questions about Subjective Well-Being

Theories are tentative answers to questions. In the case of subjective well-being, four main questions are at stake. The first question is what subjective well-being *is* precisely, and, in particular, how we distinguish subjective well-being as such from its determinants. The second question—how people *appraise* how well they are—concerns the mental processes involved. The third question is about the *conditions* for subjective well-being and is closely linked to the question of how subjective well-being can be raised. Lastly a fourth question is about the *consequences* of subjective well-being, which links up to the ideological issue of whether subjective well-being should be raised. In this chapter I give an outline of how mainstream sociology has dealt with these four questions.

What Is "Subjective Well-Being"?: Question 1

In this chapter we follow Diener's definition of subjective well-being as judging life positively and feeling good: "Thus a person is said to have high [subjective well-being] if she or he experiences life satisfaction and frequent joy, and only infrequently experiences unpleasant emotions such as sadness or anger. Contrariwise, a person is said to have low [subjective well-being] if she or he is dissatisfied with life, experiences little joy and affection and frequently feels negative emotions such as anger or anxiety" (Diener, Suh, & Oishi, 1997, p. 25).

My own definition of happiness is close to Diener et al.'s definition of subjective well-being, and I also make a distinction between cognitive and affective appraisals of life. Yet I do not see life satisfaction as a mere cognitive appraisal but as an overall judgment of life that draws on two sources of information: cognitive comparison with standards of the good life (contentment) and affective information from how one feels most of the time (hedonic level of affect). In my language "overall happiness" is synonymous with life satisfaction and subjective well-being (Veenhoven, 1984).

Most sociologists associate the term with a somewhat different matter. First, sociologists focus typically on problems. In sociology books words for subjective experiences denote negative states most of the time, such as *anomie, alienation, deprivation,* and subjective *poverty.* Second, sociological notions of subjective well-being are typically more specific and denote not only *how* well one feels but also about *what. Anomie* is discomfort about the moral climate, and in *alienation* is the feeling of being ruled by a system in which one does not take part (Beerling, 1978). This specificity is connected to still another difference: Sociological notions of subjective well-being are not only about *how* one feels about *what,* they are often also about *why* one feels so (i.e., the cause is part of the concept). Anomie is not seen as a mere state of mind, it is also believed to be a reaction to normative erosion in society. This way of thinking about subjective well-being is already visible in the work of Comte (1851–1854), the founding father of sociology. His notion of *"bonheur"* (happiness) denotes a state of intellectual enlightenment combined with sacral feelings of inclusion and consensus that result from social progress (Ple, 2000).

This way of conceptualizing subjective well-being stems from *rhetorical* use of the concept; it serves to communicate that something is beneficial and for that reason that something is connected conceptually with good feelings. Obviously, this way of conceptualization makes less sense *analytically*; if we put presumed conditions for well-being in one hat with experienced well-being, we will never be able to see what causes what. As a result, such concepts cannot be meaningfully applied in a utilitarian search for social conditions that produce the greatest happiness for the greatest number. Applied for that purpose, such concepts lead to circular reasoning. If, for example, we define subjective well-being as the feeling of connectedness that accompanies social integration, social integration is, by definition, a condition for subjective well-being. Empirical research based on such concepts will do no more than echo prepossession. This is typically the case with the indexes of well-being that are commonly used in sociology. I have discussed this matter in more detail elsewhere (Veenhoven, 2000a).

In Diener et al.'s definition, subjective well-being is seen as the product of an overall appraisal of life that balances the good and the bad. This conceptualization does not restrict itself to specific feelings and does not mix up the subjective experience with its possible causes. In the rest of this chapter I use the term *subjective well-being* in this sense.

This concept of subjective well-being is close to Bentham's (1970) classic definition of happiness as "the sum of pleasures and pains." Most sociologists know of this concept, but few have applied it, although it made a comeback in the 1960s in some pockets of sociology, in particular, in social indicators research and the sociology of aging. I was among the early readaptors (Veenhoven, 1968), but certainly not the first sociologist who harked back to Bentham; the first U.S. study on happiness in this sense had appeared in 1965 (Bradburn & Caplovitz, 1965).

How Do We Appraise How Well We Are?: Question 2

Sticking to Diener et al.'s (1997) definition of subjective well-being as being satisfied with life and feeling good, the next question is how we determine this state. What is going on in the mind when we assess how much we enjoy life? This question is of more than mere academic interest, because the answer to it has implications for how we can advance subjective well-being (Question 3) and whether it is worth advancing (Question 4).

Although sociologists are not specialized in matters of the mind, they still make psychological assumptions. They typically borrow from cognitive psychology, in which they find support for their view on humans as socially determined. In this line, sociologists see subjective well-being as a cognitive "construct" shaped by collective notions of the good life and as a result of comparisons, particularly social comparison.

Presumed Social Construction of Subjective Well-Being

Social construction theory discusses how we make sense of things. It assumes that we "construct" mental representations of reality, using collective notions as building blocks (Berger & Luckman, 1966). Social constructionism stresses human thinking and is blind to affective experience and innate drives.

In this view, subjective well-being is also a social construction and, as such, comparable to notions such as "beauty" and "fairness." A common reasoning in this line is that subjective well-being depends on shared notions about life and that these collective notions frame individual appraisals.

One of the ways this process is presumed to work is by shaping perspectives toward optimism (the glass half full) or pessimism (half empty). Optimistic cultures tend to highlight the positive aspects of life, whereas pessimistic cultures emphasize the shortcomings. Americans have been mentioned as an example of the former view and the French of the latter (e.g., Ostroot & Snyder [1985]). In that line Inglehart (1990) suggests that happiness is lower in France than in the United States because life was harder in France for earlier generations, and this experience is mirrored in a more pessimistic outlook on life today.

Another cognitive mechanism presumed to be involved is comparison with shared notions of the good life. In this view, subjective well-being is the gap between perceptions of life-as-it-is with notions of how-life-should-be (Michalos, 1985). In this line it is commonly argued that the advertisement industry reduces our well-being, because it fosters dreams of a life that is out of reach for the common person. Another example of this view is the claim that subjective well-being can be bought with resignation.

An additional mechanism that has been mentioned is the tendency to see ourselves though the eyes of others and hence also our subjective well-being. In this view, subjective well-being is a "reflected appraisal." We would be positive about our life when people around us deem us to be well off and negative when others see us as a looser. In this vein the lower happiness among singles has been explained as the result of a negative stereotype: Because singles are "labeled" as pitiful, they come to see themselves as miserable, in spite of the apparent advantages of single living (e.g., Davies & Strong, 1977).

The constructionist view implies that there is little value to subjective well-being because it is a mere idea. In addition, because notions about the good life vary across time and culture, subjective well-being is also seen to be culturally relative. A life that is deemed perfect in one idea of the good life may be seen as a failure from another point of view. For this reason this theory is popular among the critics of the utilitarian creed that we should aim at "greater happiness for a greater number"; it reduces happiness to something insignificant.

Theoretical Plausibility

It is beyond doubt that shared notions frame much of our appraisals, yet this is not to say that all awareness is socially constructed. We need no shared notions to experience pain or hunger; culture, at best, modifies our reflection on these experiences a bit. Our understanding also draws on external stimuli and inner signals. The question is thus how this process works in the case of subjective well-being.

The answer to that question depends on the definition of subjective well-being. If the term is defined as the mere belief that one's life fits the common standards for a good life, social construction is evidently involved. However, if the definition also involves affective experience, this is not so evident. In this chapter we follow Diener et al.'s (1997) definition of subjective well-being, and that definition involves a preponderance of positive affect over negative affect.

Affect and cognition are linked, but they are certainly not the same. Evaluations of life draw on both sources of information, and affective appraisals dominate. When striking the balance of their life, people appear to use their mood as the prime source of information (Schwartz & Strack, 1991), and consequently overall happiness typically correlates more strongly with hedonic levels of affect than with contentment (Veenhoven, 2006c, H6[1]). There is logic in this, because the affect system is evolutionarily older and serves to ascertain that the organism's

---

[1] The collection of "Correlational Findings" in the World Database of Happiness is sorted by subject. Subject sections are indicated with a capital letter and a number; for example, A4 for findings on happiness and Age.

basic needs are met. The cognitive system developed on top of this in *Homo sapiens*, but it did not replace the affective system. It is rather an additional device that allows planning of activities and better learning from experience. In that light it is unlikely that subjective well-being is a mere cognition.

Empirical Support

The reality value of this view cannot be tested as such, because the human mind is still a black box. Yet we can check its aptness indirectly, when we consider implications of the theory that subjective well-being is a mere social construction.

Culture Specific? One implication is that conditions for subjective well-being are variable across cultures. If subjective well-being is a culture-specific construct, its determinants will also be culturally specific. Hence empirical studies on correlates of subjective well-being must show considerable cultural variation and hardly any universal pattern. Yet the available data show otherwise. Comparison of average subjective well-being across nations reveals a common pattern. Subjective well-being is systematically higher in nations that provide a decent material standard of living, that are politically democratic and well governed, and where the cultural climate is characterized by trust and tolerance. Together these objective societal characteristics explain about 75% of the differences in subjective well-being across nations (Veenhoven & Kalmijn, 2005). Comparison of correlations within nations also shows much similarity. In all countries, the married appear to be happier than singles (Diener, 2000), and health (both physical health and mental) is also a strong correlate of happiness all over the world (Veenhoven, 2006c, P6, M7[1]). Likewise, the differences in happiness across age and gender are typically small everywhere (Veenhoven, 2006c, A4, G1).

Variable over Time? A second implication is that subjective well-being must be variable across time. If subjective well-being depends on shared notions of the good life, it will vary with fads about that matter, and this variation must reflect erratic movements in average subjective well-being in nations, comparable to changes in political preference and tastes for music. Yet again this not what the data show. Average subjective well-being appears to be very stable over time, at least in Western nations over the last 30 years, where happiness rose slightly without much fluctuations (Veenhoven, 2006b). Follow-up studies at the individual level also show considerable constancy over time (Ehrhardt, Saris, & Veenhoven, 2000).

Inconsequential? A third implication is that subjective well-being is of little consequence. If subjective well-being is sheer cognitive spin, based on fashionable ideas, it will not matter much whether it pans out positively or negatively. Subjective well-being is then a petty appraisal, such as a person's preference for one kind of wallpaper or another; nice in itself but of no consequence for anything more than that.

Once more, this appears not to be the case. Subjective well-being goes hand in hand with objective thriving. Furthermore, follow-up studies have shown that subjective well-being is a strong predictor of physical health and longevity (e.g., Danner, Friesen, & Snowdow, 2001). Together, these findings do not support the theory that subjective well-being is a mere making of the mind.

Note that these findings concern "subjective well-being-as-such" and not opinions about what adds to subjective well-being. Subjective well-being-as-such is something that we experience ourselves and which we can appraise without the help of others. Though we know *how* we feel, we often do not know *why*. In attributing grounds for our well-being, we draw more on a shared view. In this respect subjective well-being is comparable to a headache: a headache-as-such is not a social construction, it is an autonomous signal from the body. Yet our interpretations of what gives us a headache depend very much on hearsay.

Well-Being as Surpassing the Joneses

All sociologists learned in their student days about the exemplary case of "relative deprivation," described in Stouffer's (1949) classic study "The American Soldier." One of the areas assessed in this study was the satisfaction with promotion chances. Contrary to expectation, the satisfaction with this aspect of Army life appeared to be higher in units where promotion chances were low, such as the military police, than in units where promotion chances were high, such as the Air Force. This phenomenon was explained in terms of social comparison; because promotion was more common in the Air Force, Air Force personnel more often felt *entitled* to promotion. This case of satisfaction with promotion makes many sociologists think that all satisfaction depends on social comparison and thus also life satisfaction.

Social comparison theory (see Fujita, Chapter 12, this volume) is a variant of a wider comparison theory that links up with the above-mentioned notion that subjective well-being is the difference between life-as-it-is and how-life-should-be. The smaller these discrepancies are, the higher the subjective well-being is assumed to be. In this theory there can be multiple discrepancies; among other things, discrepancies between what one has and what one thinks that one could have, and discrepancies between what one has and what one feels entitled to (Michalos, 1985). Perceptions of what one could have and what would be fair to have are seen to draw on social comparison. In this view, subjective well-being is a matter of keeping up with the Joneses; we feel well if we do better and bad if we do worse.

In this theory there is little hope for achieving greater happiness for a greater number, because improving the living conditions for all will also improve the life of the Joneses, leaving the relative differences what they are. Social comparison is one of the mechanisms in the idea that we are on a "hedonic treadmill" that presumably nullifies all progress (Brickman & Campbell, 1971), and it is the main mechanism in Easterlin's (1974) theory that economic growth does not add to subjective well-being. In this view we can, at best, mitigate the effects of social comparison somewhat if we make the differences less visible. In this line Frank (1999) has advised that conspicuous consumption should be discouraged with heavy taxes on luxury goods. Limiting advertisement is also suggested in this context, in particular, commercials that use pictures of a life that is out of reach for the common person (Layard, 2005).

Theoretical Plausibility

There are several problems with this theory. First of all it is clear that social comparison does not apply to all subjective appraisal. When I hit my finger with a hammer, I feel pain—and it does not hurt less if neighbor Jones does the same. When appraising our situation, we use various sources of information, and social comparison is only one of these.

This point brings us to the question of what value social comparison provides for assessing how well one lives. Obviously, that value is limited to aspects of life in which social comparison is possible, such as your income. Social comparison is not so relevant for evaluating the less visible aspects of life, such as your sex life or the pleasure you take from watching the sunset. Where comparison with the Joneses is practicable, it informs us about what is *possible* in life but not necessarily about what is *desirable* or *enjoyable*. Looking over the fence of my neighbor, I can see that I lag behind in the number of beer cans emptied, but this does not tell me whether I would be better off if I drank more. Advocates of social comparison theory would retort that we compare only in areas that are socially valued in society, such as money and fame, and this reality links up with the assumption that notions of the good life are socially constructed. Yet even if beer boozing were highly valued in my society, and if I wholeheartedly supported that value, I would end up less well if I drank more than my dipsomaniacal neighbor. That is evident because drinking too much is bad for the body, irrespective of how I *think* about it. This example illustrates a major flaw in comparison theory: It forgets that we are *biological* organisms.

Obviously we cannot feel well if our body is harmed. Affective alarms start ringing when we do not get enough food or when our temperature falls too low. Less obvious but no less existent are psychological needs, such as the need to belong and to use and develop our potentials. We feel lousy when lonely and bored when unchallenged. Humans are not born as a tabula rasa, on which socialization imprints culture-specific wants; we are prewired to need some things and as a result feel good when these needs are met.

In this respect we are very much like our fellow animals. Dogs and cats can also feel good or bad and evidently do not calculate their subjective well-being by comparing shared standards of the good life. Evolution has simply programmed them to feel good or bad subjectively in situations that are good or bad for their survival objectively. Our affective system is not much different from that of dogs and cats, and also serves to make us do intuitively what is good for us. Human cognition has developed on top of this affective program and allows us to reflect on affective signals and even to ignore them to some extent. Yet this is not to say that cognition has replaced affective experience. Without affective information we are conatively blind; we cannot choose and cannot come to an overall judgment (Damasio, 1994).

I have discussed this alternative "need theory" of happiness elsewhere (Veenhoven, 1995, 2000a). This theory is also called "livability theory," and in this case the emphasis is on the conditions that allow for need gratification. Together with Lucas, Diener has reviewed the strong and weak points of this theory (Diener & Lucas, 2000). Though alien to mainstream sociology, this latter view on subjective well-being would fit sociobiology; to my knowledge this field of sociology has not yet considered the issue.

Fit with Facts

Social comparison is at best one piece of information in appraisals of subjective well-being, and it is an empirical question to determine how much it matters. We can see how much when considering some implications of the theory. One testable implication of social comparison theory is that people typically are neither positive nor negative about their life. If we feel good because we do better than the Joneses, then the Joneses must feel bad because they do worse. This trend must manifest in an average around neutral in general population samples. Yet survey data do not support this prediction; average subjective well-being is far above neutral in modern nations.

Another implication is that subjective well-being must be higher among people who do well on socially valued standards. This is not always the case, however. Though people in high-status jobs are typically happier than people in low-status occupations (Veenhoven, 2006c, O1), there is no correlation between subjective well-being and level of education (Veenhoven, 2006c, E1). Likewise, there is only modest correlation between subjective well-being and income, and this correlation is at least partly due to an effect of the former on the latter, happiness adding to earning chances (Veenhoven, 2006c, I1). However, subjective well-being does appear to depend on things that have little to do with social comparison, as we will see below.

What Conditions Foster Subjective Well-Being?: Question 3

Dealing with this question, sociologists first look at social conditions. At the macro level they look at characteristics of society, such as industrialization and individualization, and take particular interest in variations in state organization, such as welfare state regimes. Looking at conditions for happiness within societies, sociologists look at people's position on the social ladder, at their participation in public institutions, and at their embedding in private networks.

Modernity

Sociology developed in the turmoil of transition from an agrarian to an industrial society and this has focused attention on problems of modernization. Sociologists conducted incisive studies about the agonies of working-class people in the early phase of industrialization, about discrimination of migrants and the perils of life in growing cities. There are also insightful accounts of moral disorganization and the decline of the family. This research on modern misery has fueled the idea that life was better in the "good old days." Every year I ask my sociology students whether they think that modernization has made society more livable, and invariably the majority thinks that this is not the case.

A common theory behind this idea of withering well-being is that we humans are prewired for strong social networks, such as small communities, close-knit families, and a united church. Many sociologists were raised with Tönnies's (1979) distinction between traditional "*Gemeinschaft*" and modern "*Gesellschaft*" and heard their professors tell them that the former is more livable than the latter (though Tönnies himself saw the development to *Gesellschaft* as an improvement). Hence it is no surprise to find sociologists at the head of the communitarian movement that aims to "bring community back in society" (Etzioni, 1993).

Are we really prewired for a life in "strong" social networks? The pattern of cohesive communities, extended families, and a strong church is characteristic of agrarian societies but not of the hunter–gatherer society from which the human species has evolved. Hunter–gatherer societies are rather characterized by "weak" social ties, shifting bands being common in such societies, as is serial monogamy. Exertion of power is limited in hunter–gatherer existence, and social relations are therefore largely based on exchange and attraction. Seen in this light, modern individualized *Gesellschaft* may fit human nature better than traditional collectivist *Gemeinschaft*. Maryanski and Turner (1992) make this point convincingly in their seminal study *The Social Cage*, which documents the human preference for weak ties with findings from anthropology and ethnology. They show how the agrarian revolution forced humans into an oppressing social system (the social cage) and explain why people massively turned their back on pastoral *Gemeinschaft* once the industrial revolution provided a way out.

We cannot assess the subjective well-being of our ancestors, but anthropological archeology has found indications of their physical condition. Longevity appears not to have risen after the agrarian revolution, whereas health deteriorated (Sanderson, 1995). This shift marks a quality dip in human history. As we all know, the industrial revolution has been followed by an unprecedented rise in longevity that still goes on today and that also involves a steady rise in the number of years lived in good health. Less well known is the fact that subjective well-being has also risen. This rise appears in the comparison of more and less modern nations at the present time and also is the trend in modern nations over the last 40 years (Veenhoven, 2005a, 2006b).

So there is truth in the notion that societal development *may* go against human nature and reduce subjective well-being. Yet, contrary to what most sociologists believe, this reduction happened not after the industrial revolution, but thousands of years earlier in the wake of the agrarian revolution. In contrast, modernization appears to have boosted subjective well-being.

Welfare State

Many sociologists work for institutions of the welfare state. This context fosters a tendency among sociologists to equate public welfare with well-being. In The Netherlands they even denote these two concepts with the same word (*welzijn*). In this line it is assumed that subjective well-being is higher in extended welfare states such as Sweden than in residual welfare states such as the United States, and that this status is believed to be particularly true for "vulnerable" people, such as the aged and unemployed. This theory is not unchallenged, however; for instance, Murray (1984) argues that lavish welfare is inefficient and causes people to go "from the frying pan into the fire."

Empirical research shows no higher subjective well-being in welfare states than in otherwise comparable nations where "Father State" is less open-handed. Surprisingly there is also no difference in inequality of subjective well-being, as measured using the standard deviation of happiness. This absence of a difference appears both in a comparison of nations in the early 1990s and in a comparison over time within nations (Veenhoven, 2000b). An analysis that focused on the unemployed, in particular, yielded the same result (Ouweneel, 2000). These findings may mean that there is some truth in both theoretical positions and that the positive and negative effects of state welfare balance out.

Social Inequality

The development of sociology was also influenced by the emancipation movements of the 20th century, first of laborers and then of women and ethnic minorities. Though these movements have been successful to a great extent, inequality is a still the main issue in sociology. In this line, sociologists tend to think of subjective well-being in terms of inequality; people who feel bad are assumed to be deprived in some way, and people who are deemed to be deprived are assumed to feel bad.

Social inequality is commonly defined as differential "access to scarce resources," and the resources typically mentioned in social textbooks are income, power, and prestige. Income differences are most prominent in the discourse on social inequality, in particular, differences at the bottom of the income distribution. The tradition of poverty research in sociology stresses the adverse effects of income inequality on well-being and warns of a growing split in society between haves and have-nots.

It is evident that social inequality *can* reduce subjective well-being, particularly of the deprived. Yet it is not so evident that all inequalities *do* and that income inequality is a main thread to subjective well-being in modern society. Cocaine is a scarce resource in most Western nations, and there are clear differences in access to it, but people who can easily get cocaine do not stand out as having greater subjective well-being. Not everything that is scarce is beneficial, a point that may also apply to socially valued luxury goods such as big cars, second houses, and fancy holidays. Remember the above discussion on social comparison. It seems more plausible that inequality hurts only when it interferes with the gratification of basic needs, such as our need for food or respect.

The first sociological surveys on subjective well-being were conducted in the context of marketing research for the welfare state and were expected to show suffering among the deprived. However, this finding failed to appear in the data. As mentioned above, subjective well-being is only marginally related to socioeconomic position in modern nations. Subjective well-being is more strongly related to socio*emotional* position, that is, ties with friends, family, and clubs. Yet these are not "scarce resources," of which only limited amounts are available.

Another surprise is that there is no correlation between the degree of income inequality in nations and average subjective well-being (Berg, 2006). Apparently, we can live with big disparities in income. This accommodation does not mean that we can live equally well with all forms of inequality; for example, gender inequality in nations does go with lower average well-being. In this case it is not only the women who suffer, men are also less happy in gender-segregated nations (Chin Hon Foei, 2006).

Still another unexpected outcome is that inequality in happiness, as measured with the standard deviation, appears to have decreased in modern nations over the last 40 years (Veenhoven, 2005c). That finding is in flat contradiction with the sociological theory of the "new inequality" rising in modern society.

Social Participation

Sociologists are also concerned about the involvement of individuals in society. Many sociologists work for organizations that try to engage people in their communities and the political process. Though this work is done for the benefit of institutions in the first place, it is generally believed that individual citizens also profit from social participation (e.g., Putnam, 2000); remember the above-noted tendency of sociologists to put different varieties of the good in one hat. Several mechanisms have been mentioned in this context; one is that social participation creates "social capital" that can be used to "produce" subjective well-being. Another presumed mechanism is that social participation is rewarding in itself, not only because it involves rewarding contacts with other people, but also because it fosters a sense of having control and being part of society.

Sociological intuition fits the data better in this case. Comparative studies at the nation level show higher subjective well-being in nations with a well-functioning democracy and dense networks of voluntary associations (Veenhoven, 2004). Studies among individuals in nations show invariably that active members of clubs and churches report greater subjective well-being than nonmembers or passive members (Veenhoven, 2006c, S6-8). Unfortunately, the available data do not give us information about cause and effect, so the correlation could be due largely to effects of happiness, which would fit Fredrickson's (2004) "broaden and build" theory.

This is not to say that more participation is always better and certainly not that participation in the public sphere is most conducive to subjective well-being. We see this point in the case of work life. Paid work is often praised as required for subjective well-being, but the data show that many can live without paid work. For example, retirement does not seem to reduce subjective well-being (Veenhoven, 2006c, R2), and full-time homemakers have been found to be happier than working mothers (Veenhoven, 2006c, E2.2.1). Only among male breadwinners are the employed at an advantage (Veenhoven, 2006c, E2). Still another point to note in this context is that subjective well-being appears to be lowest in the phase of life where participation in public life is highest. Comparison of subjective well-being across age groups reveals a U-shaped pattern of people feeling best in their early 20s and after age 50, and worst in the midyears of life when they are most involved in work.

Social Support

Though private life is not the prime domain of Western sociology, there is a long tradition of research into family ties and a more recent body of research on friendship. Subjective well-being is a common theme in this context. It is generally assumed that we need such "primary" ties and that subjective well-being depends on the availability and quality of the ties. Again, several causal mechanisms have been hypothesized to be involved. One of these is that intimates "support" us materially and immaterially (e.g., Putnam, 2000) Among the immaterial kinds of support are information, emotional backing, and behavioral correction. Another theory holds that family relations protect against negative labeling as a deviant.

Empirical research has indeed shown strong relations between intimate ties and subjective well-being, and in this case there is also evidence for causal effects of the former on the latter (e.g., Lucas, Clark, Diener, & Georgellis, 2003). The causal mechanism seems to be social support rather than protection against negative stereotyping (Veenhoven, 1989), a finding that is still another indication that cognitive theories of subjective well-being fall short.

What Are the Consequences of Feeling Well or Not?: Question 4

Research on subjective well-being has focused on its *determinants* in search of an answer to the question of how it can be advanced. Another issue is the *consequences* of subjective well-being, which is relevant to answering the question of whether subjective well-being should be furthered.

This is a topic in the psychology of subjective well-being and, in particular, in the recent field of positive psychology. Together with Lyubomirsky, Diener has published a review of the literature that shows positive effects on various aspects of human functioning, such as creativity, social contacts, work performance, and physical health (Lyubomirsky, King, & Diener, 2005). The data fit well with the above-mentioned theory that subjective well-being "*broadens*" and "*builds*" (Fredrickson, 2004); *broadening* means that subjective well-being widens our perceptual horizon, and *building* means that it facilitates the formation of resources.

Sociologists have not given much thought on this topic as yet, and mainstream opinion is still largely guided by the tale of the *Brave New World* (Huxley, 1932), in which subjective well-being goes hand in hand with superficial consumerism, political apathy, and general ignorance. That story fits the theory that subjective well-being is a mere cognitive illusion that does not root in real quality of life. Sociologists see typically more value in discontent, which they regard as the seed of personal motivation and social change.

Is Subjective Well-Being a Subject for Sociology?

Some of my colleague sociologists feel that the subject of subjective well-being should be left to psychology, because it is a mental state and not a condition of society. I think they are wrong.

One reason is that the subjective well-being of individuals entails important information about the quality of the social system in which they live. If people typically feel bad, the social system is apparently not well suited for human habitation. One of the aims of sociology is to contribute to a better society, and the study of subjective well-being provides clues for a more livable society (Veenhoven, 2004). This inductive approach to the good society is also a counterpoise to the speculative theorizing about the good society and an antidote against the ideological prepossessions on that matter. There is a rising demand for information about social conditions that foster subjective well-being among policymakers because, among other reasons, the great ideologies have lost appeal.

Another reason why sociologists should be more concerned about subjective well-being is that it is one of the determinants of social behavior. Most sociologists would be surprised to learn that happy people are typically better citizens, that they are better informed about political matters, that they use their voting rights more often, that they involve themselves more in civil action and are, at the same time, less radical in their political views (Lyubomirsky & Diener, 2005). Clearly, these attributes are relevant for understanding the functioning of the democratic system. Subjective well-being is also likely to affect the functioning of other social systems, such as work organizations and friendship networks.

So, individual subjective wellbeing is both an outcome social systems and a factor in their functioning. As such the subject belongs to the core business of sociology.

References

Beerling, R. F. (1978). Vervreemding. In L. Rademarekers (Ed.), *Sociologische encyclopedie* [*Encyclopedia of sociology*] (pp. 790–792). Utrecht, The Netherlands: Aula.

Bentham, J. (1970). *An introduction into the principles of morals and legislation.* London: Athloue Press. (Original work published 1789)

Berg, M. (2006). *Income inequality and happiness in nations.* Manuscript submitted for publication, Erasmus University, Rotterdam.

Berger, P. L., & Luckman, T. (1966). *The social construction of reality: A treatise in the sociology of knowledge.* Garden City, NY: Doubleday.

Bradburn, N. M., & Caplovitz, D. (1965). *Reports on happiness: A pilot study of behavior related to mental health.* Chicago: Aldine.

Brickman, P., & Campbell, D. T. (1971). Hedonic relativism and planning the good society. In M. H. Appley (Ed.), *Adaptation level theory: A symposion* (pp. 287–302). London: Academic Press.

Chin Hon Foei, S. S. (2006). *Gender inequality and happiness in nations.* Manuscript submitted for publication, Erasmus University, Rotterdam.

Comte, A. (1921). *Système de politique positive* [*The system of positive politics*]. Paris: Siège de la sociètè positiviste. (Original work published 1851–1854)

Damasio, A. R. (1994). *Descartes' error: Emotion, reason and the human brain.* New York: Grosset-Putnam.

Danner, D. D., Friesen, W. V., & Snowdon, D. A. (2001). Positive emotions in early life and longevity: Findings from the nun study. *Journal of Personality and Social Psychology, 80,* 804–813.

Davies, A. G., & Strong, P. M. (1977). Working without a net: The *bachelos* as a social problem. *Sociological Review, 25,* 109–129.

Diener, E. (2000). Subjective well-being: The science of happiness and a proposal for a national index. *American Psychologist, 55,* 34–43.

Diener, E., & Lucas, R. E. (2000). Explaining differences in societal levels of happiness: Relative standards, need fulfilment, culture and evaluation theory. *Journal of Happiness Studies, 1,* 41–78.

Diener, E., Suh, E., & Oishi, S. (1997). Recent findings on subjective well-being. *Indian Journal of Clinical Psychology, 24,* 25–41.

Easterlin, R. A. (1974). Does economic growth improve the human lot? Some empirical evidence. In P. A. Davis & W. R. Melvin (Eds.), *Nations and households in economic growth* (pp. 98–125). Palo Alto, CA: Stanford University press.

Ehrhardt, J., Saris, W. E., & Veenhoven, R. (2000). Stability of life-satisfaction over time: Analysis of change in ranks in a national population. *Journal of Happiness Studies, 1,* 177–205.

Etzioni, A. (1993). *The spirit of community: The reinvention of American society.* New York: Simon and Schuster.

Frank, R. H. (1999). *Luxury fever: Why money fails to satisfy in an era of excess.* New York: Free Press.

Fredrickson, B. L. (2004). The broaden-and-build theory of positive emotions. *Philosophical Transactions of the Royal Society of London (Biological Sciences), 359,* 1367–1377.

Huxley, A. (1932). *Brave new world: A novel.* London: Shattow & Windus.

Inglehart, R. (1990). *Culture shift in advanced industrial society.* Princeton, NJ: Princeton University Press.

Layard, R. (2005). *Happiness: Lessons from a new science.* New York: Penguin Books.

Lucas, R. E., Clark, A. E., Diener, E., & Georgellis, Y. (2003). Reexamining adaptation and the set point model of happiness: Reaction to changes in marital status. *Journal of Personality and Social Psychology, 84,* 527–539.

Lyubomirsky, S., King, L., & Diener, E. (2005). The benefits of frequent positive affect: Does happiness lead to success? *Psychological Bulletin, 131,* 803–855.

Maryanski, A., & Turner, J. H. (1992). *The social cage: Human nature and the evolution of society*. Palo Alto, CA: Stanford University Press.

Michalos, A. C. (1985). Multiple discrepancy theory. *Social Indicator Research, 16*, 347–413.

Murray, G. (1984). *Losing ground: American social policy 1950–1980*. New York: Basic Books.

Nolan, P., & Lenski, G. (2004). *Human societies: An introduction to macro-sociology*. Boulder, CO: Paradigm Press.

Ostroot, N., & Snyder, W. W. (1985). Measuring cultural bias in a cross-national study. *Social Indicators Research, 17*, 234–251.

Ouweneel, P. (2000). Social security and well-being of the unemployed in 42 nations. *Journal of Happiness Studies, 3*, 167–192.

Ple, B. (2000). Auguste Comte on positivism and happiness. *Journal of Happiness Studies, 1*, 423–445.

Putnam, R. D. (2000). *Bowling alone: The collapse and revival of American community*. New York: Simon & Schuster.

Sanderson, S. K. (1995). *Social transformations*. London: Blackwell.

Schwartz, N., & Strack, F. (1991). Evaluating one's life: A judgmental model of subjective well-being. In F. Strack, M. Argyle, & N. Schwartz (Eds.), *Subjective well-being: An interdisciplinary perspective* (pp. 27–48). Oxford, UK: Pergamon Press.

Stouffer, S. A. (1949). *The American soldier: Adjustment during army life*. Princeton, NJ: Princeton University Press.

Tönnies, F. (1979). *Gemeinschaft und Gesellschaft: Grundbegriffe der reinen Soziologie* [Community and Society: Basic concepts of sociology]. Darmstadt: Wissenschaftliche Buchgesellschaft. (Original work published 1887)

Veenhoven, R. (1968). Geluk als onderwerp van wetenschappelijk onderzoek [Happiness as a subject of scientific research]. *Sociologische Gids, 17*, 115–122.

Veenhoven, R. (1984). *Conditions of happiness*. Boston: Reidel.

Veenhoven, R. (1989). Does happiness bind? In R. Veenhoven (Ed.), *How harmful is happiness?* (pp. 44–60). Rotterdam, The Netherlands: University Press.

Veenhoven, R. (1995). The cross-national pattern of happiness: Test of predictions implied in three theories of happiness. *Social Indicators Research, 43*, 33–86.

Veenhoven, R. (2000a). The four qualities of life: Ordering concepts and measures of the good life. *Journal of Happiness Studies, 1*, 1–39.

Veenhoven, R. (2000b). Well-being in the welfare state: Level not higher, distribution not more equitable. *Journal of Comparative Policy Analysis, 2*, 91–125.

Veenhoven, R. (2004). Happiness as a public policy aim: The greatest happiness principle. In P. A. Linley & S. Joseph (Eds.), *Positive psychology in practice* (pp. 658–678). New York: Wiley.

Veenhoven, R. (2005a). Is life getting better? How long and happy do people live in modern society? *European Psychologist, 10*, 330–343.

Veenhoven, R. (2005b). Trend average happiness in nations 1946–2004. *World Database of Happiness: Distributional findings in nations, Trend-report 2005-1*. Available at *www.worlddatabaseofhappiness.eur.nl/hap_nat/findingreports/List_of_reports.htm*.

Veenhoven, R. (2005c). Return of inequality in modern society? Test by trend in dispersion of life-satisfaction across time and nations. *Journal of Happiness Studies, 6,* 457–487.

Veenhoven, R. (2006a). Quality of life research. In C. D. Bryant & D. L. Peck (Eds.), *Handbook of 21st century sociology.* New York: Sage.

Veenhoven, R. (2006b). Rising happiness in nations 1946–2004: A reply to Easterlin. *Social Indicators Research, 79,* 421–436

Veenhoven, R. (2006c). *World database of Happiness: Correlational findings.* Available at *www.worlddatabaseofhappiness.eur.nl/hap_cor/cor_fp.htm.*

Veenhoven, R., & Kalmijn, W. (2005). Inequality-adjusted happiness in nations: Egalitarianism and utilitarianism married together in a new index of societal performance. *Journal of Happiness Studies, 6,* 421–455.

4

Evolution and Subjective Well-Being

SARAH E. HILL and DAVID M. BUSS

The scientific study of subjective well-being generally focuses on two key components related to well-being: (1) the balance of negative versus positive moods experienced by individuals on a day-to-day basis, and (2) the amount of global satisfaction individuals express about their lives (Diener, Suh, Lucas, & Smith, 1999; Diener & Emmons, 1984; Pavot, Diener, Colvin, & Sandvik, 1991). Researchers exploring these components of subjective well-being have successfully identified a number of key features of human social life that can add to or detract from one's well-being and overall life satisfaction. For instance, researchers have demonstrated links between subjective well-being and factors such as health, wealth, and marital status (Gove & Shin, 1989; George & Landerman, 1984; Diener, Gohm, Suh, & Oishi, 2000; Diener, Sandvik, Seidlitz, & Diener, 1993; Okun, Stock, Haring, & Witter, 1984). Researchers also have identified important individual differences in predispositions to the experience of happiness, many of which appear to have a substantial heritable component (Lykken & Tellegen, 1996; Tellegen et al., 1988). Personality variables such as extraversion (high) and neuroticism (low) have emerged as among the strongest and most consistent predictors of subjective well-being (Diener & Lucas, 1999). Perhaps more importantly, the scientific study of subjective well-being has moved researchers beyond looking solely at economic and sociological indicators as ways to define individuals' life quality (Diener & Suh, 1997). Although income, crime, and unemployment levels play important roles in life quality as experienced by individuals, these measures alone are not sufficient to understand how satisfied and happy people feel in their day-to-day lives. The subjective element is essential because people react differently to the same circumstances and make their evaluations of situations based on their own values, expectancies, and previous experiences (Diener et al., 1999, p. 277).

Given the importance of this emerging field of inquiry, it is surprising that few researchers have yet to explore subjective well-being from an evolutionary perspective. However, given that the underlying mechanisms that generate subjective well-being presumably have been shaped by the process of evolution by natural selection, an evolutionary perspective should offer novel insights into the nature and function of well-being in individuals' lives. In the following sections, we provide an overview of evolutionarily informed research on subjective well-being. First we use an evolutionary perspective to highlight some psychological features and environmental cues that can be detrimental to subjective well-being. These include discrepancies between modern and ancestral environments and psychological mechanisms that have been shaped by selection to induce subjective distress. We then address psychological features that have been shaped by selection and allow people to feel happy and satisfied with their lives. We close with suggestions for how to harness our evolved psychologies to better promote well-being and propose future avenues for research on subjective well-being from an evolutionary perspective.

Impediments to Subjective Well-Being

One important contribution that evolutionary psychology has added to the science of subjective well-being has been the identification of obstacles that people must overcome to improve their well-being. These obstacles include both the existence of psychological features that have been shaped by the process of natural selection to intentionally cause subjective distress, and the identification of instances of distress caused by discrepancies between our modern environment and that in which we have spent the majority of our evolutionary histories (see Buss, 2000a).

Dissatisfied by Design:
Adaptations That Cause Subjective Distress

The psychological products of the evolutionary process consist of characteristics that have played a role in solving statistically recurring adaptive problems that humans have been solving over evolutionary time. From an evolutionary psychological perspective, the emotions can be viewed as component parts of a coordinated suite of changes (cognitive, affective, physiological, etc.) shaped by selection to alert the bearers that a change has occurred in the internal or external environment that requires attention (Cosmides & Tooby, 2000). The subjective experience of emotions—such as the positive or negative affective shifts associated with emotional experiences—is not viewed as being good or bad, although experienced as such by individuals. Rather, emotions are understood to be features designed by the evolutionary process based on their ability to help our ancestors survive and reproduce over evolutionary time.

Unfortunately, many of the features that have facilitated successful survival and reproduction do not have the result of making us feel happy or satisfied with our lives. According to one evolutionary psychological hypothesis, feelings of subjective distress and discomfort are evolved psychological responses shaped by selection to signal strategic interference. Strategic interference theory (Buss, 1989) posits that many "negative" emotions, such as anger or jealousy, have been designed by the evolutionary process to signal that someone or something is impeding one's preferred behavioral strategy. Strategic interference has been hypothesized to function by (1) focusing an individual's attention on the source of strategic interference while temporarily screening out information that is less relevant to the adaptive problem being faced, (2) prompting storage of the relevant information in memory, (3) motivating action to reduce the strategic interference, and (4) motivating action to prevent future such interference.

The human mind likely contains numerous psychological adaptations that have been selected by the evolutionary process based on their ability to signal strategic interference. Some examples of these features are envy (Hill & Buss, 2006a), anxiety (Marks & Nesse, 1994), depression (Price & Sloman, 1987; Nesse, 2005, 2006), fears and phobias (Marks, 1987), sexual jealousy (Buss, 1988; Buss, Larsen, Weston, & Semmelroth, 1992; Daly, Wilson, & Weghorst, 1982), low self-esteem (Hill & Buss, 2006a; Kirkpatrick & Ellis, 2001, 2006), and anger and upset (Buss, 1989). Although upsetting to the individual experiencing them, from an evolutionary perspective, such negative emotional responses have been shaped by selection to solve recurrent adaptive problems faced by our ancestors, such as loss of status, sexual coercion, the presence of environmental hazards (e.g., poisonous snakes, spiders), and sexual infidelity. The experience of negative emotions, although subjectively unpleasant, provides the necessary wake-up call to our consciousness to recognize that there is an adaptive problem that needs to be solved, and it subsequently motivates action to solve it.

Consider the adaptive problems associated with social competition. Competing successfully against rivals in competitions for access to scarce resources requires extensive social comparisons. Whether attempting to win the heart of a desirable mate, navigate a status hierarchy, or secure a coveted new job, individuals must constantly strive for access to desirable resources or positions that others are simultaneously attempting to acquire. Over evolutionary time, selection would have favored those individuals who took note when social rivals possessed advantages they did not have and felt motivated to acquire those same advantages for themselves. Evidence supports the hypothesis that envy is one such emotional adaptation that has been shaped by selection to signal strategic interference of this nature (Hill & Buss, 2006). Envy, according to this hypothesis, functions to alert a person to a rival's possible or actual advantage and prompts action designed to (1) acquire these resources for him- or herself, (2) take these resources directly from the rival, or (3) attempt to mitigate any social damage done to him- or herself via unfavorable social comparisons with the advantaged individual.

The emotion of envy can be damaging to subjective well-being, however. No one can deny the subjective distress that sometimes follows a friend or rival gaining an advantage that we would like for ourselves. The feelings of resentment in response to another's perceived advantage have soured relationships between siblings, destroyed friendships, and chilled relations among coworkers. Feelings of upset and hostility can be so visceral and unpleasant that the individual would rather terminate the relationship than continue to experience this uncomfortable reminder of the other's advantage. Despite the damage that envy can have on subjective well-being, it serves an important function in social competitions. Individuals who experience envy in response to a social competitor's advantage would be appropriately alerted to the advantage and motivated to commence corrective action. Over the course of evolutionary time, individuals who did not feel subjective discomfort in these situations would likely have been outcompeted by their more envious counterparts. Although envy often results in subjective distress, this type of emotional distress functions to motivate adaptive action (Buss, 2000a).

The adaptive problems inherent in social competition can also shed light on some of the cognitive adaptations and decision-making processes that can have a potentially negative impact on subjective well-being. Many resources necessary for successful survival and reproduction are limited in quantity and, as such, not equally available to all who want them. For example, in the domain of mate competition, there are a limited number of men and women who embody the characteristics that men and women most desire in their mates (Buss, 2003). Because there are fewer "high-mate value" mates than there are individuals who desire them, those few individuals lucky enough to win the hearts of the desirable necessarily do so at the expense of their competition. The qualities that lead individuals to gain preferential access to desirable mates, over evolutionary time, out-reproduced their mating competitors. Modern humans possess the adaptations that led to their success.

Based on this logic, evolutionary psychologists have recently proposed that the human mind should have a "positional bias" in how success is judged in resource competition situations (Hill & Buss, 2006). That is, it is predicted that individuals will be less concerned with how much they have in an absolute sense and more concerned with how much more they have compared to their peers in a number of delimited domains (Frank, 1999). Using an evolutionary perspective, Hill and Buss (2006) proposed that humans attend to the positional rather than absolute values of (1) resources that are known to affect survival or reproduction, and (2) personal attributes that affect individuals' abilities to acquire such resources. They also hypothesized that the positional bias will be sex-differentiated in those domains where the fitness payoffs from competition have differed qualitatively for each sex throughout human evolutionary history.

One domain in which both men and women have generally been found to exhibit the positional bias is when judging the desirability of outcomes such as how much income they would like to have or their preferred amount of educational attainment (Hill & Buss, 2006; Solnick & Hemenway, 1998). Although educational attainment and income are evolutionarily novel concepts, they both correspond with access to financial resources, which can themselves be turned into goods that promote survival and reproduction. New evidence also suggests that the domains in which men and women are most likely to exhibit the positional bias may differ based on the different adaptive problems that each has had to solve over the course of evolutionary history. For instance, the domain of physical attractiveness is one in which women have historically competed more fiercely than men due to the premium that men place on appearance in selecting mates (Buss, 1989). This reasoning has led evolutionary psychologists to predict that women should exhibit the positional bias more than men when reasoning about their preferred levels of physical attractiveness. As predicted, women were found to exhibit the positional bias significantly more than men in this domain (Hill & Buss, 2006).

Because individuals appear to judge their own successes in delimited domains based on comparisons with how everyone else is performing, subjective distress and dissatisfaction with oneself can occur when encountering others who are better off in one of these domains. Furthermore, the positional bias hypothesis suggests that even if we are able to work hard enough to gain access to those things of others that we covet, it is not likely to lead to long-term satisfaction and happiness (Frank, 1999). Even though we may feel pleasure after we receive an increase in pay or move into a larger house, it is typically not long before we go back to feeling much the same as we did before the raise or move (although see Diener, Lucas, & Scollon, 2006, for important modifications of this "hedonic treadmill" theory). Even though Americans now live in larger houses that contain more color TVs, computers, and cars than they ever have at any point in our history, they are no happier now than they were previously (Frank, 1999; Myers & Diener, 1995).

Psychological processes such as the positional bias and envy guarantee that long-term satisfaction with one's income, position in the status hierarchy, or job will be difficult to achieve. These hypothesized adaptations, in addition to other adaptations designed to cause subjective distress, make the quest for well-being sometimes difficult to achieve.

Discrepancies between Ancestral and Modern Environments

The modern world, for most of us, is quite different from that in which ancestral humans spent the majority of their evolutionary history. Although we do not have a videotaped record of our evolutionary past, archaeological evidence suggests that humans spent the majority of their evolutionary history as hunter–gatherers, living in small groups that likely consisted of between 50 and 200 individuals (Dunbar, 1993). Ancestral humans did not have access to the wealth of conveniences, technologies, and extravagances that are so much a part of modern life. Our current environment offers medical technologies and advances in food procurement that have allowed our populations to grow and average lifespans to lengthen. We have access to hundreds of cable channels, all of which we can watch on our big-screen televisions in the privacy of our own 4,000-square-foot homes. We have machines that wash our clothes, sanitize our dishes, and cook our food. It is hard to argue that we aren't much better off than were our hunter–gatherer forbearers in a number of ways. However, despite the many ways in which humans have improved their conditions of living, the modern environment also differs from that of our ancestors in ways that can make us feel isolated and alone.

Our ancestors likely spent the majority of their lives surrounded by close allies and kin members. Social transactions typically occurred among individuals who engaged in regular contact. Although the current environment offers an almost overwhelming supply of conveniences not available to our ancestral counterparts, many of us do not have access to the intimate social support systems that likely characterized the conditions through which we have spent the majority of our evolutionary history (Nesse & Williams, 1994). The majority of people living in the United States live in small family units, typically consisting of between one and four individuals. Rather than being part of a large, extended community of friends and allies, many of us live in large cities where we are surrounded by thousands or millions of strangers. This anonymity is exacerbated by the fact that many of us find ourselves having to frequently relocate or travel for employment purposes, both of which make it difficult to develop and sustain meaningful relationships with others. This fact has led some evolutionary psychologists to suggest that one detriment to our subjective well-being—depression—might partly be explained by the fact that our modern living conditions are such that we live in virtual anonymity, removed from the types of social support that are so important to subjective well-being (Nesse, 1990, 2006). Humans are a very social species. Our well-being is very highly dependent on having access to people with whom we have deep, meaningful relationships.

Researchers exploring the link between well-being and sociality have demonstrated that being with others typically has the effect of improving mood, whereas being alone tends to have the opposite effect (Argyle, 1987; Lewinsohn, Redner, & Seeley, 1991; Sarason, Sarason, & Pierce, 1990).

Activities in the modern environment also differ from those in which humans historically spent their waking hours. Our ancestors had a close connection with the fruits of their labor. Food was gathered to feed one's family. Meat was procured from cooperative hunting ventures and was brought back to be shared with extended kin and social allies. People had an intimate connection with the work they performed because it had a direct impact on their survival. This connection contrasts with the types of work that most of us routinely must perform to make a living. The long hours that most of us spend in front of computers, copy machines, and hunched over filing cabinets can be socially isolating and far removed from the final product of our labor. This is not to say that most of us would prefer to go back to the days of eating only what we kill. Most of us are perfectly content to spend our daylight hours indoors, away from the "hostile forces of nature." However, the long hours in the office coupled with feelings of disconnection from the fruits of their labor that people often have can potentially have a negative impact on subjective well-being. Work-related stress and feeling that one's work is meaningless are both correlated with anxiety and depression (Maslach, Schaufeli, & Leiter, 2001), both of which are detrimental to well-being.

Competing with Unbeatable Rivals: Social Competition with the Super-Elite

Another way in which our evolved psychologies can negatively affect our subjective well-being is when those features that have been shaped by selection to facilitate successful social competition interact with our current media-saturated environments. It has been hypothesized the human mind has been shaped by selection to have a positional bias in judging the relative success of outcomes that can have an impact on fitness. Thus, men's and women's feelings of satisfaction with how attractive they or their romantic partners are, how much income they have, or how much investment they are garnering from their parents or a mate are dependent on how they stack up relative to their peers. Such biases in our social judgments have been adaptive throughout most of our evolutionary history. They would have allowed individuals to assess the optimal amount of competitive effort to put forth to outcompete rivals. However, in our current environment, not everyone to whom we are daily exposed is an actual social competitor. We need only turn on our televisions or gaze up at a billboard to be exposed to people who are, literally, the richest and most attractive in the world. Large-scale media exposure increases the size and attractiveness of our reference groups and the range and grandeur of the possible goals that we can set for ourselves. Using such a skewed reference group to form self-assessments of success and well-being make even the most successful individual feel that he or she can never succeed, despite the fact that the images we see are no more than fantasies created by the media (Sloman & Gilbert, 2000).

Because men and women judge their success with regard to how much income they have, based on where they stand relative to their rivals, for instance, it is possible that media exposure to depictions of others who have immense wealth may have an unnecessarily negative impact on one's satisfaction with one's financial holdings. Furthermore, given that most women tend to exhibit the positional bias when making judgments about their own physical attractiveness, it is likely that constant exposure to the extremely attractive women depicted on television, in film, and in magazines could make women feel unnecessarily bad about themselves in this domain.

Some empirical evidence supports this supposition. Gutierres and her colleagues have performed a variety of studies that demonstrate that such media exposure may have negative consequences on individuals' subjective well-being. Women subjected to viewing numerous photographs of highly attractive women subsequently felt less attractive themselves and showed a decrease in self-esteem (Gutierres, Kenrick, & Partch, 1999). Consumers of beauty magazines may wish to take note. Men showed a similar pattern after exposures to descriptions of highly dominant and influential men. These results are sex-differentiated in ways predicted by an evolutionary framework and demonstrate an important way in which our current environmental context can have detrimental effects on our feelings of subjective well-being. Exposures to such media also appear to affect how satisfied individuals feel with their romantic partners. In a similar series of studies, researchers discovered that men exposed to multiple images of attractive women subsequently rated their commitment to their current partner as lower than a comparable group of men exposed to images of women average in attractiveness (Kenrick, Gutierres, & Goldberg, 1989; Kenrick, Neuberg, Zierk, & Krones, 1994). Women exposed to multiple images of dominant, high-status men showed a similar decrement in commitment to and love of their regular partner, compared to a group of women exposed to less dominant men.

Psychological Features That Contribute to Well-Being

An evolutionary perspective on subjective well-being suggests that individuals may encounter a number of obstacles that impede well-being during their lifetimes. The many differences between modern and ancestral environments, coupled with the existence of psychological mechanisms designed to facilitate successful social competition and cause psychological distress, ensure that human social life will contain a fair amount of discontentment. However, an evolutionary perspective can also offer a unique perspective on the types of activities and environments that are conducive to facilitating subjective well-being, as well as insights into how individuals can harness their evolved psychologies to better promote subjective well-being in their everyday lives.

What Is Happiness, and How Can We Get More of It?

Evolutionary psychologists have suggested that happiness tracks modern manifestations of ancestral signals of evolutionary fitness (Ketelaar, 2004; Nesse, 1990). Stated differently, happiness is hypothesized to serve as a psychological reward, an internal signaling device that tells an organism that an adaptive problem has been solved successfully or is in the process of being solved successfully. The types of events and situations that are expected to have the biggest positive impact on subjective well-being are those that are related to longstanding adaptive problems humans have been solving over evolutionary time. Promoting happiness and subjective well-being is thus often merely a matter of exploiting knowledge of evolved desires and attempting to fulfill them (Buss, 2000a, 2000b). Studies of private wishes and goals reveal that the motivations behind them are often intimately correlated with fitness (Buss, 2000a). Included among these are the desires for professional success; achieving intimacy in personal relationships; being more physically attractive; helping friends and relatives; securing personal safety, health, power, and access to high-quality food; and possessing personal and financial resources (King & Broyles, 1997; Petrie, White, Cameron, & Collins, 1999).

Taking steps to fulfill desires and the goals determined by these desires makes people feel happy. The experience of positive affect serves as an internal reward and motivator, increasing the probability that the individual will continue moving toward accomplishing his or her goals. Current research suggests that the process of moving towards one's goals may actually be more important to subjective well-being than the end-goal attainment. Working toward reaching goals is correlated with feelings of satisfaction and contentment as long as adequate progress is being made toward the goals at hand (Carver, Lawrence, & Scheier, 1996; Csikszentmihalyi, 1990; Diener et al., 1999; Hsee & Abelson, 1991).

Additional support for the link between solving adaptive problems and subjective well-being can be found in the many correlations between subjective well-being and such fitness indicators as health, marital status, and access to financial resources. Researchers have found a strong correlation between subjective well-being and self-perceptions of health (George & Landerman, 1984; Okun et al., 1984), a domain that is very relevant to survival and reproductive success. Additionally, individuals who have successfully solved the adaptive problem of securing a long-term mate appear to have greater subjective well-being than their unmated counterparts. Married people report greater happiness than those who have never been married or are divorced, separated, or widowed, even when variables such as age and income are controlled for (Glenn & Weaver, 1988; Gove, Hughes, & Style, 1983). This finding has been consistently demonstrated in national and regional surveys conducted in the United States (Gove & Shin, 1989) as well as in international studies (Diener et al., 2000). Successfully solving the adaptive problem of securing a long-term mate, in short, seems to produce happiness, although causality likely runs in both directions: Happy individuals are more likely to succeed in attracting mates.

Researchers have also uncovered findings that suggest that there is a relationship between subjective well-being and amount of financial resources available to individuals. Researchers have demonstrated a strong positive relationship between the wealth of a nation and its inhabitants' average subjective well-being, although increases in income are not inevitably associated with increases in subjective well-being (Diener et al., 1993). This finding suggests that having access to sufficient financial resources to solve important adaptive problems such as securing access to food, clean water, and housing may have a significant impact on subjective well-being. Although further research needs to be done on this topic, existing research appears to suggest that solving important adaptive problems, and even the process of working toward solving them, are expected to be linked closely to happiness and subjective well-being.

Interestingly, one finding appears to contradict the evolutionary perspective articulated here: the effects of having children on marital happiness. The birth of a child is typically greeted with great joy by the parents, as one might expect. Children, after all, are the primary vehicles by which parental genes are replicated. Nonetheless, having children produces a decrement in marital happiness in most subpopulations in U.S. culture—a well-documented sociological finding (Glenn & McGlanahan, 1982). One can speculate about possible proximate causes. As effort becomes allocated toward the child, the previous flow of rewards that come from a marital partner decline. Children can add economic stress. And perhaps lacking the large network of extended kin to help ease the burdens of child care, modern nuclear families experience sources of stress unknown to their forebears. Appropriate theoretical interpretation of this apparent anomaly—that children reduce rather than enhance marital satisfaction—must await research that examines more traditional societies, such as the Ache, the Gebusi, and the !Kung San.

On a final note, it is not clear that a reduction in marital satisfaction produces an overall reduction in subjective well-being. Perhaps the specific components of subjective well-being must be differentiated—well-being around marriage; well-being around work; well-being associated with dyadic alliances; well-being associated with kin. A more domain-specific conceptual and empirical strategy may be needed to understand the apparent anomaly between having children and marital happiness.

Harnessing Our Adaptations to Promote Well-Being

An evolutionary perspective suggests a number of domains in which individuals are expected to exhibit a positional bias when making judgments about the desirability of certain social outcomes, and this bias can have a negative effect on subjective well-being. The feelings of relative deprivation that arise from unfavorable social comparisons can have the effect of lowering mood and self-esteem (Frank, 1999). However, an evolutionary perspective also predicts that there are a number of domains in which individuals will not exhibit a positional bias (Hill & Buss, 2006). Individuals choosing to focus their energies into these domains may have greater subjective well-being due to their self-perceptions of performance being more in their own control. For instance, it has been demonstrated that the positional bias is absent when individuals are reasoning about the number of years that they would like to spend happily married (Hill & Buss, 2006). Individuals appear to make judgments on this issue independent of information about the number of years their peers have been happily married. Both men and women expressed a strong preference for being happily married for an absolutely longer period of time, even though this meant that their peers have been happily married longer than themselves. Thus, it is likely that working on maintaining a harmonious marital life can have a positive effect on subjective well-being, regardless of how happy others' marriages are.

Another domain in which individuals' preferences for social outcomes appear to be relatively unaffected by comparisons with peers is the length of vacation time allotted to them in a given year (Hill & Buss, 2006; Solnick & Hemenway, 1998). Both men and women judged an absolutely longer vacation to be more desirable than a shorter one, despite the longer one being shorter than the vacations allotted to their coworkers. Shifting focus away from these domains in which the positional bias is present (e.g., income, physical attractiveness) and focusing instead on these and other domains in which it is absent may promote subjective well-being. Individuals who choose to focus their energies on maintaining a long, happy marriage and taking full advantage of available vacation time rather than passing it up may have greater control over their ability to experience subjective well-being, because feelings of success and satisfaction in these domains are less contingent on the performance of others.

Awareness that humans exhibit the positional bias and make extensive social comparisons in delimited domains could potentially assist individuals who want to set up their environments to promote subjective well-being. As described, we live in a huge world where there are an almost infinite number of people with whom we can compare ourselves. These comparisons can be made with friends, family members, coworkers, and even with people we view on our television sets or in advertisements. One potential avenue to increasing subjective well-being is to take control over our comparison groups. Most of us are not willing to cut off contact with wealthy or attractive friends, family, or coworkers. However, the much less drastic step of taking a temporary or long-term media "fast" may be a simple way for individuals to promote subjective well-being in their lives. Choosing to limit contact with, or altogether eschewing, media such as fashion magazines, catalogs, and certain television shows may positively affect self-perceptions of attractiveness, status, and wealth. Additionally, a more altruistic route to promoting subjective well-being might be found in helping others less fortunate than oneself. Doing so has the potential of not only helping others in a time of need, but also of increasing one's number of social bonds and providing balance to one's social comparison groups, both of which have a positive effect on self-perceptions and happiness.

Yet another way individuals can harness their evolved psychologies to promote subjective well-being in the current environment is through the use of modern technological advances to develop and maintain social and familial relationships. Technologies such as cellular telephones, e-mail, and airplanes have been designed—in part—to free us from the barriers of physical distance and allow easy contact with friends and families. Other technologies, such as dating and networking websites, have been created to allow individuals to develop new relationships in a way that renders geographical boundaries virtually obsolete. Twenty-first-century humans have done everything in their power to ensure that they can stay in touch with even the most distant friends and relatives. Although telephone calls and 3-day weekends spent visiting with loved ones are no substitutes for having them close at hand daily, taking full advantage of the many technologies that facilitate social relationships may enhance the number and depth of relationships and social networks and, in turn, promote subjective well-being.

Knowledge of evolutionary psychology and our evolved desires can also potentially lead to greater understanding and contentment with our individual goals and values. For instance, throughout human evolutionary history, one of the primary avenues by which men have been able to augment their reproductive success has been through gaining access to the resources necessary to secure access to desirable mates (Buss, 2003). Conversely, women's reproductive success has been more closely linked to the heavy investment in childbearing and childrearing (Trivers, 1972). Psychologists have demonstrated that women, on average, express a greater interest than men in spending time with and caring for children (Buss, 2004). Behavioral measures are consistent with these interests, with women devoting more time and energy to raising children than do men (Browne, 2002).

One of the side effects of this sex difference is that many women find the rigid schedules and huge time commitments required for many occupations at odds with their desire to spend time investing in their families. Although many women with families are deeply dedicated to their jobs away from the home, they often endure a great deal of stress trying to balance work and family life. This fact is likely responsible for the fact that increasing numbers of women, despite being more educated than ever, are choosing to opt out of the labor force to raise children (Still, 2006). This is not to suggest that the secret to a woman's subjective well-being is to quit her job and stay home with her children or tend to housework. Such a suggestion would render many women—including the first author of this chapter—miserable. Rather, women in the workforce who have families may choose to embrace their evolved desires for family life and seek alternative ways to fulfill these desires in conjunction with their career goals. Discussing flex-time schedules with their bosses and opting to work only part-time while raising children are two ways in which women have begun to better meet the demands of their careers while dedicating the amount of time they desire to their families (Still, 2006). Furthermore, merely understanding that their desires to be with their families are not signs of weakness, but rather the activation of the psychological features shaped by selection, may contribute to women's feelings of self-worth and subjective well-being.

Future Avenues for Evolutionarily-Informed Research on Subjective Well-Being

One of the hallmarks of evolutionary psychology has been its success as a metatheory, guiding researchers toward novel research questions in psychology. Using knowledge of the adaptive problems that humans have had to solve over the course of evolutionary history has heuristic value with which to derive predictions about the design of the mind, brain, and behavior. The application of evolutionary psychological principles to the study of subjective well-being should lead to the creation of new bodies of knowledge in this growing field of scientific interest.

One way that evolutionary psychologists might contribute to the scientific study of subjective well-being would be to empirically explore the nature of the relationship between the numerous domains of adaptive problems confronting humans over evolutionary time and the importance of these domains to subjective well-being. An evolutionary framework would predict a relatively strong, positive relationship between the importance of a given adaptive problem and its effect on well-being. That is, the more closely a domain's historical relevance to reproductive success, the more that individual successes and failures in that domain would be expected increase and decrease subjective well-being. We would predict, for instance, that a man's subjective well-being would be more affected by his ability to acquire economic resources than his ability to bake the perfect soufflé (unless the latter ability had a bearing on the former).

Similarly, an evolutionary account of subjective well-being would predict that the types of factors that have the greatest impact on subjective well-being will change throughout the lifetime, based on changes in the importance of solving different adaptive problems over the lifetime. Thus, the ability to attract and gain sexual access to short-term mates might weigh mightily on a man's subjective well-being when he is in his 20s and in prime "mating mode." However, 40 years later, this same man's well-being will likely be more dependent on factors such as the health of his spouse and the successes of his children and grandchildren. Future research exploring the relationship between subjective well-being and the relative importance of the different adaptive problems that must be solved at different points in development may uncover new knowledge about the different factors that influence subjective well-being throughout the lifetime.

Additional avenues of evolutionarily informed research could explore whether cultural attempts to attenuate some of the negative side effects of modern, urban living have been successful. Relocation prompted by jobs, schooling, or other social or economic factors is becoming more the rule than the exception in our modern environment. It would be interesting for researchers to explore whether having ready access to e-mail, cellular telephones, and cheap airfare attenuate this discrepancy between our modern social environment and that of our ancestors and whether this access facilitates subjective well-being. Or do these measures fail to bridge the gap between hunter–gatherer life and modern urban living? It would also be interesting to explore whether these technological advances have led to an increase in the number of people who have been willing to relocate away from their families. Future research will determine whether technology has been able to bridge one of the gaps that exists between the past and the present and that can negatively impact subjective well-being.

Another important direction centers on exploring subjective well-being in a more domain-specific manner. Just as the existence of a g or general intelligence does not negate the importance of specific cognitive abilities, such as spatial rotation and verbal fluency, the existence of a g or general factor in well-being does not negate the importance of differentiated well-being in specialized domains. One woman might be elated over the success of her children, miserable in her marriage, and feel neutrally about her job. Another might feel miserable about her difficulty in getting pregnant, yet still be delighted in her marriage and revel in her work successes. A more domain-specific approach to well-being may help to clarify apparent anomalies, such as the one that indicates that children in U.S. families reduce marital happiness.

Lastly, future research on subjective well-being from an evolutionary approach can explore whether conscious attempts to change one's perceptions of one's social competitors have the effect of keeping one's social competition mechanisms in check. Because individuals judge their own success in a number of domains based on how they perform relative to their rivals, research needs to determine whether decreasing media exposure, choosing to surround oneself with others who are similarly endowed in wealth and beauty, or helping less fortunate people has the effect of increasing subjective well-being. If conscious attempts such as these do have a positive impact on subjective well-being, this finding could potentially affect how psychologists treat those with status anxiety and eating disorders. Perhaps limiting self-comparisons to those with whom people have direct contact could make people feel better about themselves and raise their overall subjective well-being.

Conclusions

Evolutionary psychology has yielded important insights into a number of research domains within psychology, including the science of subjective well-being. Evolutionary psychology provides insights into obstacles that can have a negative effect on subjective well-being. Discrepancies between current environments and those inhabited by our distant ancestors, psychological features that have been designed to cause upset and distress, and the interaction between the two can have detrimental effects on subjective well-being. Evolutionary psychology also yields insight into the types of factors that will make us happy and makes suggestions about ways in which we might harness our evolved psychologies to facilitate subjective well-being. Little research has yet been done on subjective well-being from an evolutionary perspective.

Nonetheless, early research from this perspective appears promising (Hill & Buss, 2006). First, an evolutionary perspective serves heuristic value in leading researchers to domains likely to be of critical importance—those tributary to solving statistically recurrent problems of survival and reproduction. Second, it leads to hypotheses not produced by other perspectives. None but an evolutionary perspective, for example, would lead to the nonobvious prediction that women's well-being will rise near ovulation, when they peak in reproductive value, and that men will lack these predictable monthly variations in subjective well-being (see Buss, 2000a). Third, an evolutionary perspective provides a powerful metatheory for explaining why humans (and other organisms) have well-designed psychological systems that produce happiness and unhappiness. In at least these three ways, an evolutionary perspective can make important conceptual and empirical contributions to a domain about which all humans care deeply.

References

Argyle, M. (1987). *The psychology of happiness*. London: Routledge.

Browne, K. R. (2002). *Biology at work: Rethinking sexual equality*. New Brunswick, NJ: Rutgers University Press.

Buss, D. M. (1988). From vigilance to violence: Tactics of mate retention. *Ethology and Sociobiology, 9,* 291–317.

Buss, D. M. (1989). Conflict between the sexes: Strategic interference and the evocation of anger and upset. *Journal of Personality and Social Psychology, 56,* 735–747.

Buss, D. M. (2000a). The evolution of happiness. *American Psychologist, 55,* 15–23.

Buss, D. M. (2000b). *The dangerous passion.* New York: Free Press.

Buss, D. M. (2003). *Evolution of desire: Strategies of human mating.* New York: Basic Books.

Buss, D. M. (2004). *Evolutionary psychology: The new science of the mind.* New York: Pearson Education.

Buss, D. M., Larsen, R. J., Westen, D., & Semmelroth, J. (1992). Sex differences in jealousy: Evolution, physiology, and psychology. *Psychological Science, 3,* 251–255.

Carver, C. S., Lawrence, J. W., & Scheier, M. F. (1996). A control-process perspective on the origins of affect. In L. L. Martin & A. Tesser (Eds.), *Striving and feeling: Interactions among goals, affect, and regulation* (pp. 11–52). Mahwah, NJ: Erlbaum.

Cosmides, L., & Tooby, J. (2000). Evolutionary psychology and the emotions. In M. Lewis & J. M. Haviland-Jones (Eds.), *Handbook of emotions* (2nd ed., pp. 91–115). New York: Guilford Press.

Cosmides, L., & Tooby, J. (2004). Knowing thyself: The evolutionary psychology of moral reasoning and moral sentiments. In R. E. Freeman & P. Werhane (Eds.), *Business, science, and ethics: The Ruffin Series No. 4* (pp. 93–128). Charlottesville, VA: Society for Business Ethics.

Csikszentmihalyi, M. (1990). *Flow: The psychology of optimal experience.* New York: Harper.

Daly, M., Wilson, M., & Weghorst, S. J. (1982). Male sexual jealousy. *Ethology and Sociobiology, 3,* 11–27.

Diener, E., & Emmons, R. A. (1984). The independence of positive and negative affect. *Journal of Personality and Social Psychology, 47,* 1015–1117.

Diener, E., Gohm, C., Suh, E., & Oishi, S. (2000). Similarity of the relations between marital status and subjective well-being across cultures. *Journal of Cross-Cultural Psychology, 31,* 419–436.

Diener, E., & Lucas, R. (1999). Personality and subjective well-being. In D. Kahneman, E. Diener, & N. Schwarz (Eds.), *Well-being: The foundations of hedonic psychology.* New York: Sage.

Diener, E., Lucas, R. E., & Scollon, C. N. (2006). Beyond the hedonic treadmill: Revising the adaptation theory of well-being. *American Psychologist, 61,* 305–314.

Diener, E., Sandvik, E., Seidlitz, L., & Diener, M. (1993). The relationship between income and subjective well-being: Relative or absolute? *Social Indicators Research, 28,* 195–223.

Diener, E., & Suh, E. M. (1997). Measuring quality of life: Economic, social, and subjective indicators. *Social Indicators Research, 40,* 189–216.

Diener, E., Suh, E. M., Lucas, R. E., & Smith, H. L. (1999). Subjective well-being: Three decades of progress. *Psychological Bulletin, 125,* 276–302.

Dunbar, R. I. M. (1993). Coevolution of neocortical size, group size, and language in humans. *Behavioral and Brain Sciences, 16,* 681–735.

Frank, R. H. (1999). *Luxury fever: Why money fails to satisfy in an era of excess.* New York: Free Press.

George, L. K., & Landerman, R. (1984). Health and subjective well-being: A replicated secondary data analysis. *International Journal of Aging and Human Development, 19,* 133–156.

Glenn, N. D., & McGlanahan, S. (1982). Children and marital happiness: Further specification of a relationship. *Journal of Marriage and the Family, 44,* 63–72.

Glenn, N. D., & Weaver, C. N. (1988). The changing relationship of marital status to reported happiness. *Journal of Marriage and Family Relations, 50,* 317–324.

Gove, W. R., Hughes, M., & Style, C. B. (1983). Does marriage have positive effects on the psychological well-being of the individual? *Journal of Health and Social Behavior, 24,* 122–131.

Gove, W. R., & Shin, H. (1989). The psychological well-being of divorced and widowed men and women. *Journal of Family Issues, 11,* 4–35.

Gutierres, S. E., Kenrick, D. T., & Partch, J. J. (1999). Beauty, dominance, and the mating game: Contrast effects in self assessment reflect gender differences in mate selection. *Personality and Social Psychology Bulletin, 25,* 1126–1134.

Hill, S. E., & Buss, D. M. (2006a). Envy and positional bias in the evolutionary psychology of management. *Managerial and Decision Economics, 27,* 131–143.

Hill, S. E., & Buss, D. M. (2006b). The evolution of self-esteem. In M. H. Kernis (Ed.), *Self-esteem: Issues and answers.* New York: Psychology Press.

Hsee, C. K., & Abelson, R. P. (1991). Velocity relations: Satisfaction as a function of the first derivative of outcome over time. *Journal of Personality and Social Psychology, 60,* 341–347.

Kenrick, D. T., Gutierres, S. E., & Goldberg, L. (1989). Influence of erotica on ratings of strangers and mates. *Journal of Experimental Social Psychology, 25,* 159–167.

Kenrick, D. T., Neuberg, S. L., Zierk, K. L., & Krones, J. M. (1994). Evolution and social cognition: Contrast effects as a function of sex, dominance, and physical attractiveness. *Personality and Social Psychology Bulletin, 20,* 210–217.

Ketelaar, T. (2004). Ancestral emotions, current decisions: Using evolutionary game theory to explore the role of emotions in decision-making. In C. Crawford & C. Salmon (Eds.), *Darwinism, public policy, and private decisions* (pp. 145–168). Mahwah, NJ: Erlbaum.

King, L. A., & Broyles, S. J. (1997). Wishes, gender, personality, and well-being. *Journal of Personality, 65,* 49–76.

Kirkpatrick, L. A., & Ellis, B. J. (2001). An evolutionary approach to self-esteem: Multiple domains and multiple functions. In M. Clark & G. Fletcher (Eds.), *The Blackwell handbook of social psychology, Vol. 2: Interpersonal processes* (pp. 411–436). Oxford, UK: Blackwell.

Kirkpatrick, L. A., & Ellis, B. J. (2006). An evolutionary approach to self-esteem research. In M. H. Kernis (Ed.), *Self-esteem: Issues and answers.* New York: Psychology Press.

Lewinsohn, P. M., Redner, J. E., & Seeley, J. R. (1991). The relationship between life satisfaction and psychosocial variables: New perspectives. In F. Strack, M. Argyle, & N. Schwarz (Eds.), *Subjective well-being: An interdisciplinary perspective* (pp. 141–169). Oxford, UK: Pergamon Press.

Lykken, D., & Tellegen, A. (1996). Happiness is a stochastic phenomenon. *Psychological Science, 7,* 186–189.

Marks, I. M. (1987). *Fears, phobias, and rituals: Panic, anxiety, and their disorders.* New York: Oxford University Press.

Marks, I. M., & Nesse, R. M. (1994). Fear and fitness: An evolutionary analysis of anxiety disorders. *Ethology and Sociobiology, 15,* 247–261.

Maslach, C., Schaufeli, W. B., & Leiter, M. P. (2001). Job burnout. *Annual Review of Psychology, 52,* 397–422.

Myers, D. G., & Diener, E. (1995). Who is happy? *Psychological Science, 6,* 10–19.

Nesse, R. M. (1990). Evolutionary explanations of emotions. *Human Nature, 1,* 261–289.

Nesse, R. M. (2005). Twelve crucial points about emotions, evolution, and mental disorders. *Psychology Review, 11*(4), 12–14.

Nesse, R. M. (2006). Evolutionary explanations for mood and mood disorders. In D. J. Stein, D. J. Kupfer, & A. F. Schatzberg (Eds.), *The American psychiatric publishing textbook of mood disorders* (pp. 159–175). Washington, DC: American Psychiatric Association.

Nesse, R. M., & Williams, G. C. (1994). *Why we get sick.* New York: New York Times Books.

Okun, M. A., Stock, W. A., Haring, M. J., & Witter, R. A. (1984). Health and subjective well-being: A meta-analysis. *International Journal of Aging and Human Development, 19,* 111–132.

Pavot, W., Diener, E., Colvin, C., & Sandvik, E. (1991). Further validation of the Satisfaction with Life Scale: Evidence for the cross-method convergence of self-report well-being measures. *Journal of Personality Assessment, 57,* 149–161.

Petrie, K. J., White, G., Cameron, L. D., & Collins, J. P. (1999). Photographic memory, money and liposuction: Survey of medical students' wish lists. *British Medical Journal, 319,* 1593–1595.

Price, J. S., & Sloman, L. (1987). Depression as yielding behavior: An animal model based on Schjelderup-Ebbe's pecking order. *Ethology and Sociobiology, 8,* 85–98.

Sarason, B. R., Sarason, I. G., & Pierce, G. R. (Eds.). (1990). *Social support: An interactional view.* New York: Wiley.

Sloman, L., & Gilbert, P. (2000). *Subordination and defeat: An evolutionary approach to mood disorders and their therapy.* Mahwah, NJ: Erlbaum.

Solnick, S. J., & Hemenway, D. (1998). Is more always better? A survey on positional concerns. *Journal of Economic Behavior and Organization, 37,* 373–383.

Still, M. C. (2006). The opt-out revolution in the United States: Implications for modern organizations. *Managerial and Decision Economics, 27,* 159–171.

Tellegen, A., Lykken, D. T., Bouchard, T. J., Wilcox, K. J., Segal, N. L., & Rich, S. (1988). Personality similarity in twins reared apart and together. *Journal of Personality and Social Psychology, 54,* 1031–1039.

Trivers, R. (1972). Parental investment and sexual selection. In B. Campbell (Ed.), *Sexual selection and the descent of man: 1871–1971* (pp. 136–179). Chicago: Aldine.

5

The Pursuit of Happiness in History

Darrin M. McMahon

If the pursuit of happiness is as old as history itself, then it is surely worth asking what the sources have to say about this perennial human quest. The time to do so is now. For at no other point in human history have so many men and women believed with such unquestioned certainty that they *should* be happy, that this is their inherent state and natural right. Thomas Jefferson's proud affirmation in the Declaration of Independence that the *pursuit of happiness* is a basic human entitlement—a truth at once God-given and self-evident—has slowly evolved into a much wider assumption about its capture and attainment. We deserve to be happy, Americans and many others now tend to believe, and we should be so.

In truth, the assumption that happiness is the natural human state is a relatively recent phenomenon—the product of a dramatic shift in human expectations carried out since the 18th century. Remembering that fact and recalling, too, the received wisdom of some of the many historical observers who have pointed out the potential perils of pursuit may help us view our own search for happiness in a slightly different light. In the end, I want to suggest that perhaps the best way to find happiness, paradoxically, may well be to look for something else.

Ancient Greek Philosophy of Happiness

But let us first begin at the beginning—or at least with what scholars usually agree is the first work of history in the Western tradition, The *History*, by Herodotus (1987/circa 440 B.C.E.), set down in Ancient Greece sometime in the middle of the fifth century B.C.E. Croesus, the fabulously wealthy king of Lydia, has summoned before him the itinerant sage, Solon, lawgiver of Athens and a man who has traveled over much of the world in search of wisdom. The Lydian king lacks nothing, or so he believes, and he attempts to convince Solon of the fact, leading the wise Athenian round his stores of treasure so that he might marvel at their splendor. Ostensibly needing nothing, Croesus nonetheless reveals that he is in need, for he is overcome by a "longing" to know who is the happiest man in the world. Foolishly, Croesus believes that he himself might be that man, or that he might strive to become him.

Solon's wisdom, however, and the succession of distinctly unhappy events that follows, succeed in dispelling this illusion. When Solon observes cautiously that the "divine is altogether jealous and prone to trouble us" (Herodotus, 1987/circa 440 B.C.E., p. 47), adding that in the span of a human life "there is much to see that one would rather not see and much to suffer likewise," Croesus is unmoved. And when Solon points out further that because of the unpredictability of human affairs, he cannot yet say if Croesus is, or will ever be, happy, for "man is entirely what befalls him," the proud Lydian is openly contemptuous, dismissing Solon as "assuredly a stupid man."

No sooner has he done so than Croesus receives a great visitation of evil. His son is killed in a freak hunting accident, Croesus himself misinterprets an oracle at Delphi and is lured into a disastrous war, and his kingdom is destroyed by invading Persian armies. Only as a captive, facing imminent death atop a funeral pyre whose flames lick at his feet, does Croesus realize the wisdom of Solon's words and the folly of his own presumption. "No one who lives is happy," he exclaims, calling out his own fate for the benefit of all who "are in their own eyes happy" (Herodotus, 1987/circa 440 B.C.E., p. 74).

Now it may seem that this tragic tale of divine retribution and frustrated human aims is a particularly morbid introduction to history—any history—let alone a history of happiness. And nowhere would this seem more the case than in the contemporary United States. Since the Puritans fled the Old World intent on creating anew, we have tended to begin our tales on a brighter note, and we have long grown accustomed to ending them that way too. In a country that has come to expect happiness in all things, it is safe to say that Solon would never be elected on his platform: Call no man happy until he is dead.

But it is precisely for this reason that it is worth listening to his wisdom. For Solon's message that the relentless pursuit of happiness threatens always to subvert itself is one that resonates again and again in Western history.

Consider the very word that Herodotus (1987/circa 440 B.C.E.) employs to describe the elusive thing that his tragic hero seeks. In truth, Herodotus employs several terms—among them, the ancient Greek *olbios*, *eutychia*, and *eudaimon*—which all, like their close cousin *makarios*, signify good fortune and blessedness, divine favor and prosperity. But it is above all the adjective *eudaimon*, and the noun *eudaimonia* (happiness), that features most prominently in Herodotus's work. In the succeeding 100 years it would emerge as an absolutely critical term in the lexicon of Greek philosophy.

Comprised of the Greek *eu* (good) and *daimon* (god, spirit, demon), *eudaimonia* contains within it a notion of fortune, for to have a good *daimon* on your side, a guiding spirit, is to be lucky. It also possesses a notion of divinity, for a *daimon* is an emissary of the gods, a personal spirit who watches over each of us, acting invisibly on the Olympians' behalf. But what is most interesting is that this *daimon* is an occult power, a hidden, spiritual force that drives human beings forward, where no specific agent can be named. It is this mysterious quality that helps account for that unpredictable "something" that impels Croesus along, driving him in pursuit of he knows not what. For though to have a good *daimon* means to be carried in the direction of the divine, to have a bad *daimon*—a *dysdaimon*—is to be turned aside, led astray, or countered by another. The gods, alas, are as capricious as mortals, as that unhappy wife of Shakespeare's Othello, Desdemona, learns to her dismay. Her name is simply a variation on the Greek word for unhappy, *dysdaimon*, as Shakespeare certainly knew. He was probably also aware that *daimon* is the Greek root of the modern word "demon," a fiend or an evil spirit who haunts and threatens us, who always has the power to do us wrong (Burkert, 1985, p. 180).

Something of that vaguely sinister connotation lurks in *eudaimonia* itself. Thus, when Croesus asks, "Is the happiness (*eudaimonia*) that is mine so entirely set at naught by you . . . ?" (Herodotus, 1987/circa 440 B.C.E., pp. 46–47), Solon responds that although Croesus's life may seem good now, it is far too early to predict where his *daimon* will finally lead him. In an uncertain world, life is unpredictable, less something to be made than to be endured. Only those who do so successfully—until the very end—can be deemed fortunate, blessed, happy.

Historians of Greek philosophy will point out that this emphasis on the chance or unpredictable nature of human affairs—an emphasis so central to the entire tradition of Greek Tragedy—was challenged in the centuries that followed (Nussbaum, 1994). From Socrates, Plato, and Aristotle in the fourth and fifth centuries B.C.E. to the Epicureans and Stoics who enjoyed such favor throughout the Mediterranean world in the aftermath of the conquests of Alexander, lovers of wisdom and their devotees declared happiness (*eudaimonia*) to be the final aim of philosophical reflection and virtuous activity (Annas, 1993). To discover the secret of the flourishing life became for these men the *summum bonum*, the highest good, one that they were by no means willing to leave entirely to chance. On the contrary, they took as their point of departure the belief that human beings could exercise considerable control over the fate of their lives by living virtuously. Thus does Aristotle (1985/circa 350 B.C.E.) declare famously that happiness "is an activity of the soul expressing virtue" (p. 22). To the extent that we can learn to be good, he believed, we can learn to be happy.

All this is without question; it is also inspiring. Yet it would be wrong to assume that the classical philosophers' stress on human virtue succeeded in banishing the demons from *eudaimonia*. "Someone might possess virtue," Aristotle (1985/circa 350 B.C.E.) himself concedes, but still "suffer the worst evils and misfortunes" (pp. 7–8). He calls this the (bad) "luck of Priam," in reference to that unfortunate father of Hector in Homer's *Iliad*, who is forced, like Croesus, to endure the death of his beloved son and the destruction of his kingdom through no real fault of his own. To call such a person happy would be perverse, Aristotle insists, thereby acknowledging our inability to eradicate completely the uncertainty bound up with the pursuit of our highest end.

But Aristotle's reservations about the pursuit of happiness run deeper than this. Even if the virtuous man succeeds in running life's gauntlet without serious misfortune, he must deal with the paradoxical fact that the closer he comes to the end of life, the more cause he will have to regret the loss. According to Aristotle: "The more he has every virtue and the happier he is, the more pain he will feel at the prospect of death. For this sort of person, more than anyone, finds it worth while to be alive, and is knowingly deprived of the greatest goods, and this is painful" (1985/circa 350 B.C.E., p. 45). As the happiness of the happy man increases, so does his suffering at its loss.

Aristotle, like the Stoics, counsels bravery in the face of this contradiction—recommending, in effect, that the virtuous person look death in the eye, grin, and bear it. We may find this admirable advice, but that it was not entirely satisfying to the denizens of antiquity is confirmed by the tremendous success of the next great philosophy of happiness to sweep the ancient world: Christianity. In this new faith, the paradoxes of pursuit were only further multiplied.

Christianity's Philosophy of Happiness

"Blessed are those who mourn" (Matthew 5:3), we read in the Gospel of Matthew in the New King James Translation (NKJT), or "Happy are those who are persecuted for righteousness's sake" (Matthew 5:10). Similarly shocking to our received assumptions are the beatitudes of Luke: "Happy are you when people hate you, and when they exclude you, revile you" (Luke 6:22). Those who weep are apparently "happy," we are told, like those who are hungry or are poor.

Admittedly, the critical word in question here is no longer *eudaimon* but the Greek term *makarios*. Frequently rendered in English as "blessed," *makarios*, however, may just as validly be translated as "happy," as in fact it is in some other versions of the Bible. Many Greek authors, including Aristotle and Plato, used the two words (*eudaimon* and *makarios*) interchangeably. But this is not to deny that the evangelists themselves meant something very different from what their classical forebears intended by either term. Indeed, in some ways, their meaning is precisely the opposite. For if one can be genuinely "happy" or "blessed" in this new Christian sense, while mourning, or weeping, or starving—happy, in a manner of speaking, while sad—does it not follow that those who are "happy" in a more conventional sense are quite possibly flirting with the ultimate sorrow? The prosperous, the well-fed, those who feel good and are quick to laugh should beware, at the very least, that their earthly rejoicing is dangerously premature: God may well have other plans in store for them. Meanwhile, those who suffer unjustly in this world may take heart. "Now is your time of grief," Christ tells his disciples in the Gospel of John, "but I will see you again and you will rejoice, and no one will take away your joy" (John 16:22, NKJV).

In one sense, this counsel was simply the reassertion of the wisdom of the tragic tradition. We should call no person happy until he or she is dead, Christians might legitimately claim, because God, who through his providence controls both fate and fortune, may quickly bring our earthly striving to naught. As the monk in that classic account of Christian pilgrimage, Chaucer's *Canterbury Tales* (McMahon, 2006, p. 496), reminds his fellow travelers as late as the 14th century:

And thus does Fortune's wheel turn treacherously
And out of happiness bring men to sorrow

The same admonition is repeated throughout the Middle Ages and the early Renaissance, the very period that gave rise to the modern words for "happiness" in the principal Indo-European languages (McMahon, 2006, pp. 136–137). It is hardly surprising that every one of these words—from the German *Glück* to the French *bonheur*—is linguistically related to good fortune or luck, what the Old English called *hap*. Well after the coming of Christ, the earthly variety of "happiness" continued to depend on what *happened* to us, and this, good Christians knew, was ever prone, like fortune's wheel, to take a turn for the worse.

But if in this respect the Christian world made a place for the older, tragic understanding of happiness as divine fortune or good luck, it should also be clear that it considerably altered the meaning of the phrase "call no man happy until he is dead." Strictly speaking, happiness in the Christian conception *was* death (McMahon, 2006, p. 106). No longer considered a boundary marking off the conclusion of a life well lived, death was treated by Christians as a gateway that led from the inescapable striving and suffering of our earthly pilgrimage to the conclusion and rest of endless ecstasy, rapture, and bliss. Nothing at all will be lacking in death's everlasting life, St. Thomas Aquinas (1988/circa 1258–1264) affirms typically in the *Summa against the Gentiles*, for "in that final happiness every human desire will be fulfilled" (p. 9). In heaven, it seems, the saints will be "inebriated" by the plenty of God's house and shall drink of the "torrent" of God's pleasure. Quite literally, the saved will get drunk on God.

For all who suffer from the thirst of human dissatisfaction, this was—and remains—an inspiring prospect, providing what St. Augustine (1984/circa 412–425) termed the "happiness of hope." But as he fully appreciated, this same hope necessarily cast a dark shadow on the prospects for happiness on earth. If perfect happiness could only come in death by the grace of God, then it followed that the struggle to obtain earthly happiness was a vain one. Pouring scorn on "all these [pagan] philosophers [who] have wished, with amazing folly, to be happy here on earth and to achieve bliss by their own efforts" (p. 852), Augustine (1984/circa 412–425) argued at length in the *City of God* that "true happiness" was "unattainable in our present life." Due to the lasting consequences of "Original Sin," we are condemned to suffer on earth—to yearn and long for a satisfaction that we can never know as mere mortals.

Adding yet another paradox to this already paradoxical history, Augustine (1984/circa 412–425) and his Christian brethren thus imagined the pursuit of happiness as a form of punishment, a continual, nagging reminder of our banishment from the Garden of Eden and the consequent human inability to live contentedly without God's grace. According to this perspective, every time we long for happiness, we remind ourselves of our unworthiness and inability to attain it on our own, a vicious cycle whose necessary by-product was guilt. As Nietzsche (1994/1887) would later observe ruefully, those who came before Christ did not suffer the same pangs of conscience, did not feel "ashamed of their happiness." They do not say "It's a disgrace to be happy" (pp. 96–97). All those weighed down by Christian guilt and the strange logic of the Beatitudes, on the other hand, must at the very least experience a moment of doubt every time they smile.

This is not to suggest that there were no counter-veiling impulses in the Christian tradition. The antinomian ecstasies of the early messianic communities, who believed, with Matthew, that the kingdom of God was at hand, certainly had cause for rejoicing. And it is equally true that the Jewish tradition had always acknowledged a healthy place for the enjoyment of God's earth, giving Christian interpreters sunny precedents such as those of the Book of Ecclesiastes, which recommends that the faithful savor the milk and honey of existence. "Go, eat your bread with enjoyment, and drink your wine with a merry heart; for God has long ago approved what you do" (Ecclesiastes 9:7). In this view, to "enjoy life with the wife whom you love" (Ecclesiastes 9:9), is to honor the gifts of the creator. Similarly, St. Francis observed cheerfully that "it is not right for the servant of God to show sadness and a dismal face" (Smith, 2001, p. 132). And both

Luther and Calvin would later emphasize that happiness and good cheer may be viewed as the fruit of justification, a sign of the presence of God's redeeming grace. Whereas "sin is pure unhappiness," Luther (1983) observed, "forgiveness is pure happiness" (Vol. 5, p. 198).

Philosophy of Happiness in the Enlightenment

All this underscores the rather straightforward point that Christianity, like any religious tradition, is necessarily replete with rival tendencies and competing claims. Yet it is also fairly easy to show that this same tradition's more general misgivings about happiness succeeded in dampening human expectations for some time. It was only in the 17th century—at the dawn of the period that we now call the Enlightenment—that men and women in the West dared to think of happiness as something more than a divine gift or otherwordly reward, less fortuitous than fortune, less exalted than a millenarian dream (McMahon, 2006, p. 177) In the Enlightenment, for the first time in human history, comparatively large numbers of men and women were exposed to the novel prospect that they might not have to suffer as an unfailing law of the universe, that they could—and should—expect happiness in the form of good feeling and pleasure as a right of life.

The causes of this momentous transformation range from developments within the Christian tradition that gave greater sanction to earthly enjoyment and deemphasized the impact of Original Sin; to new secular attitudes regarding the pleasures of pleasure; to the birth of consumer cultures able to offer an ever-expanding array of luxuries to ever-widening circles (McMahon, 2006, p. 205). Fascinating in their own right, these developments must cede their place in the present discussion, however, to what they wrought. For freed to think of happiness as something other than the superior striving of the happy few, men and women granted happiness on earth the privileged place they had once afforded to happiness hereafter. "Paradise is where I am," Voltaire declared with his characteristically provocative wit in the first line of his 1736 poem "Le Mondain" (2003/1736, p. 303). By the century's end, his *bon mot* was more than just a happy phrase. Whereas scarcely a century before, rulers had been enjoined to lead in the service of the faith and morals of their subjects—to lead in the service of salvation—they were now being asked to serve a different lord. "Happiness is in truth the only object of legislation of intrinsic value," the English utilitarian Joseph Priestley observed at the end of the 18th century (Porter, 2000, p. 204), echoing Voltaire's own claim in a letter of 1729 that "the great and only concern is to be happy" (Craver, 2005, p. 258). From the greatest happiness to the greatest number, this was the voice of a new age.

There was much to applaud in this new creed. If we human beings were not required to look shamefacedly on enjoyment, we were increasingly free to seek our pleasures where we could. To dance, to sing, to enjoy our food, to revel in our bodies and the company of others—in short, to delight in a world of our own making—was not to defy God's will but to live as nature intended. This was our earthly purpose. Bringing with it a whole new range of attitudes that clashed with venerable taboos, the new bearing on happiness worked to overturn impediments to sexual pleasure, material prosperity, self-interest, and simple delight for simply standing in the way. At the same time, defenders of happiness focused their energy on "unnatural" barriers to our natural end. They assailed injustice and inhumanity, prejudice and superstition, barbarism and false belief for barring the way of the human pursuit (McMahon, 2006, p. 209). To the present day that same set of convictions remains at the heart of our closest-held humanitarian assumptions: that suffering is wrong and that it should be relieved wherever possible; that the enjoyment of life is, or ought to be, a basic human entitlement.

The liberating potential of this new creed notwithstanding, the belief that happiness was our natural condition entailed a vicious corollary. For if we *ought* to be happy, didn't it follow that when we were not, there was something wrong? For centuries Christianity had cast a pall over the prospect of happiness on earth, provoking guilt at the thought of worldly delight. But it also justified and made sense of human suffering and dissatisfaction. The long-term impact of the Enlightenment had precisely the opposite effect: creating guilt as a consequence of the failure to be happy, guilt at feeling sadness and pain (McMahon, 2006, p. 250).

It may well be that it is only now—when all must smile for the camera and sadness is treated as a disease—that human beings are experiencing the full force of this development. But even in the 18th century, keen observers were aware that the pursuit of happiness might have a dark side. "The time is already come," Samuel Johnson remarked in 1759, "when none are wretched but by their own fault" (1985, p. 87). If happiness were our natural condition, and if neither Original Sin nor the mystery of grace, the movement of the stars nor the caprice of fortune, controlled our fate, then the failure to be happy would be just that—*failure*.

Was it really so clear, Johnson (1985/1759) wondered, that human beings were intended to be happy, and that they could make themselves so? The supposition itself, he understood, involved an assumption—an article of faith—about the purpose of human existence, about the final destiny and end. And if this supposition were wrong, as he well believed, then it placed on human beings an awful burden, a responsibility that they could never entirely fulfill. "What . . . is to be expected from our pursuit of happiness," one of his characters asks in his masterpiece *Rassellas*, "when we find the state of life to be such, that happiness itself is the cause of misery?" (Johnson, 1985/1759, pp. 116–117). It was a disconcerting question, and it haunted others of the age. After the untimely death of his mistress, Madame de Châtelet, and the terrible shock of the Lisbon earthquake of 1755, which wiped out thousands in a day, Voltaire himself came to doubt his earlier optimism. In response, he penned his famous *Candide*, mocking the optimistic faith that all is for the best in the best of all possible worlds. Jean-Jacques Rousseau (1782) shared his reservations. "I doubt whether any of us knows the meaning of lasting happiness" (p. 88), he despaired after a lifetime of pursuit, confirming a suspicion he had voiced earlier in his career: "Happiness leaves us, or we leave it" (1979a/1762, p. 447).

Unlike Johnson, however, and unlike Voltaire, Rousseau refused to leave the matter at that. Child of the Enlightenment that he was, in part, he remained adamant in his faith that happiness must be our natural end. Perhaps long ago, in a primitive state of nature, he mused, when our needs and faculties coexisted in harmony as they should, human beings were readily content. But that equilibrium had been upset long ago, with the balance further swayed in the direction of discontent by forces central to life as it was lived in the modern world. Presenting us with ever-greater possibilities and ever-expanding needs, modern commercial societies multiplied human desires, which ranged steadily ahead of our ability to fulfill them, creating envy and dissatisfaction in their wake. And so, Rousseau (1979) concluded, if human nature, as constituted in the modern world, rendered us incapable of achieving happiness, the world and human nature would have to be changed. "As soon as man's needs exceed his faculties and the objects of his desire expand and multiply, he must either remain eternally unhappy or seek a new form of being from which he can draw the resources he no longer finds in himself" (Rousseau, 1994, Vol. 4, p. 82). To do that required radically altering the structure of society.

This was the task Rousseau set himself in his most famous work, *The Social Contract*, which proposed, in an infamous line, that human beings could be "forced to be free." To his credit, Rousseau never made the same claim about happiness, and in fact explicitly states elsewhere that "there is no government that can force the Citizens to live happily; the best is one that puts them in a condition to be happy if they are reasonable" (Rousseau, 1994, Vol. 4, p. 41). Such qualifications, however, went unheeded. Distorting Rousseau's original intentions, men and women at the time of the French Revolution sought to bring his new human and society into being—with terrible results. As France and much of Europe reeled from war and the ghastly slaughter of "the Terror," the Jacobin leader Saint-Just declared in the spring of 1794 that happiness was "a new idea in Europe" (1984, p. 715). His colleague and fellow "terrorist," Joseph Marie Lequinio, went further, seeing fit to utter the words that Rousseau himself had eschewed. In a secular sermon delivered in the fall of 1793, Lequinio ended with a chilling invocation. "May the sacred love of the fatherland . . . force every individual to take the only road that can lead them to the end they propose—the end of happiness" (Lequino, 1793, pp. 18–19). That "road," of course, was the road of the revolution; the "force" was provided by the guillotine; and the "end" was stated clearly in the first article of the Jacobin constitution: "the goal of society is common happiness" (McMahon, 2006, p. 261).

It is no exaggeration to say that this very same revolutionary promise—to remake human beings and their world in the service of happiness—lies behind every one of the terrible experiments in social engineering that have brought such misery to the post-Enlightenment world. It is there in Marx (1983/1843–1844), with his declaration in the *Contribution to the Critique of Hegel's Philosophy of the Right* that "the overcoming of religion as the *illusory* happiness of the people is the demand for their real happiness" (p. 115). It is there in Engels (Engels & Marx, 1975/1847), with his candid avowal in the "Communist Confession of Faith" that "there exist certain irrefutable basic principles which, being the result of the whole of historical development, require no proof"—namely, that "every individual strives to be happy" and that "the happiness of the individual is inseparable from the happiness of all" (Vol. 6, p. 96). It is there, too, in the entry "happiness" in the *Great Soviet Encyclopedia* (1973–1983) with its assertion that "through a revolutionary struggle to transform society," happiness could be secured for the masses in realizing the "ideals of communism" (Vol. 25, p. 48). Finally, it is there, haunting the graves of the tens of millions who have perished in pursuit of such tragic illusions.

The terrible history of these ventures is well known to us today. And perhaps, in the West at least, we can feel some confidence that this knowledge will help guard against similar experiments in the immediate future. To force human beings to be happy, it now seems clear, is no more practicable than to force them to be free.

The U.S. Pursuit of Happiness

But what of that other revolutionary experiment—and its liberal promise of freedom, the freedom to pursue happiness in any way we choose? Jefferson, it is worth stressing, placed the emphasis on the *pursuit* of happiness in the founding document of the United States, not its attainment—and he was enough of a realist to doubt whether we could ever firmly grasp so slippery a thing. As his collaborator Benjamin Franklin is said to have observed: "The constitution only gives you the right to pursue happiness. You have to catch it yourself." The lines are undoubtedly apocryphal—for one thing, Franklin well knew that it was the Declaration, and not the Constitution, that conferred this right. But the sentiment itself is an apt approximation of the intent of the Founding Fathers. Governments must limit themselves to providing the basic conditions for the pursuit of happiness—civil liberties, peace and security, the protection of private property, the rule of law—and allow individuals to do the rest for themselves.

It was, and remains, a noble vision. But it is worth dwelling a little longer on just what this pursuit of happiness entailed. And here we should pause to consider the neglected term: *pursuit*. As the critic and historian Garry Wills (2002) has emphasized, the word had a much harder meaning in the 18th century than it does today, retaining a close link with its cognates *prosecute* and *persecute* (p. 245). Thus, Samuel Johnson (1755/1985) listed the word in his 18th-century *Dictionary of the English Language* as:

To Pursue . . .	1. To chase; to follow in hostility.
Pursuit . . .	1. The act of following with hostile intention.

If one thinks of pursuing happiness as one pursues a fugitive (and, indeed, in Scottish law criminal prosecuters were called *pursuers*, a usage with which Jefferson was familiar), the "pursuit of happiness" takes on a somewhat different inflection. To pursue, in this sense, is to follow with hostile intention, chasing down a renegade wherever "he" might lead us, and growing ever-more frustrated as the sweat forms on our brow. Like the *daimon* who lurks in *eudaimonia*, happiness may lead us high and low, and often astray. And when it does, it is only natural to begin to resent the thing that continually eludes us.

Lest this sound too far-fetched, it is worth recalling that there were strong precedents for precisely such ambivalence toward happiness in not only the classical tradition, in which the founding fathers were so well schooled, but also in Christianity. The *desire* for happiness was, for St. Augustine and his heirs, an intimate souvenir of our separation from God, a nagging source of pain and an ever-present reminder of what we could not have in this life due to our original transgression. The unfilled yearning for happiness, in short, was a symptom of God's punishment, the restlessness we would always feel until we found our way back to "Him."

Whether Jefferson himself and the other Founding Fathers made such conscious associations is far from clear. But it is hardly surprising to find perceptive observers who arrived at similar reflections. Think of Tocqueville (1988/1835–1840), who expressed such astonishment at the impatience and agitation of Americans. "No one could work harder to be happy," (Tocqueville, 1988/1835, Vol. 1, p. 243) he observed in *Democracy in America*, marveling repeatedly at the ceaseless, restless energy he perceived Americans expending in search of a better life. Rushing from one thing to the next, an American will travel hundreds of miles in a day. He will build a house in which to pass his old age and then sell it before the roof is on. He will continually change paths "for fear of missing the shortest cut leading to happiness." Finally, though, "Death steps in . . . and stops him before he has grown tired of this futile pursuit of that complete felicity which always escapes him" (Tocqueville, 1988/1840, Vol. 2, pp. 536–537). In dogged pursuit until the end, the restless American is brought up short only by death. And that, Tocqueville (1988/1840) concluded, in reference to America's related quest for an ever-elusive equality, was "the reason for the strange melancholy often haunting inhabitants of democracies in the midst of abundance, and of that disgust with life sometimes gripping them in calm and easy circumstances" (Vol. 2, p. 538).

John Stuart Mill's Insight

As the last line implies, Tocqueville (1988/1840) intended his reflections as a commentary not only on the specific case of the United States, but on liberal democracy more generally, which he deemed rightly was the inevitable wave of the future. It is striking, then, that his correspondent and contemporary, the equally astute John Stuart Mill, observed a similar phenomenon in that other great liberal empire of the 19th century, Great Britain. Indeed, Mill even observed the phenomenon in himself. Raised to be an apostle of the philosophy of his father's friend, Jeremy Bentham, the proponent of "felicific calculus" and the "greatest happiness of the greatest number," the young Mill made the attainment of happiness his life's work. And yet in his early manhood, having suffered a debilitating breakdown and an extended bout of depression, he hit upon a strange insight. As he confessed late in life in his gripping *Autobiography* (1989/1873):

> I now thought that this end [happiness] was only to be attained by not making it the direct end. Those only are happy (I thought) who have their minds fixed on some object other than their own happiness; on the happiness of others, on the improvement of mankind, even on some art or pursuit, followed not as a means, but as itself an ideal end. Aiming thus at something else, they find happiness by the way. . . . Ask yourself whether you are happy, and you cease to be so. The only chance is to treat, not happiness, but some end external to it, as the purpose of life. . . . This theory now became the basis of my philosophy of life. (pp. 117–118)

This was a stunning avowal for one who continued throughout his life to hold happiness in the highest esteem. The way to reach it, he grasped, was to search for something else. Those who would capture happiness must pursue other things.

What are we to make of such talk from the vantage point of the early 21st century? It may be tempting to dismiss Mill's (1989/1873) reflections, along with those of many of the other thinkers examined here, as the abstractions of men of thought—fine *theories*, perhaps, but hardly grounded in solid research. And yet it is interesting to note that at least some solid research has helped to bear out Mill's reflections, echoing the wisdom of the ages that appears to suggest that those who pursue happiness directly should watch their step. In his well-known studies of the experience of "flow," the psychologist Mihaly Csikszentmihalyi (1990) has found that those engaged in purposeful, challenging activity, pursued for its own sake, are apt to live more satisfying—more satisfied—lives than those who don't, and that their reported levels of subjective well-being reflect this fact. The work of many other positive psychologists—including that of Professor Diener— would seem to confirm such findings. Csikszentmihalyi (1990) himself even goes so far as to invoke Mill directly, arguing that "we cannot reach happiness by consciously searching for it" (p. 2), but only indirectly, by the by.

Devoting ourselves to activities that we deem meaningful—whether these be hiking, writing, or playing bridge—is, of course, a long way from the classical belief that we can reach a god-like happiness by treading a single path of virtue. It falls short, too, of Mill's own unrealized dream that some other highest end— the promotion of liberty, say, or service to society—might carry us to happiness collectively. Nor will the pursuit of purposeful activity do much to surpass the limitations of our genes. This is a less exalted path, a roundabout way, that makes no claims to offer up good feeling and ready delight in the form of instant gratification—or in a pill. A long-term journey, the pursuit of purposeful activity is almost always difficult, requiring planning, sacrifice, and dedication to an end deemed worthy of devotion in and of itself.

This may not be a sensational revelation—the stuff of best-seller lists or "seven easy steps." But in an age of inflated expectations, fed by false promises and excessive claims, it is probably worth heeding some tempered advice. We could do worse than to take counsel from a man who also felt the pull of the promise of paradise on earth, but who then thought better of the prospect. When Voltaire's hero, Candide, returns from circling the globe, wiser but no happier than when he began, he concludes simply that "we must cultivate our garden." Those seeking happiness—or something like it—at the dawn of the 21st century could do worse than to take up the hoe. Horticulture might just be the answer.

References

Annas, J. (1993). *The morality of happiness.* New York: Oxford University Press.

Aquinas, T. (1988). Summa contra gentiles. In P. E. Sigmund (Ed. & Trans.), *St. Thomas Aquinas on politics and ethics.* New York: Norton.

Aristotle (1985). *Nichomachean ethics* (T. Irwin, Trans.). Indianapolis: Hackett. (Original work B.C.E.)

Augustine. (1984). *Concerning the city of God against the pagans* (H. Bettonson, Trans.). London: Penguin Books. (Original work written circa 412–425)

Burkert, W. (1985). *Greek religion* (J. Raffan, Trans.). Cambridge, MA: Harvard University Press.

Craver, B. (2005). *The age of conservatism* (T. Wangh, Trans.) New York: New York Review of Books.

Csikszentmihalyi, M. (1990). *Flow: The psychology of optimal experience.* New York: Harper & Row. (Original work written 1847)

Engels, F., & Marx, K. (1975). *Collected works.* Moscow: Progress Publishers.

Great Soviet Encyclopedia. (1973–1983). New York: Macmillan.

Herodotus. (1987). *History* (D. Grene, Trans.). Chicago: University of Chicago Press. (Original work written circa 440 B.C.E.)

Johnson, S. (1755). *A dictionary of the English language.* London: Strahan.

Johnson, S. (1985). *The history of Rasselas, prince of Abissinia* (D. J. Enright, Ed.). London: Penguin Books. (Original work published 1759)

Lequinio, J.-M. (1793). *Du bonheur.* Archives National F17 A1003, plaq. 3, no. 1263.

Luther, M. (1983). *Sermons of Martin Luther.* Grand Rapids, MI: Baker Book House.

Marx, K. (1983). *The portable Karl Marx* (E. Kamenka, Trans.). New York: Penguin Books. (Original work written 1843–1844)

McMahon, D. M. (2006). *Happiness: A history.* New York: Atlantic Monthly Press.

Mill, J. S. (1989). *Autobiography* (J. M. Robson, Ed.). London: Penguin Books. (Original work published 1873)

Nietzsche, F. (1994). *On the genealogy of morality* (K. Ansell-Pearson, Ed.; C. Diethe, Trans.). Cambridge, NY: Cambridge University Press. (Original work published 1887)

Nussbaum, M. (1994). *The therapy of desire: Theory and practice in Hellenistic ethics.* Princeton, NJ: Princeton University Press.

Porter, R. (2000). *Creation of the modern world: The untold story of the British enlightenment.* New York: Norton.

Rousseau, J.-J. (1979a). *Emile* (A. Bloom, Trans.). New York: Basic Books. (Original work published 1762)

Rousseau, J.-J. (1979b). *Reveries of a solitary walker* (P. France, Trans.). New York: Penguin Books. (Original work published 1782)

Rousseau, J.-J. (1994). *The collected writings of Rousseau* (by J. R. Bush, R. D. Masters, & C. Kelley, Eds.; R. D. Masters & C. Kelly, Trans.). Hanover, NH: University Press of New England.

Saint-Just, L. de. (1984). *Oeuvres completes de Saint-Just* [The complete work of Saint-Just] (M. Duval, Ed.). Paris: Editions Gérard Lebovici.

Smith, L. (2001). Heavenly bliss and earthly delight. In S. McCready (Ed.), *Discovery of happiness* (pp. 116–136). London: MQ Publications.

Tocqueville, A. de. (1988). *Democracy in America* (J. P. Mayer, Ed.; G. Lawrence, Trans.). New York: HarperPerennial. (Original work published 1835–1840)

Voltaire, F. (2003). Le mondain [The man of world]. In Voltaire Foundation (Ed.), *The complete works of Voltaire* (pp. 295–303). Oxford, UK: Voltaire Foundation. (Original work published 1736)

Wills, G. (2002). *Inventing America: Jefferson's Declaration of Independence.* New York: Mariner Books.

II

MEASURING SUBJECTIVE
WELL-BEING

6

The Structure of Subjective Well-Being

Ulrich Schimmack

In his highly influential *Psychological Bulletin* article "Subjective Well-Being", Diener (1984) proposed that subjective well-being has three distinct components: *life satisfaction* (LS), *positive affect* (PA), and *negative affect* (NA). More recently, Diener, Suh, Lucas, and Smith (1999) also included satisfaction in specific life domains (henceforth *domain satisfaction* [DS], e.g., satisfaction with health) in the definition of subjective well-being. Researchers often distinguish cognitive and affective components of subjective well-being (Diener, 1984; Diener et al., 1999). Life satisfaction and domain satisfaction are considered cognitive components because they are based on evaluative beliefs (attitudes) about one's life. In contrast, PA and NA assess the affective component of subjective well-being and reflect the amount of pleasant and unpleasant feelings that people experience in their lives.

This chapter examines the structural relations among these components in three sections. First, I examine the structural relations among cognitive components of subjective well-being. Specifically, I examine the relation between life satisfaction and domain satisfaction (LS–DS) as well as the relation among satisfactions in various domains (DS–DS; e.g., job satisfaction and marital satisfaction). Second, I review the controversial and inconsistent literature on the relation between the two affective components of subjective well-being (i.e., PA and NA). Finally, I examine the relation between cognitive well-being and affective well-being.

The Structure of Cognitive Well-Being

Structural research on cognitive well-being has two aims. First, it simply tries to establish general characteristics of structural relations among cognitive components of subjective well-being. The second aim of structural research is to elucidate the causal processes that produce the structure of cognitive well-being. This chapter focuses on the causal processes that produce the structure of subjective well-being. Figure 6.1 illustrates several potential causal processes that can produce a correlation between life satisfaction and domain satisfaction. Based on Diener's (1984) seminal article, a main distinction is between bottom-up and top-down theories of subjective well-being. Bottom-up theories assume that life satisfaction judgments are based on an assessment of satisfaction in a relatively small number of life domains (Andrews & Withey, 1976; Brief, Butcher, George, & Link, 1993; Heller, Watson, & Hies, 2004; Schimmack, Diener, & Oishi, 2002). Thus, these theories assume that LS–DS correlations reflect a causal influence of DS on LS. In Figure 6.1 bottom-up effects are illustrated by the direct links between DS and LS, with the causal arrow pointing to LS. For example, an individual with high marital satisfaction has high life satisfaction because his or her marital satisfaction is an important aspect of his or her satisfaction with life as a whole. In contrast, top-down theories postulate the reverse direction of causality (i.e., LS causes DS). In Figure 6.1 top-down effects are illustrated by the direct links between LS and DS with the arrow pointing to DS. Somebody who is generally satisfied with life may also evaluate life domains more positively, although general satisfaction is not based on satisfaction with particular domains.

It is noteworthy that I use the labels *top-down* and *bottom-up* only to distinguish between causal theories of the relation between LS and DS. Bottom-up

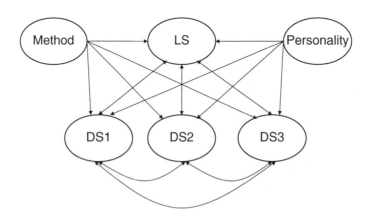

FIGURE 6.1. Causal models of the relation between life satisfaction and domain satisfaction.

theories can be further distinguished with regard to their assumptions about the determinants of DS. For example, Brief et al. (1993) proposed that domain satisfaction is also influenced by top-down processes. Specifically, the authors found that the personality trait *neuroticism* (i.e., a disposition to have more negative feelings and cognitions) predicted health satisfaction, which in turn predicted life satisfaction. Similar results have been obtained for marital satisfaction and job satisfaction (Heller et al., 2004). In the present context, these models are bottom-up because they assume that a change in domain satisfaction will result in a change in life satisfaction. In contrast, top-down models assume that changes in domain satisfaction have no effect on life satisfaction.

Top-down and bottom-up theories are not the only causal models of LS–DS relations. Another possibility is that the correlation is caused by shared method variance because life satisfaction and domain satisfaction are often assessed with the same method, typically self-reports (see, e.g., Andrews & Whithey, 1976; Schimmack & Oishi, 2005). In Figure 6.1 this model is illustrated by causal paths from a method factor to life satisfaction and domain satisfaction. According to this model, correlations between life satisfaction and domain satisfaction exaggerate the strength of the causal influence of DS on LS, or vice versa, because shared method variance inflates these correlations.

It is also possible that the correlation is due to a substantial causal effect of another variable that independently influences DS and LS. For example, neuroticism could lead to more negative evaluations of domain satisfaction (e.g., health) and life satisfaction. In Figure 6.1 this model is illustrated by causal effects of personality traits on life satisfaction and domain satisfaction. Although the correlation between LS and DS would not be a method artifact, a common influence of personality would still imply that LS–DS correlations exaggerate the strength of direct causal effects of DS on LS, or vice versa.

The nature of the causal processes that link DS and LS has great practical importance. Only bottom-up theories of subjective well-being predict that changes in domain satisfaction (e.g., an increase in financial satisfaction) produce changes in life satisfaction. All other theories make the counterintuitive prediction that changes in domain satisfaction have no consequences for individuals' life satisfaction.

Stability of the Structure of Cognitive Well-Being

Investigations of the structure of cognitive well-being assume a relatively stable structure. In contrast to this assumption, Schwarz and Strack (1999) have proposed that the relation between life satisfaction and domain satisfaction (LS–DS) is highly unstable. The authors suggest that people use simple heuristics to deal with the difficult task of evaluating their whole life. As a result, they may rely on information that is temporarily accessible at the moment of the evaluation. For example, in a phone survey at home, respondents rely on satisfaction with family, whereas in a survey at work they rely on job satisfaction to judge life satisfaction. The bleak implication of this theory is that structural research on subjective well-being would be futile.

Recent evidence suggests that this model overstates the importance of temporarily accessible information on life satisfaction judgments (Fujita & Diener, 2005; Schimmack, Diener, et al., 2002; Schimmack & Oishi, 2005). Life satisfaction judgments are much stabler than predicted by this model. Furthermore, experiments that manipulate the accessibility of different information have relatively weak effects on the correlations between DS and LS (Schimmack & Oishi, 2005). This evidence suggests that LS judgments are heavily influenced by chronically accessible information that has considerable stability over intervals of several months or a year.

Influence of Shared Method Variance

It is fairly easy to examine the potential influence of shared method variance on the correlation between DS and LS. For example, many studies have demonstrated that DS–LS correlations vary across different domains (Andrews & Withey, 1976; Schimmack, Diener, et al., 2002; Schimmack & Oishi, 2005). For example, satisfaction with family is more highly correlated with LS than satisfaction with weather or the national government. This finding is inconsistent with a pure method effect, because DS is assessed with the same method. Thus, method effects should produce the same correlations across domains. A more elaborate approach requires the assessment of LS and DS with different methods. For example, Heller, Judge, and Watson (2002) obtained significant correlations between self-reports of LS and informant reports of job satisfaction as well as between self-reports of job satisfaction and informant reports of LS ($rs = .27–.39$). The correlations were only slightly weaker than correlations between self-reports of LS and DS ($rs = .43–.48$).

A study by Schimmack, Diener, Oishi, and Suh (2006) provides further evidence on this issue. Students reported their LS and satisfaction with seven domains (romantic, finances, family, grades, social life, recreation, and housing). In addition, family members and friends provided informant ratings of students' life satisfaction. Self-reports of DS were averaged to obtain a measure of general DS. Consistent with prior studies, self-reported LS and DS were highly correlated ($r = .60$; Andrews & Withey, 1976; Schimmack & Oishi, 2005; Schimmack, Oishi, & Diener, 2002). Importantly, self-reported DS also correlated significantly with informant ratings of LS ($r = .50$). Once more, this correlation was only slightly weaker than the correlation based on self-reports of LS and DS. In short, there is consistent evidence that common method variance accounts for only a small portion of the correlation between DS and LS.

Common Influence of Personality

Numerous studies have examined the possibility that LS–DS correlations are due to the common influence of personality traits (Brief et al., 1993; Heller et al., 2002, 2004; Schimmack, Diener, & Oishi, 2002). These studies typically show that personality traits that correlate with LS also tend to be correlated with DS. For example, neuroticism is a negative predictor of LS and job satisfaction. As a result, controlling for personality traits weakens correlations between DS and LS. Nevertheless, DS typically shares unique variance with LS.

A study by Schimmack (2006d) provides further evidence on this issue. A large sample of undergraduate students ($n = 1,241$) completed measures of LS (i.e., the first three-items of the Satisfaction with Life Scale; e.g., "I am satisfied with my life"; Diener, Emmons, Larsen, & Griffin, 1985), three-item measures of satisfaction in 10 domains (academic, recreation, romantic, family/parents, friendships, health, housing, traffic, weather, and goal progress; see Schimmack & Oishi, 2005), and a short measure of the Big Five personality traits (see Schimmack, Oishi, Furr, & Funder, 2004—Study 4). Satisfactions in all domains except goal progress were averaged to obtain a measure of DS. Goal progress was excluded because it is a broad category and can reflect satisfaction in several more specific domains. The simple correlation between LS and average DS was $r = .70$ ($n = 1,241$). All personality traits were significantly correlated with LS and DS with correlations ranging from $r = .13–.27$ (sign reversed for neuroticism) for LS to $r = .15–.29$ for averaged DS. As a result, controlling for the shared variance with personality traits reduced the correlation between LS and DS, but the relation remained strong: *partial r* = .64. In sum, personality traits provide a partial explanation for LS–DS relations, but direct causal processes are likely to contribute to this relation as well.

A Simple Top-Down Model of LS–DS Correlations

It is more difficult to determine whether LS–DS relations are due to bottom-up or top-down processes (Headey, Veenhoven, & Wearing, 1991). The simplest top-down model assumes that people who are generally satisfied with life are more satisfied with everything. This model makes several predictions that are inconsistent with the literature. First, it predicts strong correlations among domain satisfactions, but DS–DS correlations are generally small to moderate (Andrews & Withey, 1976; Heller et al., 2004), and a large number of respondents who report high satisfaction in one domain report low satisfaction in other domains. For example, Schimmack (2006d) obtained an average correlation of $r = .28$ ($n = 1,241$) for the nine domains listed above. This finding also holds for changes in DS. Headey, Holmstrom, and Wearing (1984) found that most people who reported increased satisfaction in some domains also reported decreased satisfaction in other domains.

The second prediction of a simple top-down model is that LS–DS correlations should be the same across various domains. In contrast, empirical studies consistently report stronger correlations for important domains than for unimportant domains (Andrews & Withey, 1976; Schimmack, Diener, & Oishi, 2002). Schimmack (2006d) examined this issue by correlating LS with DS in nine domains. In addition, a smaller sample of students rated the importance of the nine domains. The correlation between LS–DS correlations and importance ratings of domains across the nine domains was nearly perfect: $r = .93$, $p < .01$. In short, a simple top-down model cannot account for the small-to-moderate DS–DS correlations and the systematic differences in LS–DS correlations across domains.

A Sophisticated Top-Down Model

It is possible, however, to construct more sophisticated top-down models that account for these findings. For example, a sophisticated top-down model could assume that (1) DS is substantially influenced by domain-specific factors, and (2) that general LS has a stronger impact on satisfaction in important domains (e.g., family) compared to unimportant domains (e.g., weather). The moderating effect of importance could be due to cognitive factors in the organization of beliefs about one's life. For example, the positive evaluation of life in general could spread more to central aspects of one's life than to peripheral aspects. It is possible to test this top-down model because it makes precise quantitative predictions about the correlations among domain satisfaction. For example, if LS were a strong cause of marital satisfaction ($r = .50$) and a moderate cause of job satisfaction ($r = .30$), the model predicts that the correlation between the two DSs is the product of the two effects (i.e., $r = .15$). This example illustrates two points. First, the sophisticated top-down model predicts only small-to-moderate DS–DS correlations. Second, it predicts that DS–DS correlations vary as a function of domain importance. Because important domains are more strongly influenced by LS, they also are more highly correlated with satisfaction in other domains.

Large samples are needed to conduct empirical tests of these predictions because the predicted correlations are small. Some data are available from a meta-analysis of the relation between LS, job satisfaction, and marital satisfaction (Heller et al., 2004). LS was moderately correlated with job satisfaction ($n = 19,811$; $r = .35$) and marital satisfaction ($n = 7,540$; $r = .42$). Based on these correlations, the top-down model predicts a small correlation of $r = .15$ between job satisfaction and marital satisfaction. The observed correlation in the meta-analysis is consistent with this prediction ($n = 6,248$; $r = 14$).

Stronger evidence can be obtained by examining the pattern of correlations among several domains. Schimmack (2006d) tested the predicted DS–DS correlations among nine domains (noted above) in a large undergraduate sample. First,

DSs in the nine domains were correlated with LS. Second, DS in one domain was correlated with satisfaction in the other eight domains. These correlations were averaged for each domain, producing two new variables that contained information about each domain's relation to (1) life satisfaction and (2) the other domains. A top-down model predicts a high correlation between these two variables across the nine domains—which was indeed the case: $r = .80$, $p < .05$. Both variables were also correlated with domain importance. For example, an important domain (e.g., family) had higher correlations with LS and with other domains than an unimportant domain (e.g., weather).

Schimmack (2006d) also used structural equation modeling to test how well observed DS–DS correlations conform to the DS–DS correlations predicted by the sophisticated top-down model. The model was based on 30 variables with three items for each domain and three items for LS. The first model fitted a pure measurement model, in which each of the three items for each construct loaded on a single factor. All factors were allowed to covary freely with each other. Model fit was evaluated based on Hu and Bentler's (1999) recommendation that the root mean square error of approximation (RMSEA) should be below .06, although others consider a fit of .08 as adequate (Browne & Cudeck, 1993). The standardized root mean square residual (SRMR) should be below .05 for good fit, although values up to .10 may be adequate (Hu & Bentler, 1995). Accordingly, the measurement model had a good fit to the data: χ^2 (360, $n = 1,241$) = 974, $p < .05$, SMSR = .019, RMSEA = .037. The top-down model imposed a single second-order factor with causal paths onto each of the nine domain factors. The model also included a causal path from LS to the second-order domain satisfaction factor. Overall fit of the top-down model was still good, although it did not fit the data as well as the measurement model: χ^2 (395, $n = 1,241$) = 1,284; SMSR = .046, RMSEA = .043. As predicted by the top-down model, LS was a strong predictor of the second-order factor of domain satisfaction, $r = .87$. The acceptable fit of the top-down model is remarkable and suggests that a sophisticated top-down model has the potential to account for the structure of cognitive well-being. This model would still imply that domain satisfaction has no causal effect on LS.

Empirical Tests of Bottom–Up and Top–Down Models

Correlations between LS and DS are insufficient to test the direction of causality. One solution to this problem is to include a third variable that has a direct effect on one construct but not the other. In this case, the causal direction between LS and DS can be inferred by examining whether the third variable has an indirect effect on the other construct. For example, objective income is likely to have a direct effect on financial satisfaction. A bottom-up model predicts that income also influences LS because it assumes a causal effect of financial satisfaction on LS.

In contrast, the top-down model assumes that an influence of income on financial satisfaction does not influence LS because domain satisfaction has no causal effect on LS. Subsequently, I discuss two studies that use this approach to test top-down and bottom-up models. One study includes a potential direct cause of global LS; the other study includes a potential direct cause of domain satisfaction.

Positive Illusions

One problem of the top-down model is the elusive nature of individual differences in LS when under the assumption that individual differences in LS are not caused by domain satisfaction, personality, or method artifacts. Why are some people more satisfied with their lives independent of their satisfaction with important life domains? One popular hypothesis in psychology is that individual differences in subjective well-being are based on illusory self-perceptions (Taylor & Brown, 1988). However, support for this hypothesis is often based on questionable measures of illusions (Colvin & Block, 1994). To address this limitation, Schimmack and Sidhu (2006) developed a new measure of biased self-perceptions. This measure is based on the assumption that biases can be assessed only in comparison to an objective standard. Furthermore, biases in a single domain may be inappropriate measures of self-evaluative biases for two reasons. First, most of the variance in self-reports of a single domain may be due to measurement error. Second, even a single objective measure is influenced by measurement error. As a result, it is an imperfect measure to control for valid variance in self-ratings. To solve this problem it is necessary to measure biases in self-perceptions across a variety of independent attributes. To the extent that biases are positively correlated across independent attributes, it is highly probable that they reflect general self-evaluative biases. Schimmack and Sidhu (2006) obtained self-reports for four specific attributes (facial attractiveness based on a photo, jumping, intelligence, and trivia knowledge). In addition, objective measures of the four attributes were also obtained.

Initial analysis showed that individual differences in objective attributes were unrelated to each other and unrelated to LS. The finding for attractiveness replicates a study by Diener, Wolsic, and Fujita (1995). Bias measures were obtained by regressing self-ratings onto the objective measures and retaining standardized residuals. Bias scores were significantly correlated with each other and formed a single factor. This finding reveals the influence of a general self-evaluative bias on ratings of self-attributes. To obtain a measure of general self-evaluative biases, the four specific bias measures were averaged. The general evaluative bias was significantly correlated with LS, $r = .28$ ($n = 98$). Furthermore, LS was again highly correlated with averaged domain satisfaction: $r = .60$ ($n = 98$). Based on these correlations, the top-down model predicts a correlation of $r = .17$ between the bias measure and DS. The actual correlation was very similar to this prediction: $r = .16$ ($n = 98$). However, due to the small sample size, the confidence interval for the observed correlation is large. Furthermore, in a second study that did not include the objective measures but assessed evaluative bias several months prior to the assessment of LS and DS, the correlations were identical: $r = .21$ ($n = 163$). This finding suggests that the bias measure is a direct predictor of DS. Furthermore, the strength of the correlation is weak. As a result, global evaluative biases account for only a small portion of the variance in LS and the correlation between LS and DS. Thus, the nature of the individual differences in LS remains elusive. In short, these results provide only modest support for the top-down model.

Income

Compared to the difficulty of finding direct predictors of global LS, it is easier to find objective characteristics of domains that influence DS. However, once more, large samples are needed to test the bottom-up model because a single objective characteristic will have only a small-to-moderate effect on global life satisfaction. One of the most extensively studied objective measures is income. Numerous studies show that income is correlated with financial satisfaction, and financial satisfaction correlates with LS (e.g., Diener & Oishi, 2000). However, both correlations are moderate. As a result, the bottom-up model predicts only a small effect of income on LS. Existing data are consistent with this prediction (Diener & Biswas-Diener, 2002; Hsieh, 2004). To further test this hypothesis, Schimmack (2006a) analyzed data from the 1999–2002 wave of the World Values Survey (Inglehart, Basanez, & Diez-Medrano, 2004). Over 60,000 respondents from 48 nations provided information about their LS, financial satisfaction, and relative income compared to the national average. Schimmack (2006a) standardized scores within nations to remove the influence of national differences on the results. Income was a moderate predictor of financial satisfaction ($r = .27$), and financial satisfaction was a strong predictor of LS ($r = .55$). Based on these findings, a bottom-up model predicts a correlation of $r = .15$ (.55 × .27) between income and LS. The actual correlation was close to this prediction ($r = .18$). Separate analysis for each nation showed that the results were quite consistent across nations. The largest discrepancies were obtained in Serbia and South Africa. In both countries income was a stronger predictor of LS than predicted by the bottom-up model. Only one country (Brazil) showed a notable discrepancy that failed to support the bottom-up model.

An alternative explanation of the relation between income and LS could be that happy individuals earn more money (Diener & Biswas-Diener, 2002). As a result, a top-down model would also predict a correlation between income and financial satisfaction because LS influences both income and financial satisfaction. However, this model predicts a correlation of only $r = .10$ ($.55 \times .18$) between income and financial satisfaction, whereas the actual correlation is significantly stronger, $r = .27$.

Further support for the bottom-up model stems from longitudinal evidence that income changes at least temporarily produce changes in LS (Di Tella, Heisken De New, & MacCulloch, 2006). These results suggest that LS–DS correlations are at least partially due to bottom-up processes.

An Indirect Test of Bottom-Up Models: A Dyadic Approach

Although the inclusion of objective predictors of DS can be very informative, it is often difficult to specify or measure these variables. To address this problem, I proposed a dyadic approach to indirectly estimate the effect of objective domain characteristics on DS (Schimmack, 2006b). The dyadic approach is based on the familiar logic of twin studies, which relies on dyadic similarity of twins to make inferences about genetic effects on subjective well-being (Roysamb, Harris, Magnus, Vitterso, & Tambs, 2002). Whereas dyadic similarity between twins reveals genetic influences, dyadic similarity between individuals who share the same environment but are not genetically related reveals environmental influences. The indirect approach has two advantages over the approach of directly measuring objective domain characteristics. First, it reveals effects of domain characteristics on DS without the need to know, a priori, what these objective characteristics are. Similarly, twin studies reveal genetic effects without specifying the genes that produce these effects. Second, the indirect approach reveals the combined effects of several objective characteristics. As a result, the effects are stronger and it is possible to test bottom-up and top-down theories in smaller samples. Similarly, twin studies reveal strong genetic effects, whereas single genetic markers have much weaker relations to observable individual differences (Greenberg et al., 2000).

Married couples provide an ideal opportunity to test top-down and bottom-up models of subjective well-being for several reasons. First, spouses are not genetically related (i.e., they are not blood relatives). Thus, similarity between spouses cannot be due to genetic relatedness. Second, spouses share many objective determinants of DS (e.g., household income, housing). Thus, one would expect high dyadic similarity for DS. This is indeed the case, especially for the domain of marital satisfaction (e.g., Spotts et al., 2004). The bottom-up and the top-down model make different predictions about dyadic similarity in LS. The bottom-up model predicts that the common determinants of DS that produce similarity in that arena produce spousal similarity in LS. In contrast, the top-down model assumes that DS has no causal influence on LS. As a result, the objective factors that produce similarity in DS do not produce similarity in LS. Consistent with the bottom-up model, numerous studies have reported moderate-to-high spousal similarity in LS (Bookwala & Schulz, 1996; Schimmack & Lucas, 2007; Schimmack, Pinkus, & Lockwood, 2006).

One possible alternative explanation for spousal similarity in LS is positive assortative mating, which assumes that spouses with similar traits are more likely to marry each other. However, empirical data suggest that this is an unlikely explanation for spousal similarity in LS. For example, spouses show similar changes in LS over a time interval of 20 years (Schimmack & Lucas, 2007). Although assortment can explain initial similarity, it fails to explain why changes in the LS of one spouse predict similar changes in the LS of the other spouse. Thus, spousal similarity in LS provides additional evidence for bottom-up influences of DS on LS.

A Direct Test of Bottom-Up Models: Introspective Evidence

Schimmack, Diener, and Oishi (2002) used another approach to determine the causes of LS: The authors examined what respondents were thinking when they answered questions about LS. It is plausible that satisfaction in a particular domain has a causal influence on LS if respondents think about this domain during the judgment of LS. Consistent with bottom-up theories, respondents reported thinking about important domains (e.g., family) more than about unimportant domains (e.g., weather). Furthermore, participants' thoughts about domains moderated DS–LS correlations. That is, DS predicted LS when respondents thought about a domain. This finding is consistent with bottom-up theories. In addition, the DS–LS correlations were low and not significant when participants did not think about a domain. This finding suggests weak top-down effects on DS–LS correlations because top-down effects do not require activation of domain knowledge during LS judgments.

Conclusion

In sum, studies of cognitive well-being have produced some fairly robust findings that any structural model needs to address. Most of these findings are consistent with bottom-up theories: (1) the significant effect of domain importance on LS–DS correlations; (2) the reliable effects of objective domain characteristics assessed directly or indirectly on LS; and (3) reports that people are thinking about important life domains when judging LS. However, another reliable finding is that DSs are systematically correlated, and that top-down models do a fairly good job at predicting these correlations. Thus, it is possible that a complete theory of cognitive well-being will include both bottom-up and top-down processes.

Andrews and Withey (1976) proposed that both processes operate over time in a feedback loop. For example, an increase in salary may first boost financial satisfaction and, in turn, LS. As a result of the increased LS, satisfaction in other domains may increase without objective changes in these domains. Future research needs to test this hypothesis.

The Structure of Affective Well-Being

In 1969 Bradburn published his classic book, *The Structure of Psychological Well-Being*, which laid the foundation for the distinction between PA and NA as independent components of subjective well-being (Diener, 1984; Schimmack, 2007; Schimmack, Bockenholt, & Reisenzein, 2002). Bradburn (1969) distinguished three types of independence, which I call structural, causal, and momentary independence. *Structural independence* means that "within a given period of time, such as a week or two, one may experience many different emotions, both positive and negative, and that in general there is no tendency for the two types to be experienced in any particular relation to one another" (Bradburn, 1969, p. 225). Structural independence is most often implied when PA and NA are distinguished in the subjective well-being literature. *Causal independence* means that PA and NA are influenced by different causes. Finally, *momentary independence* means that fleeting experiences of PA are independent of momentary experiences of NA.

Structural Independence of PA and NA

Bradburn (1969) provided the first evidence for structural independence of PA and NA. He assessed PA and NA with five questions about experiences of PA (e.g., "I felt on top of the world") and NA ("I felt depressed or very unhappy") over the past few weeks. Responses were made on a dichotomous yes–no scale. Correlations among these items showed a pattern that has been replicated in numerous studies: (1) positive correlations among PA items, (2) positive correlations among NA items, and (3) correlations close to zero between PA and NA items.

Diener's (1984) influential review of the literature noted several limitations of Bradburn's work. The main limitations were (1) the failure to control for the potential influence of response styles such as acquiescence biases; (2) the confounding of valence and arousal in measures of PA and NA; (3) the use of items that measure affect in specific situations rather than pure affect; and (4) the use of a dichotomous response format that records the simple occurrence of affect. In the following material I review the evidence regarding the influence of these factors on tests of the structural independence of PA and NA.

Response Styles

Some researches have argued that the independence of PA and NA is a method artifact due to the influence of response styles on affect ratings (Green, Goldman, & Salovey, 1993). Rorer (1965) defined response styles as content-free tendencies to choose certain response categories. If some respondents consistently check *yes* independent of the item content, observed correlations will be biased in a positive direction. The yes–no response format used by Bradburn may be especially susceptible to response biases. In an empirical test of this hypothesis, Green et al. (1993) observed a weak negative correlation between checklist measures of PA and NA ($r = -.25$), whereas other measures yielded much stronger negative correlations ($r = -.84$, after controlling for random measurement error). Based on these findings, Green et al. (1993) concluded that (1) checklists are heavily contaminated by response styles, and (2) PA and NA are not structurally independent.

It did not take long for Diener and colleagues to respond to this challenge. Diener, Smith, and Fujita (1995) conducted a multitrait, multimethod analysis of the structure of affective traits. The study used retrospective self-reports of affect in the past month, averaged daily diary ratings of affect over a 6-week period, and aggregated informant ratings by three or more family members and friends. The main finding of this study was that the method-free correlation between PA and NA was considerably weaker than the one obtained by Green et al. (1993), $r = -.44$. In addition, there was no evidence that self-ratings were contaminated by response styles (Schimmack, Bockenholt, & Reisenzein, 2002). Other studies have provided further evidence that response styles are too weak to account for the structural independence of PA and NA (Schimmack, 2003, 2007; Watson & Clark, 1997).

Influence of Arousal

Numerous authors have proposed that the relation between PA and NA varies as a function of the specific items that are used to measure PA and NA (e.g., Russell & Carroll, 1999). The argument is that some measures of PA and NA are limited to arousing PA (e.g., excited) and arousing NA (e.g., nervous). Structural independence for these measures is the result of a strong negative correlation for the valence component (positive vs. negative) and a strong positive correlation for the shared arousal component (Schimmack & Reisenzein, 2002). In contrast, measures that do not share a common arousal component (e.g., happy, sad) should be highly negatively correlated. Empirical support for this hypothesis is modest. Watson (1988) found that structural independence of PA and NA varied with the item content of different PA and NA measures, but the effect was moderate. This finding has been replicated in numerous studies (Diener, Smith, &

Fujita, 1995; Schimmack, Oishi, & Diener, 2002; Schimmack, 2003). For example, Schimmack (2003) averaged momentary ratings of happiness, sadness, excitement, and worry in an experience sampling study. Whereas the correlation for excitement and worry was slightly positive, $r = .12$, the correlation for happiness and sadness was slightly negative, $r = -.12$.

Additional evidence stems from a study by Schimmack (2006c), which administered the Positive and Negative Affect Schedule scales (PANAS; Watson, Clark, & Tellegen, 1988), the Hedonic Balance Scale (HBS; Schimmack, Diener, & Oishi, 2002), and the Satisfaction with Life Scale (SWLS; Diener et al., 1985). The PANAS is considered a measure of high arousal PA and NA (Watson, Wiese, Vaidya, & Tellegen, 1999). In contrast, the HBS was developed to measure the pure valence of affective experiences. The HBS assesses PA and NA with three items each (PA = positive, pleasant, good; NA = negative, unpleasant, bad). Respondents were asked to report how they typically feel (e.g., "I tend to feel distressed"). PANAS and HBS measures of PA and NA demonstrated convergent validity (PA: $r = .71$; NA: $r = .64$, $n = 111$). The PANAS scale showed perfect structural independence of PA and NA, $r = -.06$. In contrast, the HBS measures of PA and NA were slightly negatively correlated, $r = -.23$. However, the HBS scales had higher predictive validity of LS. The HBS scales accounted for 23% of the variance in LS, and the PANAS scales added 1% of unique variance, which was not significant. PANAS scales accounted for 17% of the variance, and the HBS scales added 7%, which was a significant increase. Lucas, Diener, and Suh (1996) obtained similar findings of better discriminant validity but lower predictive validity for the PANAS measure than for other measures of PA and NA. In sum, there is some support for the hypothesis that measures that include arousal provide better support for structural independence than purer measures of hedonic valence. However, even pure measures that are not contaminated with arousal support the hypothesis of structural independence of PA and NA.

Response Formats

Arguably, the most important moderator of the correlation between PA and NA is the response format that researchers use to assess the two (Schimmack, 2007; Schimmack, Bockenholt, & Reisenzein, 2002). Correlations range from $r = -.9$ with bipolar response formats (e.g., strongly disagree to strongly agree; Green et al., 1993) to $r = +.6$ for open-ended questions about absolute frequencies (Schimmack, Oishi, Diener, & Suh, 2000). The influence of response formats on structural analysis was first noticed by Meddis (1972), who distinguished symmetrical and asymmetrical response formats. He observed that symmetrical formats produce stronger negative correlations between PA and NA than asymmetrical formats. Researchers have interpreted this finding differently. Russell (1980) relied on Meddis's response format to argue that PA and NA are bipolar opposites rather than independent affective states. Others have proposed that symmetrical formats are interpreted by respondents as bipolar response formats, which renders them useless for structural analysis of affect (Russell & Carroll, 1999; Schimmack, Bockenholt, & Reisenzein, 2002).

Variations in the interpretation of response formats may also explain other findings in structural analyses of the affective component of subjective well-being. Warr, Barter, and Brownbridge (1983) changed Bradburn's original response format from a simple yes–no one to a 4-point format that asked about the proportion of time these experiences were felt (i.e., *1* = little or none of the time, to *4* = most of the time). As a result, PA and NA were negatively correlated (*r* = −.54). In contrast, Andrews and Withey (1976) changed the dichotomous format to a frequency format. If participants answered *yes*, they also were asked how often the experience occurred. This format essentially replicated Bradburn's (1969) original finding of structural independence. Similar results were obtained in a study that compared ratings of the amount of affect (*very slightly, very much*) with Warr et al.'s (1983) proportion-of-time measure (Watson, 1988). Once more the proportion-of-time measure produced a stronger negative correlation (*r* = −.48) than the other format (*r* = −.13). It is possible that some respondents interpret the proportion-of-time measure as a bipolar scale (i.e., "How much of your time do you experience positive affect *in proportion* to the time that you experience negative affect?"). As a result, the PA measure would be contaminated with NA, and the NA measure would be contaminated with PA, which would bias the correlation in a negative direction.

Even frequency formats do not guarantee pure assessments of PA and NA. Retrospective reports of affect are difficult because people do not know the objective quantity of their past affective experiences (Schimmack, 2002). As a result, most studies rely on vague quantifiers to assess frequencies (e.g., *often, rarely, very little, very much*). Schimmack, Oishi, et al. (2000) suggested that vague quantifiers produce contaminated measures of PA and NA because respondents need a comparison standard to use vague quantifiers. What does it mean to experience happiness *often*? One way to define this question is to judge the frequency of one emotion in comparison to other emotions. This comparison leads to contaminated measures of PA and NA because the rating of PA relies on the amount of NA as a standard of comparison.

Schimmack, Oishi, et al. (2000) provided some evidence for this hypothesis. Two studies examined frequency judgments of prototypical emotions (e.g., happiness, pride, affection, sadness, anger, disappointment). Some ratings were based on absolute frequency estimates (e.g., five times a week) whereas others were based on vague quantifiers (e.g., *very rarely* to *very often*). Vague quantifier ratings systematically produced more negative correlations than the absolute estimates. Additional evidence was provided by a regression analysis of retrospective ratings of emotions onto aggregated absolute daily estimates over a 3-week period. Regression analyses revealed that vague quantifier ratings were not only positively related to daily frequencies of the same affect, but also negatively related to daily frequencies of the other affect. However, this effect was weak to moderate, suggesting that it has a relatively weak effect on structural analysis of affective well-being.

The contamination of PA and NA measures may also explain cultural variation in the correlation between PA and NA (Schimmack, Oishi, & Diener, 2002). The moderate negative correlation observed in many North American studies is also observed in many collectivistic cultures, but is weaker in East Asian cultures. This difference may be due to dialectic thinking in Asian cultures. Dialectic thinking sees opposites as complementary rather than contradictory, which makes it less likely that people who think dialectically would contrast PA with NA. As a result, PA and NA measures should be less contaminated with the opposing affect, leading to weaker negative correlations. This interpretation is consistent with the finding that ratings of momentary experiences do not show the same cultural bias (Scollon, Diener, Oishi, & Biswas-Diener, 2005). In conclusion, these findings suggests that asymmetric response formats with vague quantifiers are suitable to examine the structure of trait affect, but that this method is likely to produce a negative bias. In other words, PA and NA may appear to be negatively related if they are, in fact, structurally independent.

Discrete Emotional Experiences versus Mood

Emotion researchers increasingly distinguish between emotions and moods (Frijda, 1993; Reisenzein & Schönpflug, 1992; Schimmack & Crites, 2005; Schimmack, Oishi, et al., 2000). Schimmack, Oishi, et al. (2000) suggested that structural analyses of affect may produce different results for emotions and moods. One main reason is that emotional episodes are rare and elicited by events. As a result, the times people experience positive emotions does not limit the time people can experience negative emotions.

In contrast to emotional experiences, moods are more common. This is especially true for positive moods. Most people are happy rather than unhappy, and at any moment in time, most people report being in a positive mood without unpleasant feelings (Diener & Diener, 1996). As discussed in more detail below, positive and negative moods are also inversely related at any moment in time. As a result, the amount of unpleasant moods is likely to restrict the amount of pleasant moods, which would produce an inverse relation between PA and NA for measures of pleasant and unpleasant mood. Empirical studies support this prediction. Schimmack, Oishi, et al. (2000) used a multimethod study with retrospective and daily assessments of the time participants were in a pleasant and an unpleasant mood. Eid (1995) assessed momentary ratings of pleasant mood and unpleasant moods on four different occasions several weeks apart and estimated the general tendency to be in a good or bad mood using latent variable analysis. Both studies yielded substantial negative correlations ($rs = -.58$ to $-.92$). In sum, positive mood and negative mood are not strictly independent. However, even positive mood and negative mood are distinct dimensions of affective well-being.

Structural Independence: Summary

The existing evidence leads to the following conclusions. First, response styles have a small influence on structural analyses of PA and NA. Second, item content influences the results. The more items assess pure valence and focus on pervasive moods rather than emotional episodes, the more negative is the correlation between PA and NA. Third, bipolar interpretations of response formats introduce negative biases that lead to an overestimation of the negative dependence between PA and NA. Finally, PA and NA are clearly separable components of affective well-being, although they may not be strictly independent, as originally postulated by Bradburn (1969).

Causal Independence of PA and NA

Bradburn (1969) provided the first evidence that PA and NA are related to different predictors. Illness was more strongly related to NA than to PA. In contrast, positive social interactions were positively related to PA and unrelated to NA. These findings have been replicated in numerous studies with different measures of PA and NA (e.g., Clark & Watson, 1988). In an experience sampling study, Schimmack, Coleman, and Diener (2000) found that this was also the case when PA and NA were assessed with pure indicators of hedonic tone, namely, feeling pleasant and feeling unpleasant.

Another common finding is that PA and NA are related to different personality traits. Whereas neuroticism is more strongly related to NA than PA, extraversion is often a better predictor of PA than NA (Costa & McCrae, 1980; Diener & Emmons, 1984; Schimmack, 2003; Watson, 2000; Watson & Clark, 1992), although some studies find that extraversion is equally strongly related to PA and NA (Flory, Manuck, Matthews, & Muldoon, 2004). The relations of PA and NA to extraversion and neuroticism are particularly important for subjective well-being researchers due to the extensive literature on the genetic and biological determinants of these personality traits. This literature can be useful in the search for the distinct neurological substrates of PA and NA. Behavioral genetics studies of neuroticism and extraversion reveal different genetic dispositions for extraversion and neuroticism (McCrae, Jang, Livesley, Riemann, & Angleitner, 2001). Recent studies of genetic markers suggest that a gene that influences the neurotransmitter serotonin in the brain is more strongly linked to neuroticism than extraversion (Greenberg et al., 2000). Pharmacological interventions that influence the serotonergic system often show effects on both neuroticism and extraversion, but the effect on neuroticism is stronger (Bagby, Levitan, Kennedy, Levitt, & Joffe, 1999; De Fruyt, Van Leeuwen, Bagby, Rolland, & Rouillon, 2006; Du, Bakish, Ravindran, & Hrdina, 2002).

A few studies have directly linked PA and NA to biological measures. The most comprehensive study thus far assessed levels of PA and NA in a daily diary study over 1 week (Flory et al., 2004). Serotonin levels were assessed with an indirect biological challenge. Serotonin levels predicted PA but not NA. Although this finding is consistent with causal independence of PA and NA, it is inconsistent with the hypothesis that serotonin makes a unique contribution to NA. In sum, there is considerable evidence from psychological studies for causal independence of PA and NA, but the evidence for distinct neurological substrates of PA and NA is mixed.

Momentary Independence

Momentary independence refers to the relation between PA and NA at one moment in time. Numerous authors have pointed out that structural independence and momentary independence examine different questions (Bradburn, 1969; Diener & Emmons, 1984; Russell & Carroll, 1999; Schimmack & Diener, 1997). PA and NA can be independent over extended time periods, even if they are fully dependent at each moment. For example, even if love and hate were mutually exclusive at one moment in time, some individuals could experience more love and more hate over extended periods of time than others (Bradburn, 1969; Schimmack & Diener, 1997).

Diener and Iran-Nejad (1986) conducted the first rigorous study of momentary independence. Participants reported the intensity of various emotions in response to everyday events in an event sampling study. The study revealed a pattern that has been replicated in numerous studies (e.g., Larsen, McGraw, & Cacioppo, 2001; Larsen, McGraw, Mellers, & Cacioppo, 2004; Schimmack, 2001, 2005; Schimmack, Coleman, & Diener, 2000). Participants reported PA and NA in response to the same event, but only at low-to-moderate intensities. Reports of intense PA and intense NA were virtually absent. Diener and Iran-Nejad (1986) proposed a neurobiological model to account for this pattern. Accordingly, PA and NA are based on different neurobiological processes, but momentary activation of one system momentarily inhibits activation of the other system.

Other factors may also account for the absence of intense PA and intense NA. Schimmack (2001) explained reports of concurrent pleasant and unpleasant experiences as a function of different baseline levels of the two affects. Typically people are in a moderately good mood. In response to a negative event, negative mood is elicited and the preexisting pleasant mood is reduced but not eliminated.

Another potential mechanism is attention (Schimmack & Colcombe, 1999). Intensity of affective experiences increases with attention to the eliciting stimulus (Diener, Colvin, Pavot, & Allman, 1991). As attention is limited, it is impossible to attend fully to positive and negative aspects of the same situation. As a result, conflicting responses to positive and negative aspects are less intense than responses to a single positive or negative aspect.

Finally, some affective cues are intrinsically bipolar. These cues can still elicit mixed responses if they are paired with another bipolar cue. For example, fast music elicits happiness, whereas slow music elicits sadness. Similarly, music in major mode elicits happiness, whereas music in minor mode elicits sadness. Music that combines conflicting cues (e.g., fast music in minor mode) elicits mild happiness and mild sadness (Hunter, Schellenberg, & Schimmack, 2006). However, it is impossible to elicit intense happiness and intense sadness with music, because fast tempo reduces sadness and minor mode reduces the intensity of happiness.

The postulated inhibition processes have interesting implications for subjective well-being research. Many situations are complex and may elicit PA or NA or both (e.g., having a headache at a party). In these situations, the inhibitory processes will determine whether an individual experiences relatively more PA or NA. Thus, these processes contribute to the amount of PA and NA that individuals experience over time. For example, some studies link neuroticism to a tendency to attend more to negative, especially threatening stimuli (Derryberry & Reed, 1994). Thus, one reason for the link between neuroticism and NA could be a tendency of neurotics to attend more to the negative stimuli in their environments (Diener et al., 1999).

Conclusion

Structural theories of subjective well-being assume that PA and NA are independent. Empirical research is broadly consistent with this assumption. Although PA and NA are sometimes not strictly independent or orthogonal ($r = .00$), negative correlations are often weak to moderate. Furthermore, PA and NA have distinct causes and can even co-occur at the same moment, although not at full intensity. The main implication of this finding is that an individual with high PA does not necessarily have low NA, and vice versa. Therefore, a full understanding of subjective well-being requires an assessment of PA and NA. Furthermore, interventions that influence one component may have no effect, or even opposing effects, on the other component. Future research needs to examine both the separate causes of PA and NA as well as the causes that influence both affects.

The Relation
between Cognitive and Affective Well-Being

The cognitive and affective components of subjective well-being correlate positively with each other. The magnitude of this correlation varies widely from $r = .1$ to $.8$ (Lucas et al., 1996; Schimmack, Diener, & Oishi, 2002; Schimmack, Radhakrishnan, Oishi, Dzokoto, & Ahadi, 2002; Suh, Diener, Oishi, & Triandis, 1998). Some of this variability is due to methodological factors. Less reliable scales, such as Bradburn's (1969) Affect Balance Scale, produce weaker correlations than other measures of affect, and correlations that control for random measurement error are higher than observed correlations (e.g., Schimmack, Radhakrishnan, et al., 2002; Suh et al., 1998). However, methodological factors do not fully account for the lack of a perfect correlation between the two components. Multimethod studies generally demonstrate discriminant validity of the two components of subjective well-being (Lucas et al., 1996). That is, measures of the same construct (e.g., LS and LS) correlated more highly with each other than measures of different constructs (e.g., LS and affect) across different methods (e.g., self-ratings and informant ratings).

Suh et al. (1998) provided a theoretical explanation for this finding. They proposed that people, in part, rely directly on the affective component to judge LS. In addition, people may rely on other information (e.g., cultural norms, DS) to judge LS. The correlation between the affective and cognitive components depends on the weight that people attach to the different types of information when they judge LS. This model accounts for cultural variation in the relation between the affective and cognitive components. The correlation is stronger in more individualistic, developed, and modern cultures (e.g., $r = .57$ in Western Germany) than in less individualistic, less developed, and more traditional cultures (e.g., $r = .22$ in India). This finding is consistent with evidence that development leads to a change in people's value orientation from materialism (i.e., fulfillment of basic needs) to postmaterialistic values (e.g., the maximization of subjective well-being; Inglehart, 1997).

The affective and cognitive components are also influenced by different causes. Headey et al. (1984) found that changes in DS were a better predictor of changes in the cognitive component of subjective well-being than in the affective component of it. One possible explanation for this finding could be shared method variance between judgments of domain satisfaction and life satisfaction. To explore this possibility, Schimmack (2006d) examined the relation between LS, hedonic balance, and DS in a sample of college students. Average DS was more highly correlated with LS, $r = .69$, than with hedonic balance, $r = .55$. To control for method effects, satisfaction with weather and traffic were entered before entering the other domains. This hierarchical regression analysis revealed that hedonic balance accounted for 34% of the variance, weather and traffic added 2%, and the remaining domains added 22%. This finding suggests that objective determinants of DS (e.g., income) should have a stronger influence on LS than on the affective component of well-being. Future research needs to test this hypothesis.

Other studies have identified stronger predictors of the affective than the cognitive component of subjective well-being. Schimmack, Diener, and Oishi (2002) proposed that personality traits, especially extraversion and neuroticism, primarily influence the affective component of subjective well-being. They influence the cognitive component only to the extent that people rely on the affective component to evaluate their lives. This model predicts that personality measures correlate more strongly with the affective component than the cognitive component of subjective well-being. This prediction has been confirmed in several studies (e.g., Schimmack, Diener, & Oishi, 2002; Schimmack, Radhakrishnan, et al., 2002). Further evidence stems from Schimmack's (2006d) study of a large college sample ($n = 1,241$). Neuroticism and extraversion were stronger predictors of affective balance, $r = -.54$ (neuroticism) and $r = .39$ (extraversion), than LS, $r = -.27$ (neuroticism) and .26 (extraversion).

This pattern may be explained partially by the inclusion of affective items in measures of extraversion and neuroticism (Pytlik Zillig, Hemenover, & Dienstbier, 2002). However, affective items are only included in measures of extraversion and neuroticism because these items are highly related to other indicators of these traits. Thus, the strong relationship between personality and affect is not a mere artifact. Rather it suggests that there exist stable affective dispositions. These dispositions have a direct effect on the affective component of subjective well-being, but only an indirect effect on the cognitive component of subjective well-being. This model accounts for two other findings in the subjective well-being literature. First, personality is a weaker predictor of LS in cultures that rely less on the affective component to judge LS (Schimmack, Radhakrishnan, et al., 2002). Second, the cognitive component is less stable over time than personality traits (Fujita & Diener, 2005).

Conclusion

This chapter examined the structural relations among various components of subjective well-being. These components can be divided roughly into cognitive components (LS and DS) and affective components (PA and NA). This chapter revealed numerous robust structural relations among these components. DS and LS are highly correlated even after controlling for shared method effects and common influences of personality traits. At least some of this relation is due to bottom-up influences of DS on LS. Thus, changes in DS are likely to produce changes in LS. It is also possible that top-down processes contribute to the LS–

DS correlation, although evidence for top-down effects is less conclusive. On the affective side, PA and NA are separable components of subjective well-being with distinct causes, although they may not be strictly independent, especially in momentary assessments of affect. Personality traits, especially neuroticism and extraversion, appear to have a stronger influence on the affective component of subjective well-being than the cognitive component. Indeed, the relation between personality and the cognitive component of subjective well-being is often fully mediated by the affective component, presumably because people rely on the affective component to judge LS. In contrast, DS is a stronger determinant of LS than affective well-being. The review also revealed the need for more powerful research designs to elucidate the causal processes underlying the structure of subjective well-being. Longitudinal studies that reveal changes in well-being, in combination with dyadic designs that allow separating personality/genetic from situational/environmental influences, are especially promising (Nes, Roysamb, Tambs, Harris, & Reichborn-Kjennerud, 2006; Schimmack & Lucas, 2007).

References

Andrews, F. M., & Withey, S. B. (1976). *Social indicators of well-being*. New York: Plenum Press.

Bagby, R. M., Levitan, R. D., Kennedy, S. H., Levitt, A. J., & Joffe, R. T. (1999). Selective alteration of personality in response to noradrenergic and serotonergic antidepressant medication in depressed sample: Evidence of non-specificity. *Psychiatry Research, 86*, 211–216.

Bookwala, J., & Schulz, R. (1996). Spousal similarity in subjective well-being: The cardiovascular health study. *Psychology and Aging, 11*, 582–590.

Bradburn, N. M. (1969). *The structure of psychological well being*. Chicago: Aldine.

Brief, A. P., Butcher, A. H., George, J. M., & Link, K. E. (1993). Integrating bottom-up and top-down theories of subjective well-being: The case of health. *Journal of Personality and Social Psychology, 64*, 646–653.

Browne, M. W., & Cudeck, R. (1993). Alternative ways of assessing model fit. In K. A. Bollen & J. S. Long (Eds.), *Testing structural equation models* (pp. 136–162). Newbury Park, CA: Sage.

Clark, L. A., & Watson, D. (1988). Mood and the mundane: Relations between daily life events and self-reported mood. *Journal of Personality and Social Psychology, 54*, 296–308.

Colvin, C. R., & Block, J. (1994). Do positive illusions foster mental health? An examination of the Taylor and Brown formulation. *Psychological Bulletin, 116*, 3–20.

Costa, P. T., & McCrae, R. R. (1980). Influence of extraversion and neuroticism on subjective well-being: Happy and unhappy people. *Journal of Personality and Social Psychology, 38*, 668–678.

De Fruyt, F., Van Leeuwen, K., Bagby, R. M., Rolland, J.-P., & Rouillon, F. (2006). Assessing and interpreting personality change and continuity in patients treated for major depression. *Psychological Assessment, 18*, 71–80.

Derryberry, D., & Reed, M. A. (1994). Temperament and attention: Orienting toward and away from positive and negative signals. *Journal of Personality and Social Psychology, 66*, 1128–1139.

Diener, E. (1984). Subjective well-being. *Psychological Bulletin, 95*, 542–575.

Diener, E., & Biswas-Diener, R. (2002). Will money increase subjective well-being? *Social Indicators Research, 57*, 119–169.

Diener, E., Colvin, C. R., Pavot, W. G., & Allman, A. (1991). The psychic costs of intense positive affect. *Journal of Personality and Social Psychology, 61*, 492–503.

Diener, E., & Diener, C. (1996). Most people are happy. *Psychological Science, 7*, 181–185.

Diener, E., & Emmons, R. A. (1984). The independence of positive and negative affect. *Journal of Personality and Social Psychology, 47*, 1105–1117.

Diener, E., Emmons, R. A., Larsen, R. J., & Griffin, S. (1985). The Satisfaction with Life Scale. *Journal of Personality Assessment, 49*, 71–75.

Diener, E., & Iran-Nejad, A. (1986). The relationship in experience between various types of affect. *Journal of Personality and Social Psychology, 50*, 1031–1038.

Diener, E., & Oishi, S. (2000). Money and happiness: Income and subjective well-being across nations. In E. Diener & E. M. Suh (Eds.), *Culture and subjective well-being* (pp. 185–218). Cambridge, MA: MIT Press.

Diener, E., Smith, H., & Fujita, F. (1995). The personality structure of affect. *Journal of Personality and Social Psychology, 69*, 130–141.

Diener, E., Suh, E. M., Lucas, R. E., & Smith, H. L. (1999). Subjective well-being: Three decades of progress. *Psychological Bulletin, 125*, 276–302.

Diener, E., Wolsic, B., & Fujita, F. (1995). Physical attractiveness and subjective well-being. *Journal of Personality and Social Psychology, 69*, 120–129.

Di Tella, R., Heisken De New, J., & MacCulloch, R. (2006). *Happiness adaptation to income and to status in an individual panel.* Unpublished manuscript, Harvard University, Cambridge, MA.

Du, L., Bakish, D., Ravindran, A. V., & Hrdina, P. D. (2002). Does fluoxetine influence major depression by modifying five-factor personality traits? *Journal of Affective Disorders, 71*, 235–241.

Eid, M. (1995). *Modelle der Messung von Personen in Situationen [Models of measuring individuals in situations].* Weinheim, Germany: Beltz-PVU.

Flory, J. D., Manuck, S. B., Matthews, K. A., & Muldoon, M. F. (2004). Serotonergic function in the central nervous system is associated with daily ratings of positive mood. *Psychiatry Research, 129*, 11–19.

Frijda, N. H. (1993). Moods, emotion episodes, and emotions. In M. Lewis & J. M. Haviland (Eds.), *Handbook of emotions* (pp. 381–403). New York: Guilford Press.

Fujita, F., & Diener, E. (2005). Life satisfaction set point: Stability and change. *Journal of Personality and Social Psychology, 88*, 158–164.

Green, D. P., Goldman, S. L., & Salovey, P. (1993). Measurement error masks bipolarity in affect ratings. *Journal of Personality and Social Psychology, 64*, 1029–1041.

Greenberg, B. D., Li, Q., Lucas, F. R., Hu, S., Sirota, L. A., Benjamin, J., et al. (2000).

Association between the serotonin transporter promoter polymorphism and personality traits in a primarily female population sample. *American Journal of Medical Genetics, 96,* 202–216.

Headey, B., Holmstrom, E., & Wearing, A. (1984). The impact of life events and changes
in domain satisfactions on well-being. *Social Indicators Research, 15,* 203–227.

Headey, B., Veenhoven, R., & Wearing, A. (1991). Top-down versus bottom-up theories of subjective well-being. *Social Indicators Research, 24,* 81–100.

Heller, D., Judge, T. A., & Watson, D. (2002). The confounding role of personality and
trait affectivity in the relationship between job and life satisfaction. *Journal of Organizational Behavior, 23,* 815–835.

Heller, D., Watson, D., & Hies, R. (2004). The role of person versus situation in life satisfaction: A critical examination. *Psychological Bulletin, 130,* 574–600.

Hsieh, C. M. (2004). Income and financial satisfaction among older adults in the United
States. *Social Indicators Research, 66,* 249–266.

Hu, L., & Bentler, P. M. (1995). Evaluating model fit. In R. H. Hoyle (Ed.), *Structural
equation modeling: Concepts, issues, and applications* (pp. 76–99). London: Sage.

Hu, L., & Bentler, P. M. (1999). Cutoff criteria for fit indexes in covariance structure
analysis: Conventional criteria versus new alternatives. *Structural Equation Modeling,
6,* 1–55.

Hunter, P. G., Schellenberg, E. G., & Schimmack, U. (in press). Mixed moods: Affective
responses to music with conflicting cues. *Cognition and Emotion.*

Inglehart, R. (1997). *Modernization and post-modernization.* Princeton, NJ: Princeton University Press.

Inglehart, R., Basanez, M., & Diez-Medrano, J. (Eds.). (2004). *Human beliefs and values: A
cross-cultural sourcebook based on the 1999–2002 World Values Survey.* Mexico City:
Siglo XXI Editores.

Larsen, J. T., McGraw, A. P., & Cacioppo, J. T. (2001). Can people feel happy and sad at
the same time? *Journal of Personality and Social Psychology, 81,* 684–696.

Larsen, J. T., McGraw, A. P., Mellers, B. A., & Cacioppo, J. T. (2004). The agony of
victory and thrill of defeat: Mixed emotional reactions to disappointing wins and
relieving losses. *Psychological Science, 15,* 325–330.

Lucas, R. E., Diener, E., & Suh, E. (1996). Discriminant validity of well-being measures.
Journal of Personality and Social Psychology, 71, 616–628.

McCrae, R. R., Jang, K. L., Livesley, W. J., Riemann, R., & Angleitner, A. (2001).
Sources of structure: Genetic, environmental, and artifactual influences on the
covariation of personality traits. *Journal of Personality, 69,* 511–535.

Meddis, R. (1972). Bipolar factors in mood adjective checklists. *British Journal of Social and
Clinical Psychology, 11,* 178–184.

Nes, R. B., Roysamb, E., Tambs, K., Harris, J. R., & Reichborn-Kjennerud, T. (2006).
Subjective well-being: Genetic and environmental contributions to stability and
change. *Psychological Medicine, 36,* 1033–1042.

Pytlik Zillig, L. M., Hemenover, S. H., & Dienstbier, R. A. (2002). What do we assess
when we assess a Big 5 trait? A content analysis of the affective, behavioral and cognitive processes represented in the Big 5 personality inventories. *Personality and Social
Psychology Bulletin, 28,* 847–858.

Reisenzein, R., & Schönpflug, W. (1992). Stumpf's cognitive evaluative theory of emotion. *American Psychologist, 47,* 34–45.

Rorer, L. G. (1965). The great response-style myth. *Psychological Bulletin, 63,* 129–156.

Roysamb, E., Harris, J. R., Magnus, P., Vitterso, J., & Tambs, K. (2002). Subjective well-being: Sex-specific effects of genetic and environmental factors. *Personality and Individual Differences, 32,* 211–223.

Russell, J. A. (1980). A circumplex model of affect. *Journal of Personality and Social Psychology, 39,* 1161–1178.

Russell, J. A., & Carroll, J. M. (1999). On the bipolarity of positive and negative affect. *Psychological Bulletin, 125,* 3–30.

Schimmack, U. (2001). Pleasure, displeasure, and mixed feelings: Are semantic opposites mutually exclusive? *Cognition and Emotion, 15,* 81–97.

Schimmack, U. (2002). Frequency judgments of emotions: The cognitive basis of personality assessment. In P. Sedlmeier & T. Betsch (Eds.), *ETC: Frequency processing and cognition* (pp. 189–204). New York: Oxford University Press.

Schimmack, U. (2003). Affect measurement in experience sampling research. *Journal of Happiness Studies, 4,* 79–106.

Schimmack, U. (2005). Response latencies of pleasure and displeasure ratings: Further evidence for mixed feelings. *Cognition and Emotion, 19,* 671–691.

Schimmack, U. (2006a). *Income, financial satisfaction, and life satisfaction: A test of top-down and bottom-up models of subjective well-being.* Unpublished manuscript.

Schimmack, U. (2006b). Internal and external determinants of subjective well being: Review and public policy implications. In Y. K. Ng & L. Sang Ho (Eds.), *Happiness and public policy: Theory, case studies, and implications* (pp. 67–88). Houndmills, Basingstoke, Hampshire, UK: Palgrave Macmillan.

Schimmack, U. (2006c). *Measuring the affective component of subjective well-being: Comparing the discriminant and predictive validity of the Positive and Negative Affect Schedule and the Hedonic Balance Scale.* Unpublished manuscript.

Schimmack, U. (2006d). *The structure of subjective well-being: Personality, affect, life satisfaction, and domain satisfaction.* Unpublished manuscript.

Schimmack, U. (2007). Methodological issues in the assessment of the affective component of subjective well being. In A. Ohn & M. van Dulmen (Eds.), *Handbook of methods in positive psychology* (pp. 96–110). Oxford, UK: Oxford University Press.

Schimmack, U., Bockenholt, U., & Reisenzein, R. (2002). Response styles in affect ratings: Making a mountain out of a molehill. *Journal of Personality Assessment, 78,* 461–483.

Schimmack, U., & Colcombe, S. J. (1999). *Mixed feelings: Towards a theory of pleasure and displeasure.* Retrieved July 19, 2006, from *www.erin.utoronto.ca/~w3psyuli/msMixedFeelings.pdf*

Schimmack, U., Coleman, K., & Diener, E. (2000, June). *Mixed feelings in everyday life.* Paper presented at the 12th annual convention of the American Psychological Society, Miami.

Schimmack, U., & Crites, S. L. J. R. (2005). The structure of affect. In D. Albarracin, B. T. Johnson, & M. P. Zanna (Eds.), *The handbook of attitudes* (pp. 397–435). Mahwah, NJ: Erlbaum.

Schimmack, U., & Diener, E. (1997). Affect intensity: Separating intensity and frequency in repeatedly measured affect. *Journal of Personality and Social Psychology, 73,* 1313–1329.

Schimmack, U., Diener, E., & Oishi, S. (2002). Life satisfaction is a momentary judgment and a stable personality characteristic: The use of chronically accessible and stable sources. *Journal of Personality, 70,* 345–384.

Schimmack, U., Diener, E., Oishi, S., & Suh, E. (2006). *The influence of shared method variance on the relation between life satisfaction and domain satisfaction.* Unpublished manuscript.

Schimmack, U., & Lucas, R. E. (2007). Marriage matters: Spousal similarity in life satisfaction. *Journal of Applied Social Science Studies, 127,* 1–7.

Schimmack, U., & Oishi, S. (2005). The influence of chronically and temporarily accessible information on life satisfaction judgments. *Journal of Personality and Social Psychology, 89,* 395–406.

Schimmack, U., Oishi, S., & Diener, E. (2002). Cultural influences on the relation between pleasant emotions and unpleasant emotions: Asian dialectic philosophies or individualism–collectivism? *Cognition and Emotion, 16,* 705–719.

Schimmack, U., Oishi, S., Diener, E., & Suh, E. (2000). Facets of affective experiences: A framework for investigations of trait affect. *Personality and Social Psychology Bulletin, 26,* 655–668.

Schimmack, U., Oishi, S., Furr, R. M., & Funder, D. C. (2004). Personality and life satisfaction: A facet-level analysis. *Personality and Social Psychology Bulletin, 30,* 1062–1075.

Schimmack, U., Pinkus, R. T., & Lockwood, P. (2006). *Personality and life satisfaction: A dyadic multimethod–occasion–construct study.* Manuscript submitted for publication.

Schimmack, U., Radhakrishnan, P., Oishi, S., Dzokoto, V., & Ahadi, S. (2002). Culture, personality, and subjective well-being: Integrating process models of life satisfaction. *Journal of Personality and Social Psychology, 82,* 582–593.

Schimmack, U., & Reisenzein, R. (2002). Experiencing activation: Energetic arousal and tense arousal are not mixtures of valence and activation. *Emotion, 2,* 412–417.

Schimmack, U., & Sidhu, R. (2006). *Global evaluative biases and well-being.* Manuscript submitted for publication.

Schwarz, N., & Strack, F. (1999). Reports of subjective well-being: Judgmental processes and their methodological implications. In D. Kahneman, E. Diener, & N. Schwarz (Eds.), *Well-being: The foundations of hedonic psychology* (pp. 61–84). New York: Sage.

Scollon, C. N., Diener, E., Oishi, S., & Biswas-Diener, R. (2005). An experience sampling and cross-cultural investigation of the relation between pleasant and unpleasant affect. *Cognition and Emotion, 19,* 27–52.

Spotts, E. L., Neiderhiser, J. M., Towers, H., Hansson, K., Lichtenstein, P., Cederblad, M., et al. (2004). Genetic and environmental influences on marital relationships. *Journal of Family Psychology, 18,* 107–119.

Suh, E., Diener, E., Oishi, S., & Triandis, H. C. (1998). The shifting basis of life satisfaction judgments across cultures: Emotions versus norms. *Journal of Personality and Social Psychology, 74,* 482–493.

Taylor, S. E., & Brown, J. D. (1988). Illusion and well-being: A social psychological perspective on mental health. *Psychological Bulletin, 103,* 193–210.

Warr, P. B., Barter, J., & Brownbridge, G. (1983). On the independence of positive and negative affect. *Journal of Personality and Social Psychology, 44,* 644–651.

Watson, D. (1988). The vicissitudes of mood measurement: Effects of varying descriptors, time frames, and response formats on measures of positive and negative affect. *Journal of Personality and Social Psychology, 55,* 128–141.

Watson, D. (2000). *Mood and temperament.* New York: Guilford Press.

Watson, D., & Clark, L. A. (1992). Affects separable and inseparable: On the hierarchical arrangement of the negative affects. *Journal of Personality and Social Psychology, 62,* 489–505.

Watson, D., & Clark, L. A. (1997). Measurement and mismeasurement of mood: Recurrent and emergent issues. *Journal of Personality Assessment, 68,* 267–296.

Watson, D., Clark, L. A., & Tellegen, A. (1988). Development and validation of brief measures of positive and negative affect: The PANAS scales. *Journal of Personality and Social Psychology, 54,* 1063–1070.

Watson, D., Wiese, D., Vaidya, J., & Tellegen, A. (1999). The two general activation systems of affect: Structural findings, evolutionary considerations, and psychobiological evidence. *Journal of Personality and Social Psychology, 76,* 820–838.

7

The Assessment
of Subjective Well-Being
Successes and Shortfalls

WILLIAM PAVOT

Research on happiness, or subjective well-being, has emerged as an important area of focus for psychology in the new millennium. A significant and growing number of researchers have broken away from the field's preoccupation with depression, anxiety, and disorder (Myers, 2000), choosing instead to devote their attention to "positive psychology" (Seligman & Csikszentmihalyi, 2000, p. 5). As interest in subjective well-being and related constructs has grown, so too has the demand for instruments and methodologies designed to assess these constructs.

To a large extent, progress in the development of valid measures and methodologies has kept pace with the increases in demand. Relative to the early days of subjective well-being research (Diener, 1984), the array of measures and research methods available to contemporary researchers is impressive. The sophistication and reliability of subjective well-being measures has increased substantially. Innovative methodologies now allow researchers to develop multi-method designs that overcome many of the shortcoming and weaknesses of earlier single-method studies.

In the midst of a successful period of development, however, some shortfalls must be noted as well. Despite the substantial advances in subjective well-being assessment, the development of a broadly based, consistent, and comprehensive empirical database of subjective well-being findings has been realized only partially. A number of factors, such as an overreliance on single-method, cross-sectional designs and the use of narrow measures that provide only a partial assessment of subjective well-being, have combined to limit the generality of the findings from individual studies.

In the initial sections of this chapter, general issues related to the definition and assessment of subjective well-being are discussed and examples of current measures of subjective well-being are reviewed. Later sections of the chapter focus on alternative measures and methodologies, the limitations of the current subjective well-being database, and a discussion of the future issues and directions of subjective well-being research.

Issues of Definition and Measurement

Clear definition is a necessary precursor to valid assessment, and the assessment of subjective well-being is not exempt from this imperative. Subjective well-being is most often conceptualized as a broad domain of interest rather than a specific construct (Diener, Suh, Lucas, & Smith, 1999). A (sometimes confusing) number of related constructs have been proposed by researchers approaching subjective well-being from a variety of perspectives, but these constructs generally converge with one or the other of two fundamental components of subjective well-being. The essential elements of subjective well-being include a predominant theme of positive mood and emotional states within an individual's subjective experience and a cognitive evaluation of the conditions and circumstances of his or her life in positive and satisfying terms.

Affective responses (which potentially encompass both emotions and mood states) represent ongoing or "online" (Diener, 2000, p. 34) readouts of subjective experience. These affective responses can be divided further into positive affect (PA) and negative affect (NA). A number of studies focused on these affective responses have shown PA and NA to be separable components (Bradburn & Caplovitz, 1965; Diener & Emmons, 1984; Lucas, Diener, & Suh, 1996). Thus the affective response portion of subjective well-being is most accurately depicted (and assessed) as two components, PA and NA (see Schimmack, Chapter 6, this volume).

Judgments of satisfaction with the conditions and circumstances of life as a whole represent an additional and partially distinct element of subjective well-being. Life satisfaction judgments represent broad, cognitively based evaluations of one's life as a whole. Domain satisfactions, on the other hand, represent a focused evaluation of some specific aspect of one's life, such as employment satisfaction, marital satisfaction, or satisfaction with one's housing. Generally, there is a strong relationship between domain satisfaction and life satisfaction, and therefore, at the conceptual level, domain satisfaction is often subsumed within the life satisfaction component.

Various alternative conceptualizations of subjective well-being have been offered, but the conceptualization of subjective well-being as composed of three factors, namely, PA, NA, and life satisfaction, has received consistent empirical support (Lucas et al., 1996; Arthaud-Day, Rode, Mooney, & Near, 2005). Thus, the assumption of a "tripartite" (Arthaud-Day et al., 2005) model of subjective well-being underlies the remainder of this chapter.

A fundamental assumption of subjective well-being is that it does indeed represent the subjective experience of the individual. A primary source of information on a person's subjective experience is that person's own self-report. Self-reports have an advantage in that they represent the direct report of the subjective experience of the respondent, without the need of inference or interpretation by others. Self-report data, particularly reports of subjective well-being and life satisfaction, have been periodically criticized on the grounds that they are subject to contextual influences, biases, and response styles (Schwarz & Clore, 1983; Green, Goldman, & Salovey, 1993; Schwarz & Strack, 1999). It is important to be aware of the potential influence of these factors on self-report. Still, much research (Pavot & Diener, 1993a; Schimmack, Bockenholt, & Reisenzein, 2002; Eid & Diener, 2004; Schimmack & Oishi, 2005) has demonstrated that the influence of contextual factors and response styles is limited, and that self-reports of subjective well-being and life satisfaction are generally reliable and valid. In a comparison of the self-reports of anxiety levels within a group of children with ratings of anxiety in the same children by clinicians, Joiner, Brown, Perez, Sethuraman, and Sallee (2005) found that the children's self-reports were better predictors of anxiotypic neuroendocrine profiles than were the clinicians' ratings of anxiety. Thus, self-reports can be more accurate than expert ratings when researchers are attempting to assess subjective experiences.

Self-Report Measures of PA and NA

Several measures have figured prominently in the assessment of the affective components of subjective well-being. An early and influential measure, Bradburn's (1969) Affect Balance Scale, was designed to assess affective experiences with a set of 10 questions probing the affective experiences of the respondent "during the past few weeks." Five of these items were directed toward positive affective experiences, and five toward negative affective experiences. Respondents were asked to give "yes" or "no" answers to each item. Two subscores were thus created. The score for the NA items could then be subtracted from the PA score, and the affect balance score was the result. An alternative would be to consider the scores for PA and NA separately. The Bradburn Affect Balance Scale has been widely used since its introduction, despite evidence of some psychometric concerns (Diener & Emmons, 1984). Following the same basic pattern as the Bradburn (1969) measure but using an expanded (40-item) format and a more discriminating, frequency-based response scale, Kammann and Flett (1983) introduced the Affectometer 2. Ten facets of subjective well-being (confluence, optimism, self-esteem, self-efficacy, social support, social interest, freedom, energy, cheerfulness, and thought clarity) are each assessed by four scale items. The Affectometer 2 has high internal consistency and good convergent validity with other measures of subjective well-being (Kammann & Flett, 1983).

The Positive and Negative Affect Schedule (PANAS; Watson, Clark, & Tellegen, 1988) has become a popular instrument for many researchers. The PANAS scales include 10 affective adjectives to assess PA, and 10 affective adjectives to assess NA. Examples include "interested," "enthusiastic," and "inspired" from the PA scale, and "distressed," "upset," and "afraid" from the NA scale. The respondent reports his or her experience of each of the emotions listed using a 5-point scale. The time frame can be adjusted to represent anything from immediate experience to experiences during the past year. The PANAS scales have demonstrated good psychometric characteristics (Watson et al., 1988), although their focus leans toward high-activation or high-arousal emotions.

Based upon a different conceptualization of the affective circumplex (Russell, 1980), Diener and Emmons (1984) have developed a set of affective adjectives that have been particularly useful in subjective well-being research. Originating from the pleasant affect–unpleasant affect dimension of the circumplex, examples of these adjectives, as they might appear in a simple assessment of affect, are presented in Figure 7.1. The time frame of such an assessment could be adjusted in order to reflect the respondent's current affective state or some other length of time (e.g., "today," "in the past week," "in the past month"). A more detailed description of the selection of these adjectives is presented in Diener and Emmons (1984). These adjectives tend to be more representative of subjective well-being than those derived from alternative rotations of the affective circumplex (for a detailed discussion of the affective circumplex and issues surrounding it, see Larsen & Diener, 1992).

Another approach to the assessment of the affective components of subjective well-being involves the measurement of personality traits, particularly the temperament-level traits of extraversion and neuroticism. In a noteworthy report, Costa and McCrae (1980) presented data from three studies indicating that a considerable amount of the variance of subjective well-being between people could be accounted for in terms of personality. Specifically, PA was shown to be correlated with the trait of extraversion, and NA was found to be related to the trait of neuroticism. These findings have since been replicated

EMOTION REPORT

Using the 7-point scale below, please indicate the extent to which you have
experienced the following emotions in the past week:

Not at All	Very Slightly	Somewhat	Moderately	Much	Very Much	Extremely Much
0	1	2	3	4	5	6

    ____ Happy   ____ Depressed/Blue

    ____ Worried/Anxious   ____ Joyful

    ____ Pleased   ____ Unhappy

    ____ Angry/Hostile   ____ Enjoyment/Fun

    ____ Frustrated

FIGURE 7.1. An example of a simple assessment of affect, utilizing adjectives from the pleasant–unpleasant affect dimension.

repeatedly (see DeNeve & Cooper, 1998, for an extensive review). Thus, instruments such as the revised NEO Personality Inventory—Revised (NEOPI-R; Costa & McCrae, 1992) can be used to assess the long-term affective tone of the respondent and are often moderately to strongly correlated with other measures of subjective well-being.

Self-Report Measures of Life Satisfaction

Satisfaction measures generally fall into one of two categories: global or multidimensional satisfaction with life measures, or measures of domain satisfaction. Global satisfaction measures are designed to measure an individual's level of satisfaction with life as a whole, and multidimensional measures are intended to assess a set of important life domains. Measures of domain satisfaction tend to be narrow, focusing on one particular domain or aspect of life, such as marital satisfaction, housing satisfaction, or job satisfaction. Due to their nature, domain satisfaction measures tend to be developed for use in specific research settings (e.g., a job satisfaction measure might be developed for research in work settings) and tend to be less broadly applicable as measures of life satisfaction. In an effort to maintain a broad conceptual focus, I offer examples only of life satisfaction measures.

The Satisfaction with Life Scale (SWLS; Diener, Emmons, Larsen, & Griffin, 1985; Pavot & Diener, 1993b) is a widely used measure designed to assess an individual's overall level of life satisfaction. This 5-item scale offers very good internal consistency and temporal reliability (Pavot & Diener, 1993b), yet it is brief and easily incorporated into a larger research design. The SWLS has been translated into a number of languages, and it is useful for the assessment of people across a wide range of educational levels and ages.

The Temporal Satisfaction with Life Scale (TSWLS; Pavot, Diener, & Suh, 1998) represents an adaptation of the original SWLS items into an expanded format. The TWSLS is intended to assess the respondent's past, present, and future satisfaction. Each of the five items of the original SWLS is reworded to represent the respondent's past, present, or expected future state of life satisfaction. The resulting 15-item scale has demonstrated the same favorable psychometric characteristics as the SWLS (Pavot et al., 1998) and adds the additional feature of a temporal dimension, allowing investigators to detect distinctions and changes in life satisfaction between time frames, as experienced by the respondent.

Additional measures of life satisfaction have been developed for use with specific age groups and/or populations. The Multidimensional Students' Life Satisfaction Scale (MSLSS; Huebner, 1994) is a fairly extensive (40-item) measure designed to assess the life satisfaction of preadolescent students. The MSLSS utilizes subscales focused on relevant factors such as self, friends, family, school, and living environment. More recently, Seligson, Huebner, and Valois (2003) have reported encouraging preliminary validation data for a brief version of the MSLSS, and have also demonstrated its usefulness with high school students.

For researchers interested in assessing life satisfaction in older adults, the Life Satisfaction Scale (LSS; Neugarten, Havighurst, & Tobin, 1961) is available. Variants of the LSS include the Life Satisfaction Index A (LSIA), Life Satisfaction Index B (LSIB), and the Life Satisfaction Rating (LSR). Each of these instruments uses a multifactorial approach to assess levels of satisfaction in older adults. These factors include zest versus apathy, resolution and fortitude, congruence between desired and achieved goals, self-concept, and mood tone. It should be noted that subsequent factor analyses (e.g., Adams, 1969) have sometimes indicated a factor structure different from the original.

Additional Self-Report Measures of Subjective Well-Being

Many of the instruments in current use, such as those reviewed above, are intended to assess only the affective or life satisfaction component of subjective well-being. Some instruments, however, take a broader, wholistic approach to measurement and are intended to assess all components of subjective well-being. One such type of instrument is the Oxford Happiness Inventory (OHI; Argyle, Martin, & Lu, 1995). The OHI incorporates items related to both emotional experiences and satisfaction with life. Representative items on the OHI assess the respondent's energy level, optimism, perceived control of life, perceived health, social interest, perceived congruence between desired goals and actual achievements, as well as general sense of happiness and life satisfaction. The OHI shows good convergent validity with other measures of mood and satisfaction and has good test–retest reliability and internal consistency. With an overall structure of 29 items, the OHI represents an omnibus measure of medium length, and could potentially be useful to those wishing to assess both the affective and satisfaction components of subjective well-being with a single measure.

Another omnibus measure, the Fordyce Happiness Measures (FHM; Fordyce, 1977) uses a very brief format, consisting of an 11-choice scale on which respondents rate their overall happiness, and three additional items asking respondents to estimate the percentage of time that they are happy, unhappy, and neutral. Because of its very brief format (essentially a single item), the psychometric properties of the FHM instrument cannot be completely evaluated. Further, the single response to the 11-choice scale cannot be analyzed in terms of the separate components of subjective well-being. Still, the FHM can provide a very basic assessment of subjective well-being in situations where more complex assessments are not feasible.

A number of other additional self-report measures of subjective well-being have been developed; the instruments discussed above are intended to be representative examples, and by no means do they represent a comprehensive listing. Other sources (e.g., Pavot & Diener, 2003) can provide the reader with additional examples.

Alternative Approaches to Subjective Well-Being Assessment

Although self-reported measures of subjective well-being are the most commonly used approach to assessment, it is often desirable to include additional data sources within a given research design. These additional indices can provide external validation for self-reported measures of subjective well-being, and they can potentially add unique information about an individual's subjective well-being that may not be detected when using self-report measures exclusively.

Probably the most commonly used alternative data source within the subjective well-being literature is the informant report. Informant reports, or ratings of the subjective well-being of a target individual, are typically obtained from spouses and other family members, friends, coworkers or supervisors, or others who are well acquainted with the person of interest. Informant reports of life satisfaction have been shown to have substantial correlation to self-reports of life satisfaction (Pavot, Diener, Colvin, & Sandvik, 1991). Informant reports serve to provide convergent validity for self-report measures of subjective well-being.

One approach to the use of informant data is to obtain reports from several informants for each target individual, and then aggregate the data from the separate informant reports into one composite index. This procedure has the effect of averaging the ratings made by the multiple informants, and it tends to reduce the effect of error or response differences between the various raters.

In addition to the use of informant reports, several other alternatives for the assessment of subjective well-being are possible. For example, expert ratings of facial expressions revealed in photographs or video-recorded interactions have been found to correlate with self-reports of subjective well-being. Interviews can also provide sufficient information for the assessment of subjective well-being. Other methods, such as the use of physiological measures (Dinan, 1994) and the analysis of people's memories for good and bad events (Pavot et al., 1991), have potential use as additional indices of subjective well-being.

Methodological Innovations

Several innovative methodologies for the assessment of subjective well-being have emerged in recent years. Prominent among these techniques is experience sampling methodology (ESM; Diener, 2000; Scollon, Kim-Prieto, & Diener, 2003). ESM involves the use of palm computer technology to obtain a random sampling of a person's moods and cognitions over time. The palm computer serves as both a cuing device and a data-recording instrument. With this technology, researchers can obtain a record of the ongoing subjective experiences of the respondent, without the need to rely on retrospective reports of these subjective states. Thus, several potential problems with the use of retrospective self-reports, such as memory distortions or failures or other contextual effects at the time of recall (Schwarz & Strack, 1991), can be avoided. Further, by averaging the data obtained with ESM across a large number of occasions, the effects of any transient situational factors and momentary mood fluctuations that might be attached to individual sampling occasions are cancelled out. In a multimethod study, Sandvik, Diener, and Seidlitz (1993) compared ESM data to data obtained from one-time, self-reported measures of life satisfaction and data from informant reports, and found moderate-to-strong correlations among the different methodologies.

Along with several advantages, ESM data have some limitations and can create a new set of problems for the researcher as well. One concern is the sheer amount of data that ESM can produce. Even a relatively short period of ESM sampling can produce thousands of individual data points, creating a much more complex situation at the time of analysis (Scollon et al., 2003). Strategic decisions regarding ways to summarize and interpret data become more critical with ESM. And even though ESM appears to be a very promising methodology, it may not represent a superior approach to assessing all aspects of subjective well-being. ESM appears to be most advantageous when a researcher is interested in assessing average moods, or the dynamics of mood and emotion. Conversely, in situations where researchers are interested in global judgments (e.g., life satisfaction), more traditional, multiple-item, self-report questionnaire measures may well be preferable.

Another innovative methodology was used to assess the affective component of subjective well-being in a study conducted by Danner, Snowdon, and Friesen (2001). In this study, brief, handwritten autobiographies written by 180 Catholic nuns as they entered religious life (at an average age of 22 years) were read and scored based on their emotional content. This emotion score was then found to be related to risk of mortality in late life (75–95 years). Positive emotional content in these autobiographies was found to be strongly related to greater longevity six decades after the autobiographies were written (Danner et al., 2001). Although such written material would not be available in many instances, the success of this methodology does have implications for the design of longitudinal research, suggesting an alternative to direct self-report that could be incorporated into longitudinal designs.

A promising new methodology for assessing daily life experience and subjective well-being is the day reconstruction method (DRM; Kahneman, Krueger, Schkade, Schwarz, & Stone, 2004). The DRM involves asking respondents to systematically reconstruct their experiences and activities during the preceding day, using detailed techniques intended to minimize the effects of memory biases (Kahneman et al., 2004). These responses create a record of both the amount of time spent on various activities and the affective experiences of the respondent while he or she was engaged in each activity. The DRM is more efficient and disrupts the respondent's normal pattern of activity less than the ESM method discussed above. DRM provides a somewhat more flexible alternative to intensive ESM data, while retaining many of its advantages. Perhaps the greatest of these advantages lies in the reduction of memory biases. For a more complete description of DRM and some examples of its use, the reader is directed to Kahneman et al. (2004).

The wide selection of current measures and methodologies available for the assessment of subjective well-being provides interested investigators with a good range of options. The instruments and methods reviewed in this and previous sections of this chapter represent only examples of the overall array of measures available. Although current measures and methods of subjective well-being assessment are still, in some respects, "rudimentary" (Diener & Seligman, 2004), they represent a substantial improvement over those in use a generation ago. There is every reason to believe that, as interest in well-being and quality-of-life issues grows, the development and refinement of more reliable and valid measures of subjective well-being will continue.

Shortfalls in the Assessment of Subjective Well-Being

At the same moment that a review of the positive developments in the assessment of subjective well-being is a cause for optimism, other aspects of the research in the well-being area are a cause for concern. Despite the positive evolution of subjective well-being assessment techniques, progress toward the creation of a broadly based, reliable database of findings from well-being research has been limited. The current state of well-being data is summarized by Diener and Seligman (2004) as "a haphazard mix of different measures of varying quality, usually taken from non-representative samples of respondents" (p. 4). As a consequence of this situation, it is difficult to formulate a set of summary statements or conclusions from the data that can be broadly generalized and accepted with a high degree of confidence. From the perspective of assessment, there is a "gap" between the assessment techniques that are currently available and the manner in which these techniques are actually being utilized within many research designs. A complex set of factors has likely contributed to the creation of this empirical shortfall: This section focuses on three of those factors: a tendency to assess subjective well-being too narrowly or incompletely, a predominance of cross-sectional single-method studies, and the lack of a programmatic effort to refine subjective well-being assessment.

Many studies of subjective well-being have approached assessment with too narrow a focus. As discussed in a previous section, the three components of subjective well-being (PA, NA, life satisfaction) are separable (Lucas et al., 1996) and show at least partially unique empirical patterns. For this reason, a complete assessment should include adequate measures of all three components. But a recent analysis of a large database of publications (Diener & Seligman, 2004) indicates that a very high percentage of studies mention only one or two of these components (e.g., PA and NA but not life satisfaction), indicating that assessment within those studies did not include all of the constructs subsumed by subjective well-being. This tendency toward narrow or incomplete assessment of subjective well-being becomes a problem when researchers attempt to discern general patterns from the results of a number of diverse studies. Are the results of one set of studies, within which respondents' levels of subjective well-being are represented by measures of PA and NA, precisely comparable to another cluster of studies utilizing a life satisfaction scale as the index of subjective well-being? It is likely that the results from studies using affect-based measures will have some degree of correlation with the results of studies based on measures of life satisfaction, but it is also likely that some important distinctions between these components might be obscured and overlooked by an attempt to generalize all such studies as measuring "happiness" or "subjective well-being." For these reasons, studies that include narrow or incomplete assessment of subjective well-being may not have as much value in terms of their contribution to a sound empirical basis for the field as they otherwise might, had they included a more complete measurement of all major components.

Another limitation of current research in the area of subjective well-being is an overreliance on cross-sectional research designs, particularly those using a single methodology (e.g., self-report questionnaires only). In a typical subjective well-being study using a cross-sectional design, data are gathered at one point in time, perhaps by handing out a set of questionnaires to a psychology class, a work group, or at a senior center. The respondents complete the questionnaires and return them to the researcher. The resulting data are then analyzed, and the measure of subjective well-being is perhaps found to be correlated to some other variable that has been assessed (e.g., a personality characteristic). If the correlation is large or otherwise interesting, the results are likely to be reported in some form. Depending on the outcome of the study, additional studies might be conducted. Cross-sectional studies can be very useful, particularly in the initial stages of a research program (e.g., developing a new measure). But cross-sectional research also involves some significant limitations, particularly for research on subjective well-being.

One issue involves the effects of transient mood states and other contextual factors that might influence response to the subjective well-being measure. These momentary factors can, under some circumstances, exert a significant influence on how an individual responds to a measure of SWB (Schwarz & Strack, 1999). Because data gathered using a cross-sectional design can provide information only on a respondent's experience at a single moment in time, it is possible that this response might be influenced by some transient factor at the particular moment of response and therefore be a less valid indicator of that individual's general or global level of subjective well-being. This potential threat to the validity of assessment is particularly an issue with brief, single-item subjective well-being measures, but it can also be a factor even with multiple-item scales. Although these transient mood and contextual effects appear to be limited (Pavot & Diener, 1993a; Eid & Diener, 2004; Schimmack & Oishi, 2005), it is desirable to avoid them nevertheless; with the most simple form of a cross-sectional design, this is not possible.

One potential way to avoid transient mood and contextual effects is the use ESM, as described in a previous section. But ESM is not feasible for cross-sectional designs because it requires repeated experiential reports across days or perhaps weeks. A longitudinal design is required in order to execute ESM effectively.

If a longitudinal design is impractical, an alternative approach that would allow researchers to validate self-reports of subjective well-being from a cross-sectional study would be to use a multiple-method design. Informant reports, memory measures, or other non-self-report measures of subjective well-being can be incorporated within a study to provide external validation to self-reported measures of subjective well-being. Self-reported and non-self-report measures of subjective well-being could also be combined to produce a standardized composite score of subjective well-being. Such a technique would tend to reduce the potential impact that transient mood and contextual effects might exert on the self-reported measures.

A second issue related to the use of cross-sectional designs involves the analysis and interpretation of the data. Because experimental manipulations are rarely utilized in subjective well-being research, the approach to statistical analysis of the data from these studies is predominantly correlational in nature. Most often, measures of subjective well-being are examined to determine their relation to other variables (e.g., a correlation coefficient might be computed between a measure of PA and a measure of the personality trait of extraversion). When such a correlation coefficient is computed based on data from a cross-sectional design, it can reveal the strength and direction of a relationship between the two variables, but it cannot be used to determine a causal relationship. That is, such a correlation might inform us that the relation between PA and extraversion is positive and moderately strong, but it cannot tell us whether PA is "causing" extraversion, or vice versa. A measure of extraversion can be used to predict PA, or vice-versa, but the causal dynamics of the relation cannot be determined.

In contrast, data obtained from a longitudinal design can often be used to establish the causal pathway more clearly. An example of this process can be seen in the research on the relation between subjective well-being and marital status. People who do marry typically report higher levels of subjective well-being than those widowed, divorced, or single (Mastekaasa, 1994; Diener et al., 1999). But until recently, the causal direction was unclear. Was marriage "causing" happiness, or were happier people more likely to marry? By adopting longitudinal designs, two large-scale studies (Lucas, Clark, Georgellis, & Diener, 2003; Marks & Fleming, 1999) have demonstrated that people with initially higher levels of subjective well-being are more likely to marry by the time of a later measurement occasion. Although it is a reasonable assumption that the benefits of marriage do, to some degree, contribute to subjective well-being after marriage has occurred, it is clear that those with higher levels of subjective well-being are more likely to marry. Thus, a correlational relation observed in cross-sectional research was further articulated with longitudinal data.

A third factor that has hindered the advancement of subjective well-being assessment involves the lack of a systematic effort among researchers to move toward a refinement of the measurement process. The absence of a common protocol or set of standards for the development and use of subjective well-being measures has contributed to the "haphazard" condition of the current database, as described by Diener and Seligman (2004, p. 4). The uneven psychometric quality of the measures, combined with other methodological and sampling issues, have the effect of reducing confidence in the findings. These factors make efforts to establish general conclusions about subjective well-being, by summarizing the findings of diverse studies, risky at best.

In an effort to move toward a more refined approach to subjective well-being assessment, Diener (2005) has proposed a set of guidelines and recommendations regarding the development and use of measures of both subjective well-being and ill-being, and these proposed standards have received the endorsement of many researchers involved in research related to subjective well-being. The guidelines include recommendations regarding the psychometric quality of subjective well-being measures and the methodology by which these measures might be most effectively employed, along with definitions of subjective well-being and its major components. The guidelines are intended to establish a basis for the development of national indicators of subjective well-being, but they are generally applicable to basic research settings as well.

Taken together, the three factors discussed above have combined to slow the establishment of a dependable and valid database from the findings of subjective well-being research. General conclusions regarding the causes and consequences of subjective well-being have been slow to emerge, in part because many studies have only or narrowly assessed subjective well-being, because high-quality, multiple-method longitudinal studies are rare, and because of a lack of concerted effort by researchers to refine the assessment process.

Fortunately, remedies for all of these shortcomings are at hand. Valid and reliable measures and innovative methodologies, such as ESM, are currently available. Examples of systematic longitudinal designs have been published in recent years, and these studies can serve as a basis for future efforts. At least one attempt to organize and systematize subjective well-being assessment (Diener, 2005) has been made, and this effort appears to be well received. Thus, the potential to improve the quality of subjective well-being research and to more firmly establish the database seems good. Conducting high-quality, longitudinal research is neither cheap nor easy, but its value in terms of knowledge base is high. Cross-sectional studies can clearly serve an important function, particularly at the earliest stages of a program of research, but their power to fully explain the dynamic processes related to subjective well-being is limited.

Future Directions

In addition to rectifying the shortcomings of subjective well-being research discussed above, several additional issues are of concern for the future. Prominent among these is the need to increase the use of the findings of subjective well-being research in applied settings. Efforts in this area have already begun (Linley & Joseph, 2004), but this work will need considerable further development.

The development of national indicators of subjective well-being for the United States, with the purpose of informing public policy decisions, is another likely area of future effort (Diener, 2000, 2005; Diener & Seligman, 2004). These subjective indicators are proposed as a compliment to existing objective measures (e.g., economic indices) already in use. There is some evidence that subjective indicators may be superior to the heavily used economic indicators as quality-of-life assessments, particularly in affluent societies such as the United States (Diener & Seligman, 2004).

Along with increased efforts in applied areas, additional research on the basic processes related to subjective well-being is needed. Internal processes related to subjective well-being, such as the development of temperament-level traits (e.g., extraversion and neuroticism) need further explanation, as does the interaction of these personality processes with external, environmental factors. Another powerful influence on subjective well-being is adaptation. Very little is known about adaptation or the processes that underlie it. Much work remains in the effort to more clearly articulate this powerful process, which has strong implications for the experience of subjective well-being.

In both basic and applied research settings, valid and reliable assessment instruments and innovative assessment methodologies will continue to play a key role. The creation of increasingly sophisticated and powerful measures will be required to meet the demands of future researchers. This development process has kept pace with the growing interest in subjective well-being in recent decades, and it appears likely that the evolution in subjective well-being assessment will continue.

References

Adams, D. (1969). Analysis of a life satisfaction index. *Journal of Gerontology, 24*, 470–474.

Argyle, M., Martin, M., & Lu, L. (1995). Testing for stress and happiness: The role of social and cognitive factors. In C. D. Spielberger & I. G. Sarason (Eds.), *Stress and emotion* (Vol. 15, pp. 173–187). Washington, DC: Taylor & Francis.

Arthaud-Day, M. L., Rode, J. C., Mooney, C. H., & Near, J. P. (2005). The subjective well-being construct: A test of its convergent, discriminant, and factorial validity. *Social Indicators Research, 74*, 445–476.

Bradburn, N. M. (1969). *The structure of psychological well-being*. Chicago: Aldine.

Bradburn, N. M., & Caplovitz, D. (1965). *Reports of happiness*. Chicago: Aldine.

Costa, P. T., Jr., & McCrae, R. R. (1980). Influence of extraversion and neuroticism on subjective well-being: Happy and unhappy people. *Journal of Personality and Social Psychology, 38*, 668–678.

Costa, P. T., Jr., & McCrae, R. R. (1992). *Revised NEO Personality Inventory (NEOPI-R)* and Five Factor Inventory (NEO-FFI) Professional Manual. Odessa, FL: Psychological Assessment Resources.

Danner, D. D., Snowdon, D. A., & Friesen, W. V. (2001). Positive emotions in early life and longevity: Findings from the nun study. Journal of Personality and Social Psychology, 80, 804–813.

DeNeve, K. M., & Cooper, H. (1998). The happy personality: A meta-analysis of 137 personality traits and subjective well-being. Psychological Bulletin, 124, 197–229.

Diener, E. (1984). Subjective well-being. Psychological Bulletin, 95, 542–575.

Diener, E. (2000). Subjective well-being: The science of happiness and a proposal for a national index. American Psychologist, 55, 34–43.

Diener, E. (2005). Guidelines for national indicators of subjective well-being and ill being. Social Indicators Network News, 84, 4–6.

Diener, E., & Emmons, R. A. (1984). The independence of positive and negative affect. Journal of Personality and Social Psychology, 47, 1105–1117.

Diener, E., Emmons, R. A., Larsen, R. J., & Griffin, S. (1985). The Satisfaction with Life Scale. Journal of Personality Assessment, 49, 71–75.

Diener, E., & Seligman, M. E. P. (2004). Beyond money: Toward an economy of well-being. Psychological Science in the Public Interest, 5, 2–31.

Diener, E., Suh, E. M., Lucas, R. E., & Smith, H. L. (1999). Subjective well-being: Three decades of progress. Psychological Bulletin, 125, 276–302.

Dinan, T. G. (1994). Glucocorticoids and the genesis of depressive illness: A psycho-biological model. British Journal of Psychiatry, 164, 365–371.

Eid, M., & Diener, E. (2004). Global judgments of subjective well-being: Situational variability and long-term stability. Social Indicators Research, 65, 245–277.

Fordyce, M. W. (1977). The Happiness Measures: A sixty-second index of emotional well-being and mental health. Unpublished manuscript. Edison Community College, Ft. Myers, FL.

Green, D. P., Goldman, S. L., & Salovey, P. (1993). Measurement error masks bipolarity in affect ratings. Journal of Personality and Social Psychology, 64, 1029–1041.

Huebner, E. S. (1994). Preliminary development and validation of a multidimensional life satisfaction scale for children. Psychological Assessment, 6, 149–158.

Joiner, T. E., Jr., Brown, J. S., Perez, M., Sethuraman, G., & Sallee, F. R. (2005). The illusion of mental health: In the mind of which beholder? Journal of Personality Assessment, 85, 92–97.

Kahneman, D., Krueger, A. B., Schkade, D. A., Schwarz, N., & Stone, A. A. (2004). A survey method for characterizing daily life experience: The Day Reconstruction Method. Science, 306, 1776–1780.

Kammann, R., & Flett, R. (1983). Affectometer 2: A scale to measure current level of general happiness. Australian Journal of Psychology, 35, 259–265.

Larsen, R. J., & Diener, E. (1992). Promises and problems with the circumplex model of emotion. In M. S. Clark (Ed.), Emotion (pp. 25–59). Newbury Park, CA: Sage.

Linley, P. A., & Joseph, S. (Eds.). (2004). Positive psychology in practice. Hoboken, NJ: Wiley.

Lucas, R. E., Clark, A. E., Georgellis, Y., & Diener, E. (2003). Re-examining adaptation and the set-point model of happiness: Reactions to changes in marital status. *Journal of Personality and Social Psychology, 84,* 527–539.

Lucas, R. E., Diener, E., & Suh, E. (1996). Discriminant validity of well-being measures. *Journal of Personality and Social Psychology, 71,* 616–628.

Marks, G. N., & Fleming, N. (1999). Influences and consequences of well-being among Australian young people: 1980–1995. *Social Indicators Research, 46,* 301–323.

Mastekaasa, A. (1994). Marital status, distress, and well-being: An international comparison. *Journal of Comparative Family Studies, 25,* 183–205.

Myers, D. G. (2000). The funds, friends, and faith of happy people. *American Psychologist, 55,* 56–67.

Neugarten, B. L., Havighurst, R. J., & Tobin, S. (1961). The measurement of life satisfaction. *Journal of Gerontology, 16,* 134–143.

Pavot, W., & Diener, E. (1993a). The affective and cognitive context of self-reported measures of subjective well-being. *Social Indicators Research, 28,* 1–20.

Pavot, W., & Diener, E. (1993b). Review of the Satisfaction with Life Scale. *Psychological Assessment, 5,* 164–172.

Pavot, W., & Diener, E. (2003). Well-being (including life satisfaction). In R. F. Ballesteros (Ed.), *Encyclopedia of psychological assessment* (Vol. 2, pp. 1097–1101). London: Sage.

Pavot, W. G., Diener, E., Colvin, C. R., & Sandvik, E. (1991). Further validation of the Satisfaction with Life Scale: Evidence for the cross-method convergence of well-being measures. *Journal of Personality Assessment, 57,* 149–161.

Pavot, W., Diener, E., & Suh, E. (1998). The Temporal Satisfaction with Life Scale. *Journal of Personality Assessment, 70,* 340–354.

Russell, J. A. (1980). A circumplex model of affect. *Journal of Personality and Social Psychology, 39,* 1161–1178.

Sandvik, E., Diener, E., & Seidlitz, L. (1993). Subjective well-being: The convergence and stability of self-report and non-self-report measures. *Journal of Personality, 61,* 317–342.

Schimmack, U., Bockenholt, U., & Reisenzein, R. (2002). Response styles in affect ratings: Making a mountain out of a molehill. *Journal of Personality Assessment, 78,* 461–483.

Schimmack, U., & Oishi, S. (2005). The influence of chronically and temporarily accessible information on life satisfaction judgments. *Journal of Personality and Social Psychology, 89,* 395–406.

Schwarz, N., & Clore, G. L. (1983). Mood, misattribution, and judgments of well being: Informative and directive functions of affective states. *Journal of Personality and Social Psychology, 45,* 513–523.

Schwarz, N., & Strack, F. (1991). Evaluating one's life: A judgment model of subjective well-being. In F. Strack, M. Argyle, & N. Schwarz (Eds.), *Subjective well-being: An interdisciplinary perspective* (pp. 27–47). Oxford, UK: Pergamon.

Schwarz, N., & Strack, F. (1999). Reports of subjective well-being: Judgmental processes and their methodological implications. In D. Kahneman, E. Diener, & N. Schwarz (Eds.), *Well-being: The foundations of hedonic psychology* (pp. 61–84). New York: Sage.

Scollon, C. N., Kim-Prieto, C., & Diener, E. (2003). Experience sampling: Promises and pitfalls, strengths and weaknesses. *Journal of Happiness Studies, 4,* 5–34.

Seligman, M. E. P., & Csikszentmihalyi, M. (2000). Positive psychology: An introduction. *American Psychologist, 55,* 5–14.

Seligson, J. L., Huebner, E. S., & Valois, R. F. (2003). Preliminary validation of the Brief Multidimensional Students' Life Satisfaction Scale (BMSLSS). *Social Indicators Research, 61,* 121–145.

Watson, D., Clark, L. A., & Tellegen, A. (1988). Development and validation of brief measures of positive and negative affect: The PANAS scales. *Journal of Personality and Social Psychology, 54,* 1063–1070.

┌─────┐
│   │
│ 8 │
│   │
└─────┘

Measuring the Immeasurable

Psychometric Modeling of Subjective Well-Being Data

MICHAEL EID

Many important insights into the structure, causes, and consequences of subjective well-being can be gained only by measuring something that seems to be immeasurable to many people: satisfaction and happiness. The questions of whether, and in which way, subjective well-being can be measured has interested researchers from different fields for many years. Many chapters of this handbook address themes related to measurement issues and report the results of empirical studies that all have measured subjective well-being in a certain way. Pavot (Chapter 7, this volume) gives an overview of the successes and shortfalls of the assessment of subjective well-being; his chapter discusses specific measurement devices that can be applied to assess subjective well-being. Like any other measure in the social and behavioral sciences, measures of subjective well-being have to prove their reliability and validity. This chapter demonstrates how modern psychometric models can be applied to analyze subjective well-being data. Based on a framework model of subjective well-being, I show how psychometric models can be applied to learn more about the structure of (1) general and domain-specific life satisfaction judgments and (2) the temporal structure of affect. The chapter focuses on models with latent variables that take into account that psychological constructs (such as subjective well-being) cannot be measured

141

without measurement error. Different types of latent variable models offer different insights into the measurement process and the reliability and validity of subjective well-being judgments.

Measuring Subjective Well-Being: A Framework Model

Lischetzke and Eid (2006) have developed a framework model for the measurement of subjective well-being that is depicted in Figure 8.1. This model is based on three major distinctions that have been made in the conceptualization of subjective well-being:

1. The distinction between the *cognitive* and *affective* components of life satisfaction. Whereas the cognitive component characterizes the evaluations of one's life, in general, as well as different life domains, the affective component refers to affective reactions to life events (Diener, 2000).

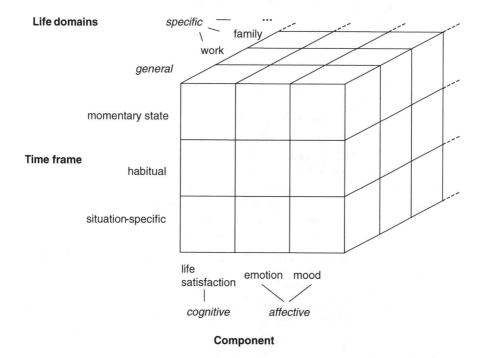

FIGURE 8.1. Framework model for the measurement of subjective well-being. Adapted from Lischetzke and Eid (2006). Copyright 2006 by Hogrefe Verlag. Adapted by permission.

2. The distinction between three different *time frames* that are based on a state–trait model of subjective well-being: The *momentary state* characterizes subjective well-being at a specific moment in time. This state depends on the subjective well-being trait (set point, general subjective well-being level) and occasion-specific influences. The *subjective well-being trait* of an individual describes the stable component of subjective well-being that does not depend on momentary or occasion-specific influences but indicates stable individual differences across situations. The *momentary occasion-specific* or *situation-specific* subjective well-being is defined as the momentary deviation of a subjective well-being state from a subjective well-being trait. It represents occasion-specific influences due to situations and the interaction between an individual and a situation. In contrast to the subjective well-being *state*, which depends on the person as well as the situation and interaction, the *occasion-specific subjective well-being* represents pure situational and interactional effects that do not depend on the habitual well-being level. It shows whether an individual feels better, the same, or worse in a specific situation compared to his or her general subjective well-being.

3. The distinction between the life as a whole (e.g., *general life satisfaction*) and different life domains (*domain-specific life satisfaction*).

All three axes of this cube can be combined. Each subcube characterizes one facet of subjective well-being that might be of interest. For example, one may be interested in how a person *generally* feels at work, how this person feels in a *momentary* situation at work (e.g., meeting with a superior), and whether or not this feeling is more positive or more negative compared to the habitual subjective well-being of this person at work (*situation-specific* subjective well-being).

Measures of subjective well-being that are chosen for assessing one selected facet should reliably and validly measure this facet. Modern psychometric models can be applied to estimate the reliability and analyze the validity of subjective well-being measures. This chapter shows how psychometric modeling can contribute to our understanding of two axes of the subjective well-being cube: the integration of general and domain-specific subjective well-being and the analysis of the different temporal facets. The integration of general and domain-specific subjective well-being has to deal with the problem that there are interindividual (*quantitative*) differences in subjective well-being but that the subjective well-being pattern for different domains might be quite individually specific (*qualitative* differences). There might be individuals who are satisfied with their job and income but not with their marriage and social life, and there might be individuals who feel high subjective well-being in their social relationships but not in their job, etc. That means that there are qualitative (typological) differences between individuals with respect to their general subjective well-being pattern but that, within each pattern, there are quantitative differences as well. The distinction of different temporal facets requires that the three components can be separated and measured, even if only measures of momentary states are available. The integration of general and specific domains is discussed and illustrated with respect to the cognitive component of subjective well-being, whereas the analysis of the different temporal facets is exemplified by the affective component of subjective well-being.

Distinguishing between Quantitative and Qualitative Differences in Life Satisfaction Measurement

The cognitive facet of subjective well-being is typically assessed by self-report items. These items refer to a person's life as a whole and/or the different life domains. Figure 8.2 shows the items of the Life Satisfaction subscale of the Freiburg Personality Inventory (FPI; Fahrenberg, Hampel, & Selg, 1984), one of the most widely applied personality questionnaires in German-speaking countries. All items are answered on a binary response scale with the categories *yes* and *no*. When analyzing the responses to life satisfaction items, one finds typically two results. (1) There are strong individual differences in life satisfaction—in other words, there are people who are more or less satisfied. (2) Items differ in their distributions: There are items that many people affirm, such as the last item in Figure 8.2, which 74% of the sample agreed with ("I am usually very confident about the future"). There are also items that only a small number of individuals agree with: Only 33% concurred with the second item in Figure 8.2 ("I am at peace with myself and have no inner conflicts"). Therefore, to enable us to analyze the interindividual as well as the interitem differences and evaluate the psychometric property of this scale, models of item response theory (IRT) were applied. In IRT models, the probability of an individual item response is a function of an individual's standing on a latent variable representing true ("error-free") individual differences in life satisfaction as well as the standing of the item on this latent variable, representing the degree of life satisfaction necessary to affirm an item with a certain probability ("difficulty" of an item).

Measuring Quantitative Differences: The Rasch Model

The simplest model of IRT is the *Rasch model* (also called the *one-parameter logistic model*; Rasch, 1960). In this model the probability of an item response depends on only two parameters: a person parameter indicating the latent (life satisfaction) value of an individual, and an item parameter indicating the difficulty of an item. The curves that describe the dependency of the response probability from the latent (life satisfaction) variable are depicted for three items in Figure 8.3. Because all items are binary, it is sufficient to present the probability curve for only one category (the probability of the first category is 1 minus the probability

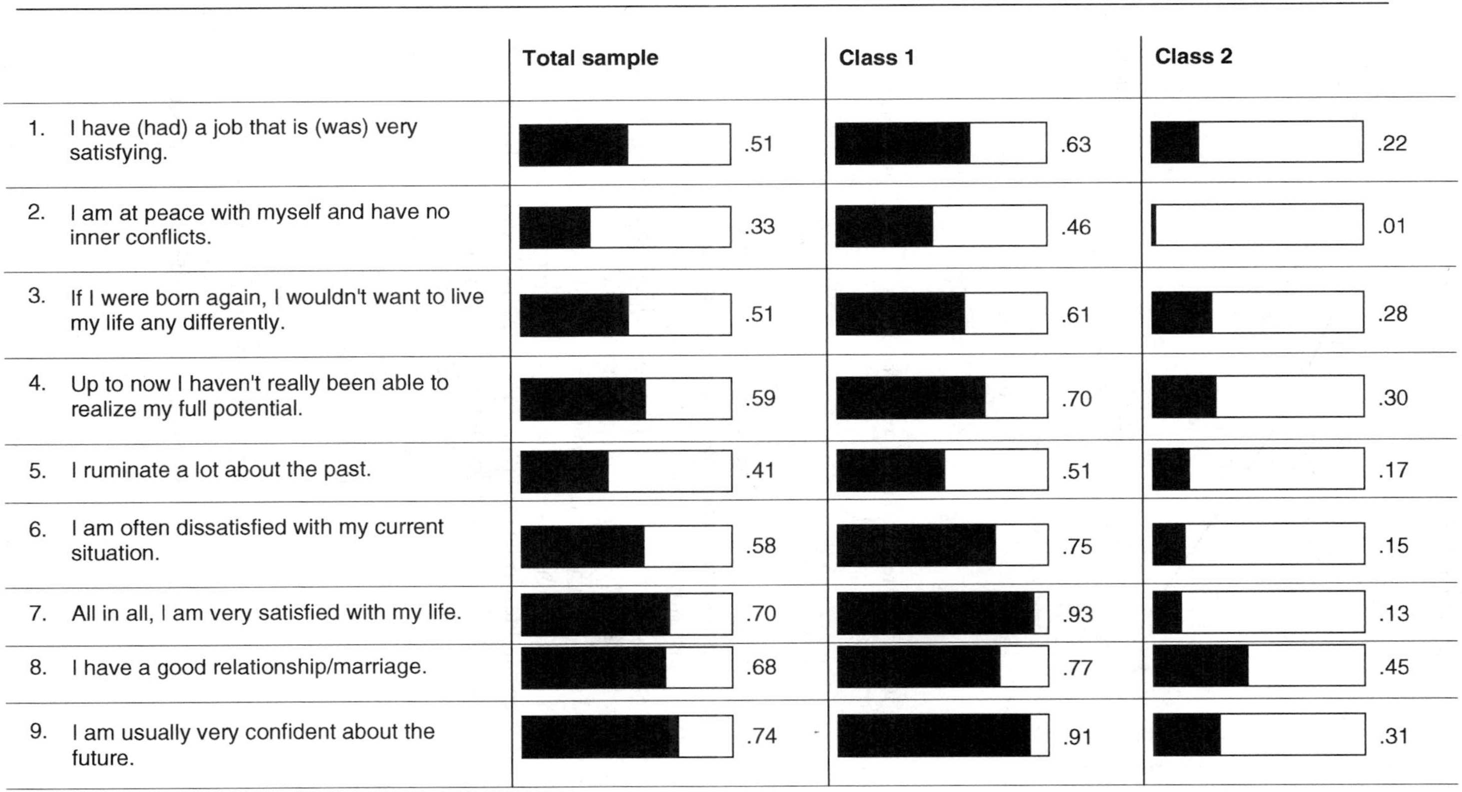

	Total sample	Class 1	Class 2
1. I have (had) a job that is (was) very satisfying.	.51	.63	.22
2. I am at peace with myself and have no inner conflicts.	.33	.46	.01
3. If I were born again, I wouldn't want to live my life any differently.	.51	.61	.28
4. Up to now I haven't really been able to realize my full potential.	.59	.70	.30
5. I ruminate a lot about the past.	.41	.51	.17
6. I am often dissatisfied with my current situation.	.58	.75	.15
7. All in all, I am very satisfied with my life.	.70	.93	.13
8. I have a good relationship/marriage.	.68	.77	.45
9. I am usually very confident about the future.	.74	.91	.31

FIGURE 8.2. Selected items of the Life Satisfaction subscale of the Freiburg Personality Inventory and item distributions in the total sample ($n = 480$) and the two latent classes (relative frequencies of the categories indicating satisfaction).

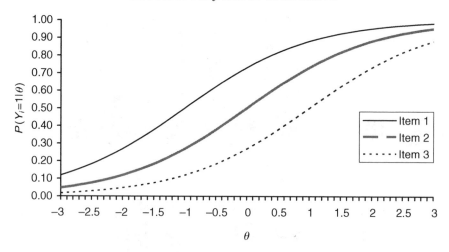

FIGURE 8.3. Item characteristic curves of three items in the Rasch model. Item parameters: $\sigma_1 = -1$, $\sigma_2 = 0$, $\sigma_3 = 1$.

of the second category). This model assumes that all items are unidimensional, meaning that they measure the same latent trait (life satisfaction). Individuals differ in their latent life satisfaction values. The higher the latent life satisfaction value of an individual, the higher is his or her probability to agree with a life satisfaction item, which simply means saying *yes* to a positively keyed item (such as the first one in Figure 8.2) and saying *no* to a negatively keyed item (such as the fourth one). All item responses are coded in such a way that a "1" indicates a response representing life satisfaction ("positive response") and a "0" represents a nonsatisfaction answer ("negative response"). The response probabilities of the categories "1" are depicted in Figure 8.3 meaning that a high value of the latent trait indicates life satisfaction. There are differences between the items: Some of the items are considered to be easy; even individuals with a comparatively low life satisfaction value have a high probability of responding positively to the item (e.g., item at the left in Figure 8.3), and some items practically require a high life satisfaction value for a positive response (difficult items, e.g., item at the right). The ordering of the difficulties of the items does not differ between individuals. All individuals have higher response probabilities for the easier items than for the more difficult items. The Rasch model is defined by the following equation

$$P(Y_i = 1|\theta) = \frac{e^{\theta - \sigma_i}}{1 + e^{\theta - \sigma_i}}$$

where a value of the conditional probability function $P(Y_i = 1|\theta)$ is the probability of positive satisfaction judgment for a value of the latent (life satisfaction) variable θ; σ_i is the item difficulty; and e is the exponential function. The probability function that describes the dependency of the response probability from the latent variable is called the *item characteristic curve*. As can be seen in the item characteristic curves shown in Figure 8.3, the shape of the item characteristic curves is always the same, but the items differ by their location on the latent variable. This location is marked by the item parameter σ_i. The value of an item parameter is the value of the latent (life satisfaction) variable, where the response probability for a category of this item equals 0.50. An item becomes easier with the decreasing value of the item parameter. Easiness means, in this context, that even individuals with a comparatively low life satisfaction value answer this item with a relatively high probability in the category that indicates life satisfaction. In addition, the assumption of local independence is made. *Local independence* means that the latent variable explains all associations between the observed variables. The items are associated because they are measuring the same trait (life satisfaction). But within a group of individuals with the same latent life satisfaction value, the different items are not related. Differences between item responses that are not determined by the latent satisfaction variable reflect unsystematic random influences that are not due to life satisfaction or another common trait.

The Rasch model has many important statistical properties. For example, it is the only psychometric model for binary items for which the sum score (the number of all affirmed items) contains all information about interindividual differences with respect to life satisfaction. However, for analyzing life satisfaction items the model has one disadvantage in its assumption that the item difficulties do not differ between individuals. This means, for example, that the difficulties of the items "I have a good relationship/marriage" and "I have (had) a job that is (was) very satisfying" have to be the same for all individuals. However, it seems to be more likely that there are qualitative (structural) differences between individuals as well. There might be individuals for whom it would be easier to say that they are satisfied with their jobs than to say that they are satisfied with their marriage, and vice versa, thus suggesting that the Rasch model is an appropriate model for analyzing individual (quantitative) differences but only in the case when there are no structural differences between individuals. When all items measure, for example, general life satisfaction, and no subgroup differences with respect to the item differences can be expected, the Rasch model would be an appropriate model to separate measurement error and random influences from true life satisfaction differences. In the current case, however, where different life domains are assessed as well, structural (qualitative) differences can be expected.

Measuring Quantitative and Qualitative Differences in Life Satisfaction Judgments: The Mixed Rasch Model

To provide researchers with the tools to consider both structural (qualitative) differences as well as individual (quantitative) differences, the Rasch model has been extended to the mixed Rasch model. This extended model assumes that the population consists of different subpopulations. For each subpopulation a Rasch model fits the data, however, the item parameters can differ between subpopulations. Thus, this model allows quantitative and qualitative individual differences. Qualitative differences are represented by different latent classes that differ in the item parameters. Quantitative differences are allowed within latent classes because individuals can have different latent life satisfaction values. If g denotes a subpopulation (latent class), the mixed Rasch model is defined by

$$P(Y_i = 1|\theta_g) = \frac{e^{\theta_g - \sigma_{ig}}}{1 + e^{\theta_g - \sigma_{ig}}}$$

(Rost, 1990). The difficulty of an item i (σ_{ig}) and the value of an individual v (θ_{vg}) can differ between classes g.

The model assumes that an individual can (and must) belong to only one latent class. However, it cannot be perfectly determined to which latent class an individual belongs. Therefore, a latent life satisfaction value will be estimated for each individual and each class. The probabilities of belonging to the different latent classes (assignment probabilities) can be estimated for each individual on the basis of his or her observed responses to the different items. Individuals can then be assigned to the latent class for which their assignment probability is maximal, and the latent satisfaction value in the latent class chosen can be taken as the best estimate of the individual's latent satisfaction. The mean of the assignment probabilities of all individuals assigned to the same class indicates the reliability of class assignments and the separability of classes.

In order to find out how many classes are necessary, a Rasch model with several latent classes must be specified and tested. The fit of the different models can be compared by information criteria such as Akaike's information criterion (AIC) or the Bayesian information criterion (BIC). These criteria weigh the fit of the model with the complexity of the model (the mixture distribution model is a more complex model). The best fitting model—that means, the most parsimonious model that explains the observed data appropriately—is the model with the smallest values of both these criteria. The BIC is superior to the AIC when the number of possible response patterns (2^K, where k is the number of items) is much larger than the sample size (Rost, 2004). The model with the lowest value of the information criteria is the best fitting model. A second possibility is to compare the observed frequencies of the different response patterns with the expected frequencies of these response patterns, given the parameters of the model. A model fits the data well when the expected frequencies of the different response patterns are close to the observed frequencies. That means that the model is able to predict reality. There are several statistical tests that can be used to determine whether the differences between the observed and the expected frequencies are significant; for example, the Pearson χ^2 test, the likelihood ratio test, or the Cressie–Read test. These statistics are asymptotically χ^2 distributed (when all expected frequencies are at least larger than 1); in cases of large item patterns and smaller samples, the distribution of the statistics can be estimated by bootstrapping analysis. Von Davier (1997) has shown that the bootstrap works well for the Pearson χ^2 test and the Cressie–Read test but not for the likelihood ratio test.

An Application of the (Mixed) Rasch Model

The Rasch model and the mixed Rasch model with different latent classes have been applied to the items presented in Figure 8.2. Because the sample size is small ($n = 480$) in relation to the number of possible response pattern (512), the selection of the model was based on the BIC. The BIC shows that the model with two latent classes fits the data best (1 class: 5170.96; 2 classes: 5131.10; 3 classes: 5172.46). Also the bootstrap fit indices indicate that the two-class model shows a good fit to the data (p values of the bootstrapped distributions: Pearson: $p = .16$, Cressie–Read: $p = .04$). The mean assignment probabilities are .96 for the first class and .91 for the second class. These assignment probabilities indicate a high reliability of class assignments and high separability of classes. The item difficulty parameters are given in Figures 8.4 and 8.5. Figure 8.4 reveals some interesting differences between the two classes. First of all, there is a strong difference with respect to item 7 ("All in all, I am very satisfied with my life"). This item is easiest in class 1 and rather difficult in class 2. Moreover, there is another strong difference with respect to item 2 ("I am at peace with myself and have no inner conflicts"). This item is the most difficult item in both classes but is much more difficult in class 2. Figure 8.5 contains the same information as Figure 8.4 but presents it in a somewhat different way. In Figure 8.5, the different ordering of the items in the two different classes is more visible than in Figure 8.4, whereas in Figure 8.4, the differences between the two classes with respect to the single items are more obvious. One very interesting difference between the two classes concerns the item "All in all, I am very satisfied with my life." This item is the easiest in class 1. People in class 1 have a generally positive view of their life (item 7) and their futures (item 9), and in order to have this generally positive view, they do not have to be satisfied with all domains of their life.

In class 2 the item "All in all, I am very satisfied with my life" is a rather difficult one. A respondent needs a rather high value on the latent life satisfaction variable to affirm this item with a comparably high probability. For people belonging to this class, it is easier for them to admit that they are satisfied with their relationship or their job than with life in general. This might also explain why it is very difficult for people in this class to be at peace with themselves without experiencing inner conflicts. Practically no one in this class is at peace

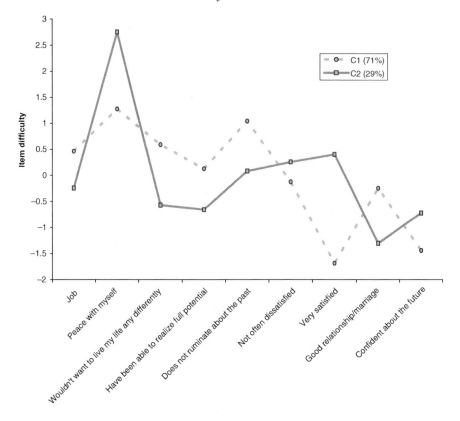

FIGURE 8.4. Item parameters for the two classes in the mixed Rasch model. C1, Class 1; C2, Class 2. The items indicating dissatisfaction were recoded for the analysis so that a high value indicates satisfaction. To facilitate the understanding of the results, the negatively keyed items were reworded.

with him- or herself (see the distribution of the item categories of the two classes in Figure 8.2).

The differences between the two classes might be explained partially by the distinction between top-down and bottom-up processes found in the theories of subjective well-being (Diener, 1984). Top-down process theories assume that there are temperamental differences in subjective well-being that exert an influence on the evaluation of different life domains: People who are generally happy evaluate their life domains in a more positive way. According to bottom-up process theories, general life satisfaction is the result of the life satisfaction in different domains. Individuals of the first class might be more top-down driven, because the general life satisfaction comes first on the latent life satisfaction dimension. People of the second class might be more bottom-up driven, which means that

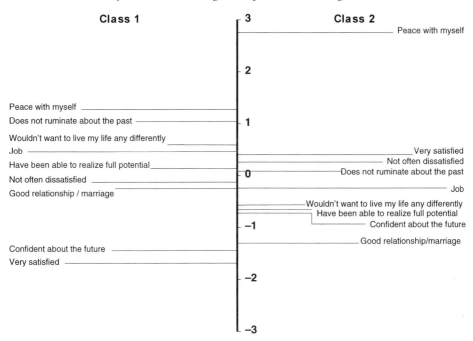

FIGURE 8.5. Comparison of the item parameters in the two latent classes.

the satisfaction with one's life might depend on the fulfillment of different expectations and aspirations, and these people might only be satisfied if all their aspirations are fulfilled. An alternative explanation would be that people belonging to the first class respond so positively to the items representing general life satisfaction because of self-deception mechanisms, whereas they have a more appropriate view of their lives when they are asked more concretely about the specific life domains.

The estimated distributions of the latent life satisfaction variables and the sum scores revealed that the first class consists primarily of individuals with high life satisfaction values (mean sum score: 6.26, *SD*: 1.66), whereas the second class is a class of relatively dissatisfied individuals (mean sum score: 2.02, *SD*: 1.26). Because of the differences between the latent classes in the distribution of the latent variables as well as the item parameters, the two latent classes also differ in the expected frequencies of the item responses in the two classes (see Figure 8.2). The frequencies of the satisfaction categories are very high in the first class and rather low in the second class. The differences are particularly strong for the item "All in all, I am very satisfied with my life": Whereas 93% of all individuals of the first class agree with this statement, only 13% of the individuals in the second class do so.

The two-class structure has some interesting consequences for the individual assessment of subjective well-being as well as for research on the determinants and consequences of individual differences in life satisfaction judgments. With respect to the individual assessment of life satisfaction, a two-step assessment procedure has to be applied. First, individuals must be assigned to latent classes based on their assignment probabilities. The latent class to which an individual is assigned characterizes his or her life satisfaction type. Then the individual life satisfaction score can be estimated. This latent value describes his or her degree of life satisfaction.

To analyze the conditions and consequences of life satisfaction differences, the two types of information (qualitative and quantitative) have to be taken into consideration. One interesting question concerns the differences between the two classes and whether class membership can be explained or predicted by other variables. In order to explain interclass differences, the point–biserial correlation between the latent class variable and the extraversion, neuroticism, and openness (social desirability) scales of the FPI were calculated. These correlations show that people belonging to class 2 respond in a less socially desirable manner ($r = -.13$, $p < .01$) and are more neurotic ($r = .44$, $p < .01$) and less extraverted ($r = -.20$, $p < .01$) than people belonging to class 1.

Within the two classes individual differences in life satisfaction are significantly negatively correlated with neuroticism (class 1: $r = -.47$, class 2: $r = -.32$). Social desirability is significantly positively correlated with life satisfaction only in class 1 ($r = .27$) but not in class 2 ($r = -.02$). Extraversion and life satisfaction are unrelated in the two classes (class 1: $r = .02$, class 2: $r = .11$). These correlation analyses revealed that personality variables are able to predict class membership (qualitative differences), and individual (quantitative) differences but the prediction structures differ between the two levels: Whereas extraversion is related to class membership, it is unrelated to individual differences within classes. Although these results are preliminary, they do show that mixture distribution Rasch models offer quite interesting possibilities for representing and predicting qualitative and quantitative differences simultaneously.

Analyzing Qualitative Differences: Latent Class Analysis

The mixed Rasch model assumes that there are quantitative and qualitative individual differences. It is a general model that not only comprises the Rasch model as a special case (when there are no qualitative differences) but also the latent class model (when there are no individual differences within classes). Latent class analysis assumes that the population consists of different subpopulations. Each subpopulation is characterized by the class-specific response probabilities of the items. In contrast to the mixed Rasch model, latent class analysis assumes that all individuals belonging to the same class do not differ in their response probabilities. If there weren't individual differences in the two classes considered in our example, the response probabilities of the two classes reported in Figure 8.2 would indicate the general response probabilities of a two-class latent class model. In this case, each individual belonging to the same class would have the same response probabilities. Eid and Diener (2001) as well as Eid, Langheine, and Diener (2003) have applied latent class analysis to analyze intercultural differences in norms for emotions and in life satisfaction judgments.

Other Models of Item Response Theory

The basic ideas of IRT have been introduced with respect to binary response variables. Analogous approaches exist for items with more than two categories. Baker, Rounds, and Zevon (2000) applied models for polytomous items to the measurement of subjective well-being. There are also IRT models in which items can differ in the form of their item characteristic curve. The handbook of van der Linden and Hambleton (1997) provides an overview of many IRT models. Recent extensions of IRT models to multidimensional models are described by Rost and Walter (2006). Von Davier and Carstensen (2007) give an overview of binary and polytomous mixed Rasch models (also called mixture distribution Rasch models) and their usefulness in different areas of research. Overviews of latent class models are provided by Hagenaars and McCutcheon (2002).

Measuring the Different Temporal Facets of Subjective Well-Being

At least three different approaches can be applied when measuring the three different temporal facets of subjective well-being depicted in Figure 8.1 (state, trait, occasion-specific deviations): (1) the direct assessment of the facets via self-report, (2) the aggregation approach, and (3) latent state–trait modeling.

Direct Assessment

According to the direct approach, an individual's current subjective well-being state ("How do you feel at this moment"), his or her general subjective well-being trait ("How do you feel in general?"), and his or her deviation to the momentary state from his or her general trait ("Do you currently feel better or worse than you generally feel?") can be rated by self-report or other report. A major advantage of this approach is that it can be easily applied and no longitudinal design is needed to measure the subjective well-being trait. Moreover, a benefit of the assessment of the momentary deviation is that this rating does not depend on the general subjective well-being trait, and the same response scale is utilized by each individual to rate situational influences. As Eid, Schneider, and Schwenkmezger (1999) have shown, floor and ceiling effects can be found in the state ratings of subjective well-being because people with a high subjective well-being trait usually use the high categories of subjective well-being state scales. Ratings of subjective well-being deviations, however, might not be affected by these ceiling and floor effects because people with generally high and generally low subjective well-being have the same room to rate situational deviations because the middle of the scale is the individual subjective well-being trait. A problem of the direct assessment is that the direct rating of one's subjective well-being trait might be affected particularly by recall biases, such as influences of current mood and other characteristics of the subjective well-being process (Kahneman, 1999; Schwarz & Strack, 1999; Stone & Litcher-Kelly, 2006).

Aggregation Approach

To avoid recall biases, all three temporal facets can be measured on the basis of repeatedly assessed subjective well-being states using the aggregation approach. A subjective well-being trait could be measured as the mean of repeatedly measured subjective well-being states. The momentary deviation is then the current state minus the trait (aggregated state) value. The aggregation approach is a reasonable and rather simple approach. Moreover, it is not limited to self-report data but can also be applied to other types of measures, such as physiological data. It also has, however, several shortcomings. One of these is found in the fact that the aggregation approach does not inform us about what we are aggregating out. If we want to measure a stable subjective well-being trait by the aggregation of several states, we have to be sure that there is, for example, no trait change. The aggregation approach does not imply a measurement model of the different temporal facets of subjective well-being that can be used to test hypotheses about the structure of subjective well-being. This can be done by models of latent state–trait theory described in more detail in the next section. Moreover, applications of this approach are presented to provide further insights into the reliability and validity of subjective well-being measures.

Separating Stable from Variable Determinants of Subjective Well-Being by Latent State–Trait Modeling

Models of latent state–trait (LST) theory (Steyer, Schmitt, & Eid, 1999) analyze repeatedly measured variables. These models are based on the idea that the current state of an individual can be decomposed in a value characterizing the general subjective well-being level (trait, setpoint) and a value representing occasion-specific influences. In addition, it as assumed that measurement error affects each measurement. Thus, to separate the different temporal facets and measurement error from each other, at least two occasions of measurement and two indicators measuring subjective well-being are needed. If the index i indicates the measure and k the occasion of measurement, an observed subjective well-being variable Y_{ik} is decomposed in the following way:

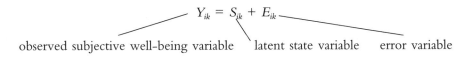

$$Y_{ik} = S_{ik} + E_{ik}$$

observed subjective well-being variable   latent state variable   error variable

Moreover, the latent state variable S_{ik} is decomposed into a latent trait variable T_{ik} and a residual O_{ik}, which represents occasion-specific influences:

$$S_{ik} = T_{ik} + O_{ik}$$

latent state variable   latent trait variable   occasion-specific residual

Occasion-specific residuals represent all influences that do not depend on the trait. These occasion-specific deviations can be caused by the fact that individuals can be in different ("inner") situations and that individuals interact in different ways in various situations. Taking both equations together—that is, by replacing the latent state variable in the first equation by the components of the latent state variable in the second equation, the basic decomposition of an observed variable in LST theory results:

$$Y_{ik} = T_{ik} + O_{ik} + E_{ik}$$

It is important to note that each observed subjective well-being measure on each occasion of measurement is decomposed into a trait variable, an occasion-specific variable, and an error variable without making any assumption about the structure of the different subjective well-being measures.

Several models have been defined to test different hypothesis about the structure of subjective well-being. A model that has often been applied is depicted in Figure 8.6 for four subjective well-being measures ($i = 1, \ldots, 4$) and two occasions of measurement k ($k = 1, 2$). In this model it is assumed that the four measures are unidimensional on the level of the occasion-specific variables but multidimensional on the level of the trait variables. The fact that measures are not unidimensional on the trait level is often found in longitudinal studies because the repeated measurement of the same items makes it possible to identify stable item-specific effects. Usually, however, the intertrait correlations are very high. The model depicted in Figure 8.6 is a model of confirmatory factor analy-

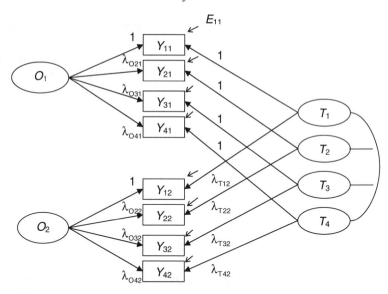

FIGURE 8.6. Latent state–trait model for four observed variables. Y_{ik}, i, indicator; k, occasion of measurement; T_i, indicator-specific trait variables; O_k, common occasion-specific variables; E_{ik}, error variables; λ_{Tik}, trait factor loadings; λ_{Oik}, occasion-specific factor loadings. For each factor one loading was fixed to 1 for identification reason. For simplicity reasons not all error variables are marked.

sis: The parameters λ_{Tik} are the loadings of the observed subjective well-being variables on the trait factors, and the parameters λ_{Oik} are the loadings of the observed variables on the occasion-specific factors. The occasion-specific factors are uncorrelated because it is assumed that the whole stability is explained by the trait factors, and occasion-specific influences of different occasions are independent. The fit of an LST model such as the one presented in Figure 8.6 can be analyzed by comparing the covariances of the observed variables with the covariances of the observed variables predicted by the model using the different fit criteria of structural equation modeling (Schermelleh-Engel, Moosbrugger, & Müller, 2003).

In the model depicted in Figure 8.6 (and also in other models of LST theory), the variance of the observed variable can be decomposed into one part that is determined by the trait variable (consistency), one part that is determined by the occasion-specific variable (occasion-specificity), and one part that is due to measurement error (unreliability). The *consistency coefficient*

$$CO(Y_{ik}) = \frac{\lambda_{Tik}^2 Var(T_i)}{Var(Y_{ik})}$$

indicates the degree of the variance of an observed variable [$Var(Y_{ik})$] that is due to interindividual trait differences [$\lambda^2_{Tik}Var(T_i)$]. A high value for this coefficient indicates that interindividual differences in subjective well-being on an occasion of measurement are mainly determined by stable interindividual (trait) differences. Trait measures of subjective well-being should have high consistency values.

The *specificity coefficient*

$$SPE(Y_{ik}) = \frac{\lambda^2_{Oik}Var(O_k)}{Var(Y_{ik})}$$

represents the proportion of variance of an observed variable that is due to occasion-specific influences and not due to trait and error influences. State measures of subjective well-being that should be sensitive to change (occasion-specific influences) ought to have rather high specificity coefficients.

The consistency and occasion-specificity coefficient add up to the *reliability coefficient*, which is 1 minus the proportion of interindividual differences that is due to measurement error:

$$Rel(Y_{ik}) = \frac{\lambda^2_{Tik}Var(T_i)}{Var(Y_{ik})} + \frac{\lambda^2_{Oik}Var(O_k)}{Var(Y_{ik})} = 1 - \frac{Var(E_{ik})}{Var(Y_{ik})}$$

All observed variables should have high reliability values.

The model presented so far is a model for continuous subjective well-being measures. It is usually applied to subjective well-being scales consisting of multiple items. In order to obtain two (or more) indicators i, a scale can be split into two test halves (e.g., each test half is the mean of the responses to one half of the items) or multiple parcels.

Eid (1996) has shown how LST models can be defined for binary and ordinal variables. These models allow the estimation of the consistency and occasion-specificity for single items. This information can be used to select items in such a way as to maximize the consistency or occasion-specificity of a scale measuring subjective well-being. Eid and Langeheine (1999) defined LST latent class models to analyze typological subjective well-being differences on the state and trait levels. Cole, Martin, and Steiger (2005) have shown how LST models can be extended to consider an additional autoregressive process on the level of the occasion-specific variables. An autoregressive process is needed when there is a change process on the level of the occasion-specific variables, which simply means that the occasion-specific deviation on one occasion of measurement depends on an occasion-specific deviation of another occasion of measurement.

Applications of Latent State–Trait Models in the Realm of Subjective Well-Being Measurement

Models of LST theory have been applied to analyze different questions concerning the reliability, validity, and structure of subjective well-being measures. The main results of these studies illustrate the different ways in which models of LST theory can be applied.

The Polarity and Dimensionality of the Affective Component of Subjective Well-Being

One of the most hotly debated issues concerning the structure of the affective component of subjective well-being is the question of whether positive and negative affects are independent or not (see Schimmack, Chapter 6, this volume). According to a bipolarity model of positive and negative affect, the two types of affect are opposite poles of one continuum. In contrast, the monopolarity model supposes that positive and negative affects cannot be ordered on a single continuum. Eid (1995) analyzed this research question in detail on the basis of LST modeling. He applied LST models for ordinal variables to analyze the structure of two pairs of semantically opposite items measuring momentary positive and negative affect (*happy, unhappy, satisfied, dissatisfied*). LST models for ordinal variables correct for differences in the distribution of positive and negative affect items. Whereas positively keyed state items usually show a symmetric distribution, negatively keyed state items are usually skewed. If items differing in their distributions are analyzed with factor models for continuous variables (as it is often done), artificially monopolar factors can be produced. Eid (1995) analyzed the structure of affect ratings by comparing the fit of several LST models. The model presented in Figure 8.6 was the only model that fit the data (Eid [1995] analyzed three occasions of measurement; the model structure was the same as the model in Figure 8.6 but contained one more occasion of measurement). According to this model, the different items measuring positive and negative affect are bipolar on the level of occasion-specific influences but monopolar on the trait level. Situational influences that make people happier are exactly those that make people less unhappy. The unidimensional structure on the occasion-specific level means that one can perfectly predict the latent deviation score of unhappiness (feeling more or less unhappy in this situation) by the latent happiness deviation score. On the trait level there were item-specific differences. However, the different trait variables are highly correlated (between $r = .67$ and $r = .92$), with the correlations between the items of the same valence being higher (between *unhappy* and *dissatisfied*: $r = .92$; between *happy* and *satisfied*: $r = .83$) than between the semantically opposite items (*happy* and *unhappy*: $r = .67$; *satisfied* and *dissatisfied*: $r = .82$). The nonperfect correlations on the trait level show that each item has a stable component (unique meaning) that is not shared with the other items.

Mood Influences on Life Satisfaction Judgments

Whereas a state–trait distinction has generally been accepted for the affective component of well-being, life satisfaction judgments are considered as a stabler subjective well-being component. Life satisfaction judgments should be sensitive to changes in the conditions in which people live, but they should not be sensitive to immediate mood fluctuations (Campbell, Converse, & Rodgers, 1976). The assumption that life satisfaction items are immune to short-time fluctuations such as mood has been questioned strongly (Schwarz & Strack, 1999). Eid and Diener (2004) analyzed mood influences on subjective well-being judgments in a longitudinal study with three occasions of measurement using LST models. They found that life satisfaction judgments are much stabler than mood judgments. Whereas the occasion-specificity coefficients were between .40 and .52 for the mood ratings, they were much lower for the life satisfaction judgments (between .12 and .16). The correlations between the occasion-specific variables of mood and life satisfaction were very low and not significant for the first two occasions (r = .13 and r = .23) and higher and significant for the third occasion of measurement (r = .55). These low correlations indicate that the occasion-specific variability of mood can only explain between 1.7 and 30% of the variability of life satisfaction judgments. Eid and Diener (2004) assumed that the higher correlation on the third occasion might be due to the fact that the last occasion of measurement was at the end of the semester (participants were college students) and that typical events at this time (e.g., exams) might have had an influence on mood and life satisfaction. In general, the much higher stability of life satisfaction judgments and the rather small correlations between the variability of mood and life satisfaction demonstrate that mood effects on life satisfaction judgments seem to be rather small in nonexperimental survey research.

Validity of Direct Assessment Methods

Eid, Notz, Steyer, and Schwenkmezger (1994) analyzed the validity of the Mood Level subscale of Underwood and Froming's (1980) Mood Survey in a longitudinal study with four occasions of measurement. An example of an item from this scale is "I usually feel quite cheerful." The consistency coefficients from the four occasions of measurement are very high (between .78 and .85) and are close to the reliability coefficients (between .89 and .92). Hence, occasion-specific influences are very small (occasion specificities: between .06 and .11), proving that this subjective well-being scale assesses very stable aspects. Moreover, the latent trait variable of this scale is highly correlated with the latent trait variable of the mood state ratings ($r = .78$), verifying high convergent validity.

Eid et al. (1999) scrutinized the validity of the direct assessment of occasion-specific deviations ("Do you feel better or worse?") and of trait assessments ("How do you feel in general?") using the same adjectives of a pleasantness–unpleasantness mood scale. Applying LST models, they found the following results: (1) The deviations ratings are uncorrelated with the trait ratings, indicating that they represent—as intended—pure situational and/or interactional effects. (2) The occasion-specific variables of the state ratings are highly correlated with those of the deviation ratings (between .70 and .90), proving their validity. (3) The consistency coefficients of the deviation ratings (between .18 and .32) are smaller then those of the state ratings (between .27 and .43), showing that deviation ratings represent mainly situational influences. However, they differ significantly from 0. This unexpected small proportion of stable differences of the deviation ratings can be explained by the fact that all participants (all were students) had been repeatedly assessed after the same lecture. The stability of deviation ratings indicates the stability of (objective) situations. The trait value of repeatedly measured deviations represents, therefore, how the students generally felt after *the lecture* compared to how they felt *in general*. Eid et al. (1999) showed that the mean of repeatedly measured deviations can be used to suppress that part of the repeatedly measured states that are due to stable situational aspects. As a consequence, the corrected correlation between the indirectly measured subjective well-being traits (on the basis of repeatedly measured states) with the directly assessed subjective well-being trait (trait self-rating) is higher ($r = .79$) than the uncorrected correlation ($r = .71$). The effect is even stronger for the Mood Level subscale of the Mood Survey (Underwood & Froming, 1980), where the corrected and uncorrected correlations are $r = .76$ and $r = .62$, respectively. These results substantiate a rather high convergent validity of direct and indirect assessment procedures. Moreover, they also demonstrate that it is useful to supplement state ratings of subjective well-being by deviations ratings in order to find out whether the subjective well-being people experience during a specific period of time is representative of their lives in general. Thus, even the indirect assessment of a subjective well-being trait by repeatedly measured states can profit from the additional direct assessment of the different temporal facets. As in other domains of the social and behavioral sciences, multimethod approaches offer deeper insights into the questions at hand than single-method designs (Eid & Diener, 2006).

Interindividual Differences in Intraindividual Variability

Subjective well-being states characterize random fluctuations of subjective well-being around the subjective well-being trait level. The degree of these fluctuations is not unsystematic but highly stable because there are strong interindividual differences in intraindividual variability. Using daily assessment data of the affective component of subjective well-being, measured each evening over a period of 52 days, Eid and Diener (1999) applied LST modeling to examine whether intraindividual variability is stable over time. They calculated the intraindividual standard deviation over all the days of 1 week for two test halves of seven scales, measuring three positive and four negative affects. The intraindividual standard deviations were the observed variables in a LST model, such as the one depicted in Figure 8.6. The estimated occasion-specificity coefficients (between .00 and .18 for the positive affects and between .07 and .57 for the negative affects) showed that the intraindividual variability of subjective well-being during 1 week is highly stable and has, particularly for positive emotions, the character of a trait.

Separating Stable from Variable and Resilient from Nonresilient Individuals with Mixture Distribution Latent State–Trait Models

Models of LST theory assume that the estimated parameters of the model characterize all individuals of the population appropriately. This means, for example, that all individuals stem from the same population in which the degree of expected variability is described by the variance of the occasion-specific factors. Interindividual differences in intraindividual variability are allowed but only to a certain degree. For example, if the variances of the occasion-specific variables are small, the expected variability is also small, and if the variances are large, there could be strong differences in the variability. The population, however, might not be homogeneous with respect to the expected variability. Given the strong interindividual differences in intraindividual variability, there is good reason to assume that some subpopulations differ in the degree of intraindividual variability they allow. Eid and Langeheine (2003, 2007) have extended LST models for categorical variables to mixture distribution models, and Courvoisier, Eid, and Nussbeck (2007) defined mixture distribution LST models for continuous variables. These models assume that the population consists of subpopulations differing in the variances of the occasion-specific variables. Courvoisier et al. (2007), for example, found that there were two latent classes. The larger class (76%) was characterized by higher intraindividual variability of subjective well-being measures and generally lower subjective well-being mean values. The smaller class (24%) was stabler and showed a high degree of subjective well-being. Most interestingly, the two latent classes differed in the influences of daily hassles and uplifts on the occasion-specific mood difference. Whereas in the first, more variable class, daily hassles had a negative and daily uplifts had a positive influence on subjective well-being, in the second class, only daily uplifts had a significant positive influence, whereas the influence of daily hassles was not significant. People in the second class seem to profit from positive daily events and to be rather resilient to the influences of negative life events.

Separating Trait Change from Occasions-Specific Variability

In the LST models presented here, the latent trait variables do not change within the time period considered. However, LST models can be extended easily to allow trait change as well. Intervention methods for enhancing subjective well-being (see Emmons, Chapter 23, this volume; Fredrickson, Chapter 22, this volume; King, Chapter 21, this volume) aim not only at changing momentary subjective well-being states but also the habitual subjective well-being level. If one measures subjective well-being states several times before an intervention and several times after an intervention, the general mood level (i.e., the mean of the different states) should be higher after the treatment than before. LST models with trait change allow distinguishing between the short-term state variability caused by situational influences and more enduring trait changes (Eid & Hoffmann, 1998). Trait change represents the degree of change on the trait level free of influences due to measurement error and occasional influences in the period before and after the treatment. Steyer (2005) provides a detailed discussion of the conclusions that can be drawn about the effect of a treatment when it is evaluated by LST trait change models.

Psychometric Modeling of Single-Case Data

Models of LST theory require a sample of individuals and a sample of occasions of measurement. The analysis of different individuals allows an examination of *inter*individual differences in subjective well-being, and the consideration of different occasions of measurement enables the analysis of *intra*individual differences over time. To apply these models, however, it is necessary that the models fit for the total population or at least for subpopulations (mixed models).

If the research interest is in a single individual, factor models for single-case data can be applied. These models focus on the structure of the occasion-specific deviation variables of a single individual. If one is, for example, interested in the structure of the four positive and negative affect items, a single-case factor model, with a factor for positive affect and a factor for negative affect, would have the form presented in Figure 8.7. This model has no trait factor because the trait is a constant for an individual, and there is only one positive and one negative affect factor because the values of the observed variable are now the different individual values at different occasions of measurement. The values of the factors are the true occasion-specific values for a single individual on the different occasions of measurement. This single-case factor model is a model of *p*-technique factor

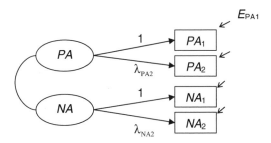

FIGURE 8.7. Single-case factor model for repeatedly measured indicators of positive and negative affect. PA_i, indicators of positive affect; NA_i, indicators of negative affect; PA, NA, occasion-specific factors representing true occasion-specific values for a single individual; E_{PA_i}, error variables. For simplicity reasons not all error variables are marked.

analysis (Nesselroade, 2001). Ong, Horn, and Walsh (2007), for example, used p-technique factor models to analyze the structure of hedonic and eudomanic well-being of nine individuals who recorded their well-being 10 times a day over a period of 61 days. They found that the two constructs showed discriminant validity for all individuals analyzed. However, the two-factor model did not fit for all individuals in the same way. Feldman (1995) explored whether the structure of affect differs between individuals. She analyzed the response to 16 affect markers that were repeatedly measured over 62–91 days. She found a two-factor structure for nine participants, a three-factor structure for 12 participants, and a three-factor structure for two participants. Moreover, the participants differed in the degree to which valence and arousal components were present in their ratings. Larsen and Cutler (1996) analyzed 21 mood adjectives with p-technique factor analysis. They found strong individual differences in emotional complexity, as indicated by the fact that the individuals differed in the number of factors needed to explain the structure of affect (between two to five factors). Emotional complexity was negatively correlated with subjective well-being for men but positively correlated for women.

Models of p-technique factor analysis are appropriate only if the repeated measurements are independent. If there is a change process, the dependency between the occasions of measurement has to be considered. For example, there can be an autoregressive process indicating that a subjective well-being state depends on the subjective well-being states measured before. In this case, single-case dynamic factor analysis that models the temporal structure can be applied (e.g., Nesselroade, 2001). Ferrer and Nesselroade (2003), for example, showed how dynamic factor analysis can be applied to examine the structure of positive and negative affect. Moreover, they showed how this approach can be used to compare the structure of affective subjective well-being between a husband and wife and how the mutual influences of affect can be tested. They found that the husband's negative affect particularly influenced the wife's positive and negative affect.

If there are nonlinear changes such as daily or weekly cycles, frequency domain analysis (spectral analysis) can be applied (Larsen, 1987). Chow, Grimm, Ram, and Fujita (2007) found, for instance, strong individual differences in the extent to which individuals' emotions follow a weekly cycle. They also show how modeling strategies of IRT and spectral analysis can be combined.

Whereas mixed models such as the mixed Rasch models and the mixed LST models follow a top-down strategy (searching for subgroup differences if the model does not hold for the population), single-case factor analysis can be applied for bottom-up strategies—that means, the search for a common structure of subjective well-being based on the comparison of single cases. In order to combine idiographic methods such as single-case analysis with nomothetic approaches for explaining individual differences, the parameters of single-case analysis can be related to other (personality) variables (Larsen, 2007).

Conclusion

This chapter focused on the psychometric models (latent variable models) that can be applied to analyze the reliability and validity of subjective well-being measures. These models offer many ways to analyze the psychometric quality of subjective well-being both on the individual level as well as on the level of individual differences. Besides the latent variable models, all other statistical methods can be applied to analyze subjective well-being data. The *Handbook of Methods in Positive Psychology*, edited by Ong and van Dulmen (2007), shows how advanced statistical approaches such as structural equation models, hierarchical linear models, IRT models, single-case methods, experimental methods, and many others can be applied to learn more about the structure, condition, and consequences of subjective well-being.

References

Baker, J. G., Rounds, J., & Zevon, M. A. (2000). A comparison of graded response and Rasch partial credit models with subjective well-being. *Journal of Educational and Behavioral Statistics, 25,* 253–270.

Campbell, A., Converse, P. E., & Rodgers, W. L. (1976). *The quality of American life: Perceptions, evaluations, satisfactions.* New York: Sage.

Chow, S.-M., Grimm, K. J., Ram, N., & Fujita, F. (2007). Exploring cyclic change in emotion using item response models and frequency-domain analysis. In A. Ong &

M. van Dulmen (Eds.), *Handbook of methods in positive psychology* (pp. 803–832). New York: Oxford University Press.

Cole, D. A., Martin, N. C., & Steiger, J. H. (2005). Empirical and conceptual problems with longitudinal trait–state models: Support for a Trait–State–occasion model. *Psychological Methods, 10*, 3–20.

Courvoisier, D., Eid, M., & Nussbeck, F. (2007). Mixture distribution latent state–trait analysis: Basic ideas and applications. *Psychological Methods, 12*, 80–104.

Diener, E. (1984). Subjective well-being. *Psychological Bulletin, 95*, 542–575.

Diener, E. (2000). Subjective well-being: The science of happiness, and a proposal for a national index. *American Psychologist, 55*, 34–43.

Eid, M. (1995). *Modelle der Messung von Personen in Situationen* [Models for measuring individuals in situations]. Weinheim, Germany: Psychologie Verlags Union.

Eid, M. (1996). Longitudinal confirmatory factor analysis for polytomous item responses: Model definition and model selection on the basis of stochastic measurement theory. *Methods of Psychological Research—Online, 1*, 65–85. Available at *www.mpr-online.de/*.

Eid, M., & Diener, E. (1999). Intraindividual variability in affect: Reliability, validity, and personality correlates. *Journal of Personality and Social Psychology, 76*, 662–676.

Eid, M., & Diener, E. (2001). Comparing norms for affect across cultures: Inter- and intranational differences. *Journal of Personality and Social Psychology, 81*, 869–885.

Eid, M., & Diener, E. (2004). Global judgments of subjective well-being: Situational variability and long-term stability. *Social Indicators Research, 65*, 245–277.

Eid, M., & Diener, E. (2006). *Handbook of multimethod measurement.* Washington, DC: American Psychological Association.

Eid, M., & Hoffmann, L. (1998). Measuring variability and change with an item response model for polytomous variables. *Journal of Educational and Behavioral Statistics, 23*, 193–215.

Eid, M., & Langeheine, R. (1999). Measuring consistency and occasion specificity with latent class models: A new model and its application to the measurement of affect. *Psychological Methods, 4*, 100–116.

Eid, M., & Langeheine, R. (2003). Separating stable from variable individuals in longitudinal studies by mixture distribution models. *Measurement, 1*, 179–206.

Eid, M., & Langeheine, R. (2007). Detecting population heterogeneity in stability and change of subjective well-being by mixture distribution models. In A. Ong & M. van Dulmen (Eds.), *Handbook of methods in positive psychology* (pp. 501–607). New York: Oxford University Press.

Eid, M., Langeheine, R., & Diener, E. (2003). Comparing typological structures across cultures by latent class analysis: A primer. *Journal of Cross-Cultural Psychology, 34*, 195–210.

Eid, M., Notz, P., Steyer, R., & Schwenkmezger, P. (1994). Validating scales for the assessment of mood level and variability by latent state–trait analyses. *Personality and Individual Differences, 16*, 63–76.

Eid, M., Schneider, C., & Schwenkmezger, P. (1999). Do you feel better or worse? On the validity of perceived deviations of mood states from mood traits. *European Journal of Personality, 13*, 283–306

Fahrenberg, J., Hampel, R., & Selg, H. (1984). *Das Freiburger Persönlichkeitsinventar* [Freiburg Personality Inventory] *FPI* (4th ed.). Göttingen, Germany: Hogrefe.

Feldman, L. A. (1995). Valence focus and arousal focus: Individual differences in the structure of affective experience. *Journal of Personality and Social Psychology, 69,* 153–166.

Ferrer, E., & Nesselroade, J. R. (2003). Modeling affective processes in dyadic relations via dynamic factor analysis. *Emotion, 3,* 344–360.

Hagenaars, J. A., & McCutcheon, A. L. (Eds.). (2002). *Applied latent class analysis.* Cambridge, UK: Cambridge University Press.

Kahneman, D. (1999). Objective happiness. In D. Kahneman, E. Diener, & N. Schwarz (Eds.), *Well-being: The foundations of hedonic psychology* (pp. 3–25). New York: Sage.

Larsen, R. J. (1987). The stability of mood variability: A spectral analytic approach to daily mood assessments. *Journal of Personality and Social Psychology, 52,* 1195–1204.

Larsen, R. J. (2007). Within-person covariation analysis: Application to the study of affect. In A. Ong & M. van Dulmen (Eds.), *Handbook of methods in positive psychology* (pp. 749–772). New York: Oxford University Press.

Larsen, R. J., & Cutler, S. (1996). The complexity of individual emotional lives: A within-subject analysis of affect structure. *Journal of Social and Clinical Psychology, 15,* 206–230.

Lischetzke, T., & Eid, M. (2006). Wohlbefindensdiagnostik [Assessment of well-being]. In F. Petermann & M. Eid (Eds.), *Handbuch der Psychologischen Diagnostik [Handbook of psychological assessment]* (pp. 550–557). Göttingen, Germany: Hogrefe.

Nesselroade, J. R. (2001). Intraindividual variability in development within and between individuals. *European Psychologist, 6,* 187–193.

Ong, A. D., Horn, J. L., & Walsh, D. A. (2007). Stepping into the light: Modeling the intraindividual dimensions of hedonic and eudamonic well-being. In A. Ong & M. van Dulmen (Eds.), *Handbook of methods in positive psychology* (pp. 12–28). New York: Oxford University Press.

Ong, A. D., & van Dulmen, M. (Eds.). (2007). *Handbook of methods in positive psychology.* New York: Oxford University Press.

Rasch, G. (1960). *Probabilistic models for some intelligence and attainment tests.* Copenhagen: Danish Institute for Educational Research.

Rost, J. (1990). Rasch models in latent classes: An integration of two approaches to item analysis. *Applied Psychological Measurement, 14,* 271–282.

Rost, J. (2004). *Testtheorie, Testkonstruktion [Test theory, test construction].* Bern, Switzerland: Huber.

Rost, J., & Walter, O. (2006). Multimethod item response theory. In M. Eid & E. Diener (Eds.), *Handbook of multimethod measurement* (pp. 249–268). Washington, DC: American Psychological Association.

Schermelleh-Engel, K., Moosbrugger, H., & Müller, H. (2003). Evaluating the fit of structural equation models: Test of significance and descriptive goodness-of-fit measures. *Methods of Psychological Research—Online, 8,* 23–74. Available at *www.mpronline.de/.*

Schwarz, N., & Strack, F. (1999). Reports of subjective well-being: Judgmental processes and their methodological implications. In D. Kahneman, E. Diener, & N. Schwarz (Eds.), *Well-being: The foundations of hedonic psychology* (pp. 61–84). New York: Sage.

Steyer, R. (2005). Analyzing individual and average causal effects via structural equation models. *Methodology, 1,* 39–54.

Steyer, R., Schmitt, M., & Eid, M. (1999). Latent state–trait theory and research in personality and individual differences. *European Journal of Personality, 13,* 389–408.

Stone, A., & Litcher-Kelly, L. (2006). Momentary capture of real world data. In M. Eid & E. Diener (Eds.), *Handbook of multimethod measurement* (pp. 61–72). Washington, DC: American Psychological Association.

Underwood, B., & Froming, W. J. (1980). The Mood Survey: A personality measure of happy and sad moods. *Journal of Personality Assessment, 44,* 404–414.

van der Linden, W. J., & Hambleton, R. K. (Eds.). (1997). *Handbook of modern item response theory.* New York: Springer.

von Davier, M. (1997). Bootstrapping goodness-of-fit statistics for sparse categorical data: Results of a Monte Carlo study. *Methods of Psychological Research—Online, 2,* 29–48. Available at *www.mpr-online.de/.*

von Davier, M., & Carstensen, C. (Eds.). (2007). *Multivariate and mixture distribution Rasch models.* New York: Springer.

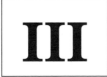

THE HAPPY PERSON

9

Personality and Subjective Well-Being

RICHARD E. LUCAS

Subjective well-being is an overarching domain that includes a broad collection of constructs that relate to individuals' subjective evaluation of the quality of their lives. Psychologists and other social scientists are interested in this topic for at least four reasons. First, the topic is important because subjective well-being is valued by laypeople. Psychologists study well-being because they hope to identify factors that will allow people to achieve permanent increases in it. Second, researchers pursue an understanding of subjective well-being because they believe such an understanding could lead to the identification of basic human needs (Veenhoven, 1995; Wilson, 1967). For instance, if research shows that strong social relationships reliably lead to higher well-being and the lack of such bonds reliably lead to lowered well-being, then such a finding might provide evidence that human beings have a *basic need* for belongingness (e.g., Baumeister & Leary, 1995). Third, psychologists study subjective well-being because it provides insight into the ways that basic affect and evaluation systems function. By studying the judgment processes that underlie well-being reports (Schwarz & Strack, 1999), psychologists can answer basic questions about the ways in which people make evaluations and judgments. Finally, by linking subjective well-being with outcomes, researchers can show how affective processes motivate action (e.g., Fredrickson, 1998).

In at least two of these four areas, researchers presume that subjective well-being can change and that it is sensitive to external circumstances. Psychologists attempt to identify correlates of well-being because they hope that these correlates will illuminate the processes that cause high well-being, which, in turn, should lead to promising interventions. Similarly, psychologists who strive to understand basic needs believe that variation in external circumstances should correlate with happiness and reveal the deficits that reliably affect mental health. Yet one of the most surprising findings that has emerged from decades of research is that subjective well-being appears to be stable over time and at least moderately strongly related to stable personality traits (Diener, Suh, Lucas, & Smith, 1999). In fact, Gilovich and Eibach (2001) suggested that the relatively weak influence of situational factors and the relatively strong influence of personality factors on well-being may be the only example of an important, counterintuitive finding that has emerged from the entire field of personality psychology.[1]

The implication of this finding is clear: If happiness is solely determined by one's personality, then research on well-being will be severely constrained. The search for external factors that promote high levels of well-being will have been conducted in vain. Programs designed to increase individuals' happiness (e.g., Lyubomirsky, Sheldon, & Schkade, 2005; Seligman, Steen, Park, & Peterson, 2005) will surely fail, and governmental policies designed to foster high levels of well-being will have no chance of success. Similarly, if happiness is not reactive to changing circumstances, attempts to use the correlates of happiness to understand basic human needs will not be fruitful. Even those researchers who use subjective well-being measures to understand the ways in which people evaluate the world may be disappointed. Well-being measures may simply reflect two dominating pieces of information: (1) a person's unchanging temperament-based outlook on life, and (2) whatever happens to be on his or her mind at the time of the judgment. Schwarz and Strack (1999) suggested as much when they argued that the literature on survey methods might lead one to conclude that "there is little to be learned from global self-reports of well-being. . . . [W]hat is being assessed, and how, seems too context dependent to provide reliable information about a population's well-being" (p. 80).

In this chapter, I review the evidence regarding the role of temperament and personality in subjective well-being. In general, researchers point to four pieces of evidence when discussing this topic. First, research has shown that external factors play only a small role in happiness. Together, demographic factors tend to explain at most (and usually much less than) 15–20% of the variance in subjective well-being (Argyle, 1999), and major life events have often been shown to lead to only small or short-lived changes in well-being (though, as I

---

[1] I do not agree, but this demonstrates the reaction that psychologists have had to these findings.

review below, more recent evidence challenges some of the standard interpretations of this research; see Diener, Lucas, & Scollon, 2006). Second, well-being is heritable and can be linked to psychophysiological structures and processes. Third, as noted well-being scores are quite stable over time, even in the face of major life changes. And finally (and perhaps most directly), well-being scores are often moderately to strongly correlated with stable personality traits. Because the first of these four pieces of evidence (the small role of external circumstances) has been addressed in quite a bit of detail elsewhere (e.g., Argyle, 1999; Diener et al., 1999), and because it is only indirectly related to the topic of personality and well-being, I focus mostly on the remaining three pieces of evidence.

The Biological Basis of Subjective Well-Being

One key source of evidence for the role of personality in subjective well-being comes from studies that link well-being to psychophysiological structures and processes. Because these biological processes are thought to be stable and to some extent inborn, any links with well-being would suggest that well-being, too, is driven by internal processes. In this section, I first review the evidence regarding the heritability of well-being. Then I examine research that links well-being to specific psychophysiological processes.

The Heritability of Well-Being Measures

In perhaps the first behavioral–genetic study of well-being measures, Tellegen et al. (1988) compared the cross-twin correlations for monozygotic twins reared together, monozygotic twins reared apart, dizygotic twins reared together, and dizygotic twins reared apart. A number of important findings emerged from this early study. First, Tellegen et al. showed that the broad heritability of well-being (as measured by various facets and higher-order factors of the Multidimensional Personality Questionnaire [MPQ]) was moderate and similar to the heritability of other personality traits. For example, the estimated heritabilities of the well-being facet and global positive emotionality factor were .48 and .40, respectively. Similarly, the heritabilities of the stress reaction facet and negative emotionality factor were .53 and .55, respectively. Thus, about half of the variance in these well-being measures could be accounted for by shared genes. Furthermore, growing up in the same household played almost no role in the similarity of twins. Shared environmental components could be removed from most models, though there was a significant effect (accounting for 22% of the variance) for positive emotionality.

Because Tellegen et al. (1988) included twins who were reared apart in their study, they could also estimate separate additive and nonadditive genetic components. If the effects of genes on subjective well-being are additive, then the more genes that two people share, the more similar they should be. Nonadditive genetic effects, on the other hand, reflect interactions among genes. In the extreme case, two people would need the exact same combination of genes to express the same phenotype. Thus, two people who were genetically related but not genetically identical could end up being no more similar than average, even if the trait in question were 100% heritable. Nonadditive effects are suggested when monozygotic twin correlations are more than twice as high as dizygotic twin correlations. Tellegen et al. found that the effects of negative emotionality were completely additive, whereas the effects of positive emotionality were completely nonadditive.

Researchers have attempted to replicate and extend Tellegen et al.'s (1988) study several times using a variety of techniques and measures. In general, the estimated contribution of broad heritability versus shared environment has held up quite well. For instance, Roysamb, Harris, Magnus, Vitterso, and Tambs (2002) examined the heritability of subjective well-being using a global well-being measure, and like Tellegen et al., they found that about 50% of the variance could be accounted for by genes. Again, models that included shared environmental factors did not fit significantly better than models without these factors.

Interestingly, Roysamb et al. (2002) found that the heritability of well-being differed across sexes. Heritability was estimated at .54 among women and .46 among men (also see Roysamb, Tambs, Reichborn-Kjennerud, Neale, & Harris, 2003, for a replication with a larger but overlapping sample). Perhaps more importantly, because Roysamb et al. included both same-sex and mixed-sex fraternal twins, they could estimate whether the same genes contributed to the happiness of men and women. If so, the correlations among same-sex dizygotic twins should be the same size as the correlations among the mixed-sex dizygotic twins. This was not the case, and Roysamb et al. estimated that the correlation between the genetic effect in men and the genetic effect in women was just .64. The authors explained this effect in terms of potential underlying mechanisms. It is possible that there is a direct temperamental effect on well-being, and that this effect is explained by the same genes across sexes. However, there may also be indirect effects, whereby genes lead individuals to select certain environments, and these environments lead to individual differences in happiness. The specific environments that promote happiness may differ for men and women. Roysamb et al. argued that the fact that the genetic effects for men and women are not perfectly correlated suggest that at least part of the effect of genes is indirect.

Because subjective well-being includes a variety of separable components that may result from different processes, it is possible that heritability may vary for the distinct components. Tellegen et al. (1988) examined the heritability of various facets and factors from the MPQ (which was intended as a measure of stable personality), and Roysamb et al. (2002) used a three-item well-being measure that incorporated questions about all three major components of subjective well-being: positive affect, negative affect, and life satisfaction. Other researchers have attempted to determine the heritability of other components, including short-term mood or long-term levels of life satisfaction. For example, Stubbe, Posthuma, Boomsma, and De Geus (2005) examined the heritability of life satisfaction using the Satisfaction with Life Scale (Diener, Emmons, Larsen, & Griffin, 1985) in a sample of over 5,000 twins from The Netherlands. Their analyses suggested that 38% of the variability in life satisfaction is heritable—a finding that is slightly lower than the estimates from Tellegen et al. or Roysamb et al. Furthermore, they estimated that almost all of these genetic effects were nonadditive. In direct contrast to the results of Roysamb et al., Stubbe et al. found that the correlation between dizygotic same-sex twins was not significantly different from the correlation between mixed-sex twins or even siblings. Although they did not model these differences in the same way that Roysamb et al. did, this pattern of correlations contradicts Roysamb et al.'s finding that the correlation among men's and women's genetic factors is substantially less than 1.

In one of the most novel behavioral–genetic studies on the heritability of well-being, Riemann, Angleitner, Borkenau, and Eid (1998) assessed monozygotic and dizygotic twins' moods across five different mood-induction conditions. Thus, in contrast to the other behavioral–genetic studies, the focus was on short-term moods rather than on long-term affective traits. Interestingly, Riemann et al. reported results that differed quite a bit from the studies reviewed above. Even when average mood levels across all five situations (which, theoretically, should be highly correlated with affective traits) were examined, estimated heritabilities were much lower than those found in previous studies. Heritabilities ranged from .18 to .19 for negative mood and from .11 to .16 for positive mood. In addition, unlike previous studies, the shared environmental component accounted for at least as much, and sometimes more, variance than did genes. The shared environment accounted for between 31 and 32% of the variance in negative mood and between 15 and 18% of positive mood. Because behavioral–genetic researchers have grown accustomed to finding moderate heritabilities and almost no shared environment for just about any personality characteristic that is examined (Turkheimer, 2000), Riemann et al.'s results are quite surprising.

Perhaps the most controversial study on the heritability of well-being is Lykken and Tellegen's (1996) paper entitled "Happiness Is a Stochastic Phenomenon." In it, the authors used a longitudinal study of twins to determine the extent to which the stable component of well-being is heritable. They found that over a 10-year period, the stability of well-being was about .50. However, the cross-twin, cross-time correlation (i.e., twin 1's time 1 score correlated with twin 2's time 2 score) was .40. Because this cross-twin, cross-time correlation is 80% as large as the stability coefficient, Lykken and Tellegen estimated that 80% of the stable component of well-being is heritable. The authors suggested that this extremely high heritability means that "trying to be happier [may be] as futile as trying to be taller" (p. 189).

However, there are a number of problems with this conclusion. First, as Lykken himself noted (Lykken & Csikszentmihalyi, 2001), even in the twin study he analyzed, only about 50% of the variance was stable over a 10-year period. Thus, even if Lykken and Tellegen's (1996) estimates are correct, then it is more accurate to say that trying to change the part of our happiness that does not change is like trying to be taller (which, of course, is tautological). However, even this qualified statement may not be completely accurate. Strong heritability on its own does not necessarily mean that something cannot be changed. Because genes may lead to happiness indirectly (e.g., through choice of environment or exposure to life events), it is possible that change can be achieved once the underlying process is understood.

Furthermore, it is important to remember that Lykken and Tellegen's (1996) conclusion is based on one study with a relatively small sample of twins (79 monozygotic twin pairs and 48 dizygotic twin pairs). Although the broad heritability of well-being has been replicated often, many of the extensions of these findings have not replicated well. And there is some reason for concern about the reliability of the estimates from this small sample. Although it is not reported in the Lykken and Tellegen paper, the time 2 correlation between monozygotic twins was only .13 (compared to a time 1 correlation of .63, and a time 2 correlation between dizygotic twins of .23; McGue, Bacon, & Lykken, 1993). The time 2 pattern of monozygotic and dizygotic correlations would actually suggest no genetic effect and a small shared environmental effect on well-being—a finding that contradicts a fairly large body of research. Furthermore, two more recent studies have reached different conclusions about the heritability of the stable component of well-being. Although Nes, Roysamb, Tambs, Harris, and Reichborn-Kjennerud (2006) replicated Lykken and Tellegen's estimates, Johnson, McGue, and Krueger (2005) found that only about 38% of the stable variance in well-being is heritable. Thus, additional replications are needed before researchers can accept the estimates from Lykken and Tellegen's study.

Overall, behavioral–genetic studies have repeatedly shown that happiness is heritable. Genes appear to account for about 40–50% of the variance in stable levels of positive affect, negative affect, life satisfaction, and other aspects of global well-being. At this point, it is unclear whether these genetic effects are additive or nonadditive, and it is unclear whether there are any reliable shared family environmental effects (though, as with most personality traits, the answer is probably "no"). Furthermore, the genes that underlie these effects may or may not vary for men and women. And finally, some evidence suggests that heritabilities are lower for state levels of mood—even when these measures are aggregated over multiple occasions—and higher for long-term levels of well-being. Taken together, the behavioral–genetic studies suggest that inborn biology plays at least some part in determining happiness.

Specific Psychophysiological Correlates

Behavioral–genetic studies show that at least some portion of the variance in well-being can be explained by genes. And, of course, genes must express themselves through some physiological process. However, the exact mechanisms by which these genetic effects are transmitted are not known. It is possible that the genetic effects are direct. Specific genes or combinations of genes may influence average hedonic tone, emotional reactivity, or emotional intensity. Alternatively, the genetic effect may be indirect. Genes may influence physiological systems that only indirectly influence well-being through their effects on environmental choice or other behaviors. Thus, behavioral–genetic studies alone cannot determine how genes and biology influence well-being. More targeted studies that examine the specific psychophysiological systems that may be involved in affective experience are required.

Perhaps the most studied neural correlate of self-reported well-being is asymmetrical hemispheric activation in the prefrontal cortex (for a review, see Davidson, 2004). For decades, Davidson and colleagues (and others) have investigated whether greater left versus right hemispheric activity is associated with approach-oriented emotions (e.g., happiness and excitement), and greater right versus left activity is associated with withdrawal-oriented emotions (e.g., fear and disgust). For instance, Davidson et al. (1990) measured brain activity during films designed to induce happiness or disgust. In accordance with their hypotheses, the happy films were associated with greater left versus right frontal and anterior temporal activity, whereas the disgust films were associated with greater right versus left activity. Thus, at a state level, this psychophysiological measure has been shown to correlate with positive versus negative emotion.

Perhaps more importantly for researchers interested in individual differences in subjective well-being, there appear to be stable individual differences in hemispheric asymmetry. For instance, Tomarken, Davidson, Wheeler, and Kinney (1992) took multiple assessments of baseline electrical activity within two occasions separated by 3 weeks. Internal consistency (calculated using multiple trials within a single session) was very high ($\alpha > .85$) and test–retest reliabilities were similar to short-term test–retest reliabilities for standard self-report measures of subjective well-being (they ranged from .65 to .75). Thus, there appear to be stable individual differences in asymmetrical activity.

These individual differences in hemispheric asymmetry have been shown to correlate with well-being. For example, Tomarken, Davidson, Wheeler, and Doss (1992) showed that individuals with relatively high left frontal activation reported more positive affect and less negative affect than individuals with relatively high right frontal activation. More recently, Urry et al. (2004) extended these results to measures of well-being beyond positive and negative affect. They showed that even measures of psychological well-being (which include scales for such constructs as self-acceptance, purpose in life, personal growth, and autonomy) were predicted by prefrontal asymmetry. Davidson and Fox (1989) showed that even among 10-month-old infants, asymmetry in prefrontal activation predicted distress in response to maternal separation. These results are also consistent with earlier studies showing that damage to the left prefrontal cortex is more likely to lead to depressive symptoms than is damage to the right prefrontal cortex (see Davidson, 2004, for a review).

Davidson and colleagues have also used additional techniques to determine exactly how these psychophysiological differences are related to subjective well-being. They believe that asymmetry does not directly influence average hedonic tone. Instead, it is thought to be a diathesis that predicts various aspects of the response to emotional challenge. For instance, in one study, Wheeler, Davidson, and Tomarken (1993) showed that baseline measures of asymmetry predicted reaction to emotional films. Greater left prefrontal activation was associated with more intense positive affect after a positive film; greater right prefrontal activation was associated with more intense negative affect after a negative film. Larson, Sutton, and Davidson (1998) showed that asymmetry may be related to emotion regulation. This group of researchers took advantage of the fact that negative emotions potentiate the startle response. By assessing this startle response at varying intervals after the presentation of a negative stimulus, they could determine how long the potentiating effects of the negative mood lasted. Larson et al. found that prefrontal asymmetry was unrelated to the magnitude of the startle response during the presentation of the stimulus, but this measure did predict startle magnitude after the offset of the stimulus. The authors interpreted this effect to mean that prefrontal asymmetry is associated with automatic recovery (a form of emotion regulation) after the emotional event.

Although much of the research that focuses explicitly on the psychophysiological underpinnings of subjective well-being has centered on hemispheric asymmetry, research in other domains is also relevant. For instance, LeDoux and colleagues (see LeDoux, 2000, and LeDoux & Phelps, 2000, for reviews) have amassed a large body of evidence showing that the amygdala is involved in emotional processing. The amygdala appears to be involved in the conditioning of fear, and LeDoux and Phelps suggested that "the amygdala plays an important role in the assignment of affective significance to sensory events" (p. 158). It is still unclear whether and how individual differences in amygdalar activity are related to subjective well-being, though Abercrombie et al. (1998) provided evidence that metabolic rate in the right amygdala does predict negative affect. Furthermore, Canli et al. (2001) were able to show that greater activation to positive relative to negative pictures in the right amygdala was associated with scores on an extraversion measures. According to the authors, this finding was the first demonstration that the amygdala—which is usually associated with the processing of negative information—is also involved in the processing of positive stimuli.

Other theories focus on general systems that may underlie broad, affective and motivational traits (e.g., Cloninger, 2004; Gray, 1970). For instance, within the context of affiliative behavior, Depue and his colleagues (Depue & Collins, 1999; Depue & Morrone-Strupinsky, 2005) have linked a variety of psychophysiological processes with emotions. Specifically, Depue and Morrone-Strupinsky suggested that affiliative behavior could be broken down into two distinct phases of activity, both of which are intimately involved with psychophysiologically based emotional processes. In an appetitive phase of affiliative behavior, dopamine systems affect the feelings of excitement as an organism approaches a potential reward. In a consummatory phase, opiate systems affect feelings of pleasure, gratification, and liking that result from the attainment of a social reward. Although Depue and Morrone-Strupinsky link individual differences in these systems to the personality trait of affiliation, the processes involved have clear relevance for well-being. Differential functioning in these systems may result in individual differences in the emotions that ultimately promote affiliative behavior.

It is tempting to conclude from this research that differences in these psychophysiological processes provide the link from genes to the observed individual differences in well-being. It is also tempting to infer that because these underlying differences are biologically based, they are difficult, if not impossible, to change. However, Davidson (2004) is careful to point out that such a conclusion would be premature. For instance, animal studies have shown that early environment can directly affect the biological systems that govern emotional response to stressors (e.g., Francis & Meaney, 1999). Furthermore, Davidson and colleagues have shown that some of the physiological indicators that have been linked with subjective well-being can change over time. For instance, an 8-week mindfulness meditation training program led to changes in asymmetry that mirror the individual differences described above (Davidson et al., 2003). Thus, it is important not to infer from these biological differences that subjective well-being cannot change.

The Stability of Subjective Well-Being

Personality is thought to reflect an enduring tendency to behave in similar ways across varying situations and over time. Thus the hallmarks of a personality characteristic are its consistency and stability. For instance, in a meta-analysis of stability estimates, Roberts and Del Vecchio (2000) showed that personality traits were stable even over long periods of time. On average, 6- to 7-year stability coefficients for personality traits ranged from .54 during the college years, to .64 at age 30, to .74 between the ages of 50 and 70. Other researchers have shown that personality characteristics are stable across situations (e.g., Epstein, 1979), though, of course, there has been debate about this issue throughout the history of the field. Nevertheless, if personality plays an important role in subjective well-being, we should also expect happiness and other related variables to be stable over time and across situations.

Numerous studies show that there are consistent and enduring patterns in people's cognitive and emotional evaluations of their lives. When people are asked to evaluate different aspects of their lives (e.g., their relationships, income, health, and environment), there are moderate to strong correlations between the various ratings, even across domains that would not be expected to correlate very strongly. Diener (1984) labeled this a "top-down" effect, and many researchers assume that it is due to the strong and pervasive impact of personality factors on people's evaluation of their lives (Heller, Watson, & Ilies, 2004). Presumably, those individuals with a temperament-based tendency to be happy also tend see the world through rose-colored glasses.

Recently, I investigated the strength of this top-down effect using domain satisfaction ratings from a long-running panel study (Lucas, 2004). Participants were asked to rate their satisfaction on a variety of domains each year for many years. By using hierarchical latent state–trait models, I could separate stable trait variance in domain satisfaction ratings from transient state variance. I was then able to determine how much of the stable variance was shared across domains. If domain satisfaction ratings are primarily determined by top-down effects, then once measurement error is removed, most of the stable variance should be shared across domains. Results showed that, at most, 53% of the stable variance in any of the latent domain satisfaction traits was shared across domains. The remaining variance (up to 72% of the total variance) was unique, stable variance that was not shared across domains. Furthermore, measures of objective variables (e.g., the number of doctors visits, a person's actual income) were related both to the unique and shared components. This finding means that even the shared top-down variance may be sensitive to external circumstances. Together, these results suggest that there are reliable and moderately strong top-down effects on domain satisfaction ratings, but in most cases, these effects do not overwhelm the specific domain variance. In addition, at least some of what appears to be a top-down effect may, in fact, be due to the actual covariation among conditions in people's lives.

Research on top-down and bottom-up processes shows that people evaluate diverse domains in similar ways. But do they actually report similar levels of happiness when they are in diverse situations? To address this question, Diener and Larsen (1984) assessed momentary affect multiple times in a variety of situations.

Cross-situational consistency coefficients were generally quite high. Positive affect at work correlated .70 with positive affect reported during recreation experiences; negative affect at work correlated .74 with negative affect in recreation situations. Similar correlations were found when comparing affect in social situations to affect reported when alone, and when comparing affect in novel situations to affect in typical situations. Even higher correlations were obtained for life satisfaction. Thus, there appear to be stable individual differences in the level of positive and negative affect that people experience, and these individual differences are apparent even in relatively diverse situations.

It is also possible to show that people are able to recognize and report on these stable affective and cognitive reactions, even as their emotions fluctuate on a day-to-day basis. Eid and Diener (2004) used multistate–multitrait–multiconstruct models to estimate how much stable trait variance there was in multiple reports of well-being over time. They asked participants to report on their mood and their global well-being three times over a 2-month period. Using structural equation modeling techniques, Eid and Diener were able to show that most of the variance in subjective well-being measures is stable trait variance. For instance, between 74 and 84% of the variance in the Satisfaction with Life Scale was stable over time. Only a small percentage was occasion-specific state variance, and this state variance tended to be only weakly related to state variance in moods. Importantly, although mood levels did fluctuate considerably over time (i.e., there was less trait variance and more occasion variance in each assessment when compared to global measures), the trait component was strongly correlated with global well-being. Thus, people can recognize and report on stable levels of well-being, and these measures are not strongly influenced by transient affective states.

Of course, showing that happiness is stable over the course of a few weeks or months is only the first step in showing that stable individual differences in well-being exist. It is possible that constructs could be very stable over the short run but still change dramatically over many years or after the experience of major life events. A number of studies have examined the long-term stability of subjective well-being measures, and most show that well-being measures exhibit a moderate degree of stability. Magnus and Diener (1991) reported that the 4-year stability of life satisfaction was .58 and that this correlation only dropped to .52 when self-reports were used to predict informant reports 4 years later. Lucas, Diener, and Suh (1996) reported stability coefficients that ranged from .56 to .61 for positive affect, negative affect, and life satisfaction over a 3-year period. Costa and McCrae (1988) found similarly high correlations between self and spouse ratings over a 6-year period. Watson and Walker (1996) examined the 3-year stability of affect ratings and found correlations that ranged from .36 to .46.

Recently, psychologists have been able to take advantage of existing data sets to examine the stability of well-being measures over even longer periods of time. Fujita and Diener (2005) used data from the German Socio-Economic Panel (GSOEP) study to assess the stability of a single-item life satisfaction measure over a 17-year period. As might be expected from the results reviewed above, year-to-year stabilities were moderately high, in the range of .50–.60. In addition, these stabilities dropped off over time. However, even over the full 17 years of the study, stability coefficients for this single-item measure were approximately .30.

Lucas and Donnellan (2006) used latent state–trait models to determine the extent to which stable trait variance contributed to measures of life satisfaction. Using 9 years of data from the British Household Panel Study, a long-running, nationally representative panel study of households in Britain, we were able to isolate variance due to (1) a stable trait, (2) an autoregressive trait, and (3) occasion-specific variance and measurement error. Consistent with Fujita and Diener's (2005) analysis, about 37% of the variance in life satisfaction in any single year was stable trait variance. This finding suggests that long-term stabilities should bottom-out around .30–.40. We were also able to show that an additional 30% of the variance was accounted for by an autoregressive trait, which accounts for the relatively high stability over shorter periods of time. It is also likely that at least some of the remaining variance within a single year is reliable variance that is unique to the specific year. This suggestion is supported by separate analyses on a multi-item measure of psychological distress. The use of multiple items allowed us to separate measurement error from reliable situation-specific variance, and similar estimates for stable trait, autoregressive trait, and occasion-specific state variance were obtained.

These studies demonstrate that there is moderate stability in subjective well-being over long periods of time. The question then arises as to whether subjective well-being itself should be considered a trait, or whether it is less stable than other trait measures. Fujita and Diener (2005) compared the stability of life satisfaction in the GSOEP to the stability of personality as estimated by Roberts and Del Vecchio (2000). Although 1-year stabilities were similar in size (at least among young samples), the stability of life satisfaction dropped much more quickly (suggesting more of an autoregressive structure). Vaidya, Gray, Haig, and Watson (2002) compared the 2.5-year stability of personality and affect in the same sample. They showed that personality traits were significantly more stable than affect. For instance, stability coefficients for the Big Five personality traits ranged from .59 to .72, whereas the stability of negative affect was .49, and the stability of positive affect was .51. Depending on the autoregressive nature of these effects, these relatively small short-term differences could translate into major differences over long periods of time.

Although the stability of subjective well-being suggests that internal factors may play a role, it is possible that stability results from unchanging external circumstances. To address this question, it is necessary to examine stability among individuals who undergo major life events, and to determine whether these life events have an impact on well-being. Early research suggested that life events do not affect stability and that people inevitably adapt back to their temperament-based well-being setpoints. For instance, Costa, McCrae and Zonderman (1987) examined the stability of well-being among individuals who had major changes in life circumstances (e.g., divorce, widowhood, or job loss) and individuals who had very few changes in life circumstances. Stability estimates were only slightly lower in the high-change group. Similarly, researchers who have investigated the impact of life events have often emphasized people's somewhat remarkable ability to adapt (e.g., Brickman, Coates, & Janoff-Bulman, 1978). These results supported the prevailing view that people inevitably return to temperament-based setpoints following major life events (see Diener et al., 2006, for a review).

However, more recent evidence challenges the idea that life events have little to no effect on well-being. As Watson (2004) has pointed out, small differences in stability can be important over the long term, and recent evidence confirms that life events do seem to affect the stability of well-being measures. In fact, these effects appear to be stronger than the effects on other personality traits. For instance, Vaidya et al. (2002) showed that life events during a 2-year period had a bigger effect on mean levels and stability coefficients for affect variables as compared to personality variables.

More importantly, recent longitudinal studies examining the effect of major life events show that such events can have strong and lasting impact on people's happiness. For instance, Lucas, Clark, Georgellis, and Diener (2003) showed that although adaptation to marriage is relatively quick (occurring within a couple of years), adaptation to widowhood is much slower (taking about 8 years). Perhaps more importantly, adaptation effects varied considerably across individuals. Some people reported large drops in satisfaction and very little recovery over time. Others reported only minor changes and/or a complete return to baseline. Thus, for some individuals, widowhood (and even marriage) was associated with lasting changes in happiness.

Furthermore, research on other life events shows that even when average trajectories are examined, adaptation is often not complete. Lucas, Clark, Georgellis, and Diener (2004) showed that unemployment has lasting effects on happiness, and Lucas (2005) showed that divorce also appears to have permanent effects. Most recently, Lucas (2007) used two nationally representative panel studies to show that the onset of a long-term disability has relatively large and lasting effects on measures of life satisfaction. For instance, people who experienced severe disabilities dropped over a full standard deviation from their own baseline levels, and these levels did not show any trends back to baseline, even though participants were followed for an average of 8 years after onset. These results are consistent with most cross-sectional studies comparing individuals with disabilities to population norms (e.g., Dijkers, 1997). In fact, Lucas (2007) and Diener et al. (2006) showed that much of the research on the effects of disability have been misinterpreted and that these conditions often have lasting effects on subjective well-being.

Together, these results have a number of important implications for research on subjective well-being. First, there is some degree of stability even over long periods of time. It appears as though this stability is not due entirely to stable life circumstances. Even those individuals who undergo major life changes report moderate stability over time. Thus, this research provides evidence for the influence of personality on well-being measures. However, stability estimates are not so high as to suggest that happiness cannot change. Even among samples who are not selected based on their experience of major life events, stabilities drop over time, bottoming out at around .30–.40. These results suggest that approximately one-third of the variance in well-being measures is stable variance that changes only slightly over time. Furthermore, these stability estimates tend to be lower (often considerably lower in the long term) than the stability of other personality traits such as extraversion, neuroticism, or conscientiousness. Finally, studies of life events show that such events affect both the mean levels and the stability of life satisfaction. Although no positive events have been found that reliably increase well-being, many negative events, including widowhood, divorce, unemployment, and the onset of disability, appear to have lasting or even permanent effects on people's happiness. These findings are consistent with the idea that personality contributes to do, but does not completely set, long-term levels of well-being.

Associations with Specific Personality Traits

If personality matters for subjective well-being, then it should be possible to identify specific personality characteristics that are reliably associated with well-being and to develop theories about the processes that link these constructs. A great deal is known about which personality traits correlate with well-being. In addition, progress in identifying the processes that are responsible for these effects is occurring.

Most research on the links between personality and well-being focuses on the personality traits of extraversion and neuroticism. Although hints about these associations had been seen in the literature for decades (see Lucas, 2000, and Watson & Clark, 1997, for reviews of the historical links between extraversion and positive affect), the first suggestion that these two factors play a primary role in subjective well-being can be traced to Costa and McCrae (1980). They noted that positive and negative affect often form two distinct factors, and they showed that extraversion predicted positive affect, whereas neuroticism predicted negative affect. Although the correlations in their study were actually quite weak (e.g., *r*s around .20), the fact that they were stable over time led Costa and McCrae to suggest that stable individual differences were important for well-being. The pattern of associations that Costa and McCrae found has been replicated often.

Yet, in perhaps the most comprehensive study of personality and subjective well-being, DeNeve and Cooper (1998) questioned whether these two traits were really that important for subjective well-being. They meta-analytically combined the results from hundreds of studies that had examined the correlations between traits and various conceptualizations of subjective well-being. Somewhat surprisingly, their estimates suggested that correlations were only weak to moderate in size. For example, after classifying the various personality traits into five categories representing the Big Five, DeNeve and Cooper found correlations with well-being ranged only from .11 (for openness to experience) to .22 (for neuroticism). Extraversion only correlated .17 with subjective well-being. These correlations were significantly different from zero but surprisingly weak, given the narrative reviews that had appeared at that time. Importantly, they are not that much larger than the correlations with some demographic characteristics, and researchers had often emphasized that effects of this size were too weak to be important.

Unfortunately, the results from DeNeve and Cooper's (1998) meta-analysis are somewhat difficult to interpret. Although it is useful to think about broad categories of traits when summarizing the results of a meta-analysis, the results may be misleading if the classification is inaccurate or too broad. If trait measures that do not really tap the extraversion dimension are included in the extraversion category, then the average correlation with well-being may be diluted. Similarly, if correlations with different forms of subjective well-being are aggregated even when those different components are only weakly correlated with one another, then strong correlations with personality traits may not emerge. Lucas and Fujita (2000) showed that these methodological factors do indeed affect the correlations that are found. They conducted an updated meta-analysis of the correlation between extraversion and positive affect, focusing only on measures that had been designed specifically to assess these two constructs. They found a much higher average correlation of .37.

Although extraversion and neuroticism have been studied most frequently, other traits also exhibit moderate to strong associations with well-being. DeNeve and Cooper (1998) found that repressive defensiveness, trust, hardiness, and some forms of locus of control and self-esteem also exhibited relatively high correlations, though most of these correlations were derived from a very small number of studies. Even within the Big Five, agreeableness and conscientiousness tend to exhibit reliable correlations with positive and negative affect. For instance, in a study involving almost 400 undergraduate students, Vaidya et al. (2002) found that agreeableness correlated −.43 with negative affect (compared to .61 for neu-

roticism) and .34 with positive affect (compared to .42 for extraversion). Similarly, conscientiousness correlated −.33 with negative affect and .42 with positive
affect. Although correlations with agreeableness and conscientiousness have often
been ignored in the literature (for an exception, see Watson & Clark, 1992), they
are often small to moderate in size and may deserve further attention. Finally,
personality traits such as optimism and self-esteem reflect general positive views
about the self and the world, and they too, have been shown to correlate with
well-being (e.g., Lucas et al., 1996; Schimmack & Diener, 2003).

Because these correlations have been shown to be reliable, it is useful to go
on to explain why these associations exist. McCrae and Costa (1991) noted that
there are two general classes of explanations: instrumental and temperamental.
According to instrumental explanations, personality traits affect subjective well-
being indirectly, through choice of situations or the experience of life events. For
example, optimists may expect good things to happen and therefore may try
harder to achieve their goals. This extra effort may actually lead to the attainment
of more beneficial outcomes, and these outcomes may affect happiness. If such a
model were correct, optimism would affect happiness only indirectly through a
number of intervening processes.

In contrast, temperament theories posit that there is a direct link between
personality and affect that does not flow through life events or life experiences.
Many of these theories link extraversion and neuroticism to affect through two
basic motivational systems (see Carver, Sutton, & Scheier, 2000; Elliott &
Thrash, 2002; Tellegen, 1985) that have been proposed and investigated by Gray
(1970, 1981, 1991). According to Gray, much of the variability in personality can
be explained by three fundamental systems: the behavioral activation system
(BAS), which regulates reactions to signals of conditioned reward and non-
punishment; the behavioral inhibition system (BIS), which regulates reactions to
signals of conditioned punishment and nonreward; and the fight–flight system
(FFS), which regulates reactions to signals of unconditioned punishment and
nonreward.

Initially, Gray (1970, 1981) argued that extraversion reflected the relative
strength of the BAS versus the BIS (extraverts were thought to have greater BAS
strength, introverts were thought to have greater BIS strength) and that neuroticism reflects the combined strength of the two systems. According to this model,
extraverts should be prone to experiencing positive, approach-oriented emotions, whereas introverts should be prone to experiencing negative, withdrawal-
oriented emotions. Neurotics should experience all emotions strongly, whereas
stable individuals should experience them less strongly. Gray later revised this
model and suggested that the extraversion–introversion dimension was more
closely aligned with individual differences in BAS strength than it was with individual differences in BIS strength (also see Tellegen, 1985). Thus, extraverts
should be more sensitive than introverts to signals of reward, and this reward sen-

sitivity should be exhibited in the form of enhanced information processing and increased positive emotions when exposed to positive stimuli. Similarly, the neuroticism dimension is now thought to be closely aligned with individual differences in BIS strength, which means that neurotic people should be more sensitive than stable people to signals of punishment. This punishment sensitivity should be exhibited in the form of enhanced information processing and increased negative emotions when exposed to negative stimuli.

Tests of these models have often proceeded by (1) ruling out simple instrumental hypotheses and (2) testing specific temperament hypotheses that can derived from Gray's model. For example, Lucas, Le, and Dyrenforth (in press) noted that there are two relatively simple instrumental hypotheses that could explain the association between extraversion and positive affect. First, because extraverts are more sociable than introverts, extraverts may participate in more social activity than introverts. If social activity tends to be pleasurable, then this increased social activity may account for extraverts' greater happiness. Alternatively, extraverts and introverts may engage in similar amounts of social activity, but because extraverts are more sociable than introverts, extraverts may enjoy these situations more than introverts do. Lucas et al. (in press) used daily- and moment-report techniques to examine the types of activities in which extraverts and introverts engaged and to examine how their positive affect changed over time. Although extraverts did engage in some types of social activities more than introverts, these differences were not large and could not account for much of the association between extraversion and positive affect. In addition, extraverts did not respond more positively to social situations than did introverts, which refutes the second explanation. Thus, even after controlling for differential participation in and reaction to social situations, extraverts were still happier than introverts.

Other researchers have tried to find more direct support for temperament-based theories. For instance, in two early studies, Larsen and Ketelaar (1989, 1991) showed that neurotics were more reactive than stable individuals to negative mood inductions, whereas extraverts were more reactive than introverts to positive mood inductions. These effects have been replicated a number of times (e.g., Gomez, Cooper, & Gomez, 2000; Gross, Sutton, & Ketelaar, 1998; Morrone, Depue, Scherer, & White, 2000; Morrone-Strupinsky & Depue, 2004; Rusting & Larsen, 1997; Zelenski & Larsen, 1999). However, a number of other studies has failed to replicate the extraversion reactivity effect, and Lucas and Baird (2004) used meta-analytic techniques to show that the effect is not robust.

One possible explanation for the discrepant results is that positive emotional reactivity may not be a reliable individual difference (at least when assessed by self-report techniques). Lucas, Baird, and Le (2006) administered four different mood-induction procedures to participants over the course of 9 months. They also asked participants to participate in two separate week-long experience sampling sessions during this period. They then calculated an index of positive emotional reactivity for each of the four mood inductions and the two experience sampling sessions. Results showed that these reactivity indexes were not only uncorrelated with extraversion, they were also only weakly correlated with one another. Therefore it is questionable whether reliable individual differences in positive emotional reactivity can be assessed using self-report techniques. However, some attempts to address this question using psychophysiological measures have been fruitful (e.g., Canli et al., 2001).

Although space constraints prevent a discussion here, researchers have begun to use a variety of paradigms to understand the processes that link personality and subjective well-being. For instance, researchers have used attentional paradigms to understand how personality and emotional factors influence attention to rewarding and punishing stimuli (e.g., Derryberry & Reed, 1994). Similarly, researchers have used a variety of paradigms from cognitive psychology to explore the processes that underlie these effects (e.g., Rusting, 1998; Robinson & Compton, Chapter 11, this volume). These cognitive and emotional processes have also been linked with specific psychophysiological processes (e.g., Canli, 2004). Thus, future multimethod research will likely provide important information about the dynamic processes that link personality and subjective well-being.

In summary, there is now a large body of research linking personality and well-being. The most studied links are those between extraversion and positive affect, and between neuroticism and negative affect. However, many other traits, including agreeableness, conscientiousness, optimism, and self-esteem, have also exhibited replicable and moderately strong associations with one or more well-being constructs. It is still unclear whether each of these traits contributes unique variance in the prediction of subjective well-being, and future multitrait–multimethod studies will be needed to resolve this issue. In addition, the processes that are responsible for the observed associations have not been clarified. But, fortunately, theoretical progress has been made, and there are now a number of detailed models that strive to explain these links. Subjective well-being researchers are getting closer to an understanding of the behavioral, cognitive, and physiological processes that are responsible for these replicable associations.

Summary

The research reviewed in this chapter shows that stable internal factors clearly play an important role in subjective well-being. Positive affect, negative affect, and life satisfaction are moderately heritable, stable over time, and moderately to strongly correlated with psychophysiological indicators and personality traits such as extraversion and neuroticism. In contrast, external factors such as income, health, and even the number of friends that a person has (Lucas & Dyrenforth, 2006) are all only weakly correlated with well-being. Thus, we can tell more about a person's subjective well-being by asking about his or her personality than by examining the conditions in his or her life.

It may be tempting to conclude from this evidence that happiness cannot change and that subjective well-being researchers can ignore external factors. If so, interventions designed to increase well-being would likely not work. However, a close examination of the research reviewed in this chapter shows that such a conclusion would almost surely be wrong. Enough research has been conducted that we can provide precise estimates of the size of the effects that were reviewed, and these estimates leave quite a bit of room for change and external influence. For instance, it seems clear that approximately 30–50% of the variance in well-being at a single occasion can be explained by genetic effects. Although these estimates may be higher for the stable component of well-being, it appears that only about 30% of the variance in well-being measures is actually stable over long periods of time. Thus, quite a bit of change occurs over time, and this change is likely related to events that occur in people's lives (even if researchers have yet to specify exactly which events are responsible). Finally, personality traits matter, but we do not know exactly what processes underlie these effects. By studying these associations, it may be possible to understand what makes extraverts happy and neurotic people unhappy, and this knowledge may lead to successful interventions. Thus, research on the links between personality and well-being fits well within a comprehensive approach to understand the factors that influence and can lead to lasting changes in subjective well-being.

References

Abercrombie, H. C., Schaefer, S. M., Larson, C. L., Oakes, T. R., Lindgren, K. A., Holden, J. E., et al. (1998). Metabolic rate in the right amygdala predicts negative affect in depressed patients. *Neuroreport: An International Journal for the Rapid Communication of Research in Neuroscience, 9*, 3301–3307.

Argyle, M. (1999). Causes and correlates of happiness. In D. Kahneman, E. Diener, & N. Schwarz (Eds.), *Well-being: The foundations of hedonic psychology* (pp. 353–373). New York: Sage.

Baumeister, R. F., & Leary, M. R. (1995). The need to belong: Desire for interpersonal attachments as a fundamental human motivation. *Psychological Bulletin, 117*, 497–529.

Brickman, P., Coates, D., & Janoff-Bulman, R. (1978). Lottery winners and accident victims: Is happiness relative? *Journal of Personality and Social Psychology, 36*, 917–927.

Canli, T. (2004). Functional brain mapping of extraversion and neuroticism: Learning from individual differences in emotion processing. *Journal of Personality, 72*, 1105–1132.

Canli, T., Zhao, Z., Desmond, J. E., Kang, E., Gross, J., & Gabrieli, J. D. E. (2001). An fMRI study of personality influences on brain reactivity to emotional stimuli. *Behavioral Neuroscience, 115,* 33–42.

Carver, C. S., Sutton, S. K., & Scheier, M. F. (2000). Action, emotion, and personality: Emerging conceptual integration. *Personality and Social Psychology Bulletin, 26,* 741–751.

Cloninger, C. R. (2004). *Feeling good: The science of well-being.* New York: Oxford University Press.

Costa, P. T., & McCrae, R. R. (1980). Influence of extraversion and neuroticism on subjective well-being: Happy and unhappy people. *Journal of Personality and Social Psychology, 38,* 668–678.

Costa, P. T., & McCrae, R. R. (1988). Personality in adulthood: A six-year longitudinal study of self-reports and spouse ratings on the NEO Personality Inventory. *Journal of Personality and Social Psychology, 54,* 853–863.

Costa, P. T., McCrae, R. R., & Zonderman, A. B. (1987). Environmental and dispositional influences on well-being: Longitudinal follow-up of an American national sample. *British Journal of Psychology, 78,* 299–306.

Davidson, R. J. (2004). Well-being and affective style: Neural substrates and bio-behavioural correlates. *Philophical Transactions of the Royal Society of London B, 359,* 1395–1411.

Davidson, R. J., Ekman, P., Saron, C. D., Senulis, J. A., & Friesen, W. V. (1990). Approach/withdrawal and cerebral asymmetry: I. Emotional expression and brain physiology. *Journal of Personality and Social Psychology, 58,* 330–341.

Davidson, R. J., & Fox, N. A. (1989). Frontal brain asymmetry predicts infants' response to maternal separation. *Journal of Abnormal Psychology, 98,* 127–131.

Davidson, R. J., Kabat-Zinn, J., Schumacher, J., Rosenkranz, M., Muller, D., Santorelli, S. F., et al. (2003). Alterations in brain and immune function produced by mindfulness meditation. *Psychosomatic Medicine, 65,* 564–570.

DeNeve, K. M., & Cooper, H. (1998). The happy personality: A meta-analysis of 137 personality traits and subjective well-being. *Psychological Bulletin, 124,* 197–229.

Depue, R. A., & Collins, P. F. (1999). Neurobiology of the structure of personality: Dopamine, facilitation of incentive motivation, and extraversion. *Behavioral and Brain Sciences, 22,* 491–569.

Depue, R. A., & Morrone-Strupinsky, J. V. (2005). A neurobehavioral model of affiliative bonding: Implications for conceptualizing a human trait of affiliation. *Behavioral and Brain Sciences, 28,* 313–395.

Derryberry, D., & Reed, M. A. (1994). Temperament and attention: Orienting toward and away from positive and negative signals. *Journal of Personality and Social Psychology, 66,* 1128–1139.

Diener, E. (1984). Subjective well-being. *Psychological Bulletin, 95,* 542–575.

Diener, E., Emmons, R. A., Larsen, R. J., & Griffin, S. (1985). The Satisfaction with Life Scale. *Journal of Personality Assessment, 49,* 71–75.

Diener, E., & Larsen, R. J. (1984). Temporal stability and cross-situational consistency of affective, behavioral, and cognitive responses. *Journal of Personality and Social Psychology, 47,* 871–883.

Diener, E., Lucas, R. E., & Scollon, C. (2006). Beyond the hedonic treadmill: Revising the adaptation theory of well-being. *American Psychologist, 61*, 305–314.

Diener, E., Suh, E. M., Lucas, R. E., & Smith, H. L. (1999). Subjective well-being: Three decades of progress. *Psychological Bulletin, 125*, 276–302.

Dijkers, M. (1997). Quality of life after spinal cord injury: A meta analysis of the effects of disablement components. *Spinal Cord, 35*, 829–840.

Eid, M., & Diener, E. (2004). Global judgments of subjective well-being: Situational variability and long-term stability. *Social Indicators Research, 65*, 245–277.

Elliot, A. J., & Thrash, T. M. (2002). Approach avoidance motivation in personality: Approach and avoidance temperaments and goals. *Journal of Personality and Social Psychology, 82*, 804–818.

Epstein, S. (1979). The stability of behavior: I. On predicting most of the people much of the time. *Journal of Personality and Social Psychology, 37*, 1097–1126.

Francis, D. D., & Meaney, M. J. (1999). Maternal care and the development of stress responses. *Current Opinion in Neurobiology, 9*, 128–134.

Fredrickson, B. L. (1998). What good are positive emotions? *Review of General Psychology: New Directions in Research on Emotion, 2*, 300–319.

Fujita, F., & Diener, E. (2005). Life satisfaction set point: Stability and change. *Journal of Personality and Social Psychology, 88*, 158–164.

Gilovich, T., & Eibach, R. (2001). The fundamental attribution error where it really counts. *Psychological Inquiry, 12*, 23–26.

Gomez, R., Cooper, A., & Gomez, A. (2000). Susceptibility to positive and negative mood states: Test of Eysenck's, Gray's, and Newman's theories. *Personality and Individual Differences, 29*, 351–366.

Gray, J. A. (1970). The psychophysiological basis of introversion–extraversion. *Behaviour Research and Therapy, 8*, 249–266.

Gray, J. A. (1981). A critique of Eysenck's theory of personality. In H. J. Eysenck (Ed.), *A model for personality* (pp. 246–276). New York: Springer-Verlag.

Gray, J. A. (1991). Neural systems, emotion, and personality. In J. Madden, IV (Ed.), *Neurobiology of learning, emotion, and affect* (pp. 273–306). New York: Raven Press.

Gross, J. J., Sutton, S. K., & Ketelaar, T. (1998). Relations between affect and personality: Support for the affect-level and affective reactivity views. *Personality and Social Psychology Bulletin, 24*, 279–288.

Heller, D., Watson, D., & Ilies, R. (2004). The role of person versus situation in life satisfaction: A critical examination. *Psychological Bulletin, 130*, 574–600.

Johnson, W., McGue, M., & Krueger, R. F. (2005). Personality stability in late adulthood: A behavioral genetic analysis. *Journal of Personality, 73*, 523–551.

Larsen, R. J., & Ketelaar, T. (1989). Extraversion, neuroticism and susceptibility to positive and negative mood induction procedures. *Personality and Individual Differences, 10*, 1221–1228.

Larsen, R. J., & Ketelaar, T. (1991). Personality and susceptibility to positive and negative emotional states. *Journal of Personality and Social Psychology, 61*, 132–140.

Larson, C. L., Sutton, S. K., & Davidson, R. J. (1998). Affective style, frontal EEG asymmetry and the time course of the emotion-modulated startle response. *Psychophysiology, 35*, S52.

LeDoux, J. E. (2000). Emotion circuits in the brain. *Annual Review of Neuroscience, 23,* 155–184.

LeDoux, J. E., & Phelps, E. A. (2000). Emotion networks in the brain. In M. Lewis & J. Haviland-Jones (Eds.), *Handbook of emotion* (2nd ed., pp. 157–172). New York: Guilford Press.

Lucas, R. E. (2000). *Pleasant affect and social behavior: Towards a comprehensive model of extraversion.* Unpublished doctoral dissertation, University of Illinois, Champaign.

Lucas, R. E. (2004, June). *Top-down and bottom-up models of life satisfaction judgments.* Paper presented at the 6th International German Socio-Economic Panel Study User Conference.

Lucas, R. E. (2005). Time does not heal all wounds: A longitudinal study of reaction and adaptation to divorce. *Psychological Science, 16,* 945–950.

Lucas, R. E. (2007). Long-term disability is associated with lasting changes in subjective well-being: Evidence from two nationally representative longitudinal studies. *Journal of Personality and Social Psychology, 92,* 717–730.

Lucas, R. E., & Baird, B. M. (2004). Extraversion and emotional reactivity. *Journal of Personality and Social Psychology, 86,* 473–485.

Lucas, R. E., Baird, B. M., & Le, K. (2006). *The role of positive emotional reactivity in the extraversion/positive affect relation.* Manuscript in preparation, Michigan State University, Lansing.

Lucas, R. E., Clark, A. E., Georgellis, Y., & Diener, E. (2003). Reexamining adaptation and the set point model of happiness: Reactions to changes in marital status. *Journal of Personality and Social Psychology, 84,* 527–539.

Lucas, R. E., Clark, A. E., Georgellis, Y., & Diener, E. (2004). Unemployment alters the set point for life satisfaction. *Psychological Science, 15,* 8–13.

Lucas, R. E., Diener, E., & Suh, E. (1996). Discriminant validity of well-being measures. *Journal of Personality and Social Psychology, 71,* 616–628.

Lucas, R. E., & Donnellan, M. B. (in press). Can happiness change? Using the STARTS model to estimate the stability of subjective well-being. *Journal of Research in Personality.*

Lucas, R. E., & Dyrenforth, P. (2006). Does the existence of social relationships matter for subjective well-being. In K. D. Vohs & E. J. Finkel (Eds.), *Self and relationships: Connecting intrapersonal and interpersonal processes* (pp. 254–273). New York: Guilford Press.

Lucas, R. E., & Fujita, F. (2000). Factors influencing the relation between extraversion and pleasant affect. *Journal of Personality and Social Psychology, 79,* 1039–1056.

Lucas, R. E., Le, K., & Dyrenforth, P. S. (in press). Explaining the extraversion/positive affect relation: Sociability cannot account for extraverts' greater happiness. *Journal of Personality.*

Lykken, D., & Csikszentmihalyi, M. (2001). Happiness—Stuck with what you've got? *The Psychologist, 14,* 470–472.

Lykken, D., & Tellegen, A. (1996). Happiness is a stochastic phenomenon. *Psychological Science, 7,* 186–189.

Lyubomirsky, S., Sheldon, K. M., & Schkade, D. (2005). Pursuing happiness: The architecture of sustainable change. *Review of General Psychology, 9,* 111–131.

Magnus, K., & Diener, E. (1991, May). *A longitudinal analysis of personality, life events, and subjective well-being*. Paper presented at the 63rd annual meeting of the Midwestern Psychological Association, Chicago.

McCrae, R. R., & Costa, P. T. (1991). Adding *Liebe und Arbeit*: The full five-factor model and well-being. *Personality and Social Psychology Bulletin, 17,* 227–232.

McGue, M., Bacon, S., & Lykken, D. T. (1993). Personality stability and change in early adulthood: A behavioral genetic analysis. *Developmental Psychology, 29,* 96–109.

Morrone, J. V., Depue, R. A., Scherer, A. J., & White, T. L. (2000). Film-induced incentive motivation and positive activation in relation to agentic and affiliative components of extraversion. *Personality and Individual Differences, 29,* 199–216.

Morrone-Strupinsky, J. V., & Depue, R. A. (2004). Differential relation of two distinct, film-induced positive emotional states to affiliative and agentic extraversion. *Personality and Individual Differences, 36,* 1109–1126.

Nes, R. B., Roysamb, E., Tambs, K., Harris, J. R., & Reichborn-Kjennerud, T. (2006). Subjective well-being: Genetic and environmental contributions to stability and change. *Psychological Medicine, 36,* 1033–1042.

Riemann, R., Angleitner, A., Borkenau, P., & Eid, M. (1998). Genetic and environmental sources of consistency and variability in positive and negative mood. *European Journal of Personality, 12,* 345–364.

Roberts, B. W., & Del Vecchio, W. F. (2000). The rank-order consistency of personality traits from childhood to old age: A quantitative review of longitudinal studies. *Psychological Bulletin, 126,* 3–25.

Roysamb, E., Harris, J. R., Magnus, P., Vitterso, J., & Tambs, K. (2002). Subjective well-being: Sex-specific effects of genetic and environmental factors. *Personality and Individual Differences, 32,* 211–223.

Roysamb, E., Tambs, K., Reichborn-Kjennerud, T., Neale, M. C., & Harris, J. R. (2003). Happiness and health: Environmental and genetic contributions to the relationship between subjective well-being, perceived health, and somatic illness. *Journal of Personality and Social Psychology, 85,* 1136–1146.

Rusting, C. L. (1998). Personality, mood, and cognitive processing of emotional information: Three conceptual frameworks. *Psychological Bulletin, 124,* 165–196.

Rusting, C. L., & Larsen, R. J. (1997). Extraversion, neuroticism, and susceptibility to positive and negative affect: A test of two theoretical models. *Personality and Individual Differences, 22,* 607–612.

Schimmack, U., & Diener, E. (2003). Predictive validity of explicit and implicit self-esteem for subjective well-being. *Journal of Research in Personality, 37,* 100–106.

Schwarz, N., & Strack, F. (1999). Reports of subjective well-being: Judgmental processes and their methodological implications. In D. Kahneman, E. Diener, & N. Schwarz (Eds.), *Well-being: The foundations of hedonic psychology* (pp. 61–84). New York: Sage.

Seligman, M. E. P., Steen, T. A., Park, N., & Peterson, C. (2005). Positive psychology progress: Empirical validation of interventions. *American Psychologist, 60,* 410–421.

Stubbe, J. H., Posthuma, D., Boomsma, D. I., & De Geus, E. J. C. (2005). Heritability of life satisfaction in adults: A twin-family study. *Psychological Medicine, 35,* 1581–1588.

Tellegen, A. (1985). Structures of mood and personality and their relevance to assessing anxiety, with an emphasis on self-report. In A. H. Tuma & J. D. Maser (Eds.), *Anxiety and the anxiety disorders* (pp. 681–706). Hillsdale, NJ: Erlbaum.

Tellegen, A., Lykken, D. T., Bouchard, T. J., Wilcox, K. J., Segal, N. L., & Rich, S.

(1988). Personality similarity in twins reared apart and together. *Journal of Personality and Social Psychology, 54,* 1031–1039.

Tomarken, A. J., Davidson, R. J., Wheeler, R. E., & Doss, R. C. (1992). Individual differences in anterior brain asymmetry and fundamental dimensions of emotion. *Journal of Personality and Social Psychology, 62,* 676–687.

Tomarken, A. J., Davidson, R. J., Wheeler, R. E., & Kinney, L. (1992). Psychometric properties of resting anterior EEG asymmetry: Temporal stability and internal consistency. *Psychophysiology, 29,* 576–592.

Turkheimer, E. (2000). Three laws of behavior genetics and what they mean. *Current Directions in Psychological Science, 9,* 160–164.

Urry, H. L., Nitschke, J. B., Dolski, I., Jackson, D. C., Dalton, K. M., Mueller, C. J., et al. (2004). Making a life worth living: Neural correlates of well-being. *Psychological Science, 15,* 367–372.

Vaidya, J. G., Gray, E. K., Haig, J., & Watson, D. (2002). On the temporal stability of personality: Evidence for differential stability and the role of life experiences. *Journal of Personality and Social Psychology, 83,* 1469–1484.

Veenhoven, R. (1995). The cross-national pattern of happiness: Test of predictions implied in three theories of happiness. *Social Indicators Research, 34,* 33–68.

Watson, D. (2004). Stability versus change, dependability versus error: Issues in the assessment of personality over time. *Journal of Research in Personality, 38,* 319–350.

Watson, D., & Clark, L. A. (1992). On traits and temperament: General and specific factors of emotional experience and their relation to the five-factor model. *Journal of Personality, 60,* 441–476.

Watson, D., & Clark, L. A. (1997). Extraversion and its positive emotional core. In R. Hogan & J. A. Johnson (Eds.), *Handbook of personality psychology* (pp. 767–793). San Diego, CA: Academic Press.

Watson, D., & Walker, L.-M. (1996). The long-term stability and predictive validity of trait measures of affect. *Journal of Personality and Social Psychology, 70,* 567–577.

Wheeler, R. E., Davidson, R. J., & Tomarken, A. J. (1993). Frontal brain asymmetry and emotional reactivity: A biological substrate of affective style. *Psychophysiology, 30,* 82–89.

Wilson, W. (1967). Correlates of avowed happiness. *Psychological Bulletin, 67,* 294–306.

Zelenski, J. M., & Larsen, R. J. (1999). Susceptibility to affect: A comparison of three personality taxonomies. *Journal of Personality, 67,* 761–791.

10

Happiness and the Invisible Threads of Social Connection

The Chicago Health, Aging, and Social Relations Study

John T. Cacioppo, Louise C. Hawkley,
Ariel Kalil, M. E. Hughes, Linda Waite,
and Ronald A. Thisted

Studies of the effects of social and psychological factors on happiness have tended to fall outside the purview of the National Institutes of Health, which are generally organized around categories of human diseases (e.g., National Institute of Allergy and Infectious Diseases; National Institute of Arthritis and Musculoskeletal and Skin Diseases; National Cancer Institute; National Heart, Lung, and Blood Institute; National Institute on Alcohol Abuse and Alcoholism). Although people's desire to achieve and maintain happiness can be a strong motivational force, research on happiness languished until Ed Diener and like-minded scientists began their seminal work in the area (e.g., see Kahneman, Diener, & Schwarz, 1999).

Our evolutionary heritage has resulted in a variety of mechanisms that motivate us to achieve or maintain pleasant affective states. Hunger, thirst, cold, and pain each alerts us to tissue needs and motivates us to act to rectify the apposite need. These motivations are so effective in resolving tissue needs, one might argue, that people have time to pursue higher goals that make them happy and contented. But happiness is not simply the opposite of pain, sadness, or discomfort (Cacioppo, Gardner, & Berntson, 1999). For instance, Diener and colleagues found that happiness, as measured with the Satisfaction with Life Scale (SWLS; Diener, Emmons, Larsen, & Griffin, 1985), is correlated inversely with negative moods, but the magnitude of these correlations is modest, suggesting that happiness is more than the absence of pain or suffering. Moreover, Pavot, Diener, Colvin, and Sandvik (1991) reported a factor analysis that shows happiness items loading separately from positive affect and negative affect.

Research over the past two decades has greatly advanced our understanding of positive emotions in general. Age, gender, ethnicity, marital status, education, and income together have been found to account for only 8–20% of the variance in happiness (e.g., Campbell, Converse, & Rodgers, 1976; DeNeve & Cooper, 1998). Although the effect is not large, levels of happiness appear to increase in older age (Carstensen, Pasupathi, Mayr, & Nesselroade, 2000; Stock, Okun, Haring, & Witter, 1983). Moreover, household income has generally been related to happiness only at low levels of income; once necessities can be afforded, the association between money and happiness appears to be quite weak (see Biswas-Diener, Chapter 15, this volume). Positive illusions such as overly positive self-evaluations or self-esteem, unrealistic perceptions of agency or control, and exaggerated optimism (Taylor & Brown, 1988) promote happiness (Myers & Diener, 1995) at the expense of reality, which in addition to adaptation and social comparison standards, may help account for the transient impact of life events on happiness (see Shmotkin, 2005). Finally, research on happiness reminds one of Garrison Keillor's Lake Woebegone (where all the children are above average): The majority of the people examined by Diener and Diener (1996) responded above the midpoint when indicating their level of happiness.

Our purpose here is to investigate the social and behavioral correlates of individual differences in happiness and the determinants of changes in happiness over time in adults 50–68 years of age living in a large metropolitan area. The 2002 U.S. Census indicates that this age group represents approximately 18% of the population, owns over half of all financial assets in the United States, accounts for more than half of the funds spent annually on new car sales, and generally drives the overall U.S. economy. Most have also spent their adult life working and are now nearing or have reached retirement.

We investigated the correlates and determinants of happiness in the Chicago Health, Aging, and Social Relations Study (CHASRS), a population-based longitudinal study of 229 English-speaking African Americans, Hispanic Americans, and European Americans born between 1935 and 1952 and living in a large metropolitan area (Cook County, Illinois) and first tested in 2002. The participants were selected using a multistage probability sampling design in which African Americans and Hispanic Americans were oversampled and gender equality maintained. First, a sample of households was selected; then sampled households were screened by telephone for the presence of an age-eligible person who was sufficiently ambulatory to come to the University of Chicago for a day-long visit to the laboratory. Age-eligible persons were then asked to participate in the study. If a household contained more than one age-eligible person, the person with the most recent birthday was selected. A quota sampling strategy was used to achieve an approximately equal distribution of respondents across the six gender by race/ ethnic group combinations.

The response rate among eligible persons was 45%, comparable to those for other well-conducted telephone surveys. This response rate assumes that households for which the presence of an eligible individual was unknown (23% of all households) were just as likely to contain an eligible individual as households that were successfully screened. Considering that participation in the CHASRS involved spending an entire day at the university each year for 5 years, the response rate was good. The final sample size for the first wave of CHASRS was 229 individuals born between 1935 and 1952; 52% female; mean age of 57.4 years; 34.4% African Americans, 28.3% Hispanic Americans, and 37.3% European Americans; 61.3% married; with a mean of 13.5 years of education and a mean household income of $67,728. Comparison of the characteristics of the CHASRS sample with those of the 2002 wave of the Health and Retirement Study (HRS), a nationally representative, longitudinal telephone study of persons born 1947 or earlier, confirmed that the CHASRS sample was representative of middle-age and older Americans living in urban settings.

Participants arrived at the laboratory at around 8:30 A.M. for approximately 8 hours of testing, including informed consent, questionnaires, interviews, lunch, and physiological and genetic assessments. As part of the testing, participants completed the five-item SWLS (Diener et al., 1985), a measure of happiness and subjective well-being, and the UCLA loneliness scale (Russell, Peplau, & Cutrona, 1980), a measure of the extent to which one's social relationships are satisfactory. Given the notion that negative and positive states are not redundant, our use of loneliness to index relationship satisfaction warrants an explanation. According to their discrepancy model of loneliness, Peplau and Perlman (1982; Perlman & Peplau, 1998) conceptualize loneliness as a mismatch between needed or desired and actual social relationships. Loneliness scores range from 20 to 80, with lower scores indicating more relationship satisfaction. The mean score in the CHASRS is 36, which reflects generally high levels of relationship satisfaction.

Diener and colleagues have investigated the association between happiness and positive and negative affect (e.g., Eid & Diener, 2004), whereas we focused on more specific mood states as measured by the Profile of Mood States (POMS; McNair, Lorr, & Droppleman, 1992) scale. As summarized in Table 10.1, we found that happiness was correlated with the subscales of Tension/Anxiety, Con-

**TABLE 10.1. Correlations between Happiness
and Positive and Negative Mood on POMS Subscales**

	Happiness (subjective well-being)
Tension/Anxiety	−.24★★ (212)
Confusion/Bewilderment	−.14★ (205)
Fatigue/Inertia	−.30★★ (210)
Depression/Dejection	−.31★★ (212)
Vigor/Activity	.30★★ (213)
Anger/Hostility	−.09, n.s. (212)

Note. POMS, Profile of Mood States. ns in parentheses.
★ p < .05; ★★ p < .001.

fusion/Bewilderment, Fatigue/Inertia, and Depression/Dejection, and happiness was positively correlated with Vigor. Interestingly, happiness was unrelated to Anger/Hostility in these older adults.

The Disposition of Happiness

Happiness, as Diener and colleagues have demonstrated, is not simply a transient mood state (Suh, Diener, & Fujita, 1996). In the CHASRS sample, the 1-year test–retest stability of measured happiness ranges from .70 to .73, and the 2-year test–retest stability is .68 (ps < .001). These test–retest reliabilities suggest that happiness has a strong dispositional component, a notion that is further evidenced by the findings that the happiness of lottery victors and that of accident victims who are left quadriplegic nearly returns to their prior levels within 2 years (Brickman, Coates, & Janoff-Bulman, 1978). If happiness is a disposition, however, it is not reducible to traditional personality constructs. Prior research has shown an association between happiness and surgency, agreeableness, emotional stability, and conscientiousness. In our study of older adults (see Table 10.2), we found that happiness was weakly correlated with agreeableness and surgency, modestly correlated with emotional stability and optimism, and more strongly correlated with loneliness and self-esteem.

Kwan et al. (1997; see also Benet-Martínez & Karakitapoğlu-Aygün, 2003) determined that personality (e.g., surgency, emotional stability) was associated

TABLE 10.2. Correlations between Happiness and Dispositional Variables

	Happiness (subjective well-being)
Agreeableness	.11, n.s. (205)
Surgency	.13, $p = .06$ (204)
Emotional stability	.21★ (207)
Optimism	.27★★ (214)
Loneliness	−.43★★ (214)
Self-esteem	.48★★ (212)

Note. ns in parentheses.
★ $p < .01$; ★★ $p < .001$.

with happiness through its effects on self-esteem and relationship satisfaction. We tested this model using measures of self-esteem and loneliness (the higher the score, the lower the relationship satisfaction) to determine if this structure would be found in a population-based urban sample of older adults, as well. Our results replicated the prior research in this area: (1) When surgency, agreeableness, and emotional stability were entered simultaneously to predict happiness, the coefficient for emotional stability remained statistically significant; and (2) when loneliness and self-esteem were next entered, both predicted happiness, and these variables fully mediated the association between personality (extraversion, agreeableness, and emotional stability) and happiness (see Table 10.3).

TABLE 10.3. Standardized Regression Coefficients for Dispositional Variables Predicting Happiness

	Model 1	Model 2
Agreeableness	0.039	−0.001
Surgency	0.066	−0.11
Emotional stability	0.177★	0.027
Loneliness		0.368★★★
Self-esteem		−0.251★★

Note. n = 201.
★ $p < .05$; ★★ $p < .01$; ★★★ $p < .001$.

We generally replicated the work of Kwan, Bond, and Singelis (1997) and Benet-Martínez and Karakitapoğlu-Aygün (2003), showing that happiness is a stable individual difference that is predicted distally by emotional stability primarily and by both relationship satisfaction/loneliness and feelings of self-worth more proximally. Leary's sociometer theory (Leary & Baumeister, 2000; Leary, Tambor, Terdal, & Downs, 1995) suggests that self-esteem is an internal, psychological system that gauges the degree to which an individual feels included versus excluded by other people. Accordingly, self-esteem and loneliness are strongly associated ($r = -.57$), making noteworthy the fact that they both significantly predict happiness.

These analyses do not specify whether satisfying social relationships make people happy, happy people are more likely to perceive or develop satisfying relationships, or a third variable (e.g., optimism) contributes to both perceptions of satisfying relationships and happy states. To test whether optimism might be operating as a third variable that contributes to both happiness and positive perceptions of self and others, we extended the analyses described above by including optimism in the first stage of the model to determine if it contributed additionally to dispositional influences on happiness. The results indicated that when optimism was entered with surgency, agreeableness, and emotional stability, only optimism was significantly associated with individual differences in happiness ($\beta = .28$, $p < .01$). That is, the Big 5 personality traits were no longer related to happiness. As before, however, when we added self-esteem and relationship satisfaction (loneliness) to the models, none of the personality variables, including optimism, predicted happiness, whereas both relationship satisfaction and self-esteem were significantly related to happiness.

In sum, individual differences in happiness appear to be solidly anchored in the invisible threads of connections to others.

Social Circumstances and Happiness

Demographic factors such as ethnicity, household income, and material wealth have not been found to be strongly related to happiness (e.g., see Biswas-Diener, Chapter 15, this volume). Other demographic factors, such as age and marital status, have been associated with happiness, however. According to Carstensen's socioemotional selective theory (Carstensen, Isaacowitz, & Charles, 1999; Carstensen & Fredrikson, 1998), people have a sense of their time left in life, and perceived boundaries on time direct attention to emotionally meaningful aspects of life. When time is perceived as abundant, an individual's motivation and goals center on acquiring new information, expanding horizons, and pursuing achievements. When time is perceived to be limited, positive emotional experience becomes the preeminent motivation, and the individual tunes attentional, cognitive, and social investments to enhance emotional closeness and positive affect. In an illustrative study, Nolen-Hoeksema and Ahrens (2002) investigated the levels of depressive symptoms in 25- to 35-year-old, 45- to 55-year-old, and 65- to 75-year-old adults. These groups were selected to represent different life circumstances and social histories. Results indicated that as a group, the older adults reported the lowest levels of depressive symptomatology. We recently replicated the inverse association between age and depressive symptomatology in the CHASRS (Cacioppo, Hughes, Waite, Hawkley, & Thisted, 2006). But happiness and depressive symptomatology are not simply mirror opposites. What is the association between demographic factors such as age and happiness in the CHASRS?

Bivariate analyses confirm that age was associated with happiness, but so were household income and marital status (see Table 10.4). When the demographic characteristics of age, gender, ethnicity, marital status, and household income were entered simultaneously, only age (β = .21, p < .01) and household income (β = .18, p < .02) predicted happiness. Contrary to expectations, the association between household income and happiness indicates that this association was not limited to the very poor (see Figure 10.1).

It may be that a person with higher household income also has more social network roles (e.g., spouse, relative, friend, neighbor, volunteer, group member, coworker), and it is the diversity of social roles rather than income per se that is associated with happiness. To test this reasoning, we next entered Cohen's social diversity index (the number of social network roles; Cohen, Doyle, Skoner, Rabin, & Gwaltney, 1997) into the multiple regression equation. The results indicated that age (β = .22, p < .001) and household income (β = .17, p < .02) net of education and other demographic characteristics continued to be associated with happiness, whereas the social diversity index was only weakly related to happiness (β = .13, p < .08).

Social networks can be quantified not only in terms of social diversity but also in terms of network size (number of persons with whom participants speak at

TABLE 10.4. Standardized Regression Coefficients for Demographic Variables Predicting Happiness

Age	0.210**
Female gender	−0.076
Black race/ethnicity	−0.143
Hispanic race/ethnicity	0.002
Married or living with a partner	0.105
Household income	0.164*

Note. n = 201.
* p < .05; ** p < .01.

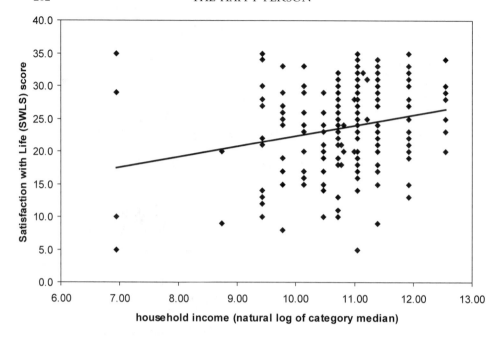

FIGURE 10.1. Happiness is associated with household income across a range of incomes from less than $5,000/year to more than $200,000/year.

least once every 2 weeks) and network integration (e.g., marital status, church attendance, voluntary group memberships, frequency of contact with friends and family). We repeated our analyses using each of these social network indices in place of Cohen's social diversity index. The results were unchanged: Both measures of social network predicted happiness, but the inclusion of these network measures did not substantively reduce the association between happiness and age *or* household income.

Finally, we examined the role of wealth in predicting happiness. Although wealth and household income tend to covary, wealth may act as an additional buffer from unexpected financial stressors. Moreover, debt may tax psychological resources, perhaps especially in a sample that is transitioning to retirement. Inspection of the overall means on measures of wealth revealed that only 30% of the respondents in our population-based sample of middle-age and older adults was debt free, the median debt was under $5,000, and 7.9% carried more than $25,000 in debt. Home equity was the primary source of wealth in this sample, with the median home equity being from $50,000 to $100,000, the median car value falling between $2,000 and $10,000, the median bank deposit being between $1,000 and $5,000, and the majority of respondents indicating that they possessed no stocks, pension, or retirement investments. As summarized in Table

**TABLE 10.5. Correlations between Happiness
and Wealth and Debt Variables**

	Happiness (subjective well-being)
Home equity	.18* (180)
Car value	.18* (187)
Stock value	.22* (175)
Defined pension plan value	.29* (190)
Bank account value	.28* (185)
Debt	−.19* (192)

Note. ns in parentheses.
★ $p < .01$.

10.5, regression analyses confirmed that happiness was negatively associated with debt and positively associated with home equity, car value, stock value, defined pension plan, and bank account value. Multiple regression analyses indicated that (smaller) accrued debt predicted happiness net of demographic characteristics ($\beta = -.16$, $p < .04$). When household income was added to the model, the coefficient for debt was reduced ($\beta = -.12$, $p < .09$), whereas income remained related to happiness ($\beta = .27$, $p < .01$). When defined pension plan was added, however, the pension plan emerged as a significant association ($\beta = .23$, $p < .001$), and the association between happiness and household income was eliminated ($\beta = .11$, $p > .15$). These data raise the interesting hypothesis that happiness is not as much about what can be purchased with current income as it is about having future prospects free of significant financial concerns.

The first year of data collection in the CHASRS was 2002. With the economic downturn and the September 11 attacks in 2001, the first year of CHASRS occurred during a difficult time in this country. Thirty-five percent of the respondents reported a negative financial life event during the prior year, and 11% reported a negative life event in the work domain (e.g., involuntary unemployment). Each of these categories of life events was related to happiness, and it is possible that income emerged as an important predictor of happiness in the first wave of CHASRS because the 12 months prior to subjects' participation in 2002 was such a difficult year for the U.S. economy. However, when cross-sectional data from the most recent year were examined (i.e., 2004), the multiple regression for happiness indicated that income and age were again significantly related to happiness (βs = .32 and .19, ps < .01, n = 182). Thus, the prediction of happiness by household income net other demographic variables were not unique to 2002.

In sum, age and household income were related to individual differences in happiness. As in prior research, these associations were small but significant. Loneliness was also predictive of happiness, and social network measures did not account for this relationship. This finding is consistent with prior research showing that it is the quality rather than quantity of the interpersonal relationships that is important.

Stress and Happiness

Exposure to stressful life events is known to make people unhappy, and the participants in the CHASRS were no exception. We found that the number of negative life events the prior year (expressed as a log score to normalize the distribution) was negatively related to happiness. We additionally found that the total number of objective chronic stressors to which participants had been exposed was negatively related to happiness. Although all of the subscales were negatively related to happiness, the happiness of middle-age to older adults in urban U.S. settings appears to be most damaged by money and financial stressors, followed in order of magnitude by problems with their social life and recreation, love and marriage, residence/housing, work, family and children, health, and general stressors.

Individual differences in coping styles have also been found to relate to health (Carver, Scheier, & Weintraub, 1989). To investigate whether coping styles were related to happiness, we calculated the associations between happiness and the Coping Inventory for Stressful Situations (CISS; Cosway, Endler, Sadler, & Deary, 2000) subscales of Task-Oriented Coping, Emotion-Focused Coping, and Avoidance Coping. None of these coping styles was related to happiness (see Table 10.6). We also calculated associations between happiness and four coping styles measured by the COPE instrument (Carver et al., 1989). Active coping and instrumental support seeking were not associated with happiness, but emotional support seeking and behavioral withdrawal were significantly related to happiness (see Table 10.6). Support-seeking behavior is an adaptive response to stress, whereas behavioral withdrawal is generally considered maladaptive. These results are consistent with prior results showing that happiness is associated with good coping responses (reviewed in Lyubomirsky, King, & Diener, 2005) and may point to important risk factors or points of intervention for low subjective well-being in older adults.

We next examined the strength of the association between stress hormones and happiness to determine whether these putative indices of allostatic load

TABLE 10.6. Correlations between Happiness and Measures of Stress and Coping

	Happiness (subjective well-being)
Number of negative life events	−.22*** (214)
Number of chronic stressors	−.37*** (215)
Money and financial stressors	−.45*** (208)
Social life and recreation stressors	−.33*** (209)
Love and marriage stressors	−.32*** (181)
Residence/housing stressors	−.29*** (209)
Work stressors	−.27*** (203)
Family and children stressors	−.23*** (161)
Health stressors	−.18** (208)
General stressors	−.17** (213)
Overnight urinary epinephrine	−.14 (178)
Task-oriented coping	.05 (211)
Emotion-oriented coping	−.12 (215)
Avoidance coping	−.01 (213)
Active coping style	.02 (213)
Instrumental support seeking coping style	.07 (214)
Emotional support seeking coping style	.14* (214)
Behavioral withdrawal coping	−.15* (211)

Note. ns in parentheses.
* $p < .05$; ** $p < .01$; *** $p < .001$.

might relate to happiness. Among our measures were overnight levels of epinephrine, norepinephrine, and cortisol (creatinine residualized to equate for differences in concentration), mean salivary cortisol over a 3-day period, mean bedtime salivary cortisol, mean morning salivary cortisol, and mean morning rise in salivary cortisol. These measures in the CHASRS have proven to be sensitive and related to various demographic and psychosocial variables, such as perceived stress (Masi, Rickett, Hawkley, & Cacioppo, 2004; Hawkley, Masi, Berry, & Cacioppo, 2006; Adam, Hawkley, Kudielka, & Cacioppo, 2006). The only association to approach statistical significance was overnight epinephrine levels ($p <$ .07), however. Stressors may have short- to intermediate-term effects on happiness, but happiness reflects much more than the inverse of a unitary stress response.

The historic and traditional model of stress holds that qualitatively different sources of psychological stressors may differ in their intensity, duration, frequency, or controllability/predictability but are in other respects quite equivalent (e.g., McEwen, 1998; Selye, 1956). According to this model, perceived stress, depressive symptoms, loneliness, poor social support, and hostility are simply alternative manifestations of stress, and their relief or absence contributes comparably to happiness. Are these psychosocial factors comparably related to happiness, or is perceived stress the common feature of these factors that is most strongly related to happiness? Bivariate analyses in the CHASRS indicated similar associations between each of these factors and happiness: perceived stress, depressive symptoms, loneliness, social support, and hostility (see Table 10.7). When these five variables were entered simultaneously to predict happiness, however, only loneliness remained significantly associated with happiness ($\beta = -.20$,

TABLE 10.7. Correlations between Happiness and Psychosocial Variables

	Happiness (subjective well-being)
Perceived stress	−.40* (212)
Depressive symptoms	−.41* (213)
Loneliness	−.43* (214)
Social support	.36* (215)
Hostility	−.26* (205)

Note. *n*s in parentheses.
* $p < .001$.

$p < .03$), again attesting to the importance of satisfaction with our social relationships to our subjective well-being. When loneliness was added to the list of demographic characteristics to predict happiness, the positive associations between happiness and age ($\beta = .18$, $p < .01$) and household income ($\beta = .13$, $p < .07$) remained relatively intact, and the negative association between happiness and loneliness remained significant ($\beta = -.40$, $p < .001$).

In sum, individuals who reported high levels of objective chronic stressors during the prior year also reported lower levels of happiness. Different sources of psychological stress were also associated with diminished happiness, and of these, loneliness proved to be the most robust correlate of happiness.

Health and Happiness

Prior research suggests that happiness is strongly related to measures of perceived health and weakly related to objective measures of health (e.g., Brief, Butcher, George, & Link, 1993). Participants in the CHASRS, like middle-age and older adults generally in the United States, varied in health but were generally able to function with few significant disabilities. The median self-rating of health was "good" (43%), and a full 83% rated their health as good, very good, or excellent. Correspondingly, using the Charlson comorbidity index to assess chronic health conditions, 67% reported no serious chronic health conditions (e.g., heart failure, stroke, diabetes, cirrhosis) for which they took medications or regularly saw their doctor, 18% reported only one such condition, and the remaining 15% reported 2–14 conditions. As summarized in Table 10.8, self-rated health, symptoms of

TABLE 10.8. Correlations between Happiness
and Health Variables

	Happiness (subjective well-being)
Self-rated health	.27★ (212)
Charlson comorbidity index	−.12 (216)
Energy	.32★ (211)
Chronic pain	−.22★ (211)
Global sleep quality	−.27★ (198)

Note. ns in parentheses.
★ $p < .001$.

energy/fatigue (higher numbers indicate greater energy and lower fatigue), and chronic pain typically attributable to back problems or arthritis (higher numbers reflect more chronic pain) were associated with happiness. However, the association between the Charlson comorbidity index and happiness was weaker, and in this middle-age and older adult sample, only approached, but did not reach, statistical significance. As chronic health conditions worsen and impact more dramatically on daily symptoms and abilities, one would expect this association to strengthen. Alternatively, people may adapt to changes in objective health status, rendering the association between objective health and happiness rather weak.

A healthy lifestyle is one of the best means available for maintaining health into older age, so it is interesting that there were no significant associations between happiness and smoking (whether a person smokes or the number of cigarettes smoked per week), alcohol consumption (whether a person drinks or the number of drinks per week), physical exercise or activity, daily caloric intake, percent of calories from fat, percent of calories from protein, percent of calories from carbohydrates, or percent of calories from sweets or desserts ($rs \leq .1$).

Sleep is the quintessential restorative behavior, and impairments in sleep have implications for health if not well-being. In an experimental study, for instance, Spiegel, Leproult, and Van Cauter (1999) found that sleep deprivation lowers glucose tolerance, elevates evening cortisol concentrations, and increases sympathetic tonus—effects thought to mark an increased wear and tear on the organism. According to the *2001 Sleep in America* poll by the National Sleep Foundation, adults in the United States reported spending less time sleeping than they did 5 years before, with 63% of respondents reporting less than the recommended 8 hours of sleep per night and 22% reporting being so sleepy during the day that it interfered with daily activities a few days or more a week (National Sleep Foundation, 2001). The *2005 Sleep in America* poll revealed that this situation has worsened: 71% of respondents reported getting less than 8 hours of sleep per night, 50% reported feeling tired, fatigued, or not up to par at least 1 day per week, and 17% said they feel this way almost every day (National Sleep Foundation, 2005). Given these statistics, one might expect poor sleep quality to be associated with lower levels of happiness.

Sleep was quantified in the CHASRS using the Pittsburgh Sleep Quality Index (Buysse, Reynolds, Monk, Berman, & Kupfer, 1989), a questionnaire that assesses the sleep quality over a 1-month time frame. A global score was calculated for all participants by summing the scores to produce a scale score with a range of 0 (good sleep quality) to 21 (poor sleep quality). As expected, poor sleep quality was negatively associated with happiness (see Table 10.8).

In sum, perceived measures of health were modestly related to happiness, whereas objective measures were only weakly related. Health behaviors, including exercise and the number of hours sleeping, were unrelated to happiness. Sleep quality, and in particular daytime fatigue, were related to happiness, consistent with the findings from the POMS and the self-rated health measures indicating that fatigue is inversely related to happiness.

Intimacy and Happiness

Sexual intimacy continues in middle-age and older adults. Our finding in the CHASRS that interaction quality as a marker of happiness in a population-based middle-age sample in an urban U.S. city raises the question of the possible role of intimacy in everyday life and happiness. Approximately 65% of the participants in the CHASRS reported being in a current sexual relationship, and those who were in such a relationship reported higher levels of happiness than those who were not (*M*s: 24.84 and 21.56, respectively; $t[200] = -3.47$, $p < .001$). As designated in Table 10.9, happiness was also positively associated with the frequency of sexual activity over the prior 12 months, physical pleasure associated with the current sexual partner, emotional satisfaction with the current sexual partner, and negatively associated with their lack of interest in having sex during the past 12 months. The frequency with which physical problems or pain interfered with sexual activity was not related to happiness, but the frequency with which emo-

TABLE 10.9. Correlations between Happiness and Intimacy Variables

	Happiness (subjective well-being)
Frequency of sexual activity	.18* (205)
Physical pleasure with current sexual partner	.27*** (185)
Emotional satisfaction with current sexual partner	.42*** (187)
Lack of interest in having sex during the past 12 months	−.15* (183)
Frequency with which physical problems interfered with sexual activity	−.06 (193)
Frequency with which pain interfered with sexual activity	−.03 (175)
Frequency with which emotional problems interfered with sexual activity	−.19** (214)
Frequency with which stress interfered with sexual activity	.21** (214)

*Note. n*s in parentheses.
* $p < .05$; ** $p < .01$; *** $p < .001$.

tional problems or stress interfered with sexual activity was inversely related to happiness.

In sum, intimacy is an important component of feeling connected to others (Hawkley, Browne, & Cacioppo, 2005), and analyses of the CHASRS data confirmed that feeling connected to others is an important contributor to happiness. Accordingly, intimacy was also related to happiness in both male and female middle-age and older adults. That it is intimacy and not simply sexual activity is suggested by the strength of the association between happiness and the emotional satisfaction associated with one's sexual partner ($r = .42$) versus the physical pleasure associated with one's sexual partner ($r = .27$). Also consistent with this reasoning is the finding that happiness is not diminished in individuals for whom sexual activity is lower due to physical problems or pain, but happiness *is* diminished in individuals for whom sexual activity is lower due to emotional problems or stress. Individual differences in happiness again appear to be solidly anchored in the threads of connections to others.

Religiosity and Happiness

Finally, we examined the association between religiosity and happiness. Among the earliest researchers to examine such a relationship were St. George and McNamara (1984), who reported the relationship between psychological well-being (e.g., happiness, excitement in life, subjective health) and religious beliefs (e.g., strength of religious affiliation) and behaviors (e.g., church attendance), using the 1972–1982 National Opinion Research Center (NORC) General Social Survey. Results suggested that religiosity was positively associated with psychological well-being. Diener and Clifton (2002; cf. Myers, 2000) focused more specifically on happiness using the SWLS and found that religiosity was a poor predictor of happiness. Analyses of the data from CHASRS, which also focused on happiness as measured by the SWLS, replicated Diener and Clifton (2002): Neither church attendance ($r = .05$) nor religious well-being ($r = .03$) was associated with happiness in middle-age and older adults.

Longitudinal Analyses

The cross-sectional analyses of dispositional variables indicated that emotional stability, relationship satisfaction, and self-esteem were associated with happiness in an urban sample of middle-age adults, and analyses of objective social circumstances revealed that age, household income, social network size or integration, and sexual intimacy were associated with happiness. Examination of psychosocial variables suggest that happiness is not simply the absence of stress, and that loneliness, depressive symptoms, hostility, perceived stress, and social support are not simply reducible to the absence of happiness or psychological stress. Finally, multiple regression analyses indicated that age, loneliness (i.e., dissatisfaction with one's current social relationships), and household income remained significantly associated with happiness.

Cross-sectional analyses may provide useful information on dispositional characteristics of happy people as well as risk factors for unhappiness, but the causal influences of social and situational factors on happiness require longitudinal analyses. To determine predictors of changes in happiness in the CHASRS, we next conducted regression models in which happiness in the most recent year for which complete data were available (year 3) served as the criterion measure, happiness in year 1 served as the first predictor, and other measures from year 1 were then entered as predictors.

To begin, a multiple regression model was specified to examine associations between year 3 happiness and year 1 age, gender, ethnicity, income, and marital status, holding constant year 1 happiness. Replicating cross-sectional analyses, age approached significance as a predictor of changes in happiness between years 1 and 3 ($\beta = 0.11$, $p = .06$). However, in contrast with results of cross-sectional analyses, income in year 1 did *not* predict changes in happiness between years 1 and 3 ($\beta = -0.06$, $p > .3$), whereas marital status in year 1 did predict changes in happiness independent of income and remaining demographic covariates ($\beta = 0.14$, $p < .05$). These findings suggest that although concurrent associations between marital status and happiness are explicable by household income, the effects of marital status on changes in happiness are independent of income and speak to the benefits of relational connectedness afforded by an intimate partner.

Income appears to have only a contemporaneous and transient association with happiness. The association between household income and happiness was robust in year 1 of the CHASRS, and this association was replicated in a cross-sectional association between income and happiness in year 3 ($r = .30$, $p < .01$). The layperson's persistent belief that money can buy happiness (Myers, 2000) may receive some support from simultaneous measures of the two, but data from the CHASRS indicate that current household income did not predict changes in happiness between years 1 and 3—an association more difficult to intuit than the association between concurrent events.

Changes in marital status have also been shown to affect happiness (Lucas, Clark, Georgellis, & Diener, 2003). Marital change was not related to changes in happiness in the CHASRS possibly because only 8% of participants experienced a change in marital status between years 1 and 3.

Accrued debt was associated with concurrent happiness net of demographic variables, and household income only slightly reduced the impact of debt on happiness. Year 1 debt did not predict changes in happiness between years 1 and 3, however, when age, gender, ethnicity, marital status, and household income were held constant. Similarly, none of the year 1 measures of wealth (i.e., home equity, car value, stock value, defined benefit plan, bank account value) was a significant predictor of changes in happiness, holding constant income and demographic variables.

Prior research by Diener and colleagues showed that only recent life events (i.e., during the previous 3 months) influenced happiness (Suh et al., 1996). Consistent with this work, we found that life events experienced in the 12 months prior to the year 1 assessments did not predict changes in happiness between years 1 and 3. As would be expected given the transient nature of the measure, we also found that year 1 urinary epinephrine, a transient indicator of stress, was unrelated to changes in happiness between years 1 and 3.

We saw earlier that chronic stress was inversely associated with concurrent happiness, and that financial stress was the most potent chronic stress in this regard. Chronic stress in year 1 also influenced changes in happiness between years 1 and 3: The greater the number of domains in which individuals experienced chronic stress in year 1, the lower their year 3 happiness ($\beta = -0.12$, $p < .05$, $n = 172$), an effect that persisted net of income and other demographic covariates. However, no single chronic stress domain, including chronic financial stress, predicted subsequent happiness, suggesting that the cumulative load of stress is responsible for dampening subsequent happiness levels.

Life events, income, debt, and wealth have relatively short-lasting effects on happiness and are unrelated to 2-year changes in levels of happiness, but what about the effects of social network diversity, size, and integration? Longitudinal analyses indicated that none of these social network measures predicted changes in happiness between years 1 and 3 (net of age, gender, ethnicity, marital status, and income; $ps > .3$).

As noted earlier, social network size and diversity are not as important to social satisfaction (e.g., as manifested in low levels of loneliness using the UCLA scale) as are good quality social relationships (Hawkley, Burleson, Berntson, & Cacioppo, 2003). In our cross-sectional analyses, for example, relationship satisfaction/loneliness was associated with happiness independent of income. In the longitudinal analyses, year 1 loneliness predicted changes in happiness between years 1 and 3 net of age, gender, ethnicity, and income ($\beta = -0.11$, $p < .05$, one-tailed, $n = 172$), and this prediction was reduced only somewhat by the addition of marital status to the regression model ($\beta_{loneliness} = -0.10$, $p < .06$, one-tailed). Age and marital status remained predictors of changes in happiness ($\beta s \geq 0.13$, $ps < .05$). Notably, even though loneliness and chronic stress were correlated—$r (219) = .36$, $p < .01$—the effect of relationship satisfaction/loneliness on subsequent happiness was not explained by chronic stress.

The longitudinal nature of the CHASRS also permitted us to test the reverse causal direction: Do happy people perceive or develop more satisfying relationships (i.e., experience lower loneliness)? Prior research has demonstrated that people who feel happy act more positively toward others, which promotes reciprocal influences between positive affect and higher quality social interactions (Hawkley, Preacher, & Cacioppo, 2007). Holding constant year 1 loneliness, year 1 happiness predicted lower levels of loneliness in year 3 independent of age, gender, ethnicity, and income ($\beta = -0.23$, $p < .01$), indicating a reciprocal causal relationship between these variables. Income changes, on the other hand, did not predict loneliness over and above the year 1 predictors ($\beta = -0.11$, $p > .1$). The reciprocal nature of the temporal associations between happiness and relationship satisfaction indicate that each feeds forward to foster spirals of positivity (Fredrickson & Joiner, 2002; Hawkley et al., 2007) in terms of ongoing happiness and good quality social relationships.

One of the ways happiness fosters general positivity is in its success-promoting effects in a variety of life domains (Lyubomirsky et al., 2005). For instance, longitudinal studies have shown that happiness predicts greater increases in income (Diener & Biswas-Diener, 2002; Diener, Nickerson, Lucas, & Sandvik, 2002; Marks & Fleming, 1999), increased likelihood of getting married (Lucas et al., 2003; Marks & Fleming, 1999), and greater relationship satisfaction, particularly marital satisfaction (Headey & Veenhoven, 1989; Ruvolo, 1998). Analyses of data from the CHASRS produced a consistent set of findings that is graphically illustrated in Figure 10.2. Briefly, happiness in our CHASRS sample in year 1 predicted changes in income between years 1 and 3 (i.e., year 3 income statistically holding constant year 1 income) net of age, gender, ethnicity, and marital status ($\beta = 0.15$, $p < .01$). Loneliness in year 1 also predicted year 3 income net of year 1 income and demographic covariates ($\beta = -0.15$, $p < .01$), and furthermore, loneliness helped to explain the effect of happiness on year 3 income ($\beta_{\text{loneliness}} = -0.12$, $p < .05$; $\beta_{\text{happiness}} = 0.10$, $p > .1$). The reverse causal

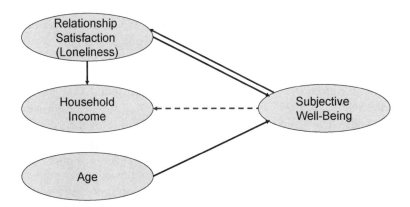

FIGURE 10.2. Model of longitudinal associations among happiness (subjective well-being), relationship satisfaction, household income, and age. Solid lines represent positive associations, and broken lines represent negative associations.

direction—that year 1 income predicted subsequent (i.e., year 3) loneliness net of year 1 loneliness—was not supported ($\beta = p > .4$). Further inspection of the cases that showed changes in household income revealed that the changes were not due to changes in marital status, nor were the changes related to year 1 happiness or loneliness.

In sum, longitudinal analyses revealed a reciprocal relationship between changes in happiness and relationship satisfaction (as measured by loneliness), an effect of age on changes in happiness, and an effect of happiness on changes in household income that was mediated by relationship satisfaction.

Conclusion

In physiology, *catabolic process* refers to the phase of metabolism in which complex molecules are broken down into simpler ones, often resulting in a release of energy (e.g., stress reactivity). The *anabolic process*, in contrast, refers to the phase of metabolism in which simple substances are synthesized into the complex materials of living tissue. Catabolic and anabolic processes both promote the survival and reproduction of the organism, but they work in a complementary rather than reciprocal or redundant fashion (cf. Cacioppo & Berntson, 2007). A comparable distinction is emerging in psychology between negative and positive psychology. Although the emphasis for years was on negative states such as stress, anxiety, sadness, anger, fear, and illness, positive conditions such as happiness and satisfaction have been found to be both statistically and functionally distinguishable from these negative states.

Consistent with Kwan et al. (1997) and Benet-Martínez and Karakitapoğlu-Aygün (2003), we found that happiness was temporally stable (1-year reliability ranging from .70 to .73 and a 2-year test–retest reliability of .68); emotional stability was distally related to happiness; personality variables no longer predicted happiness once self-esteem and relationship satisfaction (loneliness) were introduced as additional predictors in the regression analyses; and self-esteem and relationship satisfaction served as independent, proximal predictors of happiness.

As in prior research with healthy samples, we found that self-reported health was related to happiness and that objective measures of health were only nominally related to happiness. A healthy lifestyle is one of the best means of maintaining one's objective health, but we found no relationship between happiness and various measures of health behavior. This latter finding raises the interesting possibility that one of the obstacles to the adoption of a healthy lifestyle is that neither health nor healthy behaviors are associated with happiness.

If people are motivated to be happy, what may be most apparent and be encoded in memory are the life events that are correlated over short periods of time with happiness. Cross-sectional analyses revealed that age, satisfying social relationships, and household income were modest but reliable correlates of happiness in the CHASRS. Objective chronic stressors (especially objective financial stressors), coping by behavioral withdrawal, and daytime fatigue were associated with lower levels of happiness. Of these correlates, satisfying relationships, objective stressors, and money are the most likely to meet the prerequisite conditions for producing memorial effects that extend well beyond the actual lifespan of these correlates. Finding a coin in a pay phone, for instance, is sufficient to make a person happy (Isen, 2000), so in some sense people are correct when they think that money can make them happy. However, people are such poor affective forecasters that the very transient nature of such effects is ignored (Wilson & Gilbert, 2005), contributing to erroneous beliefs, for instance, that a high income will make one happier.

Stubbe, Posthuma, Boomsma, and De Geus (2005) measured happiness in 5,668 participants in The Netherlands Twin Registry using a Dutch version of the SWLS. As might be expected, given the transient influence of life events on happiness, Stubbe et al. calculated that individual differences in happiness were, in part, heritable. However, 62% of the variance in happiness was found to be attributable to persistent and transitory *environmental* factors, whereas only 38% was estimated to be heritable. Concurrent associations do not imply causal influences, of course, so longitudinal analyses were performed using data from the CHASRS to investigate the effects of factors such as relationship satisfaction, household income, and demographics on changes in happiness over a 2-year period as well as to examine the effects of happiness on changes in these variables over this 2-year period.

Three variables emerged as noteworthy. First, the age of participants in year 1 predicted changes in happiness net of other demographic factors. Carstensen et al.'s (1999) socioemotional selectivity theory provides a possible explanation for this effect, although age-related changes in amygdalar function may also play a role (Berntson, Bechara, Damasio, Tranel, & Cacioppo, 2006). Second, household income in year 1 did not predict the subsequent changes in happiness, but happiness in year 1 did predict subsequent changes in household income. Third, relationship satisfaction in year 1 predicted subsequent changes in happiness, and vice versa. When various mediational models were examined, the prediction by happiness in year 1 of subsequent changes in household income appeared to be mediated by relationship satisfaction (see Figure 10.1).

How might lower levels of loneliness transform happiness into greater income? One possibility is that happy people form good relationships in the workplace, as elsewhere (Lyubomirsky et al., 2005), and these relationships, rather than happiness per se, improve job performance, positively influence the likelihood of receiving good performance reviews and promotions, and provide better "networking" opportunities that lead in financially productive directions.

Alternatively, happiness may promote creative decision making (Isen, 2000), which in turn improves one's station in social and work domains.

In sum, results of both cross-sectional and longitudinal analyses indicated that happiness is *anchored in and contributes to* the invisible threads of connections to others. The positive feedback loop between relationship satisfaction and happiness, with its benefits for problem solving, self-efficacy motivation, decision making, and health (e.g., Isen, 2000; Hawkley et al., 2006), may serve as a foundational component of the psychological equivalent of anabolic physiology.

Acknowledgments

Funding was provided by the National Institute of Aging Grant No. PO1 AG18911 and the John Templeton Foundation.

References

Adam, E. K., Hawkley, L. C., Kudielka, B. M., & Cacioppo, J. T. (2006). Day-to-day dynamics of experience–cortisol associations in a population-based sample of older adults. *Proceedings of the National Academy of Sciences, 103,* 17058–17063.

Benet-Martínez, V., & Karakitapoğlu-Aygün, Z. (2003). The interplay of cultural syndromes and personality in predicting life satisfaction. *Journal of Cross-Cultural Psychology, 34,* 38–60.

Berntson, G. G., Bechara, A., Damasio, H., Tranel, D., & Cacioppo, J. T. (in press). Amygdala contribution to selective dimensions of emotion. *Social, Cognitive, and Affective Neuroscience.*

Brickman, P., Coates, D., & Janoff-Bulman, R. (1978). Lottery winners and accident victims: Is happiness relative? *Journal of Personality and Social Psychology, 36,* 917–927.

Brief, A. P., Butcher, A. H., George, J. M., & Link, K. E. (1993). Integrating bottom-up and top-down theories of subjective well-being: The case of health. *Journal of Personality and Social Psychology, 64,* 646–653.

Buysse, D. J., Reynolds, C. F., Monk, T. H., Berman, S. R., & Kupfer, D. J. (1989). The Pittsburgh Sleep Quality Index: A new instrument for psychiatric practice and research. *Psychiatry Research, 28,* 193–213.

Cacioppo, J. T., & Berntson, G. G. (2007). The brain, homeostasis, and health: Balancing demands of the internal and external milieu. In H. S. Friedman & R. Cohen Silver (Eds.), *Foundations of health psychology* (pp. 73–91). New York: Oxford University Press.

Cacioppo, J. T., Gardner, W. L., & Berntson, G. G. (1999). The affect system has parallel and integrative processing components: Form follows function. *Journal of Personality and Social Psychology, 76,* 839–855.

Cacioppo, J. T., Hughes, M. E., Waite, L. J., Hawkley, L. C., & Thisted, R. (2006). Loneliness as a specific risk factor for depressive symptoms in older adults: Cross-sectional and longitudinal analyses. *Psychology and Aging, 21,* 140–151.

Campbell, A., Converse, P. E., & Rodgers, W. L. (1976). *The quality of American life: Perceptions, evaluations, and satisfactions.* New York: Sage.

Carstensen, L. L., & Fredrickson, B. L. (1998). Socioemotional selectivity in healthy older people and younger people living with the human immunodeficiency virus: The centrality of emotion when the future is constrained. *Health Psychology, 17,* 1–10.

Carstensen, L. L., Isaacowitz, D. M., & Charles, S. T. (1999). Taking time seriously: A theory of socioemotional selectivity. *American Psychologist, 54,* 165–181.

Carstensen, L. L., Pasupathi, M., Mayr, U., & Nesselroade, J. R. (2000). Emotional experience in everyday life across the adult life span. *Journal of Personality and Social Psychology, 79,* 644–655.

Carver, C. S., Scheier, M. N., & Weintraub, J. K. (1989). Assessing coping strategies: A theoretically based approach. *Journal of Personality and Social Psychology, 56,* 267–283.

Cohen, S., Doyle, W. J., Skoner, D. P., Rabin, B. S., & Gwaltney, J. M., Jr. (1997). Social ties and susceptibility to the common cold. *Journal of the American Medical Association, 277,* 1940–1944.

Cosway, R., Endler, N. S., Sadler, A. J., & Deary, I. J. (2000). The Coping Inventory for Stressful Situations: Factorial structure and associations with personality traits and psychological health. *Journal of Applied Biobehavioral Research, 5,* 121–143.

Diener, E., & Biswas-Diener, R. (2002). Will money increase subjective well-being? *Social Indicators Research, 57,* 119–169.

Diener, E., & Clifton, D. (2002). Life satisfaction and religiosity in broad probability samples. *Psychological Inquiry, 13,* 206–209.

Diener, E., & Diener, C. (1996). Most people are happy. *Psychological Science, 7,* 181–185.

Diener, E., Emmons, R. A., Larsen, R. J., & Griffin, S. (1985). The Satisfaction with Life Scale. *Journal of Personality Assessment, 49,* 71–75.

Diener, E., Nickerson, C., Lucas, R. E., & Sandvik, E. (2002). Dispositional affect and job outcomes. *Social Indicators Research, 59,* 229–259.

Eid, M., & Diener, E. (2004). Global judgments of subjective well-being: Situational variability and long-term stability. *Social Indicators Research, 65,* 245–277.

Fredrickson, B. L., & Joiner, T. (2002). Positive emotions trigger upward spirals toward emotional well-being. *Psychological Science, 13,* 172–175.

Hawkley, L. C., Browne, M. W., & Cacioppo, J. T. (2005). How can I connect with thee? Let me count the ways. *Psychological Science, 16,* 798–804.

Hawkley, L. C., Burleson, M. H., Berntson, G. G., & Cacioppo, J. T. (2003). Loneliness in everyday life: Cardiovascular activity, psychosocial context, and health behaviors. *Journal of Personality and Social Psychology, 85,* 105–120.

Hawkley, L. C., Masi, C. M., Berry, J. D., & Cacioppo, J. T. (2006). Loneliness is a unique predictor of age-related differences in systolic blood pressure. *Psychology and Aging, 21,* 152–164.

Hawkley, L. C., Preacher, K. J., & Cacioppo, J. T. (2007). Multilevel modeling of social interactions and mood in lonely and socially connected individuals: The MacArthur social neuroscience studies. In A. D. Ong & M. van Dulmen (Eds.), *Oxford handbook of methods in positive psychology* (pp. 559–575). New York: Oxford University Press.

Headey, B., & Veenhoven, R. (1989). Does happiness induce a rosy outlook? In R.

Veenhoven (Ed.), *How harmful is happiness? Consequences of enjoying life or not* (pp. 106–127). Rotterdam, The Netherlands: Universitaire Pers Rotterdam.

Isen, A. M. (2000). Positive affect and decision making. In M. Lewis & J. M. Haviland-Jones (Eds.), *Handbook of Emotion* (2nd ed., pp. 417–435). New York: Guilford Press.

Kahneman, D., Diener, E., & Schwarz, N. (1999). *Well-being: The foundations of hedonic psychology.* New York: Sage.

Kwan, V. S. Y., Bond, M. H., & Singelis, T. M. (1997). Pancultural explanations for life satisfaction: Adding relationship harmony to self-esteem. *Journal of Personality and Social Psychology, 73,* 1038–1051.

Leary, M. R., & Baumeister, R. F. (2000). The nature and function of self-esteem: Sociometer theory. In M. P. Zanna (Ed.), *Advances in experimental social psychology* (Vol. 32, pp. 1–62). San Diego, CA: Academic Press.

Leary, M. R., Tambor, E. S., Terdal, S. K., & Downs, D. L. (1995). Self-esteem as an interpersonal monitor: The sociometer hypothesis. *Journal of Personality and Social Psychology, 68,* 518–530.

Lucas, R. E., Clark, A. E., Georgellis, Y., & Diener, E. (2003). Reexamining adaptation and the set point model of happiness: Reactions to changes in marital status. *Journal of Personality and Social Psychology, 84,* 527–539.

Lyubomirsky, S., King, L., & Diener, E. (2005). The benefits of frequent positive affect: Does happiness lead to success? *Psychological Bulletin, 131,* 803–855.

Marks, G. N., & Fleming, N. (1999). Influences and consequences of well-being among Australian young people: 1980–1995. *Social Indicators Research, 46,* 301–323.

Masi, C. M., Rickett, E. M., Hawkley, L. C., & Cacioppo, J. T. (2004). Gender and ethnic differences in urinary stress hormones: The population-based Chicago Health, Aging, and Social Relations Study. *Journal of Applied Physiology, 97,* 941–947.

McEwen, B. S. (1998) Protective and damaging effects of stress mediators. *New England Journal of Medicine, 338,* 171–179.

McNair, D. M., Loor, M., & Droppleman, L. (1992). Profile of mood states. *Test Critiques, 1,* 522–529.

Myers, D. G. (2000). The funds, friends, and faith of happy people. *American Psychologist, 55,* 56–67.

Myers, D. G., & Diener, E. (1995). Who is happy? *Psychological Science, 6,* 10–19.

National Sleep Foundation. (2001). Less fun, less sleep, more work: An American portrait. Available at *www.sleepfoundation.org/NSAW/execsum3.8.ppt.*

National Sleep Foundation. (2005). *2005 Sleep in America Poll.* Available at *www.sleepfoundation.org/.*

Nolen-Hoeksema, S., & Ahrens, C. (2002). Age differences and similarities in the correlates of depressive symptoms. *Psychology and Aging, 17,* 116–124.

Pavot, W. G., Diener, E., Colvin, C. R., & Sandvik, E. (1991). Further validation of the Satisfaction with Life Scale: Evidence for the cross-method convergence of well-being measures. *Journal of Personality Assessment, 57,* 149–161.

Peplau, L. A., & Perlman, D. (Eds.). (1982). *Loneliness: A sourcebook of current theory, research, and therapy.* New York: Wiley.

Perlman, D., & Peplau, L. A. (1998). Loneliness. In H. Friedman (Ed.), *Encyclopedia of mental health* (Vol. 2, pp. 571–581). San Diego, CA: Academic Press.

Russell, D., Peplau, L. A., & Cutrona, C. E. (1980). The revised UCLA loneliness scale: Concurrent and discriminant validity evidence. *Journal of Personality and Social Psychology, 39,* 472–480.

Ruvolo, A. P. (1998). Marital well-being and general happiness of newlywed couples: Relationships across time. *Journal of Social and Personal Relationships, 15,* 470–489.

Selye, H. (1956). *The stress of life.* New York: McGraw-Hill.

Shmotkin, D. (2005). Happiness in the face of adversity: Reformulating the dynamic and modular bases of subjective well-being. *Review of General Psychology, 9,* 291–325.

Spiegel, K., Leproult, R., & Van Cauter, E. (1999). Impact of a sleep debt on metabolic and endocrine function. *Lancet, 354,* 1435–1439.

St. George, A., & McNamara, P. H. (1984). Religion, race and psychological well-being. *Journal for the Scientific Study of Religion, 23,* 351–363.

Stock, W. A., Okun, M. A., Haring, M. J., & Witter, R. A. (1983). Age differences in subjective well-being: A meta-analysis. In R. J. Light (Ed.), *Evaluation studies: Review annual* (Vol. 8, pp. 279–302). Beverly Hills: Sage.

Stubbe, J. H., Posthuma, D., Boomsma, D. I., & De Geus, E. J. C. (2005). Heritability of life satisfaction in adults: A twin-family study. *Psychological Medicine, 35,* 1581–1588.

Suh, E., Diener, E., & Fujita, F. (1996). Events and subjective well-being: Only recent events matter. *Journal of Personality and Social Psychology, 70,* 1091–1102.

Taylor, S. E., & Brown, J. D. (1988). Illusion and well-being: A social psychological perspective on mental health. *Psychological Bulletin, 103,* 193–210.

U.S. Census Bureau. (2002). *Demographic trends in the 20th century.* Washington, DC: U.S. Department of Commerce.

Wilson, T. D., & Gilbert, D. T. (2005). Affective forecasting: Knowing what to want. *Current Directions in Psychological Science, 14,* 131–134.

11

The Happy Mind in Action

The Cognitive Basis of Subjective Well-Being

MICHAEL D. ROBINSON and REBECCA J. COMPTON

Ed Diener devoted the majority of his research career to understanding what is of utmost importance to all human beings, namely their levels of happiness or subjective well-being. High levels of subjective well-being not only feel good but are also beneficial in a variety of other ways as well (Lyubomirsky, King, & Diener, 2005). Therefore, there is little doubt that it is beneficial to experience high levels of subjective well-being. However, human beings are puzzling in relation to this important goal. Although we may all desire to experience high levels of subjective well-being, many individuals do not. Furthermore, seeking to be happy may be among the least successful strategies in actually *being* happy (Csikszentmihalyi, 1997). Being happy, therefore, is not something that we can easily will upon ourselves. Rather, it is something that naturally emerges from a life well lived.

What is a life well lived? This is clearly a difficult question to answer, and readers of this volume will encounter many excellent answers to this question. Here we present one sort of answer to this question, one that relies on a cognitive analysis of subjective well-being. Cognition may seem like a dry, unemotional field of inquiry, but one goal of the present chapter is to convince the reader that this is not true. Cognition, it turns out, is not something that just "happens," but rather something that is intimately related to our motivations and goals. Moreover, our success in achieving the goals that we have set for ourselves is very much dependent on our cognitive skills and information-processing tendencies. The latter point is substantiated multiple times.

If cognition is important to subjective well-being, what *is* cognition? Broadly speaking, cognition concerns three operations that we highlight here. First, cognition involves the prioritization of certain classes of information over others, a point that will be made in our discussion of selective attention. Second, cognition involves categorization tendencies—that is, processes responsible for assigning meaning to stimuli. Third, cognition involves self-regulation, which can be defined in various ways but is generally important in attempts to maintain or change cognitive-processing tendencies in the service of an active goal. Throughout our discussion, we seek to demonstrate both the benefits and limitations of a cognitive analysis of subjective well-being in relation to the information-processing operations of (1) selective attention, (2) categorization, (3) priming, (4) implicit associations, (5) cognitive conflict, and (6) self-regulation.

Selective Attention

James (1950/1890) characterized the infant's subjective life as a "blooming, buzzing confusion" (p. 462). Here, he was suggesting that with increasing age and experience, we learn to simplify a complex world by focusing on particular classes of information relative to other classes of information. Clearly, this hypothesis has been supported from a cognitive perspective (Pashler, 1998). Because attention is often referred to as the "gateway to consciousness," it is easy to see how individual differences in selective attention may either support or undermine tendencies toward subjective well-being. Indeed, some recent studies have explored such links.

Some of this research has explored links between basic (i.e., nonaffective) attention-related processes and variables linked to subjective well-being. Gasper and Clore (2002) found that positive affect was associated with an attentional focus favoring global rather than local aspects of visual stimuli. Studies such as these imply that higher levels of subjective well-being engender a wider attentional focus. In addition to the global focus characteristic of higher levels of subjective well-being, it is also appears that higher levels of subjective well-being are associated with superior abilities to disengage attention from nonvalid (or nonpredictive) spatial cues (e.g., Compton, Wirtz, Pajoumand, Claus, & Heller, 2004). Thus, higher levels of subjective well-being are generally associated with attentional flexibility, defined in terms of wider spatial attention and abilities to shift attention quickly. Such results are compatible with Isen's (2004) suggestion that positive affect promotes a greater degree of cognitive flexibility, here in relation to spatial attention processes.

Other studies have examined affect-specific selective biases. Along these lines, a large body of work demonstrates that anxious individuals selectively attend to threatening relative to nonthreatening stimuli (e.g., Mogg & Bradley, 1998). Beyond such correlational results, recent data indicate that manipulations of attention, either toward or away from threatening stimuli, influence subsequent reactions to ambiguously threatening events (e.g., MacLeod, 1999). The latter result is important in showing that selective attention biases contribute to, or cause, emotional vulnerabilities to negative affect (MacLeod, 1999).

Because almost all of the prior studies focused on relations between negative affect and attention to threat, Tamir and Robinson (in press) recently addressed the question of whether positive affect might be associated with, and cause, selective biases favoring rewarding information (e.g., words such as *love*) over nonrewarding information (e.g., words such as *desk*). In a first study, daily experiences of high-arousal positive affect (e.g., states of excitement) were associated with tendencies to selectively attend to rewards relative to nonrewards in a spatial attention task. Three additional studies provided support for the idea that momentary experiences of positive affect alter selective attention such that it favors rewards in spatial attention tasks (Tamir & Robinson, in press).

Thus, it generally appears that what people feel reflects that to which they selectively attend. If they selectively attend to threats, they feel anxiety (MacLeod, 1999). By contrast, if they selectively attend to rewards, they feel excitement (Tamir & Robinson, 2006). Such links appear to be bidirectional in that manipulations of selective attention alter mood states (MacLeod, 1999), and manipulations of mood states alter selective attention performance (Tamir & Robinson, in press). This said, it is important to note that the clinical literature typically focuses on intense experiences of anxiety, such as those typical of generalized anxiety disorder (MacLeod, 1999). By contrast, the Tamir and Robinson (in press) studies focused on relatively normal dimensional tendencies toward positive affect. Therefore, there is a great deal of future research necessary to extend attentional biases—either favoring threat or reward—to dimensional views of subjective well-being.

In addition, it is important to point out that theoretical models related to emotion and attention often highlight different stages of selective attention. For example, Öhman's (1997) influential model has suggested that anxiety relates to early, pre-attentive processes of attention, whereas Fox, Russo, Bowles, and Dutton (2001) have concluded that anxiety relates to later, postengagement processes of attention. As pointed out by Fox et al. (2001), many spatial attention paradigms may be relatively incapable of separating early from late attention-related processes. Therefore, it seems likely that future studies will be increasingly concerned with differentiating pre-attentive and postattentive processes, leading to the development of new and potentially more reliable measures of individual differences (e.g., Wilkowski, Robinson, & Meier, 2006).

Categorization

Although selective attention is surely relevant to subjective well-being, it is arguable that subjective well-being relates more strongly to the process of assigning *meaning* to stimuli. For example, imagine that Happy Harry and Sad Sam go to a restaurant and find out that their preferred menu item (roasted chicken) is no longer available from the kitchen. Happy Harry may treat this event as an opportunity to explore new, more adventurous culinary options, whereas Sad Sam may decide that the meal is ruined. In other words, the same event may give rise to different categorization tendencies depending on levels of subjective well-being: either optimistic (Happy Harry) or pessimistic (Sad Sam).

Do categorization tendencies directly reflect and predict levels of subjective well-being? Results from several studies have supported this idea (for reviews, see Robinson, 2004; Robinson & Neighbors, 2006). In one series of studies, Robinson, Vargas, Tamir, and Solberg (2004) sought to examine whether categorization tendencies related to negative meaning predict subjective well-being in daily life. To examine this question, the authors designed a task in which participants were asked to quickly and accurately evaluate stimuli as either neutral (e.g., *straw*, *pencil*) or negative (e.g., *dirt*, *insect*) in connotation. The neutral category was necessary to create a choice reaction time (RT) task, which requires two categories. In support of the idea that negative categorization tendencies undermine levels of subjective well-being, Robinson et al. (2004) found that faster negative evaluations were associated with more negative appraisals of daily life, more negative affect in daily life, and lower levels of life satisfaction. However, negative evaluation speed did not predict levels of positive affect.

A wider conclusion of this research, whether pertaining to go/no-go (e.g., Tamir, Robinson, & Solberg, 2006) or choice RT (e.g., Robinson, Solberg, Vargas, & Tamir, 2003) paradigms, is that categorization tendencies frequently interact with affective traits such as extraversion and neuroticism in the prediction of daily experiences. Indeed, interactions of this type have been so pronounced that we have concluded that categorization tendencies only rarely predict subjective well-being variables in "main effect" terms (Robinson, 2004). For example, Meier and Robinson (2004) found that fast blame tendencies (i.e., fast RT to categorize words such as *malpractice* as blameworthy in nature) predicted anger and aggression, but only at low levels of agreeableness. This pattern was subsequently replicated in experimental studies focused on the interactive prediction (Meier, Robinson, & Wilkowski, 2006).

Thus, categorization tendencies interact with emotion-related traits in determining everyday experience and behavior, although categorization tendencies and self-reported traits are not correlated in a zero-order fashion. This general conclusion, which has emerged from a fairly large body of work, suggests two more specific conclusions. One, the common-sense idea that trait–state relations are mediated by affective categorization tendencies is most definitely not supported by the data, in that self-reported traits do not predict categorization tendencies based on choice RT (Robinson, 2004; Robinson & Neighbors, 2006). Two, it appears that an implicit categorization approach to personality, to some extent advocated by Kelly (1963), cannot replace a personality science related to self-reported traits, in particular because the correlates of implicit categorization tendencies vary by traits (Robinson, 2004; Robinson & Neighbors, 2006).

Nevertheless, it is important to point out that our measures of categorization tendencies have tended to focus on unambiguous events, such as the relation between *cancer* and *threat*. This approach differs from the implicit motivation literature, which has tended to examine implicit motivation in response to ambiguous stimuli (McClelland, 1987). Moreover, the social judgment literature, too, has typically used ambiguous stimuli, which are believed to be most sensitive to chronic accessibility processes (Higgins, 1996). These considerations suggest that it may be useful to extend the categorization perspective on personality by focusing on categorization judgments in relation to ambiguous events. It is possible that this alternative judgment-related approach may yield different results, and we encourage future work along these lines.

Priming

One of the best ways to study the happy mind is to study how it organizes information. For example, it has long been apparent that repressors do not elaborate on negative emotional material, resulting in the relative inaccessibility of such material when intentionally recalled (Davis, 1987). Similarly, Showers (e.g., 1992) has shown that the structure of the self-concept, over and above the content of the self-concept, influences subjective well-being variables. People who isolate negative aspects of the self-concept within small clusters (or "baskets") tend to be happier than people who integrate positive and negative knowledge concerning the self. This is because most people have self-concepts that are positively valenced. Thus, *on average*, a more differentiated self-structure will result in positive self-aspects priming other positive self-aspects more than negative self-aspects priming other negative self-aspects.

To study the organization of emotion memories, Robinson and Kirkeby (2005) designed a task in which people judged the intensity of their positive and negative emotions on computer. Their interest was in priming across trials. A positive affect priming effect occurs when positive targets (on trial n) are judged faster following positive relative to negative "primes" on the previous trial (i.e., trial $n - 1$). A negative affect priming effect is defined similarly (i.e., a greater degree of facilitation with two negative emotion judgments in a row). The researchers found that the positive affect priming effect was stronger than the negative affect priming effect, which suggests that people have more integrated knowledge concerning their positive emotions. The authors also found that higher levels of life satisfaction correlated with stronger positive affect priming effects. Accordingly, the happy mind not only has happy thoughts but also organizes them together in such a way that one happy thought primes another one. It is easy to see why this mental organization would be beneficial to one's life satisfaction.

In a recent extension of this work, Ready, Robinson, and Weinberger (2006) examined age differences in the magnitude of positive and negative affect priming effects, as defined in terms of the emotion judgment task developed by Robinson and Kirkeby (2005). Ready et al. (2006) hypothesized that age brings more knowledge concerning the self's experience of positive and negative emotions. This greater knowledge, in turn, should support long-term memory networks related to stronger interconnections between different positive emotions, on the one hand, and stronger interconnections between different negative emotions, on the other (cf. Smith, 1998).

On the basis of such considerations, Ready et al. (2006) predicted that both positive and negative affect priming effects would be more robust with the increasing age of the individual. Ready et al. found support for this hypothesis in that older, relative to younger, adults displayed stronger positive *and* negative priming effects in the emotion judgment task developed by Robinson and Kirkeby (2005). Following the general theory of Showers (1992), Ready et al. suggested that the greater degree of differentiation of positive and negative emotional memories, among older adults, could result in a higher level of subjective well-being in this population. Because most of our emotions are positive ones, a greater differentiation of positive and negative emotions would result in a greater likelihood of one positive emotion triggering another one (Ready et al., 2006).

The scope of this priming work can be broadened to consider whether associations between life satisfaction and affective priming are specific to tasks involving self-judgments; if so, then they may have limited importance in explaining *in vivo* reactions to affective stimuli, which are unlikely to involve the self-concept to any large extent (Robinson & Clore, 2002; Robinson & von Hippel, 2006). For these reasons, Robinson and von Hippel recently sought to extend the affective priming perspective of life satisfaction by examining affective priming tendencies in tasks not requiring the explicit retrieval of self-knowledge. The first study involved emotional reactions to slides, the second study involved word categorizations, and the third study involved a simple word perception task.

Robinson and von Hippel (2006) quantified positive affect priming in terms of RT facilitation with two positive stimuli in a row, and quantified negative affect priming in a parallel manner. Life satisfaction predicted affective priming effects related to slide evaluations (Study 1), word evaluations (Study 2), semantic categorizations (Study 2), and word identifications (Study 3). In all studies, the pattern was the same: Namely, the magnitude of the negative priming effect was stronger at lower levels of life satisfaction, whereas the magnitude of the positive priming effect was stronger at higher levels of life satisfaction. Thus, being happy, defined in terms of high levels of life satisfaction, seems to depend on the relative interconnectivity of positive versus negative affective concepts in memory (Robinson & von Hippel, 2006).

Implicit Self-Esteem

Greenwald and Banaji (1995) argued that many social constructs—such as attitudes, self-esteem, and prejudice—have a significant implicit component. Three years later, Greenwald and colleagues (Greenwald, McGhee, & Schwartz, 1998) developed the Implicit Association Test (IAT) as a means to measure such implicit associations. The literature has taken off substantially since then, so much so that Fazio and Olson (2003) had to report that, although they desired to review the literature in a complete fashion, they could not do so given the staggering number of papers presented at conferences and in professional journals (with IAT studies appearing almost every week).

What is the IAT? It is an RT-based measure that borrows from, but significantly extends, related work from the perception and performance literature (De Houwer, 2003). The self-esteem version of the IAT requires individuals to perform two simultaneous choice categorization tasks related to *not me* (e.g., *other*) versus *me* (e.g., *self*) categorizations, on the one hand, and *unpleasant* (e.g., *vomit*) versus *pleasant* (e.g., *caress*) connotation, on the other (for more complete details, see Greenwald & Farnham, 2000). To the extent that individuals are high in implicit self-esteem, they should be faster in a condition in which *me* and *pleasant* share a response key compared to a condition in which *me* and *unpleasant* share a response key.

Consistent with the idea that explicit and implicit self-esteem are different constructs, there are typically very small correlations between these two measures (Hofmann, Gawronski, Gschwendner, Le, & Schmitt, 2005), even though implicit self-esteem is a very reliable implicit construct (Greenwald & Farnham, 2000). More controversial has been the suggestion that implicit self-esteem is relevant in the prediction of individual differences in subjective well-being. Bosson,

Swann, and Pennebaker (2000) report very few correlations along these lines, and Schimmack and Diener (2003) also reported that implicit self-esteem (based on a letter-preference task) did not predict subjective well-being to any major or minor extent.

More recent investigations have shown that implicit self-esteem predicts (1) everyday experiences of negative emotion (Conner & Barrett, 2005), (2) displays of negative emotion to others (Robinson & Meier, 2005), and (3) somatic symptoms (Robinson, Mitchell, Kirkeby, & Meier, 2006). Moreover, implicit self-esteem often interacts with traits to predict negative affect and somatic symptoms (Robinson & Wilkowski, 2006). These recent data suggest that there may be an intimate relation between implicit self-esteem, as measured by the IAT, and experiences and displays of negative emotion (Robinson & Meier, 2005).

The specific relation between IAT self-esteem and negative affect, but generally not positive affect (e.g., Conner & Barrett, 2005), deserves further explanation. One possibility is that high levels of implicit self-esteem constitute a type of "protective shield" that is differentially used to ward off negative self-associations but not positive ones (Robinson, Mitchell, et al., 2006). Other data, too, highlight possible relations between implicit self-esteem and the defensive operations of the self-concept (Jordan, Spencer, Zanna, Hoshino-Browne, & Correll, 2003). We add that this general, defense-related account of implicit self-esteem also comports with data reported by Pelham and colleagues (e.g., Jones, Pelham, Mirenberg, & Hetts, 2002). Thus, there are now intriguing hints that implicit self-esteem serves a defensive purpose and operates mainly in the area of protecting the self from ego threats (Conner & Barrett, 2005; Jones et al., 2002; Robinson & Meier, 2005).

Cognitive–Motivational Conflict

Psychodynamic theories have been important in suggesting that the mind can often be divided, with different components of it wishing different things (e.g., Freud, 1962). Furthermore, a conclusion of these clinicians was that motivational conflict, between different components of mind, often undermines subjective well-being (Freud, 1962; Horney, 1945). Behavioral theories of motivation have suggested the same point. For example, Miller's (1944) fascinating analysis of approach–avoidance conflicts demonstrates their pernicious effects in relation to a spatial location associated with both reward (e.g., a piece of cheese) and threat (e.g., an electrified grid). In Miller's research, rats placed in this approach–avoidance situation displayed behavioral manifestations of distress such as vacillation and defecation.

This general perspective on cognitive–motivational conflict has recently been extended in studies focused on RT-related measures. Along these lines,

Robinson, Vargas, and Crawford (2003) reported several studies revealing that explicit and implicit measures of personality interact. For example, explicit and implicit measures of femininity interacted, such that a greater degree of "match" (i.e., high explicit + high implicit or low explicit + low implicit) was associated with higher levels of subjective well-being in everyday life. Robinson, Vargas, et al. also reported that mismatches between implicit and explicit self-esteem were associated with lower levels of subjective well-being (see also Jordan et al., 2003).

Additional recent studies have focused on what we term the "threat comparator" skills of the individual (e.g., Tami et al., 2006). Briefly, prominent theories of self-regulation (Carver, 2004; Powers, 2004) posit that the successful self-regulation of behavior requires a "comparator" that is capable of categorizing stimuli in terms of active goals. For Carver (2004) and others (e.g., Meier & Robinson, 2005), the most fundamental goals of the individual relate to locomotion toward rewards and away from threats. In our studies, we have been particularly concerned with measuring threat comparator function. Therefore, we designed a go/no-go task and asked individuals to press the space bar whenever the word in question represents a significant threat to the self (e.g., *gun*, *criticism*). Individuals differ in the speed and accuracy with which they identify threatening words when told to do so, and the resulting scores operationalize threat comparator skills across individuals.

In one investigation, we focused on interactive predictions related to trait agreeableness (Robinson, Meier, & Solberg, 2005). Because agreeable individuals report a trusting, open approach to others, we posited that higher levels of threat comparator function might conflict with an open, trusting approach to social interaction. If so, higher threat comparator skills would be associated with *lower* subjective well-being among agreeable individuals. On the other hand, disagreeable individuals report a distrusting, suspicious approach to others, so we posited that higher levels of threat comparator function might be hedonically beneficial at low levels of agreeableness.

To investigate these predictions, we (Robinson et al., 2005) measured levels of subjective well-being using various common assessment instruments. As predicted, agreeableness and threat comparator function interacted to predict subjective well-being variables in all studies. Of particular importance here, higher levels of threat comparator function were associated with lower levels of subjective well-being among agreeable (but not disagreeable) individuals, consistent with the idea that cognitive tendencies to rapidly identify threats conflict with high levels of agreeableness, thereby undermining subjective well-being. Or, in more general terms, explicit/implicit "matches" are hedonically beneficial, whereas explicit/implicit "mismatches" are hedonically costly.

A subsequent investigation (Tamir et al., 2006) examined perhaps the most interesting case for our match–mismatch principles. Specifically, it is often thought that neurotic individuals are victims of their own vigilance for threats.

Clearly, this hypothesis would suggest that higher levels of threat comparator skills would undermine subjective well-being at higher levels of neuroticism. Yet, if people are generally well served when their comparator skills are suited to their trait dispositions (Robinson et al., 2003b), then higher levels of threat comparator skills could be beneficial to subjective well-being at higher levels of neuroticism.

Tamir et al. (2006) investigated such predictions in the context of tendencies to experience distress in everyday life. As predicted, neuroticism and threat comparator skills interacted to predict distress. Moreover, consistent with the match–mismatch principles, the authors found that threat comparator skills were beneficial to subjective well-being (here, defined in terms of less distress) at higher levels of neuroticism. Tamir et al. therefore concluded that neurotic individuals are actually served by, rather than victimized by, by tendencies to quickly and accurately recognize threatening stimuli.

In another series of studies (Robinson & Wilkowski, 2006), we were specifically interested in testing Horney's (1945) theory of neurotic conflict. For Horney, like Freud (1962), neurotic conflict was due to mismatches between conscious and unconscious motivation. However, Horney's theory, in contrast to Freud's, emphasized interpersonal motivation. She specifically encountered patients who consciously sought to accommodate to others (conscious high affiliation), yet unconsciously sought distance from them (unconscious low affiliation). She also encountered patients of the opposite type, who sought to be independent from others (conscious low affiliation), yet unconsciously seemed dependent on them (unconscious high affiliation). Such dynamics are reminiscent of the approach–avoidance conflicts documented by Miller (1944), with the goal-object here being personally important others.

To test Horney's (1945) theory, we (Robinson & Wilkowski, 2006) needed measures tapping conscious and unconscious affiliation tendencies. To measure conscious affiliation, we assessed agreeableness. Agreeable people self-report high levels of prosocial affect and behavior, whereas disagreeable people report that they place their own goals ahead of harmony in personal relationships. To measure unconscious affiliation, we used the IAT self-esteem task, which contrasts affective associations to the self versus others. Our thinking was that tendencies toward unconscious self-favoritism (i.e., high IAT self-esteem scores) would be subjectively beneficial at low levels of agreeableness, but subjectively costly at high levels of agreeableness specifically due to the match–mismatch principles mentioned above and so prominent in clinical theory (e.g., Horney, 1945).

In the Robinson and Wilkowski (2006) studies, neurotic conflict was measured in terms of trait neuroticism, negative affect, and psychopathological symptoms of anxiety. As predicted, agreeableness and implicit self-esteem interacted to predict these negative affect measures. At low levels of agreeableness, high implicit self-esteem was associated with *less* negative affect. However, at high

levels of agreeableness, high implicit self-esteem was associated with *more* negative affect. The studies therefore support Horney's (1945) theory in the sense that
mismatches between conscious and unconscious self-favoring tendencies (e.g.,
high agreeableness + high IAT self-esteem) are associated with a greater deal of
neurotic distress, specifically relative to the matching personality configurations
(e.g., high agreeableness + low IAT self-esteem). Such match–mismatch principles may help to provide an empirical basis for psychodynamic theories of subjective well-being.

Self-Regulation

Although theories of self-regulation (e.g., Carver, 2004; Powers, 2004) differ in
many respects, they share some important points. At a general level, self-
regulation involves both goals and cognitive skills. For example, Carver (2004)
and Powers (2004) highlight the importance of comparator processes in linking
higher-level goals to stimuli as they occur. As reported above, we have created
several comparator tasks, and the results of these studies are broadly consistent
with the idea that trait-matched comparator skills are hedonically beneficial,
likely because they are associated with a more efficient personality system of self-
regulation (e.g., Tamir et al., 2006).

An additional important aspect of self-regulation is the ability to monitor
one's own performance and to compensate for errors by bringing behavior in
line with desired goals (Lieberman, 2003). Error-monitoring and self-correction
processes are known to involve the frontal lobes; for example, a scalp potential
originating from the cingulate cortex in the frontal lobe is especially evident following errors in performance and predicts subsequent behavioral compensation
(Holroyd & Coles, 2002). Several studies have shown that chronic worriers
exhibit stronger evoked potentials following errors (e.g., Hajcak, McDonald, &
Simons, 2003). Thus, there is an intriguing relationship between negative affect
and the operation of the error self-regulation system (Luu, Collins, & Tucker,
2000).

However, such results leave it uncertain whether increased tendencies
toward error self-regulation contribute to subjective distress, or, alternatively,
may be helpful in reducing it among distress-prone individuals (Luu, Collins, &
Tucker, 2000). To investigate this question, a recent series of studies examined
relations between neuroticism, error-correction processes, and daily negative
affect (Robinson, Ode, Wilkowski, & Amodio, in press). The researchers found
that neuroticism and error self-regulation tendencies, measured in terms of
slower RT following errors, interacted in predicting daily negative affect. Specifically, higher tendencies toward error self-regulation were associated with *less*
daily distress at high levels of neuroticism. This was not true at low levels of neu-

roticism. Thus, it appears that neurotic individuals, but not non-neurotic ones, subjectively benefit from skills related to error self-regulation. This is likely true because error self-regulation processes support the defensive, avoidant sorts of motivations that characterize individuals high in neuroticism (Robinson et al., in press).

Another important function of self-regulatory processes is to inhibit activated but inappropriate cognitive routines (e.g., Lieberman, 2003). The tendency to repeat, rather than switch, activated response tendencies is often known as *perseveration*, and has long been reported in patients with frontal lobe damage (Milner, 1995). However, tasks sensitive to frontal lobe damage (e.g., the Wisconsin Card Sorting Task: Milner, 1995) are relatively insensitive to normal variations in perseveration (Pennington, Bennetto, McAleer, & Roberts, 1996). Therefore, to measure perseverative tendencies in normal populations, it may be useful to develop more sensitive assessment instruments, such as those based on RT.

The cognitive literature provides some guidelines. Specifically, Baddeley (1996) reports that cognitive responses have a tendency to reenact themselves in the absence of top-down control, specifically due to cognitive inertia. Therefore, in designing a cognitive assessment instrument of perseveration, we sought to build on this literature. In several studies, we (Robinson & Cervone, 2006; Robinson, Wilkowski, Kirkeby, & Meier, 2006) have used choice RT paradigms, such as the Stroop task, with two response options (e.g., red vs. green). Response perseveration is scored across consecutive trials and involves the relative speed to switch (e.g., red–green) versus repeat (e.g., green–green) primed response tendencies. A higher perseveration score indicates greater difficulties when responses must be switched across trials.

Although perseveration that is associated with frontal lobe damage may be pathological (Milner, 1995), this may not be the case for normal variations in perseveration among individuals without brain damage. Indeed, we predicted that perseverative tendencies would reinforce trait-linked experiences. From this perspective, if one is lucky enough to possess high levels of self-esteem and low levels of neuroticism, perseveration may tend to support higher levels of subjective well-being. By contrast, if one is unlucky enough to possess low levels of self-esteem and high levels of neuroticism, perseveration may tend to support lower levels of subjective well-being.

In support of such interactive predictions, we have found that perseverative tendencies are associated with higher levels of subjective well-being among those predisposed to high levels of subjective well-being, but lower levels of subjective well-being among those predisposed to low levels of subjective well-being (Robinson & Cervone, 2006; Robinson, Wilkowski, et al., 2006). For example, one series of studies found that perseverative tendencies were beneficial at high levels of self-esteem, but costly at low levels of self-esteem (Robinson &

Cervone, 2006). Therefore, we suggest that a tendency to repeat the past rein-forces trait-linked experiences, whether for hedonic good (e.g., high self-esteem) or bad (e.g., low self-esteem).

In discussing the hedonic correlates of perseverative tendencies, it is also important to present a complementary perspective on this data. Specifically, it is important to point out that the interactions reported in these studies indicated that trait-related variables were *less predictive* of the subjective well-being variables at lower levels of perseveration (Robinson & Cervone, 2006; Robinson, Wilkowski, et al., 2006). For example, self-esteem predicted subjective well-being outcomes at high, but not low, levels of perseveration (Robinson & Cervone, 2006). This finding comports with other data from our lab indicating that traits are less relevant among individuals who are more responsive to events as they occur (e.g., Robinson, Goetz, Wilkowski, & Hoffman, 2006; Robinson et al., 2003b).

The Happy Mind: Summary and Analysis

Having presented our major sources of data, it is now useful to adopt a wider perspective. In relation to the cognitive processes examined, it is straightforward to suggest that the happy mind might be characterized in terms of (1) attentional biases favoring positive information, (2) categorization tendencies favoring posi-tive information, (3) priming tendencies favoring positive information, (4) higher levels of implicit self-esteem, (5) a relative absence of cognitive–motivational conflict, and (6) superior self-regulation abilities. To what extent do our studies support this conception of the happy mind?

In relation to selective attention, we have found robust relations between positive affect and a tendency to selectively attend to positive information in attentional probe tasks (e.g., Tamir & Robinson, in press). However, such tasks may be more useful to the extent that they incorporate explicit evaluations and focus on spatial disengagement difficulties. Such modifications are designed to produce larger attention-related priming effects in relation to a stage of attention—disengagement—that appears to be especially sensitive to the motiva-tions of the individual (Wilkowski et al., 2006).

In relation to categorization tendencies, we have reported evidence that negative evaluation tendencies can *undermine* levels of subjective well-being (Robinson et al., 2004). However, in numerous investigations along these lines, we have yet to devise a categorization task that is associated with *higher* levels of subjective well-being. Perhaps positive affect and well-being emerge from differ-ent processes than those tapped by categorization tasks of the type reviewed here. This explanation is plausible in light of suggestions that there is an intimate relation between negative affect and encoding processes (Öhman, 1997). Positive affect, on the other hand, may be more dependent on elaborative cognitive operations, a suggestion that seems consistent with Fredrickson's (1998) "broaden-and-build" model of positive affect.

Indeed, we have found robust evidence for the idea that happy individuals display more pronounced affective priming facilitation when asked to rate the intensity of one of their positive emotions when it follows another positive emotion (Robinson & Kirkeby, 2005). This finding suggests that happy individuals have more interconnected knowledge concerning their positive emotions. To extend this effect to the organization of affective knowledge more generally, it seems useful to examine whether happy individuals also have more pronounced positive priming effects in tasks not dependent on retrieving self-knowledge. Robinson and von Hippel (2006) report data along these lines, and it therefore seems sound to suggest that subjective well-being relates to the relative magnitude of positive and negative priming effects in affective priming tasks.

In relation to IAT self-esteem, some recent reports have linked low levels of implicit self-esteem to higher levels of negative affect (e.g., Conner & Barrett, 2005; Robinson & Meier, 2005). However, none of these studies has linked implicit self-esteem to higher levels of positive affect. We therefore suggest that implicit self-esteem may be of more relevance in predicting negative affect than positive affect, probably because implicit self-esteem serves a defensive function in warding off threats to the self (Jordan et al., 2003; Robinson et al., 2006).

In relation to an absence of cognitive–motivational conflict, our results were also generally focused on negative affective outcomes. That is, the presence of cognitive–motivational conflict may be associated with higher levels of subjective distress, but the absence of such conflict may not be associated with higher levels of positive affect. We therefore suggest that cognitive–motivational conflicts may have more relevance to the prediction of negative affect than positive affect, a conclusion that seems consistent with the prior literature on approach–avoidance conflicts and their capacity to induce distress (e.g., Miller, 1944).

Finally, in relation to cognitive operations hypothesized to be associated with self-regulation, we have found little evidence for the commonsense idea that self-regulation is necessarily beneficial, here as defined in terms of higher levels of subjective well-being. For example, error self-regulation tendencies were associated with less daily distress at high, but not low, levels of neuroticism (Robinson, Ode, et al., 2006). Similarly, tendencies toward perseveration were associated with more daily distress at high, but not low, levels of neuroticism (Robinson, Wilkowski, et al., 2006). What emerges from this data, in general, is the suggestion that cognitive tendencies indicative of self-regulation are especially beneficial at high levels of neuroticism (Robinson, Ode, et al., 2006; Robinson, Wilkowski, et al., 2006). This conclusion seems broadly consistent with clinical theory (e.g., Freud, 1962) and data (e.g., Borkovec & Sharpless, 2004).

In further summary, we suggest that processes related to selective attention and priming appear to be promising in predicting positive affect in a zero-order correlational manner. By contrast, we suggest that the processes associated with categorization tendencies, implicit self-esteem, cognitive–motivational conflict, and cognitive self-regulation have more relevance to the prediction of negative affect. Even in relation to this conclusion, however, it is worthwhile to reiterate that the general picture is one in which self-reported traits and cognitive processing measures often *interact* in the prediction of subjective well-being outcomes, whether related to positive affect, negative affect, or life satisfaction. Such interactions are consistent with a broader perspective on personality that recognizes the fact that outcome variables ultimately reflect the integrative personality system of the individual, including both its explicit and implicit components.

Conclusions

The present chapter was concerned with the cognitive correlates of subjective well-being. Given the apparent productivity of this approach, further research is recommended. However, it is important to note that cognition consists of a large variety of processes, which in turn serve different functions and purposes for the individual. Moreover, these functions and purposes themselves depend on traits, temperament, and the more molar goals of the individual. Therefore, it is important to investigate the cognitive correlates of subjective well-being in a creative and systematic manner. Doing so will lead to exciting developments in the future.

Finally, we would like to conclude by paying a small tribute to Ed Diener, who played such a major role in the scientific study of subjective well-being. It seems likely to us that without Ed's ground-breaking work in this area, the present chapter would not exist. Moreover, we note that Ed Diener embraced multiple perspectives on subjective well-being in the belief that a multiplicity of perspectives would bring us closer to understanding the truth of this important, even crucial, construct. We feel indebted to him for his appreciation of a cognitive perspective of subjective well-being and hope that the present chapter provides some insights along these lines.

Acknowledgment

Michael D. Robinson acknowledges support from the National Institute of Mental Health (Grant No. MH 068241).

References

Baddeley, A. D. (1996). Exploring the central executive. *Quarterly Journal of Experimental Psychology: Human Experimental Psychology, 49,* 5–28.

Borkovec, T. D., & Sharpless, B. (2004). Generalized anxiety disorder: Bringing cognitive-behavioral therapy into the valued present. In S. C. Hayes, V. M. Follette, & M. M. Linehan (Eds.), *Mindfulness and acceptance: Expanding the cognitive-behavioral tradition* (pp. 209–242). New York: Guilford Press.

Bosson, J. K., Swann, W. B., Jr., & Pennebaker, J. W. (2000). Stalking the perfect measure of implicit self-esteem: The blind men and the elephant revisited? *Journal of Personality and Social Psychology, 79,* 631–643.

Carver, C. S. (2004). Self-regulation of action and affect. In R. F. Baumeister & K. D. Vohs (Eds.), *Handbook of self-regulation: Research, theory, and applications* (pp. 13–39). New York: Guilford Press.

Compton, R. J., Wirtz, D., Pajoumand, G., Claus, E., & Heller, W. (2004). Association between positive affect and attentional shifting. *Cognitive Research and Therapy, 28,* 733–744.

Conner, T., & Barrett, L. F. (2005). Implicit self-attitudes predict spontaneous affect in daily life. *Emotion, 5,* 476–488.

Csikszentmihalyi, M. (1997). *Finding flow: The psychology of engagement with everyday life.* New York: Basic Books.

Davis, P. J. (1987). Repression and the inaccessibility of affective memories. *Journal of Personality and Social Psychology, 53,* 585–593.

De Houwer, J. (2003). A structural analysis of indirect measures of attitudes. In J. Musch & K. C. Klauer (Eds.), *The psychology of evaluation: Affective processes in cognition and emotion* (pp. 219–244). Mahwah, NJ: Erlbaum.

Fazio, R. H., & Olson, M. A. (2003). Implicit measures in social cognition research: Their meaning and uses. *Annual Review of Psychology, 54,* 297–327.

Fox, E., Russo, R., Bowles, R., & Dutton, K. (2001). Do threatening stimuli draw or hold visual attention in subclinical anxiety? *Journal of Experimental Psychology: General, 130,* 681–700.

Fredrickson, B. L. (1998). What good are positive emotions? *Review of General Psychology, 2,* 300–319.

Freud, S. (1962). *The ego and the id.* New York: Norton.

Gasper, K., & Clore, G. L. (2002). Attending to the big picture: Mood and global versus local processing of visual information. *Psychological Science, 13,* 34–40.

Greenwald, A. G., & Banaji, M. R. (1995). Implicit social cognition: Attitudes, self-esteem, and stereotypes. *Psychological Review, 102,* 4–27.

Greenwald, A. G., & Farnham, S. D. (2000). Using the implicit association test to measure self-esteem and self-concept. *Journal of Personality and Social Psychology, 79,* 1022–1038.

Greenwald, A. G., McGhee, D. E., & Schwartz, J. L. K. (1998). Measuring individual differences in implicit cognition: The implicit association test. *Journal of Personality and Social Psychology, 74,* 1464–1480.

Hajcak, G., McDonald, N., & Simons, R. F. (2003). Anxiety and error-related brain activity. *Biological Psychology, 64,* 77–90.

Higgins, E. T. (1996). Knowledge activation: Accessibility, applicability, and salience. In E. T. Higgins & A. W. Kruglanski (Eds.), *Social psychology: Handbook of basic principles* (pp. 133–168). New York: Guilford Press.

Hofmann, W., Gawronski, B., Gschwendner, T., Le, H., & Schmitt, M. (2005). A meta-analysis of the correlation between the implicit association test and explicit self-report measures. *Personality and Social Psychology Bulletin, 31*, 1369–1385.

Holroyd, C. B., & Coles, M. G. H. (2002). The neural basis of human error processing: Reinforcement learning, dopamine, and the error-related negativity. *Psychological Review, 109*, 679–709.

Horney, K. (1945). *Our inner conflicts*. Oxford, UK: Norton.

Isen, A. M. (2004). Some perspectives on positive feelings and emotions: Positive affect facilitates thinking and problem solving. In A. S. R. Manstead, N. Frijda, & A. Fischer (Eds.), *Feelings and emotions: The Amsterdam symposium* (pp. 263–281). New York: Cambridge University Press.

James, W. (1950/1890). *The principles of psychology*. New York: Dove. (Original work published 1890)

Jones, J. T., Pelham, B. W., Mirenberg, M. C., & Hetts, J. J. (2002). Name letter preferences are not mere exposure: Implicit egotism as self-regulation. *Journal of Experimental Social Psychology, 38*, 170–177.

Jordan, C. H., Spencer, S. J., Zanna, M. P., Hoshino-Browne, E., & Correll, J. (2003). Secure and defensive high self-esteem. *Journal of Personality and Social Psychology, 85*, 969–978.

Kelly, G. A. (1963). *A theory of personality: The psychology of personal constructs*. New York: Norton.

Lieberman, M. D. (2003). Reflexive and reflective judgment processes: A social cognitive neuroscience approach. In J. P. Forgas, K. D. Williams, & W. von Hippel (Eds.), *Social judgments: Implicit and explicit processes* (pp. 44–67). New York: Cambridge University Press.

Luu, P., Collins, P., & Tucker, D. M. (2000). Mood, personality, and self-monitoring: Negative affect and emotionality in relation to frontal lobe mechanisms of error monitoring. *Journal of Experimental Psychology: General, 129*, 43–60.

Lyubomirsky, S., King, L., & Diener, E. (2005). The benefits of frequent positive affect: Does happiness lead to success? *Psychological Bulletin, 131*, 803–855.

MacLeod, C. (1999). Anxiety and anxiety disorders. In T. Dalgleish & M. J. Power (Eds.), *Handbook of cognition and emotion* (pp. 447–477). New York: Wiley.

McClelland, D. C. (1987). *Human motivation*. New York: Cambridge University Press.

Meier, B. P., & Robinson, M. D. (2004). Does quick to blame mean quick to anger?: The role of agreeableness in dissociating blame and anger. *Personality and Social Psychology Bulletin, 30*, 856–867.

Meier, B. P., & Robinson, M. D. (2005). The metaphorical representation of affect. *Metaphor and Symbol, 20*, 239–257.

Meier, B. P., Robinson, M. D., & Wilkowski, B. M. (2006). Turning the other cheek: Agreeableness and the self-regulation of aggressive-related primes. *Psychological Science, 17*, 136–142.

Miller, N. E. (1944). Experimental studies of conflict. In J. Hunt (Ed.), *Personality and the behavior disorders* (pp. 431–465). Oxford, UK: Ronald Press.

Milner, B. (1995). Aspects of frontal lobe function. In H. H. Jasper & S. Riggio (Eds.), *Epilepsy and the functional autonomy of the frontal lobe* (pp. 66–84). New York: Raven Press.

Mogg, K., & Bradley, B. P. (1998). A cognitive–motivational analysis of anxiety. *Behaviour Research and Therapy, 36,* 809–848.

Öhman, A. (1997). As fast as the blink of an eye: Evolutionary preparedness for preattentive processing of threat. In P. J. Lang, R. F. Simons, & M. Balaban (Eds.), *Attention and orienting: Sensory and motivational processes* (pp. 165–184). Mahwah, NJ: Erlbaum.

Pashler, H. E. (1998). *The psychology of attention.* Cambridge, MA: MIT Press.

Pennington, B. F., Bennetto, L., McAleer, O., & Roberts, R. J. (1996). Executive functions and working memory: Theoretical and measurement issues. In G. R. Lyon & N. A. Krasnegor (Eds.), *Attention, memory, and executive function* (pp. 327–348). Baltimore, MD: Brookes.

Powers, W. T. (2004). *Making sense of behavior: The meaning of control.* New Canaan, CT: Benchmark.

Ready, R. E., Robinson, M. D., & Weinberger, M. (2006). Age differences in the organization of emotion knowledge: Effects involving valence and time frame. *Psychology and Aging, 21,* 726–736.

Robinson, M. D. (2004). Personality as performance: Categorization tendencies and their correlates. *Current Directions in Psychological Science, 13,* 127–129.

Robinson, M. D., & Cervone, D. (2006). Riding a wave of self-esteem: Perseverative tendencies as dispositional forces. *Journal of Experimental Social Psychology, 42,* 103–111.

Robinson, M. D., & Clore, G. L. (2002). Belief and feeling: Evidence for an accessibility model of emotional self-report. *Psychological Bulletin, 128,* 934–960.

Robinson, M. D., Goetz, M. C., Wilkowski, B. M., & Hoffman, S. J. (2006). Driven to tears or to joy: Response dominance and trait-based predictions. *Personality and Social Psychology Bulletin, 32,* 629–640.

Robinson, M. D., & Kirkeby, B. S. (2005). Happiness as a belief system: Individual differences and priming in emotion judgments. *Personality and Social Psychology Bulletin, 31,* 1134–1144.

Robinson, M. D., & Meier, B. P. (2005). Rotten to the core: Neuroticism and implicit evaluations of the self. *Self and Identity, 4,* 361–372.

Robinson, M. D., Meier, B. P., & Solberg, E. C. (2005). What shields some can shackle others: The approach-related consequences of threat categorizations vary by agreeableness. *European Journal of Personality, 19,* 1–20.

Robinson, M. D., Mitchell, K. A., & Kirkeby, B. S., & Meier, B. P. (2006). The self as a container: Implications for implicit self-esteem and somatic symptoms. *Metaphor and Symbol, 21,* 147–167.

Robinson, M. D., & Neighbors, C. (2006). Catching the mind in action: Implicit methods in personality research and assessment. In M. Eid & E. Diener (Eds.), *Handbook of multimethod measurement in psychology* (pp. 115–126). Washington, DC: American Psychological Association.

Robinson, M. D., Ode, S., Wilkowski, B. M., & Amodio, D. M. (in press). Neurotic contentment: A self-regulation view of neuroticism-linked distress. *Emotion.*

Robinson, M. D., Solberg, E. C., Vargas, P. T., & Tamir, M. (2003). Trait as default: Extraversion, subjective well-being, and the distinction between neutral and positive events. *Journal of Personality and Social Psychology, 85,* 517–527.

Robinson, M. D., Vargas, P. T., & Crawford, E. G. (2003). Putting process into personality, appraisal, and emotion: Evaluative processing as a missing link. In J. Musch & K. C. Klauer (Eds.), *The psychology of evaluation: Affective processes in cognition and emotion* (pp. 275–306). Mahwah, NJ: Erlbaum.

Robinson, M. D., Vargas, P. T., Tamir, M., & Solberg, E. C. (2004). Using and being used by categories: The case of negative evaluations and daily well-being. *Psychological Science, 15,* 521–526.

Robinson, M. D., & von Hippel, W. (2006). Rose-colored priming effects: Life satisfaction and affective priming. *Journal of Positive Psychology, 1,* 187–197.

Robinson, M. D., & Wilkowski, B. M. (2006). Loving, hating, vacillating: Agreeableness, implicit self-esteem, and neurotic conflict. *Journal of Personality, 74,* 935–978.

Robinson, M. D., Wilkowski, B. M., Kirkeby, B. S., & Meier, B. P. (2006). Stuck in a rut: Perseverative response tendencies and the neuroticism–distress relationship. *Journal of Experimental Psychology: General, 135,* 78–91.

Schimmack, U., & Diener, E. (2003). Predictive validity of explicit and implicit self-esteem for subjective well-being. *Journal of Research in Personality, 37,* 100–106.

Showers, C. (1992). Compartmentalization of positive and negative self-knowledge: Keeping bad apples out of the bunch. *Journal of Personality and Social Psychology, 62,* 1036–1049.

Smith, E. R. (1998). Mental representation and memory. In D. T. Gilbert, S. T. Fiske, & G. Lindzey (Eds.), *The handbook of social psychology* (4th ed., pp. 391–445). New York: McGraw-Hill.

Tamir, M., & Robinson, M. D. (in press). The happy spotlight: Positive mood and selective attention to positive information. *Personality and Social Psychology Bulletin.*

Tamir, M., Robinson, M. D., & Solberg, E. C. (2006). You may worry, but can you recognize threats when you see them?: Neuroticism, threat identifications, and negative affect. *Journal of Personality, 74,* 1481–1506.

Wilkowski, B. M., Robinson, M. D., & Meier, B. P. (2006). Agreeableness and the prolonged spatial processing of antisocial and prosocial information. *Journal of Research in Personality, 40,* 1152–1168.

12

The Frequency of Social Comparison and Its Relation to Subjective Well-Being

FRANK FUJITA

I never compare myself to Coach Knight because I don't need to put any more pressure on myself. When you stop and look at Coach Knight's incredible numbers, you will overwhelm yourself.

—MIKE DAVIS (in Licandro, 2001)

I always compare myself to my twin sister. We're completely different people. [But] I used to be like her. We were just messy people, don't keep ourselves organized. Now I can't live without my calendar, I can't live without my journal. I just can't go without it. Her, it's like, *"I'll remember." I say, "trust me, you're not gonna remember."*

—MAYA (*Whatkidscando.org*, 2003)

I always compare myself to girls in the street or at work; they're always prettier and better dressed with nicer hair than me; I hate feeling this way and this year I'm determined to change.

—ALASIA (2006)

i live a life of opulence compared with many on this globe. yet i want more. because i never compare myself to the have nots—who does?—i always think of what i don't have.

—BETTON (2006)

Diener and Fujita (1997) outline various ways that social comparisons may or may not affect subjective well-being. They coined the term *"forced comparison hypothesis,"* which is the theory that the most propinquitous others are salient (Festinger, 1954) and will therefore serve as the primary standard for judgment. The forced comparison hypothesis predicts that one will be happier when those closest to oneself are the least fortunate. There is little evidence to support the forced comparison hypothesis. For example, Fujita (1993) found that the financial status, physical attractiveness, and academic achievement of randomly assigned roommates had no effect on participants' satisfaction with their own standing on those domains, and that the social relationships of randomly assigned roommates had a positive effect on their satisfaction with their own social relationships, such that if their roommates had very good social relationships, they were more satisfied with their own social relationships. There is evidence, however, that the larger environment, such as a school for a student assessing his or her academic ability (Marsh, 1987; Marsh & Hau, 2003; Marsh & Parker, 1984), a standard metropolitan statistical area for a person assessing his or her income (Hagerty, 2000), or a nation for a person assessing his or her individualism–collectivism (Heine, Lehman, Peng, & Greenholtz, 2002) provides a useful comparison standard. This larger environment may affect happiness via Parducci's (1984) range–frequency theory (Hagerty, 2000; Smith, Diener, & Wedell, 1989). Thus, the evidence seems to support the idea that the larger environment can affect subjective well-being through social comparisons perhaps by providing information about the distribution of attributes in the environment, but that naturalistic social comparisons with those closest to us, such as a roommate, do not affect our satisfaction.

In contrast to the forced comparison hypothesis, the *coping personality model* (Diener & Fujita, 1997) emphasizes the active construction of comparison targets and avoidance of unwanted comparisons for mood enhancement, self-motivation, and self-evaluation. For example, optimists and nondepressives will experience a more positive affective reaction to a forced comparison, whereas pessimists and depressives will experience a more negative affective reaction to a forced comparison, as the size of the comparison group increases (McFarland & Miller, 1994) because the increase produces more options in the choice of a comparison target. Optimistic and nondepressive people can cope by reducing social comparisons when performing poorly (Gibbons, Benbow, & Gerrard, 1994), but depressed people *increase* social comparisons when performing poorly (Swallow & Kuiper, 1992). People can also cope by modifying their goals and the importance of those goals to reflect their resources and recent successes and failures (Diener & Fujita, 1995). To illustrate, someone who does not possess the social graces necessary to succeed in a particular social group is likely to devalue the acceptance of that group as a goal.

There are other indicators that the relationship between social comparison and subjective well-being is a complex one. For example, more than half of the relationship between social comparison (with "other people") and income satisfaction is mediated by desires (Solberg, Diener, Wirtz, Lucas, & Oishi, 2002), such that the social comparisons are used to inform us about the types of entertainment, travel, clothes, etc., that are available to desire, and that those desires are important in determining whether we are satisfied with our income, in addition to the simple relation of "other people have more, therefore I am less satisfied." In addition, when a dimension is highly important to us, social comparison information does not affect our mood as much as when the dimension is less important (Pachnowska, 1996). Also it is important to note that either upward or downward comparisons may result in increasing or decreasing happiness (Buunk, Collins, Taylor, Van Yperen, & Dakof, 1990).

How Do Happy and Unhappy People Differ in How They Engage in Social Comparison?

Many social psychologists consider social comparison to be something that happens to an individual. From this perspective, when we are presented with another person who is obviously better or worse off, we have no choice but to make a social comparison. "It can be hard to hear an extremely intelligent person on the radio, or see an extremely handsome one in the grocery store, or participate on a panel with an expert without engaging in social comparison no matter how much we would like not to" (Goethals, 1986, p. 272). We can, however, consider social comparison to be a particular type of social cognition that we can choose either to engage in—or not.

> We hypothesize that people make these biased estimates through *constructive social comparison*. Constructive social comparison is social comparison "in the head," with little regard for actual social reality and is comprised of a number of processes, including the manufacturing of self-serving consensus estimates. (Goethals, Messick, & Allison, 1991, p. 150, emphasis in the original)

Even if we do not choose whether or not to make a comparison, we can choose whether or not to let that comparison affect our mood or self-perceptions. Thus, happy people increased their anagram ability rating, whether the peer next to them completed the task more quickly or more slowly, but unhappy people only increased their anagram ability rating if the peer next to them completed the task more slowly than they did (Lyubomirsky & Ross, 1997). A similar pattern was found with mood, except that when happy people completed the anagram task more slowly than the peer next to them, their mood increased nonsignificantly. When solving anagrams in teams that were manipulated to lose, happy people were unaffected by comparisons, indicating that they performed best in their losing team—their mood was relatively unaffected either way. Unhappy people, however, experienced decreases in positive mood when their team lost, but not if they were informed that they had performed best among their losing team (Lyubomirsky, Tucker, & Kasri, 2001; Study 1). A similar pattern was found in self-ratings of current and future performance. These findings suggest that unhappy people are more likely to depend on passive social comparison, that is, they will let whatever social comparisons are readily available in the environment affect their mood and self-concept, whereas happy people are more likely to engage in an active social comparison process, sometimes determining that social comparisons are not relevant to their mood and self-concept.

Frequency of Social Comparison

To investigate individual differences in the frequency of social comparison, Gibbons and Buunk (1999) developed the *Iowa–Netherlands Comparison Orientation Measure* (INCOM). The INCOM shows good psychometric properties, and its use has led to the beginnings of an understanding of how those high in *social comparison orientation* (SCO) who frequently make social comparisons differ from those low in SCO who make less frequent social comparisons. For example, compared with those low in SCO, those high in SCO are (1) higher in neuroticism (Buunk, Nauta, & Molleman, 2005; Gibbons & Buunk, 1999), (2) more attracted to others with dissimilar attitudes (Michinov & Michinov, 2001), (3) more satisfied with their relationships when they engage in downward comparison (Buunk, Oldersma, & de Dreu, 2001), and (4) respond with more jealousy when a romantic rival has more desirable attributes (Dijkstra & Buunk, 2002).

But the INCOM has also led to some confusing results. For example, among Dutch nurses, those high in SCO experienced more negative affect when presented with a downward comparison target but not more positive affect when presented with an upward comparison target (Buunk, Van der Zee, & Van Yperen, 2001), but among Spanish physicians, those high in SCO reported more positive affect when they saw downward comparison targets and more negative affect when they saw upward comparison targets (Buunk, Zurriaga, Peiro, Nauta, & Gosalvez, 2005). In Dutch samples, those high in SCO were lower in openness to experience (Buunk, Nauta, & Molleman, 2005; Gibbons & Buunk, 1999), but in a U.S. sample the relation was not significant and in the opposite direction (Gibbons & Buunk, 1999). It is encouraging to see that the INCOM is being used with therapists experiencing various levels of burnout (Buunk, Ybema, Gibbons, & Ipenburg, 2001), with individuals experiencing various levels of depression (Buunk & Brenninkmeijer, 2001), and with people who were being treated or had been treated for cancer (Van der Zee, Oldersma, Buunk, & Bos, 1998), but the results of these investigations are not yet coalescing into an understanding of how SCO affects emotional experience.

Others have looked at the frequency of social comparison without using the INCOM. Wheeler and Miyake (1992) found that people with high self-esteem engage in more frequent downward lifestyle comparisons than people with lower self-esteem. Schwartz and colleagues (2002) have found that "maximizers—those who want to make sure to make the very best choices—engage in more frequent upward and downward social comparisons than "satisficers"—those who want to make good enough choices. Satisficers are happier, more optimistic, and have higher levels of self-esteem and life satisfaction than maximizers.

The Relation between Subjective Well-Being and the Frequency of Social Comparison

There are several possible relationships between subjective well-being and the frequency of social comparison. Because people are able to choose whether or not to engage in social comparison, and if they do choose to compare, they can choose with whom to compare, and because people are motivated to feel good, we might expect that, all things being equal, those people who do engage in frequent social comparison would experience more positive affect and higher life satisfaction. As an analogy, because people are able to choose whether or not to refinance a home mortgage, and if they do choose to refinance, they can choose with which lender to refinance, and because people are motivated to pay the least amount of money for a product or service, we might expect that, all things being equal, those people who do refinance their home mortgage would pay a lower interest rate. Unfortunately for this social comparison hypothesis, the strong empirical relationship between the INCOM and neuroticism (Buunk, Nauta, & Molleman, 2005; Gibbons & Buunk, 1999) would present a difficult obstacle to this line of reasoning.

There are some indications that frequent social comparison may lead to negative affect. At lease one negative emotion, envy, requires an upward social comparison (Smith, Parrott, Diener, Hoyle, & Kim, 1999). But it is also possible that frequent social comparison, even frequent upward social comparison, could have enough positive emotional outcomes to outweigh the occasional experience of envy or other negative emotions. Upward comparisons can have positive emotional outcomes, especially when we draw inspiration from the target of the upward comparison. Downward comparisons can have negative effects on our mood, especially if we see our own future in the target of the downward comparison. Because social comparison frequency includes both upward and downward comparisons, and because both upward and downward comparisons can have either positive or negative emotional outcomes (Buunk et al., 1990), there may be no relationship between social comparison frequency and subjective well-being.

Another line of reasoning suggests that because uncertainty is a major cause of the desire to engage in social comparison (Festinger, 1954; Marsh & Webb, 1996), those people who frequently engage in social comparison are probably less certain in their attitudes and in their self-concept. Most people with low self-esteem don't actually disagree with items such as "I feel that I have a number of good qualities," but they do average close to the midpoint of the scale, indicating uncertainty. Thus we might expect those people who have low self-esteem to be more frequent social comparers. From this perspective, self-selected social comparisons partially remediate the negative affect that is precipitated from low self-esteem.

Empirical Study: Frequency of Social Comparison Scale

It would be useful to investigate the personality of the person who is a frequent social comparer. Although we cannot logically generalize from relationships between individual difference variables to the social cognition processes within a single individual, a personality picture of the frequent social comparer, nevertheless in addition to being interesting in its own right, can lead to some hypotheses about the within-person processes involved in social comparison and how they may affect subjective well-being.

Although the INCOM measures social comparison orientation, it may be useful to develop a new scale that focuses more directly on the *frequency* of social comparisons. Thus, whereas the INCOM asks participants to agree or disagree with statements such as "I always like to know what others in a similar situation would do," the current study directly asks participants how often they compare themselves with others.

Method

Participants and Procedures

The participants were 222 college students (110 men and 112 women) drawn from a larger sample of 259 students enrolled in a semester-long course on subjective well-being research at a large Midwestern university, the University of Illinois, Urbana–Champaign (U of I). Participants were enrolled in the course in either the fall semester of 1991 or the spring semester of 1992. The respondents completed a number of self-report personality and affect scales as class exercises either in laboratory sessions or at home. The students received lectures on well-being and also completed questionnaires and received personal feedback on many of the measures. In addition, they gathered reports from friends and family members and provided daily reports of their emotions and experiences for 52 days. Data provided by 37 individuals were omitted before the data analyses because these individuals admitted to being careless with, or faking part of, their data. Some analyses included slightly fewer individuals because of scattered missing data.

Measures

Frequency of Social Comparison Scale. Social comparison is a cognitive act. In theory, it would be possible to count each time we made a social comparison. Although no single-administration self-report measure will provide an accurate count of any behavior, it may be desirable to base a self-report scale on the number of times that we engage in social comparison. Such a scale would allow the discovery of relationships between an individual difference variable of frequent social comparison and other personality characteristics and allow us to distinguish these relationships from effects of situationally imposed social comparisons. Because both upward and downward social comparisons may have either positive or negative emotional outcomes, it was decided to focus on acts of comparison and to ignore the direction of comparison.

Informal questioning with a focus group produced a wide variety of social comparison frequency estimates, ranging from "I don't think I've ever done that" to "I can't count how many times a day I compare my looks to beautiful women." The response scale attempted to address this wide range of responses. Social comparisons can be analyzed along two dimensions: (1) who is the comparison target and (2) what is the attribute being compared. Smaller environmental targets, such as family and friends, as well as larger environmental targets, such as the average University of Illinois undergraduate, were included. A sampling of attributes was chosen, mostly to represent the attributes that are most important to our participants, such as grades, social skill, and physical attractiveness. The Frequency of Social Comparison Scale (FSCS) was designed to facilitate an understanding of the relationship between social comparisons and subjective well-being; no items were included to specifically measure social comparisons of attitudes, although those comparisons could be included in the items that asked about social comparisons by target.

The 15 items of the scale, as it was used with this sample, are presented in Table 12.1. Items should be modified or deleted to be relevant comparison targets and domains for the sample being measured. Correlation coefficients among the 15 items were transformed using Fisher's r to z transformation, averaged, and then retransformed back into the correlation metric. The average correlation of the items with each other was .59. A principle components analysis of the 15-item scale produced two eigenvalues greater than one. The first eigenvalue explains 56% of the variance in the correlation matrix of the items, the second factor explains an additional 9% of the variance. The items that loaded highest on the second factor were the domain items of spending money, moral character, financial status, and family relationships. Before rotation, all items loaded higher on the first component than on the second component. A direct oblimin rotation was performed; the two factors correlated with each other .61. Given the high explanatory power of the first eigenvalue and the high correlation between the factors, it is useful to consider the FSCS as if it were unidimensional. Cronbach's

TABLE 12.1. The Frequency of Social Comparison Scale with Means for Each Item

DIRECTIONS: Answer the following questions using the scale below. Don't just think of the last couple of days, but how often you do these things in general.

    10)—Always;
     9)—Almost always;
     8)—More than twice a day;
     7)—Once or twice a day;
     6)—Three to six times a week;
     5)—Once or twice a week;
     4)—Once or twice a month;
     3)—Once or twice a year;
     2)—Once or twice in my life;
     1)—Never

How often do you compare yourself (on anything) with:

    1) Your friends? (6.25)
    2) Your nuclear family? (4.79)
    3) The average U of I undergraduate? (5.40)
    4) The person or group you most often compare yourself with? (6.49)
    5) Anybody else? (4.83)

How often do you compare yourself with others (anybody) on:

    6) Grades? (5.74)
    7) Social skill? (5.59)
    8) Intelligence? (5.55)
    9) Spending money? (4.92)
    10) Moral character? (4.82)
    11) Financial status? (4.69)
    12) Family relationships? (4.52)
    13) Social relationships? (5.52)
    14) Physical attractiveness? (5.82)
    15) How often do you compare yourself to others on anything? (6.43)

alpha for the 15-item scale was 0.94. The 2-week, 5-week, 7-week, and 9-week test–retest reliability coefficients were 0.83, 0.64, 0.58, and 0.55, respectively. The most frequent social comparison target was friends and the least frequent social comparison target was family. The most frequent social comparison attribute was physical attractiveness and the least frequent social comparison attribute was family relationships.

Other Scales. The *NEO Personality Inventory—Revised* (Costa & McCrae, 1992) measures five dimensions of personality: neuroticism, extraversion, openness to experience, agreeableness, and conscientiousness. The Eysenck Personality Inventory (EPI; Eysenck & Eysenck, 1964) measures extraversion and neuroticism. The emotion frequency scales of the *Intensity and Time Affect Survey* (ITAS; Diener, Fujita, & Seidlitz, 1991), which is described in more detail by

Schimmack and Diener (1997), measures positive and negative emotion. The *Rosenberg Self-Esteem Scale* (Rosenberg, 1965) measures self-esteem. The Satisfaction with Life Scale (SWLS; Diener, Emmons, Larsen, & Griffin, 1985) measures life satisfaction. *The California Q-Set* (Block, 1961) can be considered to be 100 single-item personality scales.

    Peer reports of social comparison frequency, life satisfaction (SWLS), and emotional experience (ITAS) were collected. Also, daily reports of social comparison frequency, emotional experience (ITAS) and a variety of events and time spent on various activities were collected.

Results

Descriptive statistics for the measures are presented in Table 12.2. Like the INCOM, the FSCS is positively correlated with neuroticism (Buunk, Nauta, & Molleman, 2005; Gibbons & Buunk, 1999), and like Gibbons and Buunk's (1999) U.S. sample, there is no correlation with openness. The FSCS is negatively correlated with self-esteem, consistent with the hypothesis that social com-

TABLE 12.2. Descriptive Statistics Including Correlation with Social Comparison Frequency Scale

Measure	M	SD	r
Social Comparison Frequency Scale	5.42	1.54	—
Satisfaction with Life Scale	22.41	6.34	−.10
Rosenberg Self-Esteem Scale	32.59	4.92	−.27★
NEO PI–R			
Neuroticism	90.95	21.68	.42★
Extraversion	118.29	18.99	.01
Openness	116.58	20.29	.02
Agreeableness	44.88	8.25	−.20★
Conscientiousness	42.13	10.07	−.01
Eysenck Personality Inventory			
Extraversion	14.52	4.00	−.05
Neuroticism	12.96	4.71	.48★
Intensity and Time Affect Survey			
Positive Affect	36.72	7.65	−.01
Love	18.63	4.43	−.03
Joy	18.09	4.02	.01
Negative Affect	42.49	10.31	.39★
Anger	10.59	3.17	.31★
Fear	12.14	3.58	.36★
Sadness	10.44	3.06	.31★
Shame	9.32	2.73	.29★
Surprise	9.56	2.79	.06

Note. $n = 219$; correlations marked with★ are nominally significant at $p < .05$.

parison partially remediates low self-esteem. More than 4% of the sample reported comparing "once or twice a year" or less frequently with the person or group with which they most frequently compared themselves, and more than 21% of the sample reported comparing either "always" or "almost always" with the person or group with which they most often compare themselves.

In order to better understand the personality of the frequent social comparer, significant correlations with California Q-Set items are presented in Table 12.3. Note that under the complete null hypothesis with 100 independent items, we would expect the correlation of five of these items with the FSCS to be significant. Forty-five of the items reach significance, and more importantly, they present an interesting pattern. The validity check item, number 89, which reads, "Compares self to others; is alert to real or fancied differences between self and other people," has the highest correlation. Also of note, item number 84, "Is cheerful," is negatively related to the FSCS. Because of the strong relation between the FSCS and neuroticism, it is instructive to see to what extent these relations can be considered to be due to the shared relation with neuroticism. Partial correlations controlling for the NEO neuroticism scale are presented in Table 12.4. Only 15 items are still significantly correlated with the FSCS.

Peer reports were collected with an average of 4.95 peer reports per participant. A reduced peer FSCS was collected with four targets (friends, roommate, average U of I undergraduate, and anybody else) and four domains (grades, physical appearance, financial status, and social relationships) with an alpha of 0.89. The peer FSCS correlated significantly, but modestly, with the FSCS ($.24$; $n = 218$, $p < .05$). This modest relationship reduced only slightly when controlling for the NEO-PI-R (partial $r = .18$, $p < .05$). The FSCS correlated with average peer ITAS ratings of fear, anger, shame, and sadness ($.25$, $.24$, $.26$, and $.22$, respectively; all $p < .05$), but not with peer ITAS ratings of love, joy, or surprise, ($-.04$, $-.10$, $.12$, respectively; all $p > .05$) or with a peer SWLS measure ($-.12$; $p > .05$).

Hierarchical regression analyses were used to see if the FSCS could add predictive power to the personality scales when trying to predict positive affect, negative affect, and life satisfaction. The FSCS did not add significantly to the prediction of life satisfaction when added to a base model that consisted of either the five scales of the NEO PI-R or the two EPI scales ($F_{NEO(1,218)} < 1$, $p > .05$; $F_{EPI(1,218)} < 1$, $p > .05$), but the FSCS did add significantly to the prediction of negative affect ($F_{NEO(1,218)} = 4.13$, $p < .05$; $F_{EPI(1,218)} = 5.06$, $p < .05$). The FSCS did not add significantly to the prediction of positive affect when added to a base model that consisted of the five scales of the NEO PI-R ($F_{NEO(1,218)} = 2.67$, $p > .05$) but did add significantly to a base model that consisted of the two EPI scales ($F_{EPI(1,218)} = 4.28$, $p < .05$). Because there was no prediction that the FSCS would be related to positive affect, and the hierarchical regression results were mixed, further analyses were restricted to the four ITAS subscales of Negative Affect,

TABLE 12.3. Significant Correlations of Social Comparison Frequency with California Q-Set Items

r	Item no.	Item
−.29	75	Has a clear-cut, internally consistent personality
−.25	33	Is calm, relaxed in manner
−.25	92	Has social poise and presence; appears socially at ease
−.23	83	Able to see to the heart of important problems
−.23	96	Values own independence and autonomy
−.21	57	Is an interesting, arresting person
−.20	74	Is subjectively unaware of self-concern; feels satisfied with self
−.19	77	Appears straightforward, forthright, candid in dealing with others
−.18	35	Has warmth; has the capacity for close relationships; compassionate
−.17	56	Responds to humor
−.17	2	Is a genuinely dependable and responsible person
−.17	88	Is personally charming
−.16	21	Arouses nurturant feelings in others
−.15	100	Does not vary roles; relates to everyone in the same way
−.15	70	Behaves in an ethically consistent manner; is consistent with own personal standards
−.15	54	Emphasizes being with others; gregarious
−.15	60	Has insight into own motives and behavior
−.15	98	Is verbally fluent; can express ideas well
−.14	3	Has a wide range of interests
−.14	17	Behaves in a sympathetic or considerate manner
−.14	18	Initiates humor
−.13	84	Is cheerful
−.13	48	Keeps people at a distance; avoids close interpersonal relationships
.13	47	Has a readiness to feel guilty
.13	61	Creates and exploits dependency in people
.14	23	Extrapunitive; tends to transfer or project blame
.14	46	Engages in personal fantasy and daydreams, fictional speculations
.14	79	Tends to ruminate and have persistent, preoccupying thoughts
.14	7	Favors conservative values in a variety of areas
.15	59	Is concerned with own body and the adequacy of its physiological functioning
.15	40	Is vulnerable to real or fancied threat; generally fearful
.15	49	Is basically distrustful of people in general; questions their motivations
.15	19	Seeks reassurance from others
.15	38	Has hostility toward others
.16	82	Has fluctuating moods
.16	55	Is self-defeating

(continued)

TABLE 12.3. *(continued)*

r	Item no.	Item
.16	50	Is unpredictable and changeable in behavior and attitudes
.16	91	Is power oriented; values power in self or others
.18	78	Feels cheated and victimized by life; self-pitying
.20	37	Is guileful and deceitful, manipulative, opportunistic
.21	13	Is sensitive to anything that can be construed as criticism or an interpersonal slight
.22	12	Tends to be self-defensive
.27	68	Is basically anxious
.29	63	Judges self and others in conventional terms such as "popularity," "the correct thing to do," social pressures, etc.
.42	89	Compares self to others; is alert to real or fancied differences between self and other people

Note. $n = 219$.

TABLE 12.4. Significant Correlations of Social Comparison Frequency with California Q-Set Items Controlling for NEO Neuroticism

r	Item no.	Item
−.18	75	Has a clear-cut, internally consistent personality
−.18	96	Values own independence and autonomy
−.15	56	Responds to humor
−.14	21	Arouses nurturant feelings in others
−.14	92	Has social poise and presence; appears socially at ease
−.14	100	Does not vary roles; relates to everyone in the same way
.15	12	Tends to be self-defensive
.15	53	Various needs tend toward relatively direct and uncontrolled expression; unable to delay gratification
.16	9	Is uncomfortable with uncertainty and complexities
.16	59	Is concerned with own body and the adequacy of its physiological functioning
.17	7	Favors conservative values in a variety of areas
.17	91	Is power oriented; values power in self or others
.20	37	Is guileful and deceitful, manipulative, opportunistic
.30	63	Judges self and others in conventional terms such as "popularity," "the correct thing to do," social pressures, etc.
.35	89	Compares self to others; is alert to real or fancied differences between self and other people

Note. $df = 209$.

Anger, Fear, Sadness, and Shame. The FSCS was added to base models of personality with anger, fear, sadness, and shame as the dependent variables, but the FSCS only added significantly to the prediction of shame ($F_{NEO(1,218)}$ = 4.92, $p <$ .05; $F_{EPI(1,218)}$ = 4.41, $p <$ .05). In all cases where the FSCS added significantly to the prediction, it did so with a positive regression coefficient, such that we would predict that those people who socially compare frequently would experience more negative emotion, in general, and more shame, specifically.

Daily reports are not as subject to memory biases as global self-reports. Daily reports were collected for 52 days, with an average of 47.8 daily reports per participant. All items were averaged across all days prior to further analysis. The daily measure of social comparison frequency consisted of two target items (friends and other U of I students; Ms = 3.1 and 2.75, respectively) and four domain items (intelligence, physical attractiveness, financial status, and social relationships; Ms = 2.54, 2.82, 2.17, and 2.69, respectively). The response scale ranged from "1 = Not at all—I'm sure, 2 = I don't think I did at all, 3 = Once, 4 = Twice," to "9 = Twenty to fifty times, and 10 = Over fifty times." Thus the means of these items can be interpreted as being fewer than one social comparison per day, except for the friends item. There was great variability on the daily items, such that some people reported an average of over six social comparisons per day on each item, whereas others reported no social comparisons during the 7 weeks of daily measurement. The alpha reliability coefficient of the daily measure of social comparison frequency was 0.95. The FSCS correlated with daily reports of social comparison frequency (r = .48; $p <$ .05). The FSCS correlated with the daily ITAS fear, anger, shame, and sadness (r = .42, .36, .34, and .36, respectively; all $p <$ .05) and did not correlate with ITAS love and joy (r = −.03 and −.08, respectively; both $p >$ .05) but did correlate with daily ITAS surprise (r = .29; $p <$ .05), unlike the global self-report and peer-report measures of ITAS surprise.

Other daily events were correlated with the FSCS, but these relationships are post hoc and should be interpreted as exploratory findings. People who scored high on the FSCS were more likely to shout in anger (r = .31, $p <$ .05), argue with someone (r = .32, $p <$ .05), change their mind or opinion (r = .25, $p <$ .05), lie or deceive someone (r = .32, $p <$ .05), be late for class (r = .18, $p <$ .05), forget something (r = .31, $p <$ .05), assert their rights (r = .25, $p <$ .05), feel too shy to say something they wanted to (r = .41, $p <$ .05), cry (r = .17, $p <$ .05), be upset by someone's careless remark (r = .35, $p <$ .05), talk with someone they hadn't met before (r = .19, $p <$ .05), back down when they knew they were right (r = .34, $p <$ .05), and notice that someone complimented them in their presence (r = .17, $p <$ .05). They spent more time watching television (r = .17, $p <$ .05), less time sleeping (r = −.15, $p <$ .05), more time worrying about tests or papers (r = .29, $p <$ .05), more time planning (r = .20, $p <$ .05), more time worrying about their social life (r = .31, $p <$ .05), and more time exercising or participating in sports ($r = .16$, $p < .05$). Some of the many things that people who score high on the FSCS do not differ on from those who score low on the FSCS include the frequency of laughing, speaking in a class discussion, learning something new, missing class, trying something new, consuming caffeinated beverages, consuming alcoholic beverages, using analgesics such as aspirin or Tylenol, and using other nonprescription medications (all $-.12 < r < .12$; $p > .05$). They also spent no more or less time alone, shopping, studying for class, engaged in personal maintenance, socializing with family, socializing with friends, socializing on a date, working for money, listening to music, engaged with hobbies or a pet, or in religious activities (all $-.12 < r < .12$; $p > 05$).

Correlations between the daily measure of social comparison frequency and the daily ITAS were computed within subjects across days and then averaged across participants; significance was evaluated using a single-sample z-test. Social comparisons were more frequent on the days when participants experienced more fear ($r = .15$, $p < .05$), anger ($r = .11$, $p < .05$), shame ($r = .13$, $p < .05$), sadness ($r = .10$, $p < .05$), and surprise ($r = .13$, $p < .05$), but not love ($r = .00$, $p > .05$) or joy ($r = .02$, $p > .05$). These results are important because they control for neuroticism, agreeableness, self-esteem, and all other individual differences variables. Averaged within-subject correlations between the daily social comparison items and the ITAS emotion scales showed some interesting variations from the correlations with the six-item scale. For example, social comparisons on intelligence showed a different pattern of correlations than social comparisons on physical attractiveness. Daily fear was highly related to social comparisons on intelligence ($r = .16$, $p < .05$) but much less highly related to social comparisons on physical attractiveness ($r = .04$, $p < .05$). Daily joy was negatively correlated with social comparisons on intelligence ($r = -.05$, $p < .05$) but positively correlated with social comparisons on physical attractiveness ($r = .06$, $p < .05$). Daily love showed a similar pattern, correlating negatively with social comparisons on intelligence ($r = -.05$, $p < .05$) and positively with social comparisons on physical attractiveness ($r = .05$, $p < .05$). Thus the zero correlation between daily social comparison and daily love or joy may be a result of the mixing of these two opposite relationships. An examination of the trait FSCS items on intelligence and physical attractiveness did not show this divergent pattern of correlations with positive emotion items.

Discussion

There are reliable and valid individual differences in social comparison frequency. The FSCS has high internal and test–retest consistency, and it correlates well with daily reports of social comparison, and with the California Q-Set item of social comparison. The construct validation of the FSCS is off to a good start, showing negative correlations with self-esteem and agreeableness and positive correlations with neuroticism, a daily measure of social comparison, and some interesting correlations and noncorrelations with other daily behaviors and time spent in various activities. It is not surprising that the two domains on which a traditionally college student sample compare most frequently are grades and physical attractiveness. It is interesting, given the effect of the larger environment but not the smaller environment on satisfaction, that these students report comparing more frequently with their friends than with the larger group of other undergraduates at their university.

The California Q-Set description of the frequent social comparer presents an intriguing picture. In addition to a general pattern associated with neuroticism, the frequent comparer seems to favor conservative values, lack social poise, be inconsistent and unpredictable, change behavior in response to others, be concerned with popularity, be deceitful, and be power oriented. Social comparison seems to be a very private behavior; peers were not able to judge the social comparison frequency of our sample very well.

Frequent social comparison appears to be related to subjective well-being primarily through negative affect. There is more to this relationship than just an association with the personality trait of neuroticism. Social comparison frequency adds predictive power over and above the Big Five to the prediction of negative affect, in general, and shame, specifically. The relationship of social comparison with negative affect has been found both across people at the trait level and within people at the daily level. People who engage in social comparison more frequently tend to experience more negative affect, and people are more likely to engage in social comparison on days when they are experiencing more than average negative affect.

There was an important difference between daily affect and global self-reported affect, however. Global self-reported surprise didn't have any relationship with the frequency of social comparison, but daily-reported surprise was positively correlated with social comparison frequency. This was true with both the FSCS and within person, such that people reported more social comparisons on days when they experienced more than average surprise. It may be the case that events that precipitate an experience of surprise also increase uncertainty, thus increasing the motivation to engage in social comparisons.

There was also an important difference between daily social comparison frequency and global self-reported social comparison frequency. At the trait level, there was no differentiation between social comparisons on intelligence and social comparisons on physical attractiveness, but within people at the daily level, social comparisons on intelligence were more strongly related with fear and negatively related with love and joy, whereas social comparisons on physical attractiveness were less strongly related with fear and positively related to love and joy.

This finding may indicate that there isn't a simple relationship between social comparison frequency and affect, but that the attribute on which one compares mediates the relationship.

We don't yet know the causal relation between social comparison frequency and negative affect. Mild negative affect may simply serve as indication that an individual needs to think more about his or her situation, thus triggering more frequent social comparisons. It may be that the social comparisons themselves more often lead to negative emotions than positive emotions. Another possible explanation is that people who are too worried about the opinions and attitudes of others are both more likely to experience negative emotions and to engage in frequent social comparisons. The FSCS gives us a tool to start analyzing question of causal direction, by identifying the frequent comparers.

Level 1 Summary

Social comparisons can make us happy or unhappy. Upward comparisons can inspire or demoralize us, whereas downward comparisons can make us feel superior or depress us. In general, however, frequent social comparisons are not associated with life satisfaction or the positive emotions of love and joy but are associated with the negative emotions of fear, anger, shame, and sadness. One avenue for future research is the replication of the within-person findings on a more representative sample. Because of the strong relation of the frequency of social comparison with neuroticism, all future research needs to be able to separate the effects of social comparison frequency from the effects of neuroticism. It will be fruitful to focus our future efforts on the cognitive aspects of shame, to see if it is possible to untangle the causal arrow between frequent social comparison and the experience of shame.

References

alasia. (2006, January 1). My biggest goal. . . . Message posted to *www.43things.com/things/view/22327*. Retrieved March 21, 2006.

Betton, Q. (2006, February 9). The problem with. . . . Message posted to *my.opera.com/makeqfit/blog/?startidx=30*. Retrieved March 21, 2006.

Block, J. (1961). *The Q-sort method in personality assessment and psychiatric research*. Springfield, IL: Thomas.

Buunk, B. P., & Brenninkmeijer, V. (2001). When individuals dislike exposure to an actively coping role model: Mood change as related to depression and social comparison orientation. *European Journal of Social Psychology, 31*, 537–548.

Buunk, B. P., Collins, R. L., Taylor, S. E., Van Yperen, N. W., & Dakof, G. A. (1990). The affective consequences of social comparison: Either direction has its ups and downs. *Journal of Personality and Social Psychology, 59*, 1238–1249.

Buunk, B. P., Nauta, A., & Molleman, E. (2005). In search of the true group animal: The effects of affiliation orientation and social comparison orientation upon group satisfaction. *European Journal of Personality, 19,* 69–81.

Buunk, B. P., Oldersma, F. L., & de Dreu, C. K. W. (2001). Enhancing satisfaction through downward comparison: The role of relational discontent and individual differences in social comparison orientation. *Journal of Experimental Social Psychology, 37,* 452–467.

Buunk, B. P., Van der Zee, K., & Van Yperen, N. W. (2001). Neuroticism and social comparison orientation as moderators of affective responses to social comparison at work. *Journal of Personality, 69,* 745–763.

Buunk, B. P., Ybema, J. F., Gibbons, F. X., & Ipenburg, M. (2001). The affective consequences of social comparison as related to professional burnout and social comparison orientation. *European Journal of Social Psychology, 31,* 337–351.

Buunk, B. P., Zurriaga, R., Peiro, J. M., Nauta, A., & Gosalvez, I. (2005). Social comparisons at work as related to a cooperative social climate and to individual differences in social comparison orientation. *Applied Psychology: An International Review, 54,* 61–80.

Costa, P. T., Jr., & McCrae, R. R. (1992). *Revised NEO Personality Inventory and Five-Factor Inventory Professional Manual.* Odessa, Fl: Psychological Assessment Resources.

Diener, E., Emmons, R. A., Larsen, R. J., & Griffin, S. (1985). The Satisfaction with Life Scale. *Journal of Personality Assessment, 49,* 71–75.

Diener, E., & Fujita, F. (1995). Resources, personal strivings, and subjective well-being: A nomothetic and idiographic approach. *Journal of Personality and Social Psychology, 68,* 926–935.

Diener, E., & Fujita, F. (1997). Social comparisons and subjective well-being. In B. Buunk & R. Gibbons (Eds.), *Health, coping, and social comparison* (pp. 329–357). Mahwah, NJ: Erlbaum.

Diener, E., Fujita, F., & Seidlitz, L. (1991). *Manual for the intensity and time affect survey (ITAS).* Unpublished manuscript, University of Illinois at Urbana–Champaign.

Dijkstra, P., & Buunk, B. P. (2002). Sex difference in the jealousy-evoking effect of rival characteristics. *European Journal of Social Psychology, 32,* 829–852.

Eysenck, H. J., & Eysenck, S. (1964). *Manual of the Eysenck Personality Inventory.* London: Hodder & Stoughton.

Festinger, L. (1954). A theory of social comparison processes. *Human Relations, 7,* 117–140.

Fujita, F. (1993). *The effects of naturalistic social comparison on satisfaction with life domains.* Unpublished doctoral dissertation, University of Illinois, Urbana–Champaign.

Gibbons, F. X., Benbow, C. P., & Gerrard, M. (1994). From top dog to bottom half: Social comparison strategies in response to poor performance. *Journal of Personality and Social Psychology, 67,* 638–652.

Gibbons, F. X., & Buunk, B. P. (1999). Individual differences in social comparison: Development of a scale of social comparison orientation. *Journal of Personality and Social Psychology, 76,* 129–142.

Goethals, G. R. (1986). Social comparison theory: Psychology from the lost and found. *Personality and Social Psychology Bulletin, 12,* 261–278.

Goethals, G. R., Messick, D. M., & Allison, S. T. (1991). The uniqueness bias: Studies of constructive social comparison. In J. Suls & T. A. Wills (Eds.), *Social comparison: Contemporary theory and research* (pp. 149–176). Hillsdale, NJ: Erlbaum.

Hagerty, M. R. (2000). Social comparisons of income in one's community: Evidence from national surveys of income and happiness. *Journal of Personality and Social Psychology, 78,* 764–771.

Heine, S. J., Lehman, D. R., Peng, K., & Greenholtz (2002). What's wrong with cross-cultural comparisons of subjective likert scales?: The reference-group effect. *Journal of Personality and Social Psychology, 82,* 903–918.

Licandro, J. (2001, December 4). Men's basketball: Irish run into reeling Hoosiers. *The Observer Online.* Retrieved March 21, 2006, from *www.nd.edu/~observer/12042001/Sports/11.html.*

Lyubomirsky, S., & Ross, L. (1997). Hedonic consequences of social comparison: A contrast of happy and unhappy people. *Journal of Personality and Social Psychology, 73,* 1141–1157.

Lyubomirsky, S., Tucker, K. L., & Kasri, F. (2001). Responses to hedonically conflicting social comparisons: Comparing happy and unhappy people. *European Journal of Social Psychology, 31,* 511–535.

Marsh, H. W. (1987). The big-fish-little-pond effect on academic self-concept. *Journal of Educational Psychology, 79,* 280–295.

Marsh, H. W., & Hau, K. (2003). Big-fish-little-pond effect on academic self-concept: A cross-cultural (26-country) test of the negative effects of academically selective schools. *American Psychologist, 58,* 364–376.

Marsh, H. W., & Parker, J. W. (1984). Determinants of student self-concept: Is it better to be a relatively large fish in a small pond even if you don't learn to swim as well? *Journal of Personality and Social Psychology, 47,* 213–231.

Marsh, K. L., & Webb, W. M. (1996). Mood uncertainty and social comparison: Implications for mood management. *Journal of Social Behavior and Personality, 11,* 1–26.

McFarland, C., & Miller, D. T. (1994). The framing of relative performance feedback: Seeing the glass as half empty or half full. *Journal of Personality and Social Psychology, 66,* 1061–1073.

Michinov, E., & Michinov, N. (2001). The similarity hypothesis: A test of the moderating role of social comparison orientation. *European Journal of Social Psychology, 31,* 549–555.

Pachnowska, B. (1996). Affective consequences of social comparisons: Paradox of excessive importance of self-evaluation. *Polish Psychological Bulletin, 27,* 325–341.

Parducci, A. (1984). Value judgments: Toward a relational theory of happiness. In J. R. Eiser (Ed.), *Attitudinal measurement* (pp. 3–21). New York: Springer-Verlag.

Rosenberg, M. (1965). *Society and the adolescent child.* Princeton, NJ: Princeton University Press.

Schimmack, U., & Diener, E. (1997). Affect intensity: Separating intensity and frequency in repeatedly measured affect. *Journal of Personality and Social Psychology, 73,* 1313–1329.

Schwartz, B., Ward, A., Monterosso, J., Lyubomirsky, S., White, K., & Lehman, D. R. (2002). Maximizing versus satisficing: Happiness is a matter of choice. *Journal of Personality and Social Psychology, 83,* 1178–1197.

Smith, R. H., Diener, E., & Wedell, D. H. (1989). Intrapersonal and social comparison determinants of happiness: A range–frequency analysis. *Journal of Personality and Social Psychology, 56,* 317–325.

Smith, R. H., Parrott, W. G., Diener, E., Hoyle, R. H., & Kim, S. H. (1999). Dispositional envy. *Personality and Social Psychology Bulletin, 25,* 1007–1020.

Solberg, E. C., Diener, E., Wirtz, D., Lucas, R. E., & Oishi, S. (2002). Wanting, having, and satisfaction: Examining the role of desire discrepancies in satisfaction with income. *Journal of Personality and Social Psychology, 83,* 725–734.

Swallow, S. R., & Kuiper, N. A., (1992). Mild depression and frequency of social comparison behavior. *Journal of Social and Clinical Psychology, 11,* 167–180.

Van der Zee, K., Oldersma, F., Buunk, B. P., & Bos, D. (1998). Social comparison preferences among cancer patients as related to neuroticism and social comparison orientation. *Journal of Personality and Social Psychology, 75,* 801–810.

Whatkidscando.org. (2003). Student learning in small schools: An online portfolio. Retrieved March 21, 2006, from *www.whatkidscando.org/portfoliosmallschools/met/commentaryreal.html.*

Wheeler, L., & Miyake, K. (1992). Social comparison in everyday life. *Journal of Personality and Social Psychology, 62,* 760–773.

13

Regulation of Emotional Well-Being

Overcoming the Hedonic Treadmill

RANDY J. LARSEN and ZVJEZDANA PRIZMIC

In theoretical terms, subjective well-being is a complex construct consisting of several components, such as evaluative judgments, positive memories, meaning-fulness, optimism, and the relative amounts of positive and negative affect over time (Kim-Prieto, Diener, Tamir, Scollon, & Diener, 2005). Empirically, how-ever, the construct coalesces into three distinct components: (1) a cognitive com-ponent comprising judgments of life satisfaction, and an emotional component consisting of (2) high levels of positive affect and (3) low levels of negative affect (Arthaud-Day, Rode, Mooney, & Near, 2005). In population studies these three components emerge as distinct but related factors (Arthaud-Day et al., 2005). Life satisfaction correlates moderately with high positive affect (PA) and low neg-ative affect (NA), but is nevertheless a judgment process that is at least conceptu-ally distinct from affective processes. Judgments of life satisfaction show high lev-els of stability in adulthood (Diener & Larsen, 1984; Diener, Lucas, & Scollon, 2006; Eid & Diener, 2004) and are most likely difficult, though not impossible (Lucas, Clark, Georgellis, & Diener, 2004), to influence directly (Fujita & Diener, 2005). The emotional components of positive and negative affect, on the other hand, are much more reactive to situational influences and more amenable to efforts to manage or remediate these affective states (Chow, Ram, Fujita, Boker, & Clore, 2005).

In this chapter we focus on emotional well-being and argue that global subjective well-being can be influenced by regulating two out of its three main components: positive and negative affect. Moreover, we argue that due to "negativity bias" (e.g., Cacioppo & Gardner, 1999), the down-regulation of negative affect may be more important to global subjective well-being than the up-regulation of positive affect. We review a variety of strategies and behaviors known to influence ongoing PA and NA.

Emotional Well-Being

Emotional well-being can be thought of as a composite of PA and NA that ebbs and flows and has a momentary character reflecting a person's emotional status quo at any given time. As these momentary states accumulate over time, they aggregate into something like a running average, such that they begin to reflect a central tendency or characteristic level of emotional well-being, around which the person fluctuates. As such, trait measures of emotional well-being always inquire about some time period (e.g., "How have things been over the past several years?") rather than about some moment in time (e.g., "How are you feeling right now?"; Larsen & Prizmic, 2006).

There are interesting questions about how people integrate their momentary states into an aggregated judgment of their long-term subjective well-being (Kahneman, Krueger, Schkade, Schwarz, & Stone, 2004). For example, recent emotional states appear to be weighted more heavily in such integration than states more distal in time (Redelmeier & Kahneman, 1996). Nevertheless, people do make this integration when asked "over time" questions, and their answers to such questions conform to typical psychometric standards of reliability for trait measures. Moreover, their answers also appear to have construct validity; that is, they converge with concurrent subjective well-being measures, predict future measures, correlate with related constructs such as self-esteem and peer reports, and show discriminant validity (Larsen & Diener,1985).

Almost all of measures of subjective well-being correlate highly with emotional well-being, defined as the ratio of PA to NA in a person's life over a representative time span. For example, Larsen and Diener (1985) had subjects keep records of the emotions they were feeling every day for a period between 30 and 90 days. They then calculated the ratio of total positive to total negative affects for each subject over the entire period of daily reporting. This measure correlated moderately to strongly with a wide variety of questionnaire measures of subjective well-being that are widely used in surveys and psychological research. The authors concluded that, although different theorists define subjective well-being differently, most subjective well-being measures correlate highly with the ratio of PA to NA assessed over time, suggesting an emotional core to global well-being.

Even life satisfaction judgments are highly correlated with the ratio of PA to NA assessed over time (Diener, Emmons, Larsen, & Griffin, 1985). The following formula depicts the emotional core of well-being:

$$\text{Emotional well-being} = \Sigma(PA)/\Sigma(NA)$$

This formula for emotional well-being has several important implications. The first implication is that, in order for the ratio to convey maximum information, the numerator (PA) and the denominator (NA) must be uncorrelated. To date, there is a great deal of evidence that, when assessed over time (i.e., as traits or average tendencies), the amount of PA in people's lives is uncorrelated with the amount of NA (e.g., Diener & Emmons, 1985; Schmukle, Egloff, & Burns, 2002). This independence of trait PA and trait NA is important because the ratio of highly correlated scores would provide redundant information with the components, making the emotional well-being ratio less useful. Moreover, the basic finding that trait PA and trait NA are uncorrelated has led researchers to investigate the specific mechanisms that give rise to each (Larsen, in press). For our purposes here, it leads us to consider separately the regulation of PA and NA as discrete processes.

To understand the differential contributions of PA and NA, it is useful to consider the correlates of global well-being. In terms of personality predictors of well-being, two broad variables consistently emerge as correlates: extraversion and neuroticism (Diener, Oishi, & Lucas, 2003). The personality variables of extraversion and neuroticism are themselves uncorrelated. We now know that these correlations with extraversion and neuroticism emerge precisely because they differentially predict the emotional components of PA and NA. Extraversion correlates highly with long-term trait PA (but not trait NA), and neuroticism correlates highly with long-term trait NA (but not trait PA). Moreover, Larsen and his colleagues (e.g., Larsen & Ketelaar, 1989, 1991; Rusting & Larsen, 1997, 1998; Zelenski & Larsen, 1999) have shown, in experimental studies of mood inductions, that extraversion predicts reactivity to positive (but not negative) mood inductions, and that neuroticism predicts reactivity to negative (but not positive) mood inductions. Studying the behavioral and cognitive components of extraversion and neuroticism may shed important light on the processes responsible for enhanced PA and NA, respectively. More specifically, we might gain insight into the differential regulation of PA and NA by studying the behaviors associated with the personality variables of extraversion and neuroticism.

In a fascinating study along these lines, Fleeson, Malanos, and Achille (2002, Study 3) manipulated extraversion levels by having participants act in an extraverted fashion ("Act bold, talkative, energetic, and assertive") or in an introverted way ("Act reserved, quiet, passive, and compliant"). Participants then engaged in several discussions on topics of interest to college students. Self- and observer reports of PA were gathered during and after the discussions. The acting-extraverted participants displayed more PA and rated themselves as happier than those subjects instructed to act in an introverted fashion. The conclusion is that even acting extraverted may induce PA in a manner similar to trait levels of extraversion. Although the study has yet to be done, we can assume that similar effects would be found with neuroticism and NA.

Another important conclusion from the above ratio formula is that it implies two routes to increasing emotional well-being: by maximizing the numerator (PA) through the pursuit of frequent pleasures, or by minimizing the denominator (NA) through the remediation of unpleasant emotions. This conception is similar to William James's notion of happiness as the ratio of our aspirations to our accomplishments in life, wherein he suggested that we could increase happiness by either decreasing our aspirations or increasing our accomplishments (or both). Moreover, the ratio formulation assumes equality between the numerator and the denominator, such that efforts geared toward increasing the numerator could be redirected toward decreasing the denominator, and the overall effect on subjective well-being would be the same.

Asymmetry between PA and NA

Most researchers assume that PA and NA contribute equally to emotional well-being. However, there are reasons to suspect that this is not the case. Many researchers have pointed to an asymmetry in PA and NA, with the NA system being more reactive than the PA system. Baumeister, Bratslavsky, Finkenauer, and Vohs (2001) review a great deal of data, from a variety of sources, all of which converge on the general idea that "bad is stronger than good." In general, a negative event of value $-x$ will produce a stronger affective response than a positive event of value $+x$. In other words, there appears to be a gain function built into the NA system such that this system produces a larger response, per unit input, than the PA system. Cacioppo and colleagues (Cacioppo & Gardner, 1999; Ito & Cacioppo, 2005), as well as others (e.g., Rozin & Royzman, 2001), have termed this gain function the *negativity bias*.

Larsen (2002) reported on several studies that directly compare NA and PA in terms of reactivity, duration, and cognitive involvement. For reactivity, he had subjects ($n = 62$) record their daily emotions and life events every day for 56 consecutive days. Each day, in the evening, subjects rated how much they felt each of a variety of different emotions (e.g., sad, happy, enthusiastic, distressed, hostile, calm, content) during that day. These emotions were scored for global PA and NA and then standardized across all days for all subjects to $M = 0$ and $SD = 1$. Subjects also answered the following open-ended question: "What event most influenced your positive affect today?" and "What event most influenced your negative affect today?" The written event descriptions were transcribed and given to a team of raters. In all, 3,064 good event descriptions were rated and 2,907 bad event descriptions were rated. The raters were asked to judge: "How objectively good or bad is this event for the average college student?" Raters used a scale from 1 to 9, with the midpoint (5) anchored with *neutral*, and points 6 to 9 anchored with *slightly, moderately, very, and extremely good*, and points 4 to 1 anchored with *slightly, moderately, very, and extremely bad*.

Days with good event ratings greater than 1 standard deviation above the mean were aggregated, as were days with bad event ratings. This procedure has the effect of selecting a large number of days for which the good and bad events were, on average, equivalently extreme but opposite in valence. Larsen (2002) then examined self-reported PA on the good days and NA on the bad days to see whether these differ on days that are, on average, equivalent in severity. A total of 490 occasions were averaged for the positive event scores and 465 occasions were averaged for the negative event scores. Results are presented in Figure 13.1. Expressed in standard scores, average PA on the positive days was .78, whereas average NA on the bad days was 1.33. The difference is significant and consistent with the idea that NA reactivity has a gain function, such that equivalent levels of

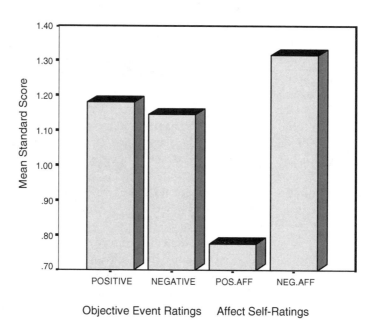

FIGURE 13.1. Mean self-reported positive and negative affect on days that had equivalent levels of objectively rated good and bad events.

objectively bad and good events produce relatively higher levels of NA than PA, respectively.

In terms of duration, it has long been argued that people adapt to good events at a faster rate than they adapt to bad events (Brickman, Coates, & Janoff-Bulman, 1978), suggesting that positive emotions habituate or return to baseline faster than negative emotions. Larsen (2002) examined this question using an experience sampling data set very similar to what was reported above, wherein subjects reported on their emotions three times a day (morning, afternoon, and evening) for 28 consecutive days. Each subject's PA and NA scores were (1) standardized within subjects; (2) all those occasions where PA was greater than 1 *SD* above the subject's mean (call this time T) were lagged; and (3) PA on the following three occasions was examined, at time T+1, T+2, and T+3. The same was done for occasions where NA exceeded 1 *SD* for each subject. This procedure allowed us to see the return toward baseline following somewhat extreme (+1 *SD*) positive and negative emotions. Results are presented in Figures 13.2 and 13.3 and show that PA dropped to baseline fairly quickly after an extreme PA occasion, being not significantly different from the expected value (the subject's own mean) at T+1; NA, on the other hand, remained higher than

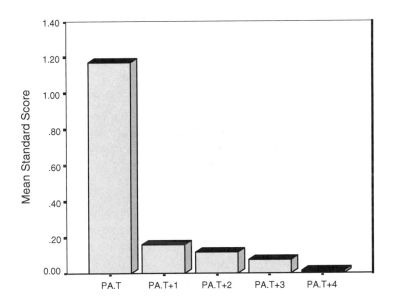

Positive Affect at Extreme Times (T) and Subsequently

FIGURE 13.2. Positive affect decay curve following occasions of extreme positive affect.

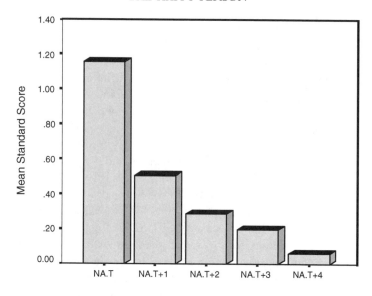

FIGURE 13.3. Negative affect decay curve following occasions of extreme negative affect.

expected for two occasions (T+1 and T+2) into the future following an extreme NA occasion. This result is consistent with the hypothesis that the rate of adaptation, defined as a return toward baseline, is steeper for PA than for NA.

In terms of cognitive activity, negative events, compared to positive events, capture more attentional resources and are stored in memory in a more accessible manner (Musch & Klauer, 2003). Due to length limitations, we give only a few brief examples of how attentional resources are more involved in the processing of negative than positive events. The first example draws on the so-called emotional Stroop task. In Stroop's original version of the task, subjects are presented with color words that are in colored ink (e.g., *BLUE* in green ink). Their task is to name the ink color as quickly as possible and ignore the word. In the emotion version of the Stroop task, the stimuli are emotion words that appear in colored ink (e.g., *DISEASE* in green). The instructions are similar: to ignore the word and name the color as quickly as possible. The dependent variable is the reaction time to name the ink color to emotional words (e.g., *MURDER, CANCER, AGONY*) compared to control words (e.g., *TALLER, SIGNAL, WHATEVER*). Most researchers using the emotional Stroop task investigate only negative words, and the typical finding is that people, on average, are slower for negative than neutral words. The few studies that have investigated positive words (e.g., Pratto & John, 1991; Dalgleish, 1995; White, 1996) typically do not find any attentional capture effects.

Another cognitive task used in investigations of cognition and emotion is the affective Simon task developed by De Houwer and colleagues (De Houwer & Eelen, 1998; De Houwer, Crombez, Baeyens, & Hermans, 2001). The original Simon task is a location interference task that uses left and right arrows as the relevant feature, to which the subject responds "left" or "right." However, the arrows pop up on the left or right side of the computer display, which interferes with the judgments. In one of De Houwer's affective Simon tasks, a word appears on a computer display, and it is in either upper case (e.g., *MURDER*) or lower case (e.g., *murder*). The subject is instructed to respond "positive" if the word is in upper case and negative if in lower case (or vice versa, depending on assignment to conditions). However, the words themselves are valenced, and hence the positivity or negativity of the word can be congruent or incongruent with the correct response. When the valence of the word is incongruent with the response (e.g., *MURDER*, to which the subject has to respond "positive"), interference is created, and reaction time is slower compared to congruent trials (e.g., *MURDER* and "negative"). However, the interference effects are not symmetric for positive and negative stimuli. Having to say "positive" to a word that is negative produces a much larger interference effect than having to say "negative" to a word that is positive (Larsen & Yarkoni, 2006).

Another cognitive paradigm useful for studying emotion and cognition is emotional priming. Here, an affective prime (e.g., an emotion-laden word such as *failure*) is presented briefly (e.g., for 200 ms), then followed by another word, the target, that is either emotionally consistent with the prime (e.g., *hatred*) or inconsistent (e.g., *flower*). The subject's task is to categorize the target as positive or negative as quickly as possible. In this task, the subject is instructed to ignore the prime and respond only to the target. However, the response to the target is facilitated (i.e., is faster) when the prime is emotionally congruent with the target, producing the priming effect. But, again, the effects of positive and negative emotional primes are not symmetric; stronger priming effects are observed for negative primes than positive primes (Hietanen & Korpela, 2004; Smith et al., 2006).

Returning to the topic of subjective well-being, the asymmetry between PA and NA in terms of the above-mentioned dimensions (i.e., reactivity, duration, cognitive involvement) has important implications. In order to maintain a positive hedonic valence (the ratio of PA to NA), we would need fewer or less intense negative experiences than positive experiences. To give one more example of how PA and NA do not contribute equally to subjective well-being, we turn to a report on results of an experiment on physiological reactivity to pleasant and unpleasant stimuli (Larsen, Cruz, Ketelaar, Welsh, & Billings, 1990). Here the authors recorded skin conductance, heart rate, and facial muscle contractions while subjects viewed pleasant and unpleasant photographic images. They predicted that a questionnaire measure of subjective well-being would correlate with diminished NA reactivity and enhanced PA reactivity in terms of physiological responses to the hedonic stimuli. However, they found only the former. That is, happy people did *not* exhibit increased autonomic activation to the positive images; rather, they exhibited diminished autonomic reactivity to the negative images. In more than a metaphorical sense, happy people did not smile more, they mainly frowned less, that is, were less reactive to the negative stimuli.

How Much Stronger Is NA Than PA?

Although many researchers have documented that NA is stronger than PA, few have taken up the question of just *how much* stronger. There are inherent difficulties in any empirical attempt to quantify an answer, such as the precision of manipulation and measurement reliability of the response. On the surface, it appears to be a dose–response type of question: How much larger must the "dose" of positive stimulation be to evoke a positive response that is equivalent in size, but opposite in valence, to a given negative response? Or, alternatively, what is the degree of difference between PA and NA responses to equivalent "doses" of hedonic stimulation? We might be tempted to approach the question with psychophysical methods. After all, emotions are internal representations of events in the external world, just as sensations are internal representations of the physical world. Psychophysical methods yielded great advances in our understanding of sensory processes. However, in sensory psychophysics, great utility was achieved by the ability to precisely control, manipulate, and objectively measure a physical stimulus (e.g., light intensity, weight, sound waves). We do not, however, have equivalent manipulation precision in the area of emotional stimulation. It is simply impossible, at this point, to equate or manipulate emotional inputs with enough precision to allow precise comparison of emotional outputs.

Despite these inherent difficulties, a few researchers have made statements about just how much stronger NA is compared to PA. Usually the statements are in the form of the critical ratio of PA to NA necessary to maintain some global state. Perhaps the first researcher to venture such a statement was the marital researcher John Gottman (e.g., 1994). In this research program Gottman examined differences between couples whose marriages were satisfying and long-lasting and couples whose marriages were dissatisfying and in dissolution (i.e., they had filed for divorce). Gottman (1994) had partners engage in a conversation on a topic of conflict in their marriage, as he videotaped them. Later the videotapes were coded for positivity and negativity expressed both verbally and in observable expressions of emotion. Among the couples in satisfying marriages, the ratio of positive to negative emotions was 5.1 to 1 for verbal content and 4.7

to 1 for emotional expressions. Among the couples in marital dissolution, the ratio of positive to negative emotions was 0.9 to 1 for verbal content and 0.7 to 1 for emotional expressions.

Larsen (2002), using two different experience sampling data sets, with daily emotion ratings gathered over 30–90 consecutive days, calculated the percentage of days when PA exceeded NA over all subjects: 73% in one sample and 76% in the other. In other words, the average person could expect to have 3 good days for each bad day. Positive emotions must prevail over negative emotions by a force of 3 to 1 if a person is to maintain an average level of subjective well-being. Viewed this way, 1 negative day has the countervalent force of 3 positive days. Larsen (2002) also examined the beta weights using average daily PA and average daily NA in regression equations predicting questionnaire measures of subjective well-being. Across a number of global subjective well-being reports, the standardized beta weights for NA are approximately three times the size of the standardized beta weights for PA. So, although average daily PA and NA are uncorrelated with each other, and although they do both contribute to, or significantly correlate with, global subjective well-being measures, the overlap between subjective well-being and NA nevertheless exceeds the overlap of subjective well-being and PA by a factor of approximately 3.0.

Schwartz and colleagues (Schwartz, 1997; Schwartz et al., 2002) examined the question of the ratio of PA to NA in a study of psychotherapy for depression. PA and NA were measured both before and after treatment in a sample of 66 depressed men. Before treatment, the ratio of PA to NA averaged 0.5 for the entire sample. After treatment, participants showing typical levels of remission in their depressive symptoms ($n = 23$) were found to have a PA-to-NA ratio of 2.3, whereas those participants showing optimal remission (judged by self-report and clinical ratings, $n = 15$) were found to have a PA-to-NA ratio of 4.3. Those subjects who showed no remission of their depressive symptoms were found to have a PA-to-NA ratio of 0.7, a value not significantly different from pretreatment baseline.

Fredrickson and Losada (2005) explicitly took up the question of the critical value of PA-to-NA ratio necessary for flourishing, and they put this question to several different data sets. In one data set they examined the interpersonal behaviors of business teams as they worked on their annual strategic plans. The verbal behaviors of each team member were coded for expressed PA (e.g., showing support, encouragement, or appreciation) and NA (e.g., expressing disapproval, sarcasm, or cynicism). Objective indicators of performance (e.g., profitability, customer satisfaction, evaluations by superiors) were used to derive an index of overall quality of the team. Without going into the complex dynamical analysis, Fredrickson and Losada concluded that a PA-to-NA ratio of 2.9 divided those teams who were flourishing from those teams that were languishing.

Using another data set, Fredrickson and Losada (2005) reported the results of an experience sampling study on college students covering 28 consecutive days of emotion reports. For each participant they calculated a PA-to-NA ratio over the month of daily reporting. They divided the samples into participants who were flourishing versus those who were not, using a measure of positive social and psychological functioning. The authors reported that, in the two samples, the participants who were flourishing had a PA-to-NA ratio of 3.2 and 3.4, whereas those participants who were not flourishing had PA-to-NA ratios of 2.3 and 2.1.

What can we conclude about how much stronger NA is compared to PA from studies such as these? One conclusion is that the estimates for the magnitude difference between PA and NA have a wide range, going from 2.3 to 5.1 among well-adjusted persons in the studies reviewed here. The precise value of this function is likely to be influenced by the nature of the measures that go into calculating PA and NA, as well as by the specific life domains in which the measures are obtained (e.g., marital behaviors, affect displayed during team work). Moreover, any estimated value will always fall within a range determined by the reliability of the measures of the component indices (i.e., the measures of PA and NA). In the absence of a precise value, we might consider what value provides a good first estimate. Because the estimates we reviewed average slightly over 3.0, we suggest that a good first estimate would be the value of pi (π, or 3.14).

The negativity bias, or the degree to which bad is stronger than good, can thus be defined mathematically as

$$|PA| \star \pi = |NA|$$

Consequently, the equation for affect balance necessary to achieve minimal levels of emotional well-being can be restated as

$$\text{Emotional well-being} = \Sigma(PA)/(\Sigma(NA/\pi))$$

Negativity Bias and the Hedonic Treadmill

A theory of well-being relevant to the negativity bias concept is the hedonic treadmill theory, originally proposed by Brickman and Campbell (1971). This theory holds that people adapt to both good and bad events and return, over time, to their hedonic setpoints. For example, after an extremely good event, such as marriage to the person of his or her dreams, a person initially reacts with strong PA but eventually adapts and returns to his or her baseline level of PA. A similar adaptation process occurs for negative events; after a bad event a person initially reacts with strong NA but eventually adapts and returns to his or her baseline level of NA. The hedonic treadmill theory received some support in Brickman et al. (1978) classic study of lottery winners and paraplegics. Studying both lottery winners and persons who had lost their ability to walk, Brickman et al. (1978) concluded that both groups were not substantially different from control groups 1 year after the good (winning the lottery) or bad (becoming paraplegic) events.

In a reanalysis of the Brickman et al. (1978) data, Diener et al. (2006) reported that the paraplegic subjects were actually 0.75 standard deviation units lower in subjective well-being than the control group after 1 year, suggesting that full adaptation to this negative event had not yet occurred. This finding is consistent with the negativity bias concept: that negative events produce relatively more intense and longer-lasting affective reactions than positive events. This finding adds a twist to the hedonic treadmill theory by implying that adaptation rates to good and bad events are not identical; we adapt more quickly to good events than equally hedonic (but opposite in sign) bad events. This notion was implied in Brickman et al.'s (1978) conclusions, lending an especially pernicious quality to the hedonic treadmill model. That is, not only do we adapt to good events, but we do so at a faster rate than we do to bad events. If we assumed that good and bad events in life happened randomly, and in equal proportions, then human life would be doomed to a preponderance of misery and NA.

In a rarely cited commentary on Brickman and Campbell's (1971) introduction of hedonic treadmill theory, McClelland (1971) reacted to the deterministic nature of the theory, which, as portrayed, acts as a universal law forcing all into the role of victim of hedonic principles. McClelland urged an alternative view on the ubiquity and power of the hedonic treadmill: "But surely there must be some element of choice here. A man can be taught the laws of hedonic relativism and learn how to gain greater satisfaction from life. He can choose his own goals and comparison groups and use all that we know about how to minimize dissatisfaction or maximize satisfaction to make a better life for himself and others" (McClelland, 1971, p. 304). In a more recent review of hedonic treadmill theory, Diener et al. (2006) came to a similar conclusion. Although agreeing with the basic facts of hedonic adaptation, Diener et al. offered several revisions to the hedonic treadmill theory to account for the fact that people are not doomed to unhappiness. One important revision, consistent with McClelland's observation, is that there are wide individual differences in adaptation rates. Diener et al. presented data that adaptation is not nearly so inevitable or automatic as is implied by the original theory. The rate and extent of adaptation to various events show wide variability across individuals.

Diener et al. (2006) reviewed two research traditions that shed light on individual differences in adaptation. One is the personality literature, in which various traits have been investigated in terms of reactivity to life events. Traits such as neuroticism and pessimism have been related to less effective adaptation to stress-ful life events. At least one study has shown that neuroticism is related to longer duration of NA episodes (Bolger & Schilling, 1991). Optimism, on the other hand, is related to faster adaptation to NA events (Scheier et al., 2003). A second literature relevant to individual differences in adaptation is the coping literature. To this we would also add the literature on emotion regulation (Gross, 1999, 2001; Larsen, 2000a, 2000b; Larsen & Prizmic, 2004). Much has been learned in recent years about specific strategies that promote coping or emotion regulation (Parkinson, Totterdel, Briner, & Reynolds, 1996). For example, cognitive reap-praisal is a strategy that some individuals use to effectively remediate the effects of negative events. In the remainder of this chapter we review a number of such strategies especially, in light of how they operate with reference to the hedonic treadmill notion.

Overcoming the Hedonic Treadmill

The hedonic treadmill really has two tracks: One concerns PA and how we react and adapt to good events; the second concerns NA and how we react and adapt to bad events. The major problem is that we tend to get over good events faster than we get over bad events. One solution to this problem would be to construct a life wherein most events were positive and few, if any, bad events occurred. Because life cannot be so completely engineered, a second, more realistic, solu-tion would be to find ways to speed up adaptation to negative events and to slow down adaptation to positive events.

Portions of the literature in positive psychology, especially that part empha-sizing interventions to increase PA (e.g., Emmons, Chapter 23, this volume), provide clues on ways to slow adaptation to positive events. Much of the litera-ture on mood regulation (Catanzaro, 2000; Larsen & Prizmic, 2004) concerns speeding up adaptation to negative events. Because of the negativity bias, pro-cesses that speed adaptation to negative events may be more fundamental to overall well-being than processes that promote lengthening of reactions to good events, although both are clearly important to global emotional well-being. As such, we start first with a consideration of behaviors and strategies that speed up adaptation to negative events.

Speeding Up Adaptation to Negative Events

Cognitive Reappraisal: Finding Meaning in Negative Events

This strategy involves the attempt to find meaning in, or develop a positive inter-pretation of, a problematic situation. It speeds up adaptation by essentially turning a bad event into a neutral or good event. Many terms have been used to describe this strategy, including positive reappraisal, cognitive restructuring, and cognitive reframing (Tamres, Janicki, & Helgeson, 2002). Tennen and Affleck (2002) use the term "benefit finding" to refer to the search for benefits in adversity, the so-called silver lining in every dark cloud. They review an impressive amount of research showing that perceiving benefits in otherwise negative experiences is associated with more adaptive long-term outcomes. For example, Davis, Nolen-Hoeksema, and Larson (1998) asked people who had lost a loved one recently whether they could find anything positive in the experience. Seventy-three percent of the subjects reported that something positive could be found, such as finding supportive others, strengthening family bonds, or providing a new perspective on life. Six months later, those who had found some benefit to their loss were less distressed than those who did not find such benefits.

The self-disclosure research by Pennebaker and colleagues (e.g., Niederhoffer & Pennebaker, 2002) is also relevant to this strategy. Pennebaker and others (e.g., Lyubomirsky, Sousa, & Dickerhoof, 2006) have shown that persons who are induced to write, talk, or think about a bad event over a period of time tend to fare better—in terms of psychological and physical health—than those who spend the same period of time being concerned about a mundane or even positive experience. Pennebaker's original explanation for this effect concerned the effort it takes to inhibit a traumatic experience, something akin to keeping a secret. His more recent interpretation of the effect, however, is along the lines of cognitive reappraisal. By writing about a negative experience, he argues, people construct a story, a reinterpretation of the event that facilitates a sense of resolution. After taking part in his writing experiments, participants recount their experience with phrases such as "coming to terms with," "understanding," and "getting past" the particular event about which they chose to write (Niederhoffer & Pennebaker, 2002, p. 578).

Downward Social Comparison

The downward social comparison strategy for speeding adaptation to negative events concerns comparing oneself to others who are worse off; if the comparison is favorable to the self, then negative affect is lessened. After a negative event, comparing oneself to others who have had a more severe negative event can serve to put one's problem into perspective. So, if a professor receives poor teacher ratings, it might be seen as a bad event. But if he or she can find other professors who have received worse ratings, then his or her rating might not seem so bad.

Social comparison research occupies a very large domain within social psychology (see Suls, Martin, & Wheeler, 2002, for a review), and so generalizations are risky. Nevertheless, research shows that people play an active role in using comparison information, and that they do so in part for emotional reasons (Fujita, Chapter 12, this volume; Suls & Wheeler, 2000). Correlational studies have shown that dispositionally happy persons are less affected by unfavorable social comparison information (Lyubomirsky & Ross, 1997; Lyubomirsky, Tucker, & Kasri, 2001). Researchers are actively mapping out the phenomenon and the boundary conditions that limit the effects of social comparison information on emotional state. For example, Lockwood (2002) has demonstrated that the impact of downward comparison on self-evaluation is dependent on such factors as similarity to the comparison other and the likelihood that the other's fate might become one's own (perceived vulnerability). Although there is much to learn about social comparison processes, it is clear that people often look for worse-off others with whom to compare fates and thereby enhance their affective states.

Problem-Directed Action
or Planning to Avoid Problems in the Future

This action-oriented strategy involves thinking about and acting on the bad event to change the situation and thereby speed adaptation. The change might involve situational selection, whereby an effort is made to actively select oneself into or out of specific activities, relationships, or places in an effort to avoid the situational aspect responsible for the negative affect. For example, asking to be transferred to a different unit at work to avoid an unpleasant coworker would be a problem-directed action. Or the situation, if it cannot be selected out of, could be modified with an effort toward changing the problematic part. For example, if one could not transfer to a different unit, then efforts could be expended toward modifying how one interacted with the troublesome coworker. A third way to control the situation is to control how one directs one's attention, picking and choosing which parts of the situation receives attention. This strategy would suggest simply not paying attention to the troublesome coworker.

Problem-focused and emotion-focused coping have been distinguished for several decades in the coping literature (e.g., Lazarus & Folkman, 1984). Whereas *emotion-focused coping* refers to any attempt to reduce negative emotion, *problem-focused coping* involves concrete actions designed to solve the problem causing the person to feel unpleasant. The emphasis in this distinction lies on the actions taken to solve the *problem* in problem-focused but not emotion-focused coping. However, Larsen (1993) reported that planning for how to avoid similar problems in the future was a frequently used strategy. Moreover, this strategy was associated with concurrent and subsequent improvements in mood. Because some problems, like "water under the bridge," cannot be recalled and fixed, it would seem that efforts expended on planning to *avoid* similar problems in the future would be useful. As such, after an unpleasant event, an improvement in mood might follow on the heels of explicitly planning how to avoid such events in the future.

Self-Reward: Thinking about or Doing Pleasant Activities

One feature of behavioral approaches to self-management is the use of self-reward. These techniques are based in a tradition that views emotion disorders, especially depression, as being caused by a lack of appropriate reinforcing experiences, especially self-administered positive reinforcement. Along these lines, researchers have found that depressed persons display a low frequency of self-reinforcing activities (Heiby, 1983). Experimental studies, in which some subjects are encouraged to increase the number of positive experiences they provide for themselves and to focus on the pleasantness of those experiences, find that doing so is associated with decreased depression (Dobson & Joffe, 1986).

Studies of daily experience have also shown similar patterns; that frequency of pleasurable activities is correlated with increased PA (Parkinson et al., 1996), though the causal direction (i.e., mood causing the selection of more pleasant activities, or vice versa) is still unknown. Nevertheless, in another study of daily experience, Fichman and colleagues (Fichman, Koestner, Zuroff, & Gordon, 1999) found that engaging in pleasant, rewarding activities was the most successful strategy for reducing NA. For the remediation of negative states, it would seem that self-reward is an obvious response. Self-rewarding experience can be an actual event (e.g., going shopping, reading a chapter in an interesting novel) or a more cognitive pleasure (e.g., taking a few minutes off to recall some pleasant experience or think about some pleasant activity planned for the future). One strategy is to imagine the future when the current problem has faded. Pleasant anticipations and pleasant memories may serve the same purposes. Josephson, Singer, and Salovey (1996) demonstrate how, after being induced to a sad mood and then required to list two memories, many participants listed positive memories. Moreover, when asked why they elected memories of that valence, most mentioned mood repair as their motivation. Similar results on using positive memories to regulate negative moods are reported by Rusting and DeHart (2000).

Fredrickson's (1998, 2000) theory of PA holds that the function of PA is, in part, to hasten recovery from negative events. In experimental studies she has shown that, following a stressor, persons induced to a positive mood show faster cardiovascular recovery than those in a control condition (Fredrickson & Levenson, 1998). Such results suggest that the deliberate attempt to self-induce PA through self-reward may be especially useful in speeding recovery from negative events (Tugade & Fredrickson, 2004).

Exercise, Relaxation, Eating, and Other Physical Manipulations

Thayer (2001) provides an important review and integration of information on the affective consequences of exercise and eating. The empirical literature is large, is dispersed across differing disciplines, and is replete with ostensibly contradictory findings. For example, moderate exercise appears positively correlated with pleasant affect in some samples but not in others. Nevertheless, Thayer's own research (e.g., 1987) indicates that moderate exercise, such as taking a 20-minute brisk walk, is a reliable method for the average person to change a bad mood and obtain a boost in felt energy.

It may seem ironic that the use of energy (to exercise) actually elevates energy, but the impact of exercise on affect and felt energy has been reliably demonstrated in a number of studies (e.g., Ekkekakis, Hall, Van Landuyt, & Petruzzello, 2000). In other research (Stevens & Lane, 2001), exercise was rated by a group of athletes as the most effective strategy for regulating anger, depression, fatigue, and tension. One possible explanation why exercise might be so effective at regulating NA is that it not only serves as a distraction from the NA but it can also be seen as a reinforcing, positive behavior in its own right, independent of its affect-regulating impact.

When it comes to food, emotional effects are complicated by a variety of factors, including gender, culture, obesity, and psychopathology. There is a great deal of research on the effects of prior mood on subsequent eating (reviewed in Thayer, 2001). Of the studies on the other causal direction, there appears to be reliable support for the intake of sweets (refined sugar) to lead to increased fatigue and NA (Thayer, 1987). Also, people appear to use stimulants, such as coffee, tea, or nicotine, in explicit attempts to self-regulate energy level (Adan, 1994). Research that directly examines the effects of ingesting various substances on mood is relatively sparse. It seems likely, however, that substances that influence blood glucose, hormones, or neurotransmitters (especially dopamine and serotonin) are likely to produce alterations in affective state. Similarly, activities such as exercise, meditation (Davidson, 2002), or even napping or going to sleep earlier than usual (Parkinson et al., 1996) can influence these important biochemicals and thus be associated with consequent changes in affective states.

Socializing: Seeking Comfort, Help, or Advice from Others

One characteristic that is almost always found to correlate with subjective well-being is the number, quality, and frequency of relationships (Diener & Seligman, 2002). Happy people spend time with others; they join groups, have many friends, have loving relationships, build social support networks, and generally find the presence of others to be both a satisfaction and a motive for further social activity (Lyubomirsky, Sheldon, & Schkade, 2005). Although such correlational evidence does not prove that spending time with others causes one to be happy, such findings are at least consistent with such a conclusion.

In a daily study of affect regulation in salespersons (who have frequent disappointments), Larsen and Gschwandtner (1995) found that social activity was among the most frequently used regulation strategies among female salespersons. As pointed out by Tice and Baumeister (1993), an important aspect of socializing for mood regulation concerns *not* socializing with persons who are in the same mood. That is, a bunch of angry people would probably not be a good group with which to socialize if one were trying to get over one's anger. This outcome would most likely hold for all negative emotions.

Socializing may work to relieve NA through a variety of processes. For example, telling one's story to someone else provides the opportunity to cognitively reframe the situation, allowing for a reappraisal and reinterpretation. It also provides distraction and changes the situation. And it potentially elicits positive emotions through the other's efforts to change how one is feeling.

Venting: Expressing NA and Catharsis

Freud's catharsis theory holds that negative emotions, when not expressed, build up tension and ultimately produce symptoms. Consequently, the discharge of negative emotions through expression was thought to rid the psychological system of tension. Psychoanalysis is sometimes viewed as a form of venting therapy because patients are encouraged to reexperience the emotions associated with past unpleasant events.

Catharsis theory is most often associated with the management of anger. However, reviews of relevant research (e.g., Geen & Quanty, 1977) conclude that venting or expressing anger *does not* reduce aggressive behavior. In recent studies, Bushman (2002; Bushman, Baumeister, & Phillips, 2001) provides strong experimental evidence that angered participants are more, not less, aggressive if they are encouraged to "let off steam" by hitting a punching bag between being angered and having an opportunity to aggress against the person who angered them. What about venting as a regulation strategy for other negative emotions? In a daily experience sampling study, when subjects reported on their moods and affect regulation behaviors three times a day, Larsen (1993) found that venting was not an effective strategy for regulating sadness. In fact, occasions when a person expressed or vented sadness (e.g., by having a "good cry") tended to be followed by occasions of elevated sadness.

Emotion feedback theories (e.g., facial feedback) suggest that the outward expression of an emotion serves to amplify the subjective impact or feeling of the emotion. Larsen, Kasimatis, and Frey (1992) demonstrated how inducing a furrowed brow produces stronger NA in response to unpleasant images compared to looking at the same images with relaxed brow muscles. The authors argued that facial expressions serve to amplify ongoing emotion. From this perspective, venting, at least in the short term, would work to amplify subjective feelings. As such, venting would probably be more useful in the up-regulation of positive emotions. That is, according to this line of thinking, smiling, laughing, or even postural adjustments, such as sitting up tall or holding one's shoulders back, could be used to increase positive feelings. We discuss this point further below.

Suppression: Keeping the NA from Being Expressed

In contrast to venting, suppression involves inhibiting the expression of the negative emotion. Emotional containment or suppression has been examined in a series of studies by Gross (e.g., Gross & Levenson, 1993, 1995; Gross, 1998a, 1998b; John & Gross, 2004). In the typical experiment, participants watch an emotion-inducing film (e.g., an arm amputation), and some are instructed to suppress outward signs of any emotion they might experience. Subjects in the suppression condition do report less disgust than the control group; however, the suppression group also exhibits increased physiological activation compared to the control group. Using a similar paradigm (viewing emotionally loaded slides), Buck (1977; Buck, Miller, & Caul, 1974) reported conceptually similar findings two decades earlier. Buck and colleagues reported that, when looking at the emotional images, less expressive subjects exhibited the most autonomic arousal. Buck argued then, as Gross does now, that the act of suppression takes effort and thus is associated with increased physiological arousal. Gross and Levenson (1993, 1997) report that the suppression of sadness and amusement is also associated with increases in physiological activation.

Although suppression does appear to diminish the subjective impact of the emotional stimulus, it does so at the cost of increasing physiological arousal. This arousal is most likely due to the conflict between the impulse to express the emotion and the effort to inhibit that expression—an outlay of energy that may interfere with adaptive functioning. Gross (2001) reviews several of his experiments demonstrating the cognitive and social consequences of the suppression of negative emotions. For example, instructions to suppress affective expressions while viewing unpleasant images were associated with poorer memory for information presented during viewing. In general, Gross views suppression as a somewhat crude emotion regulation strategy; one that takes energy to deploy and produces maladaptive side effects.

Distraction

The strategy of distraction involves disengagement from, or avoidance of, the problematic situation. The avoidance may involve an automatic shift of attention from threatening events or information (Robinson, Meier, & Vargas, 2005) or behaviors directed toward engaging in low-effort preoccupying activities (e.g., watching TV, listening to music) or engaging in more difficult preoccupying activities (e.g., working on a hobby, reading an involving book). A somewhat different slant on this strategy is to focus on the future when this problem will be resolved. In short, one can reallocate cognitive resources to other activities or by thinking about other times.

In his study of emotion regulation in everyday life, Larsen (1993) reported that, among a sample of college students who rated their moods and affect regulation behaviors three times a day for a month, distraction was the single most frequently mentioned mood regulation strategy. Out of all occasions when mood regulation strategies were used, distraction was mentioned 14% of the time. However, the effects of distraction were short-lived; mood on the occasion of distraction was slightly better than expected, though on the next report period (between 6 and 12 hours later), mood was no different from average.

To the extent that distraction is effective for negative affect relief, it most likely works by interrupting or preventing rumination (Davidson et al., 2002). Whereas most people respond to a negative life event with a negative mood, those who are prone to depression or other emotion disorders have difficulty "getting over" or recovering from negative events (Larsen & Cowan, 1988). Rumination involves turning the event over and over in one's mind, reliving the feelings it caused, imagining different outcomes, regretting what one did, and so forth. It is viewed as a breakdown in NA regulation, caused by focusing on feelings and enhancing negative cognitions, and it predicts depressive disorders, the onset of depressive episodes, and anxiety symptoms (e.g., Nolen-Hoeksema & Morrow, 1993; Nolen-Hoeksema, Morrow, & Fredrickson, 1993). Being able to control one's own attention and thoughts, through volitional effort or through automatic processes related to individual differences (Robinson et al., 2005), is the way to avoid rumination.

Withdrawal: Isolation and Spending Time Alone

It may seem contradictory that both socializing and isolation might be useful affect regulation strategies. Nevertheless, isolation appears on the list of strategies presented by several researchers (Larsen & Prizmic, 2004; Morris & Reilly, 1987; Parkinson et al., 1996; Tamres et al., 2002). This strategy refers to removing oneself from social activities during a negative emotion. We've all heard someone say, "Leave me alone, I'm in a bad mood," or "I just want to be by myself." Larsen (1993), in his study of daily mood regulation patterns, reported that this strategy is not uncommon, but that it is also not very successful in remediating negative affect. This basic finding was replicated by Fichman et al. (1999), who reported that spending time alone correlated with dispositional self-criticism (a component of depressive style) and was unrelated to mood improvement in their study of daily mood. Thus, spending time alone is often employed or endorsed as a mood regulation strategy, yet its overall effectiveness for general NA relief remains doubtful.

Perhaps the one type of NA for which withdrawal or self-isolation is adaptive is anger. It would seem that when one is angry, especially when on the verge of "flooding" or losing self-control, then withdrawal from the situation is an appropriate strategy. For example, if a parent becomes so angry at a child that he or she is on the verge of abusive physical action, then leaving the scene can be an adaptive response. However, for most other negative emotions, including sadness, anxiety, or shame, findings in the literature suggest that spending time alone may not be adaptive.

Slowing Down Adaptation to Positive Events

In a study of affect regulation strategies used in daily life, 91% of the subjects reported that they have tried effortful strategies in order to induce or maintain a positive mood (Prizmic, 1997). Some of the strategies used in regulating NA, discussed above, were also mentioned in maintaining and prolonging PA states. Other strategies were more unique to the maintenance of PA. Most of the strategies can be considered efforts to prolong PA states and to delay the process of adaptation that produces the hedonic treadmill effect. Many of the strategies we discuss are topics central to the positive psychology movement (e.g., Snyder & Lopez, 2002).

Gratitude: Counting One's Blessings or Focusing on Areas of Life That Are Going Well

This strategy takes the form of ruminating on the positive. It involves keeping a focus on one's strengths or the events in life for which one can be thankful. Emmons and McCullough (2003) reported two experiments wherein participants were randomly assigned to one of three conditions: listing their hassles, listing things for which they were thankful, or listing mundane daily activities. They made these listings either weekly for 10 weeks (Study 1) or daily for 21 days (Study 2). Participants also kept records of their moods, coping behaviors, health behaviors, and physical symptoms. Across the studies, the gratitude-outlook group exhibited heightened well-being on most of the outcome measures, relative to the control groups. The effect of counting one's blessings was particularly strong for measures of PA, but also produced interpersonal and self-reported health benefits.

Emmons and Shelton (2002) provided an interesting review of philosophical and spiritual perspectives on gratitude, as well as the small but growing scientific literature on this topic. The "examined life" would be one wherein a person regularly inventories those things for which he or she is thankful. Researchers have also considered gratitude as a stable personality trait (McCullough, Tsang, & Emmons, 2004). Others have constructed measures of individual differences in the tendency to be grateful and have found that they correlate substantially with overall well-being (Watkins, Woodward, Stone, & Russel, 2003).

Gratitude may work to slow adaptation to good events by consistently reminding oneself, or refreshing one's experience, of the good event. Another potential mechanism whereby gratitude may work is through reminding the person that there are areas of his or her life that are going well. The process may be similar to Linville's (1985) self-complexity notion. That is, by reminding oneself of the areas in life for which to be thankful, one may develop a more complex self-concept—which Linville has shown buffers the effects of stress or failure in any one area of the self-concept.

A concept related to gratitude is that of sharing positive events, called "capitalization," or telling others about one's good news (Gable, Impett, Reis, & Asher, 2004). In two studies Gable et al. (2004) showed that communicating positive events to others was associated with increased daily PA, above and beyond the effects of the positive events themselves. Sharing one's good fortunes with others may be a very effective way to slow adaptation to good events, may cultivate prolonged PA, and may enhance social bonds.

Helping Others: Committing Acts of Kindness

Altruism and emotion have been widely studied by social psychologists. However, in most experiments the causal direction of interest has examined the effects of emotion on subsequent helping. A few studies have indirectly investigated the effects of helping on the emotional state of the helper. For example, Wegener and Petty (1994) examined the anticipated consequences of helping and found that persons in a happy mood (compared to sad) based their decision to help on the anticipated positive emotional consequences of helping. Another example is the work of Rosenhan, Salovey, and Hargis (1981), which found that happy persons were more likely to help and to anticipate positive consequences for helping. However, actual measures of affect following the helping behavior were not obtained. Nevertheless, many psychologists assume it is a foregone conclusion that helping produces or maintains PA (e.g., Millar, Millar, & Tesser, 1988; Salovey, Mayer, & Rosenhan, 1991).

Much indirect evidence suggests that helping may influence PA. For example, Simmons, Hickey, and Kjellstrand (1971) showed that persons who donated a kidney to a relative were more likely to be happier than other relatives who did not donate. In a daily experience sampling study, Lucas (2000) found a substantial correlation between the percentage of time participants spent helping other people and their scores on a global well-being measure. And several researchers have demonstrated a link between dispositional happiness and the propensity to be generous, altruistic, and charitable (e.g., Feingold, 1983; Williams & Shiaw, 1999).

A concept related to helping is that of "committing random acts of kindness" (Sheldon & Lyubomirsky, 2004), which has been shown to have positive effects on the mood of the person committing the act (Lyubomirsky, Sheldon, & Schkade, 2005). Regardless of how effective this behavior is in raising the mood of the kind person, random acts of kindness are typically met with suspicion on the part of the persons receiving the undeserved act of kindness (Baskerville et al., 2000).

How is it that helping and committing acts of kindness promote more PA? Egoistic explanations hold that acts of kindness might promote expectations of reciprocity and increased liking by others, and pull for expressions of gratitude and appreciation from others. Other explanations concern how acts of helping promote a broader view of the self in social relatedness and community, as part of an interdependent social fabric, wherein what is good for one person is viewed as good for many. Also, acts of kindness may promote changes in self-perception, wherein the kind person sees him- or herself as more in control, generous, and optimistic about his or her abilities, in general, and his or her ability to be helpful, in particular. And finally, there may be social comparison effects that occur in helping, wherein generally the person needing the help provides a favorable downward social comparison target for the person doing the helping.

Humor: Laughter and Expressing Positive Emotions

Most researchers agree that there are several different forms of humor, including derisive/disparaging, self-depreciating, and self-directed or mature humor, wherein people laugh at their own failings or those of human nature in general. This latter form of humor is thought to be the most positive and beneficial form in terms of psychological adjustment (Vaillant, 1977) and the facilitation of social relationships (Lefcourt, 2002).

Much of the research on humor focuses on how it buffers during periods of stress. For example, Bonanno and Keltner (1997) reported that bereaved persons who could smile and laugh as they spoke about their deceased spouse were rated as more attractive and appealing by the interviewers. The researchers interpreted this finding to mean that laughing and smiling after a traumatic event serves as a social signal that the stressed individual is ready to reengage in normal social interaction. Correlational studies show that people with a sense of humor are better at coping with stress and illnesses, recover faster from illnesses, and appear to have enhanced immune system responses compared to low-humor individuals (Lefcourt, 2002). Of the few true experiments conducted on the topic in which laughter was induced in one group but not another (the control), results also suggested that laughter attenuates certain physiological responses to stress (e.g., Newman & Stone, 1996). Others also focus on how self-conscious attempts at humor overcome the deleterious effects of stress (e.g., Taylor, Kemeny, Reed, Bower, & Gruenewald, 2000).

The key to how laughter works may lie in the fact that it is an overt expression of a pleasant state, and expression may be the key. Kuiper and Martin (1998) demonstrated that it was laughter, not unexpressed pleasant emotions, which moderated the relation between stress and distress. The expression (laughter) may amplify or extend the effects of the positive emotion. Duclos and Laird (2001) argue that emotional experiences can be influenced through the deliberate control of emotional expressions, such as smiling and laughing. The facial feedback hypothesis—that muscles involved in emotional expressions feed back to emotion centers in the brain to amplify the ongoing emotion—would suggest that expressions of PA would act to produce longer or more intense experiences of PA (Strack, Martin, & Stepper, 1988).

Summary

In this chapter we reviewed definitions of subjective well-being and focused on its emotional core, which we consider to be the ratio of positive to negative affect over time. We review evidence that the NA system produces stronger affective output, per unit input, than the PA system, a phenomenon known as negativity bias. After reviewing the evidence, we venture so far as to speculate that negativity exceeds positivity by a factor of pi (3.14). The fact that negativity is stronger than positivity, combined with the notion of differential adaptation (we adapt faster to good events than to bad events), creates the conditions that drive the hedonic treadmill. However, most people are able to overcome the psychological forces of the hedonic treadmill and maintain at least a modicum of emotional well-being (Biswas-Diener, Vitterso, & Diener, 2005). We argue that happy persons are especially adept at speeding their emotional recovery from negative events and at slowing their hedonic adaptation to positive events. We review a number of strategies and behaviors geared toward altering hedonic adaptation rates (speeding adaptation to bad events, slowing adaptation to good events). For example, gratitude can serve to prolong the hedonic effects of positive events. In most cases we imply that the behavior (e.g., gratitude) can modify the affective state. However, it is also becoming clear that affective states (e.g., PA) can promote the specific behaviors (e.g., gratitude; Lyubomirsky, King, & Diener, 2005). The causal relationships may be bidirectional, in which case strategies for influencing affect may themselves be influenced, in a positive feedback fashion, by the affects they engender. This causal relationship may be one way to trigger upward spirals toward emotional well-being (Fredrickson & Joiner, 2002).

References

Adan, A. (1994). Chronotype and personality factors in the daily consumption of alcohol and psychostimulants. *Addiction, 89*, 455–462.

Arthaud-Day, M. L., Rode, J. C., Mooney, C. H., & Near, J. P. (2005). The subjective well-being construct: A test of its convergent, discriminant, and factorial validity. *Social Indicators Research, 74*, 445–476.

Baskerville, K., Johnson, K., Monk-Turner, E., Slone, Q., Standley, H., Stansbury, S., et al. (2000). Reactions to random acts of kindness. *Social Science Journal, 37*, 293–298.

Baumeister, R. F., Bratslavsky, E., Finkenauer, C., & Vohs, K. D. (2001). Bad is stronger than good. *Review of General Psychology, 5*, 323–370.

Biswas-Diener, R., Vitterso, J., & Diener, E. (2005). Most people are pretty happy, but there is cultural variation: The Inughuit, the Amish, and the Maasai. *Journal of Happiness Studies, 6*, 205–226.

Bolger, N., & Schilling, E. A. (1991). Personality and the problems of everyday life: The role of neuroticism in exposure and reactivity to daily stressors. *Journal of Personality, 59*, 355–386.

Bonanno, G. A., & Keltner, D. (1997). Facial expressions of emotion and the course of conjugal bereavement. *Journal of Abnormal Psychology, 106*, 126–137.

Brickman, P., & Campbell, D. T. (1971). Hedonic relativism and planning the good society. In M. H. Appley (Ed.), *Adaptation-level theory: A symposium* (pp. 287–302). New York: Academic Press.

Brickman, P., Coates, D., & Janoff-Bulman, R. (1978). Lottery winners and accident victims: Is happiness relative? *Journal of Personality and Social Psychology, 36*, 917–927.

Buck, R. (1977). Nonverbal communication of affect in preschool children: Relationships with personality and skin conductance. *Journal of Personality and Social Psychology, 35*, 225–236.

Buck, R., Miller, R. E., & Caul, W. F. (1974). Sex, personality, and physiological variables in the communication of affect via facial expression. *Journal of Personality and Social Psychology, 30*, 587–596.

Bushman, B. J. (2002). Does venting anger feed or extinguish the flame? Catharsis, rumination, distraction, anger, and aggressive responding. *Personality and Social Psychology Bulletin, 28*, 724–731.

Bushman, B. J., Baumeister, R. F., & Phillips, C. M. (2001). Do people aggress to improve their mood? Catharsis beliefs, affect regulation opportunity, and aggressive responding. *Journal of Personality and Social Psychology, 81*, 17–32.

Cacioppo, J. T., & Gardner, W. L. (1999). Emotion. *Annual Review of Psychology, 50*, 191–214.

Catanzaro, S. J. (2000). Mood regulation and suicidal behavior. In T. E. Joiner & M. D. Rudd (Eds.), *Suicide science: Expanding the boundaries* (pp. 81–103). New York: Kluwer.

Chow, S., Ram, N., Fujita, F., Boker, S. M., & Clore, G. (2005). Emotion as a thermostat: Representing emotion regulation using a damped oscillator model. *Emotion, 5,* 208–225.

Dalgleish, T. (1995). Performance on the emotional Stroop task in groups of anxious, expert, and control subjects: A comparison of computer and card presentationformats. *Cognition and Emotion, 9,* 341–362.

Davidson, R. J. (2002). Toward a biology of positive affect and compassion. In R. J. Davidson & A. Harrington (Eds.), *Visions of compassion: Western scientists and Tibetan Buddhists examine human nature* (pp. 107–130). London: Oxford University Press.

Davidson, R. J., Lewis, D. A., Alloy, L. B., Amaral, D. G., Bush, G., Cohen, J. D., et al. (2002). Neural and behavioral substrates of mood and mood regulation. *Biological Psychiatry, 52,* 478–502.

Davis, C. G., Nolen-Hoeksema, S., & Larson, J. (1998). Making sense of loss and benefiting from the experience: Two construals of meaning. *Journal of Personality and Social Psychology, 75,* 561–574.

De Houwer, J., Crombez, G., Baeyens, F., & Hermans, D. (2001). On the generality of the affective Simon effect. *Cognition and Emotion, 15,* 189–206.

De Houwer, J., & Eelen, P. (1998). An affective variant of the Simon paradigm. *Cognition and Emotion, 12,* 45–61.

Diener, E., & Emmons, R. A. (1985). The independence of positive and negative affect. *Journal of Personality and Social Psychology, 47,* 1105–1117.

Diener, E., Emmons, R. A., Larsen, R. J., & Griffin, S. (1985). The Satisfaction with Life Scale. *Journal of Personality Assessment, 49,* 71–75.

Diener, E., & Larsen, R. J. (1984). Temporal stability and cross-situational consistency of affective, cognitive, and behavioral responses. *Journal of Personality and Social Psychology, 47,* 871–883.

Diener, E., Lucas, R. E., & Scollon, C. N. (2006). Beyond the hedonic treadmill: Revising the adaptation theory of well-being. *American Psychologist, 61,* 305–314.

Diener, E., Oishi, S., & Lucas, R. E. (2003). Personality, culture, and subjective well-being: Emotional and cognitive evaluations of life. *Annual Review of Psychology, 54,* 403–425.

Diener, E., & Seligman, M. E. P. (2002). Very happy people. *Psychological Science, 13,* 81–84.

Dobson, K. S., & Joffe, R. (1986). The role of activity level and cognition in depressed mood in a university sample. *Journal of Clinical Psychology, 42,* 264–271.

Duclos, S. E., & Laird, J. D. (2001). The deliberate control of emotional experience through control of expressions. *Cognition and Emotion, 15,* 27–56.

Eid, M., & Diener, E. (2004). Global judgments of subjective well-being: Situational variability and long-term stability. *Social Indicators Research, 64,* 245–277.

Ekkekakis, P., Hall, E. E., Van Landuyt, L. M., & Petruzzello, S. J. (2000). Walking in (affective) circles: Can short walks enhance affect? *Journal of Behavioral Medicine, 23,* 245–275.

Emmons, R. A., & McCullough, M. E. (2003). Counting blessings versus burdens: An experimental investigation of gratitude and subjective well-being in daily life. *Journal of Personality and Social Psychology, 84,* 377–389.

Emmons, R. A., & Shelton, C. M. (2002). Gratitude and the science of positive psychology. In C. R. Snyder & S. J. Lopez (Eds.), *Handbook of positive psychology* (pp. 459–471). New York: Oxford University Press.

Feingold, A. (1983). Happiness, unselfishness, and popularity. *Journal of Psychology, 115,* 3–5.

Fichman, L., Koestner, R., Zuroff, D. C., & Gordon, L. (1999). Depressive styles and the regulation of negative affect: A daily experience study. *Cognitive Therapy and Research, 23,* 483–495.

Fleeson, W., Malanos, A. B., & Achille, N. M. (2002). An intraindividual process approach to the relationship between extraversion and positive affect: Is acting extraverted as "good" as being extraverted? *Journal of Personality and Social Psychology, 83,* 1409–1422.

Fredrickson, B. L. (1998). What good are positive emotions? *Review of General Psychology, 2,* 300–319.

Fredrickson, B. L. (2000). Cultivating positive emotions to optimize health and well-being. *Prevention and Treatment, 3,* Article 1. Retrieved November 11, 2002, from *journals.apa.org/prevention/volume3/pre0030001a.html.*

Fredrickson, B. L., & Joiner, T. (2002). Positive emotions trigger upward spirals toward emotional well-being. *Psychological Science, 13,* 172–175.

Fredrickson, B. L., & Levenson, R. W. (1998). Positive emotions speed recovery from the cardiovascular sequelae of negative emotions. *Cognition and Emotion, 12,* 191–220.

Fredrickson, B. L., & Losada, M. F. (2005). Positive affect and the complex dynamics of human flourishing. *American Psychologist, 60,* 678–686.

Fujita, F., & Diener, E. (2005). Life satisfaction set point: Stability and change. *Journal of Personality and Social Psychology, 88,* 158–164.

Gable, S. L., Impett, E. A., Reis, H. T., & Asher, E. R. (2004). What do you do when things go right? The intrapersonal and interpersonal benefits of sharing positive events. *Journal of Personality and Social Psychology, 87,* 228–245.

Geen, R. G., & Quanty, M. B. (1977). The catharsis of aggression: An evaluation of a hypothesis. In L. Berkowitz (Ed.), *Advances in experimental social psychology* (Vol. 10, pp. 1–37). New York: Academic Press.

Gottman, J. M. (1994). *What predicts divorce?: The relationship between marital processes and marital outcomes.* Hillsdale, NJ: Erlbaum.

Gross, J. J. (1998a). The emerging field of emotion regulation: An integrative review. *Review of General Psychology, 2,* 271–299.

Gross, J. J. (1998b). Antecedent- and response-focused emotion regulation: Divergent consequences for experience, expression, and physiology. *Journal of Personality and Social Psychology, 74,* 224–237.

Gross, J. J. (1999). Emotion regulation: Past, present, future. *Cognition and Emotion, 13,* 551–573.

Gross, J. J. (2001). Emotion regulation in adulthood: Timing is everything. *Current Directions in Psychological Science, 10,* 214–219.

Gross, J. J., & Levenson, R. W. (1993). Emotional suppression: Physiology, self-report, and expressive behavior. *Journal of Personality and Social Psychology, 64,* 970–986.

Gross, J. J., & Levenson, R. W. (1995). Emotion elicitation using films. *Cognition and Emotion, 9*, 87–108.

Gross, J. J., & Levenson, R. W. (1997). Hiding feelings: The acute effects of inhibiting negative and positive emotion. *Journal of Abnormal Psychology, 106*, 95–103.

Heiby, E. M. (1983). Assessment of frequency of self-reinforcement. *Journal of Personality and Social Psychology, 44*, 1304–1307.

Hietanen, J. K., & Korpela, K. (2004). Do both negative and positive environmental scenes elicit rapid affective processing? *Environment and Behavior, 36*, 558–577.

Ito, T. A., & Cacioppo, J. T. (2005). Variations on a human universal: Individual differences in positivity offset and negativity bias. *Cognition and Emotion, 19*, 1–26.

John, O. P., & Gross, J. J. (2004). Healthy and unhealthy emotion regulation: Personality processes, individual differences, and life span development. *Journal of Personality, 72*, 1301–1333.

Josephson, B. R., Singer, J. A., & Salovey, P. (1996). Mood regulation and memory: Repairing sad moods with happy memories. *Cognition and Emotion, 10*, 437–444.

Kahneman, D., Krueger, A. B., Schkade, D. A., Schwarz, N., & Stone, A. A. (2004). A survey method for characterizing daily life experience: The day reconstruction method. *Science, 306*, 1776–1780.

Kim-Prieto, C., Diener, E., Tamir, M., Scollon, C., & Diener, M. (2005). Integrating the diverse definitions of happiness: A time-sequential framework of subjective well-being. *Journal of Happiness Studies, 6*, 261–300.

Kuiper, N. A., & Martin, R. (1998). Laughter and stress in daily life: Relation to positive and negative affect. *Motivation and Emotion, 22*, 133–153.

Larsen, R. J. (1993, August). Mood regulation in everyday life. In D. M. Tice (Chair), *Self-regulation of mood and emotion*. Symposium conducted at the 101st annual convention of the American Psychological Association, Toronto.

Larsen, R. J. (2000a). Toward a science of mood regulation. *Psychological Inquiry, 11*, 129–141.

Larsen, R. J. (2000b). Maintaining hedonic balance: Reply to commentaries. *Psychological Inquiry, 11*, 218–225.

Larsen, R. J. (2002). Differential contributions of positive and negative affect to subjective well-being. In J. A. Da Silva, E. H. Matsushima, & N. P. Riberio-Filho (Eds.), *Annual Meeting of the International Society for Psychophysics* (Vol. 18, pp. 186–190). Rio de Janeiro, Brazil: Editora Legis Summa Ltda.

Larsen, R. J. (in press). Independence of positive and negative affect. In R. F. Baumeister & K. D. Vohs (Eds.), *Encyclopedia of social psychology*. Newbury Park, CA: Sage.

Larsen, R. J., & Cowan, G. S. (1988). Internal focus of attention and depression: A study of daily experience. *Motivation and Emotion, 12*, 237–249.

Larsen, R. J., Cruz, M., Ketelaar, T., Welsh, W., & Billings, D. (1990). Individual differences in trait happiness and physiological response to emotional stimuli. *Psychophysiology, 27*(Suppl. 4A), 47.

Larsen, R. J., & Diener, E. (1985). A multitrait–multimethod examination of affect structure: Hedonic level and emotional intensity. *Personality and Individual Differences, 6*, 631–636.

Larsen, R. J., & Gschwandtner, L. B. (1995). A better day. *Personal Selling Power, 2,* 41–49.

Larsen, R. J., Kasimatis, M., & Frey, K. (1992). Facilitating the furrowed brow: An unobtrusive test of the facial feedback hypothesis applied to unpleasant affect. *Cognition and Emotion, 6,* 321–338.

Larsen, R. J., & Ketelaar, T. (1989). Extraversion, neuroticism, and susceptibility to positive and negative mood induction procedures. *Personality and Individual Differences, 10,* 1221–1228.

Larsen, R. J., & Ketelaar, T. (1991). Personality and susceptibility to positive and negative emotional states. *Journal of Personality and Social Psychology, 61,* 132–140.

Larsen, R. J., & Prizmic, Z. (2004). Affect regulation. In R. Baumeister & K. Vohs (Eds.), *Handbook of self-regulation research* (pp. 40–60). New York: Guilford Press.

Larsen, R. J., & Prizmic, Z. (2006). Multimethod measurement of emotion. In M. Eid & E. Diener (Eds.), *Handbook of measurement: A multimethod perspective* (pp. 337–352).Washington, DC: American Psychological Association.

Larsen, R. J., & Yarkoni, T. (2006). *Negative is stronger than positive in producing interference effects in the affective Simon task.* Unpublished manuscript, St. Louis, MO.

Lazarus, R. S., & Folkman, S. (1984). *Stress, appraisal, and coping.* New York: Springer.

Lefcourt, H. M. (2002). Humor. In C. R. Snyder & S. J. Lopez (Eds.), *Handbook of positive psychology* (pp. 619–631). New York: Oxford University Press.

Linville, P. W. (1985). Self-complexity and affect extremity: Don't put all of your eggs in one basket. *Social Cognition, 3,* 94–120.

Lockwood, P. (2002). Could it happen to you? Predicting the impact of downward comparisons on the self. *Journal of Personality and Social Psychology, 82,* 343–358.

Lucas, R. E. (2000). *Pleasant affect and sociability: Towards a comprehensive model of extraverted feelings and behaviors.* Unpublished doctoral dissertation, University of Illinois at Urbana–Champaigne.

Lucas, R. E., Clark, A. E., Georgellis, Y., & Diener, E. (2004). Unemployment alters the set point for life satisfaction. *Psychological Science, 15,* 8–13.

Lyubomirsky, S., King, L. A., & Diener, E. (2005). The benefits of frequent positive affect: Does happiness lead to success? *Psychological Bulletin, 131,* 803–855.

Lyubomirsky, S., & Ross, L. (1997). Hedonic consequences of social comparison: A contrast of happy and unhappy people. *Journal of Personality and Social Psychology, 73,* 1141–1157.

Lyubomirsky, S., Sheldon, K. M., & Schkade, D. (2005). Pursuing happiness: The architecture of sustainable change. *Review of General Psychology, 9,* 111–131.

Lyubomirsky, S., Sousa, L., & Dickerhoof, R. (2006). The costs and benefits of writing, talking, and thinking about life's triumphs and defeats. *Journal of Personality and Social Psychology, 90,* 692–708.

Lyubomirsky, S., Tucker, K. L., & Kasri, F. (2001). Responses to hedonically conflicting social comparisons: Comparing happy and unhappy people. *European Journal of Social Psychology, 31,* 511–535.

McClelland, D. C. (1971). Comment on "hedonic relativism and planning the good society." In M. H. Appley (Ed.), *Adaptation-level theory: A symposium* (pp. 303–304). New York: Academic Press.

McCullough, M. E., Tsang, J., & Emmons, R. A. (2004). Gratitude in intermediate affective terrain: Links of grateful moods to individual differences and daily emotional experience. *Journal of Personality and Social Psychology, 86,* 295–309.

Millar, M. G., Millar, K. U., & Tesser, A. (1988). The effects of helping and focus of attention on mood states. *Personality and Social Psychology Bulletin, 14,* 536–543.

Morris, W., & Reilly, N. (1987). Toward the self-regulation of mood: Theory and research. *Motivation and Emotion, 11,* 215–249.

Musch, J., & Klauer, K. C. (2003). *The psychology of evaluation.* Mahwah, NJ: Erlbaum.

Newman, M. G., & Stone, A. A. (1996). Does humor moderate the effects of experimentally-induced stress? *Annals of Behavioral Medicine, 18,* 101–109.

Niederhoffer, K. G., & Pennebaker, J. W. (2002). Sharing one's story: On the benefits of writing or talking about emotional experiences. In C. R. Snyder & S. J. Lopez (Eds.), *Handbook of positive psychology* (pp. 573–583). New York: Oxford University Press.

Nolen-Hoeksema, S., & Morrow, J. (1993). Effects of rumination and distraction on naturally occurring depressed mood. *Cognition and Emotion, 7,* 561–570.

Nolen-Hoeksema, S., Morrow, J., & Fredrickson, B. L. (1993). Response styles and the duration of episodes of depressed mood. *Journal of Abnormal Psychology, 102,* 20–28.

Parkinson, B., Totterdell, P., Briner, R. B., & Reynolds, S. (1996). *Changing moods: The psychology of mood and mood regulation.* London: Longman.

Pratto, F., & John, O. P. (1991). Automatic vigilance: The attention-grabbing power of negative social information. *Journal of Personality and Social Psychology, 61,* 380–391.

Prizmic, Z. (1997). [Mood regulation strategies for positive mood]. Unpublished data.

Redelmeier, D. A., & Kahneman, D. (1996). Patients' memories of painful medical treatments: Real-time and retrospective evaluations of two minimally invasive procedures. *Pain, 66,* 3–8.

Robinson, M. D., Meier, B. P., & Vargas, P. T. (2005). Extroversion, threat categorizations, and negative affect: A reaction time approach to avoidance motivation. *Journal of Personality, 73,* 1397–1436.

Rosenhan, D. L., Salovey, P., & Hargis, K. (1981). The joys of helping: Focus of attention mediates the impact of positive affect on altruism. *Journal of Personality and Social Psychology, 40,* 899–905.

Rozin, P., & Royzman, E. B. (2001). Negativity bias, negativity dominance, and contagion. *Personality and Social Psychology Review, 5,* 296–320.

Rusting, C. L., & DeHart, T. (2000). Retrieving positive memories to regulate negative mood: Consequences for mood-congruent memory. *Journal of Personality and Social Psychology, 78,* 737–752.

Rusting, C. L., & Larsen, R. J. (1997). Extraversion, neuroticism, and susceptibility to positive and negative affect: A test of two theoretical models. *Personality and Individual Differences, 22,* 607–612.

Rusting, C. L., & Larsen, R. J. (1998). Personality and cognitive processing of affective information. *Personality and Social Psychology Bulletin, 24,* 200–213.

Salovey, P., Mayer, J. D., & Rosenhan, D. L. (1991). Mood and helping: Mood as a motivator of helping and helping as a regulator of mood. In M. S. Clark (Ed.), *Prosocial behavior* (pp. 215–237). Thousand Oaks, CA: Sage.

Scheier, M. F., Matthews, K. A., Owens, J. F., Magovern, G. J. S., Lefebvre, R. C., Abbott, R. A., et al. (2003). Dispositional optimism and recovery from coronary artery bypass surgery: The beneficial effects on physical and psychological well-being. In P. Salovey & A. J. Rothman (Eds.), *Social psychology of health* (pp. 342–361). New York: Psychology Press.

Schmukle, S. C., Egloff, B., & Burns, L. R. (2002). The relationship between positive and negative affect in the Positive and Negative Affect Schedule. *Journal of Research in Personality, 36,* 463–475.

Schwartz, R. M. (1997). Consider the simple screw: Cognitive science, quality improvement and psychotherapy. *Journal of Consulting and Clinical Psychology, 65,* 970–983.

Schwartz, R. M., Reynolds, C. F., III, Thase, M. E., Frank, E., Fasiczka, A. L., & Haaga, D. A. F. (2002). Optimal and normal affect balance in psychotherapy of major depression: Evaluation of the balanced states of mind model. *Behavioural and Cognitive Psychotherapy, 30,* 439–450.

Sheldon, K., & Lyubomirsky, S. (2004). Achieving sustainable new happiness: Prospects, practices, and prescriptions. In P. A. Linley & S. Joseph (Eds.), *Positive psychology in practice* (pp. 127–145). Hoboken, NJ: Wiley.

Simmons, R. G., Hickey, K., & Kjellstrand, C. M. (1971). Donors and non-donors: The role of the family and the physician in kidney transplantation. *Seminars in Psychiatry, 3,* 102–115.

Smith, N. K., Larsen, J. T., Chartrand, R. L., Cacioppo, J. T., Katafiasz, H. A., & Moran, K. E. (2006). Being bad isn't always good: Affective context moderates the attention bias toward negative information. *Journal of Personality and Social Psychology, 90,* 210–220.

Snyder, C. R., & Lopez, S. J. (Eds.). (2002). *Handbook of positive psychology.* London: Oxford University Press.

Stevens, M. J., & Lane, A. M. (2001). Mood-regulating strategies used by athletes. *Athletic Insight: Online Journal of Sport Psychology, 3,* Issue 3. Retrieved October 12, 2000, from *www.athleticinsight.com/Vol3Iss3/MoodRegulation.htm.*

Strack, F., Martin, L. L., & Stepper, S. (1988). Inhibiting and facilitating conditions of the human smile: A nonobtrusive test of the facial feedback hypothesis. *Journal of Personality and Social Psychology, 54,* 768–777.

Suls, J., Martin, R., & Wheeler, L. (2002). Social comparison: Why, with whom, and with what effect? *Current Directions in Psychological Science, 11,* 159–163.

Suls, J., & Wheeler, L. (Eds.). (2000). *Handbook of social comparison.* New York: Kluwer Academic/Plenum.

Tamres, L. K., Janicki, D., & Helgeson, V. S. (2002). Sex differences in coping behavior: A meta-analytic review and an examination of relative coping. *Personality and Social Psychology Review, 6,* 2–30.

Taylor, S. E., Kemeny, M. E., Reed, G. M., Bower, J. E., & Gruenewald, T. L. (2000). Psychological resources, positive illusions, and health. *American Psychologist, 55,* 99–109.

Tennen, H., & Affleck, G. (2002). Benefit-finding and benefit-reminding. In C. R. Snyder & S. J. Lopez (Eds.), *Handbook of positive psychology* (pp. 584–597). New York: Oxford University Press.

Thayer, R. E. (1987). Energy, tiredness, and tension effects of a sugar snack versus moderate exercise. *Journal of Personality and Social Psychology, 52,* 119–125.

Thayer, R. E. (2001). *Calm energy: How people regulate mood with food and exercise.* London: Oxford University Press.

Tice, D. M., & Baumeister, R. F. (1993). Controlling anger: Self-induced emotion change. In D. M. Wegner & J. W. Pennebaker (Eds.), *Handbook of mental control* (pp. 393–409). Upper Saddle River, NJ: Prentice-Hall.

Tugade, M. M., & Fredrickson, B. L. (2004). Resilient individuals use positive emotions to bounce back from negative emotional experiences. *Journal of Personality and Social Psychology, 86,* 320–333.

Vaillant, G. E. (1977). *Adaptation to life.* Boston: Little, Brown.

Watkins, P. C., Woodward, K., Stone, T., & Russel, L. (2003). Gratitude and happiness: Development of a measure of gratitude and relationships with subjective well-being. *Social Behavior and Personality, 31,* 431–452.

Wegener, D. T., & Petty, R. E. (1994). Mood management across affective states: The hedonic contingency hypothesis. *Journal of Personality and Social Psychology, 66,* 1034–1048.

White, M. (1996). Anger recognition is independent of spatial attention. *New Zealand Journal of Psychology, 25,* 30–35.

Williams, S., & Shiaw, W. T. (1999). Mood and organizational citizenship behavior: The effects of positive affect on employee organizational citizenship behavior intentions. *Journal of Psychology, 133,* 656–668.

Zelenski, J. M., & Larsen, R. J. (1999). Susceptibility to affect: A comparison of three personality taxonomies. *Journal of Personality, 67,* 761–791.

14

Two New Questions about Happiness

"Is Happiness Good?" and "Is Happier Better?"

SHIGEHIRO OISHI and MINKYUNG KOO

Historically three broad questions have dominated subjective well-being research: "What is happiness?" "Who is happy?" and "What makes people happy?" (Diener, 1984; Diener, Suh, Lucas, & Smith, 1999; Wilson, 1967). Philosophers have debated the first question for millennia without reaching any consensus (see Sumner, 1996, for review). This lack of agreement on the definition led to an impoverished state of empirical research on happiness. Indeed in 1948, Henry Murray and Clyde Kluckhohn lamented that "Aristotle's assertion that the only rational goal of goals is happiness has never been successfully refuted as far as we know, but, as yet, no scientist has ventured to break ground for a psychology of happiness" (p. 13). In 1984, however, Ed Diener broke the ground for the psychology of happiness and legitimized it for the rest of us psychologists and social scientists, with his *Psychological Bulletin* article entitled "Subjective Well-Being."

Since breaking the ground, Ed Diener has successfully built one of the most extensive nomological nets of any research programs in psychology (which must have made his intellectual hero, Paul Meehl, proud). First, Ed Diener painstakingly established the validity of subjective well-being (Diener, Emmons, Larsen, & Griffin, 1985; Pavot & Diener, 1993). In so doing, he created the foundation for the scientific inquiry into this complex phenomenon and answered the first major question, "What is happiness?" (answer: Happiness is a latent construct best indicated by a general sense of life satisfaction). Second, he documented the cross-situational consistency of subjective well-being (Diener & Larsen, 1984) and the contribution of personality to subjective well-being (e.g., Diener, Sandvik, Pavot, & Fujita, 1992; Magnus, Diener, Fujita, & Pavot, 1993), contrary to the then-fashionable social constructionism movement. In this process, he also provided the answer to the second major question, "Who is happy?" (answer: extraverts, optimists, and persons with great social relationships; see also Diener & Seligman, 2002; Myers & Diener, 1995). Third, he investigated the effect of external factors, such as resources (Diener & Fujita, 1995) and life events, on happiness (Suh, Diener, & Fujita, 1996), thereby answering the third question, "What makes people happy?" (answer: not so much positive life events per se, but rather goal attainment made possible by the match between individuals' talents, resources, and their goals; see also Oishi, Diener, Suh, & Lucas, 1999). Finally, while recognizing the significance of temperament and personality traits, he called attention to the importance of culture to the meaning and construal of well-being (e.g., Diener & Diener, 1995; Diener, Diener, & Diener, 1995).

Now that the first three questions are properly answered by Ed Diener, we can delve into other important research questions, including this chapter's main topic: What are the consequences of happiness (e.g., Do happy people make more money than unhappy people? Are they healthier than unhappy people?)? We will summarize the current state of knowledge on the consequences of happiness first, followed by the discussion of the optimal levels of happiness. Finally, we will explore cultural similarities and differences in the consequences of happiness.

The Consequences of Happiness

When Ruut Veenhoven published the article entitled "The Utility of Happiness" in 1988, he stated that "no empirical investigations have yet focused on consequences of happiness" (p. 333). Indeed, despite the fact that Veenhoven's 1988 article and 1989 edited book, *How Harmful Is Happiness?*, called attention to this important issue earlier, the consequences of happiness had not been systematically investigated until Lyubomirsky, King, and Diener's (2005) seminal meta-analysis. The relative lack of research attention to the consequences of happiness might be due to the fact that Aristotle, as well as 19th-century utilitarian philosophers, persuasively argued that happiness is the ultimate goal and ultimate good (i.e., something that can be pursued for its own sake, not for other purposes; Nussbaum, 2000). Many researchers must have felt that if happiness is the ultimate goal, why should we care about the *consequences* of this ultimate goal? We argue that even though normative analyses by moral philosophers often placed happiness as the ultimate goal, the consequences of happiness should be of great interest to well-being researchers, for several reasons. First, as Veenhoven (1989) eloquently maintained, if happiness harms us in some ways, the normative analysis on happiness becomes irrelevant in real life as the ultimate goal. Thus, the empirical evaluation of this issue is essential. Second, philosophical discussions about happiness often lack any consideration of individual and cultural differences. The consequences of happiness might vary systematically across individuals and cultures that differ in the eagerness with which they pursuit happiness (see Suh & Koo, Chapter 20, this volume). Below, we briefly summarize key review articles in this area: Veenhoven (1988, 1989), Lyubomirsky et al. (2005), and Pressman and Cohen (2005).

Veenhoven's Findings

The purpose of Veenhoven's (1988, 1989) review was to evaluate some of the negative views of happiness. Veenhoven asked a number of intriguing questions about the consequences of happiness. The first question was "Does happiness reduce sensitivity to others?" Empirical evidence indicates otherwise. For example, Wessman and Ricks' (1966) daily diary study showed that persons in good moods felt more "concerned about peers" than those in bad moods. The second question was "Does happiness lead into idleness?" Earlier daily diary studies (Flugel, 1925; Hersey, 1932; Johnson, 1937) all found that people were more active on the day when they felt happy. Experimental studies also indicate that people are more likely to help others (Isen & Levin, 1972), perform better on cognitive tasks (Fisher & Marrow, 1934), and show more expansive writing movements (Hale & Strickland, 1976) when they are in a happy mood. The third question was "Does happiness breed voting dummies?" The answer was again "no," because political participation was not associated with life satisfaction. The next question was "Does happiness loosen intimate ties?" Again, the answer was "no," because participants in a happy mood behaved more generously toward others (Bryant, 1983) and felt more positively toward others (Johnson, 1937). Also, longitudinal studies showed that happy people were more likely to remarry than unhappy people (Spanier & Furstenberg, 1982). The final question was "Is happiness healthy?" Here, the answer is "yes," because happy people had slightly better health as assessed by physicians (Veenhoven, 1984). In terms of longevity, one study found that happy people died earlier than unhappy people (Janoff-Bulman & Marshall, 1982), and one study found no difference (Palmore & Cleveland, 1976), but eight other studies found that happy people lived longer than unhappy ones.

Veenhoven's (1989) edited book asked similar questions. Two questions were not asked in Veenhoven (1988): "Does happiness buffer stress?" and "Does happiness heal cancer?" The answers to these questions were "no" and "no convincing evidence" at that time (see below for more recent review). In sum, Veehoven deserves credit for raising a number of important questions with regard to the consequences of happiness and demonstrating that negative views of happiness do not have much empirical basis. Because the number of studies reviewed in these articles was limited and effect sizes were not reported, however, definitive conclusions cannot be drawn based on these reviews alone.

Lyubomirsky, King, and Diener (2005) and Pressman and Cohen (2005) Meta-Analyses

The landscape of subjective well-being research has changed dramatically in the 17 years since Veenhoven's (1988, 1989) first reviews on this topic. Subjective well-being research has blossomed into one of the most widely researched topics in all of the social sciences (thanks to Ed Diener and other pioneers of the field, such as Carol Ryff, Ruut Veenhoven, Michael Argyle, Ed Deci, Richard Ryan, Norbert Schwarz, Fritz Strack, Martin Seligman, and Daniel Kahneman). Lyubomirsky et al.'s meta-analysis is monumental both in terms of the number of studies analyzed (225 papers) and the diversity of outcome measures. This article will most likely become a citation classic in the area of subjective well-being. Effect sizes of happiness vary widely across different outcome measures and research methods. The effect size was almost never negative, suggesting that harmful effects of subjective well-being are extremely rare. However, the effect size was modest at best ($r = .20–.30$), with a great deal of heterogeneity, suggesting that important moderators (particularly individual differences) remain to be discovered in the future.

Work and Love

Most people list success in work and love as their major life goals (Roberts & Robins, 2000). Thus, success in these two domains indicates that a person is leading a flourishing life. The key question, then, is "Do happy people have more success at work and love?" According to Lyubomirsky et al. (2005), the answer is again yes. For instance, individuals who reported having experienced more positive affect (PA) at age 18 had more prestigious jobs at age 26 than those who reported having experienced less PA ($r = .16$; Roberts, Caspi, & Moffitt, 2003). In addition, happy people received higher job performance assessments from their supervisors ($r = .17–.47$; Cropanzano & Wright, 1999; Wright & Staw, 1999). Not surprisingly, then, happy people later earned higher incomes ($r = .03$ both in Diener, Nickerson, Lucas, & Sandvik, 2002, and Marks & Fleming, 1999). Although the correlation coefficient is small, the actual effect size on the monetary sense is far from insignificant, as described in detail below. In addition, recent longitudinal studies generally confirmed Veenhoven's earlier review, in that happy people were more likely to get married at a later time ($r = .09$, Marks & Fleming, 1999; $r = .20$, Lucas, Clark, Georgellis, & Diener, 2003) and were more satisfied with their marriage at a later time (e.g., $r = .15–.40$, Ruvolo, 1998). Whereas the aforementioned studies uniformly relied on self-reported happiness, Harker and Keltner (2001) found that genuine smiles in college yearbook pictures predicted marital status 6 years later ($r = .19$) and marital satisfaction even 31 years later ($r = .20$). Finally, Staw, Sutton, and Pelled (1994) showed that workers with high PA later received more social support from colleagues than those with low PA ($r = .25$), suggesting that the positive benefit of PA is evident in friendships as well.

Experimental studies converge nicely with the aforementioned longitudinal findings. For example, positive moods led to a more positive perception of interaction partners (e.g., $r = .44$, Baron, 1987), greater interest in friendship, social activities, leisure activities, and self-disclosure (e.g., $r = .20–.44$, Cunningham, 1988), and more collaborative conflict resolution (e.g., $r = .29–.50$, Baron, Rea, & Daniels, 1992)—all of which, translated into ongoing relationships, should be associated with positive outcomes. These experimental studies indicate that not only happy predisposition but also momentary happiness mood generate positive interpersonal outcomes.

Health and Mortality

Although people do not list health as a major life goal, health is essential for individuals to be successful at work and love. Thus, health is another important life outcome. Mortality is widely considered the ultimate health outcome, because illness often leads to death. According to Lyubomirsky et al. (2005), subjective well-being predicted later mortality rate in seven studies ($r = -.06$ to $-.31$), indicating the positive association between higher subjective well-being and longevity. In seven studies subjective well-being also predicted survival rate ($r = .08–.36$), heart disease and heart attacks ($r = -.07$ to $-.12$), and stroke incidence ($r = -.05$ to $-.13$). These associations are thought to be mediated by healthier life styles of happy people. Indeed, individuals with high PA smoke cigarette less ($r = -.24$) and drink alcohol less ($r = -.22$), as well (Pettit, Kline, Genocoz, Genocoz, & Joiner, 2001; see Watson, 2000, for review).

Pressman and Cohen (2005) conducted a comprehensive meta-analysis on the link between PA and health outcomes, some of which overlap with Lyubomirsky et al. (2005). Here we briefly summarize the findings that do not overlap. In addition to mortality, survival, and various accidents, people with high-trait PA were less likely to develop a cold when exposed to a virus (Cohen et al., 2003) and less likely to be rehospitalized (Middleton & Byrd, 1996). Furthermore, all eleven studies reviewed found that both experimentally induced

PA and daily self-reported PA were associated with an increase in secretory immunoglobulin A (SIgA), the main immunological defense of mucosal surfaces. Experimental studies in which PA was induced also found a decrease in cortisol (e.g., Berk et al., 1989; Hubert & de Jong-Meyer, 1991). However, studies in which participants collected cortisol samples repeatedly in their daily environments produced mixed findings, some finding a negative association between trait PA and cortisol levels (Cohen et al., 2003), and others finding no association (Ryff, Singer, & Dienberg Love, 2004). Pressman and Cohen also reported results showing state PA leading to poorer pulmonary function (Wright, Rodriguez, & Cohen, 1998).

As Pressman and Cohen (2005) caution, the literature on PA and health is still limited in scope and methodology. In addition, the effect of PA on health is not unequivocal. However, these two meta-analyses present an overall picture that happiness is generally associated with healthier life styles, health behaviors, and outcomes.

Optimal Levels of Happiness: Is Happier Always Better?

As summarized above, happiness has more beneficial than harmful outcomes. Happiness does not lead to laziness but to industriousness. Happiness does not lead to insensitivity but to greater concern for others. Happiness does not lead to indulgence but rather to health. It should be emphasized again, however, that the effect size is modest at best. Earlier we suggested that the modest effect size of happiness on various important life outcomes may be due to moderators: namely, the effect of happiness might be strong for some individuals but weak for others. Another possibility is that the relation between happiness and outcome variables is not linear. After all, all the effect sizes calculated in Lyubomirsky et al. (2005) are correlation coefficients that assume a linear relationship. In this section, we explore the possibility that the effect of happiness is curvilinear, peaking at the moderate level of happiness as opposed to the extreme level of happiness (see Oishi, Diener, & Lucas, in press, for more details).

Our speculation that the effect of happiness on important life outcomes is nonlinear comes from Diener et al. (2002), in which they analyzed a large set of longitudinal data on Americans who entered one of 25 elite colleges in 1976. In this study, participants reported their cheerfulness, when they were incoming college freshman, on a 5-point scale (1 = lowest 10%; 2 = below average, 3 = average, 4 = above average, 5 = highest 10%) in 1976. In 1995, these participants reported their annual income. Although the correlation between cheerfulness in 1976 and annual income in 1995 was merely .03, the difference between the most cheerful ($65,023) and the least cheerful ($49,770) was not trivial. More important, they found a curvilinear relation between cheerfulness in 1976 and annual income in 1995, such that participants who rated themselves as "above average" on cheerfulness in 1976 earned $65,573 in 1995, slightly more than those who rated themselves as "highest 10%" in cheerfulness. Thus, if we use income as a criterion, the optimal level of "cheerfulness" was not the highest possible level but rather the "above-average" level.

Because Marks and Fleming (1999) reported the longitudinal correlation between life satisfaction and income, we contacted these authors and obtained data for the 1961 birth cohorts and analyzed the data in a way analogous to Diener et al. (2002). The Australian Youth in Transition study is a longitudinal study of nationally representative cohorts of young people. The respondents in this study indicated their life satisfaction ("satisfaction with life as a whole") when they were 18 years old, in 1979. They also reported their gross income in 1994, when they were 33 years old ($n = 1,166$). Consistent with Diener et al., Australians who were satisfied with their lives when they were 18 years old earned, on average, more money than those who were dissatisfied with their lives when they were 18 (see Figure 14.1). Also consistent with the findings of Diener et al., those who fell in the second highest category of life satisfaction earned more money than those in the highest category.

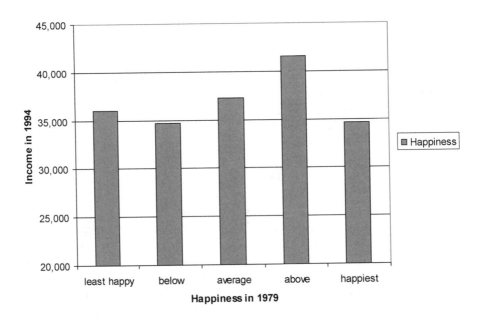

FIGURE 14.1. Optimal level of happiness for future income. X-axis indicates the level of happiness assessed in 1979, when participants were 18 years old. Y-axis indicates gross income in 1994, when participants were 33 years old, in Australian dollars.

In addition to income, we examined the longitudinal association between life satisfaction and educational attainment (the number of years of schooling they completed beyond high school in 1987, when they were 26 years old). Similar to the income findings, the second- and third-most satisfied groups completed more education than did the most satisfied group (see Figure 14.2). Finally, we examined the longitudinal relation between life satisfaction at age 18 in 1979 and the length of their intimate relationships in 1994. In contrast to the income and education findings, the most satisfied group in 1979 were, on average, involved in a longer intimate relationship in 1994 than the second and third satisfied groups (see Figure 14.3). In short, the Australian Youth in Transition study indicates that the optimal level of happiness is not the highest level of happiness in terms of educational achievement and income later in life. However, the highest level of satisfaction may, in fact, be optimal in terms of relationship stability.

It is interesting to note that World Value Survey (WVS) data converge with the findings from the Australian Youth in Transition data (see Oishi et al., in press, for details). Respondents in the WVS rated their overall life satisfaction on a 10-point scale ("All things considered, how satisfied are you with your life as a whole these days?"), and also indicated their income (in deciles from the lowest 10% in the nation to the highest 10% of the nation), highest education completed, their relationship status (i.e., whether they were currently in a stable, long-term relationship), and political actions they have taken (e.g., signing a peti-

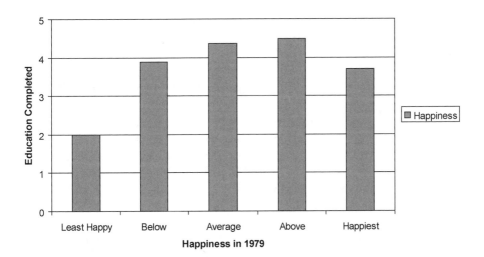

FIGURE 14.2. Optimal level of happiness for future education. *X*-axis indicates the level of happiness in 1979, when participants were 18 years old. *Y*-axis indicates years of post-high-school education completed by 1987, when they were 26 years old.

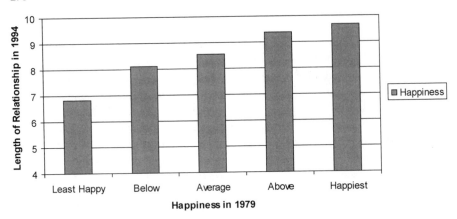

FIGURE 14.3. Optimal level of happiness for future relationship stability. X-axis indicates the level of happiness in 1979, when participants were 18 years old. Y-axis indicates the length (years) of the current romantic relationship measured in 1994, when they were 33 years old.

tion, joining in boycotts). Replicating Diener et al. (2002) and the Australian Youth in Transition data, respondents who were most satisfied with their lives did not earn as much income as respondents who rated their life satisfaction as a "9." In addition, those who were most satisfied did not have as high of educational attainment as those who were somewhat less satisfied with their lives. Furthermore, respondents who were most satisfied did not engage in political activity as much as those who were less satisfied. In contrast, the highest possible level of life satisfaction was "optimal" in terms of relationship status.

Culture and Consequences of Happiness

Most of the longitudinal studies reviewed above were conducted in the United States and other Western developed nations. Thus, the question remains whether the findings on the consequences and optimal levels of happiness will hold across cultures. Unfortunately, we were unable to locate any longitudinal data that directly address this issue. Instead we review previous research on cultural differences in the desirability of happiness, and the relations between happiness and later choice/decision making.

The desirability of happiness is important in the present context because happiness might not be associated with positive outcomes in a society where happiness is not as cherished as it is in the United States and Australia. Diener, Suh, Smith, and Shao (1995) found that U.S. college students viewed life satisfaction, happiness, joy, and contentment as more important than Chinese college students (but there were no differences between U.S. and Korean college students). Furthermore, U.S. college students viewed both feeling and expressing positive affect as more desirable and appropriate than did Korean and Chinese college students. Interestingly, Chinese students conversely thought that experiencing and expressing negative affect were more desirable and appropriate than did U.S. students. Eid and Diener (2001) took these findings one step further, using a latent class analysis to show that there was a class of Chinese college students who deemed positive emotions as neither desirable nor undesirable and negative emotions as desirable. This class existed only among Chinese college students (not among Taiwanese, Australians, or Americans). The existence of this subgroup in China suggests that correlates and consequences of happiness might be different between Chinese and U.S. populations.

If PA is not viewed as valuable and functional among Asian Americans as it is by European Americans, then the actual experiences of PA might not predict Asian Americans' future choices and decisions as well as those of European Americans. To test this idea, Oishi and Diener (2003) had participants solve anagram tasks (Study 1) and play a basketball game (Study 2) while assessing their actual enjoyment of the task. After the completion of the task, participants were asked to indicate whether they would like to repeat the same task or perform another task. As predicted, actual enjoyment of the task predicted the choice of the task among European American but not among Asian American participants (see Heine et al., 2001, for similar results). To summarize the results, European Americans who enjoyed the anagram (basketball) chose the anagram (basketball) at time 2, whereas European Americans who did not enjoy the anagram (basketball) chose the word fragment task (darts game) at time 2. Among Asian American participants, we did not find such a straightforward relation between actual enjoyment and subsequent choice. Together, these findings suggest that PA has a more direct consequence for choice and decision making for European Americans than for Asian Americans. It is interesting to note, then, that European American findings are perfectly in line with the influential affect-as-information theory (Schwarz & Clore, 1988), which assumes that PA is an internal signal that things are going well and no change is required, whereas NA is a signal that things are not going well and some change is required. In contrast, Asian American findings are not consistent with the affect-as-information theory.

If PA signals that no change is required, then when feeling PA, individuals should treat the current level of life satisfaction as a good indicator for future life. In contrast, if NA signals that a change is required, then when feeling NA, people should not treat the current level of life satisfaction as a good indicator of their future life. Oishi, Wyer, and Colcombe (2000) examined this relation. In the first two studies, Oishi et al. showed that, as predicted by the affect-as-information theory (Schwarz & Clore, 1988), current life satisfaction predicted the likelihood estimates of future positive life events for European Americans, when positive mood was induced. In contrast, life satisfaction predicted future life events when negative mood was induced among Asian Americans, as if negative moods signaled that the current state is a good estimate of the future. In the final study, Oishi et al. replicated the first two studies using a subliminal priming procedure. Specifically, life satisfaction predicted the likelihood estimates of positive life events happening to participants in the future, when in a positive mood subliminally primed with the concepts associated with individualism (e.g., self, alone, freedom). In contrast, life satisfaction predicted the likelihood estimates when in a negative mood among participants primed with the concepts associated with collectivism (e.g., team, sharing, loyalty). In sum, these earlier studies provide indirect evidence that the link between happiness and important life outcomes might be more direct among European Americans than others, and that the optimal level of happiness for these life outcomes might be different across cultures. Thus, the investigation of cross-cultural similarities and differences in the consequences and optimal levels of happiness is an important future direction in subjective well-being research.

Discussion

Our analyses give rise to two broad conclusions: (1) happiness has positive benefits in diverse areas, ranging from health and longevity to job performance, income, and close relationships; and (2) the optimal levels of happiness vary across domains: the highest possible level of happiness was associated with later relationship success, whereas the second- or third-highest levels of happiness were associated with higher income, education, and civic engagement.

Consequences of happiness have been the weakest link in the nomological net of subjective well-being. Thanks to Lyubomirsky et al. (2005), the connection between happiness and important life outcomes was firmly established. However, theoretical understanding of this phenomenon is still in its infancy. There are many well-being theorists proposing the importance of motivation in happiness (Csikszentmihalyi, 1997; Emmons, 1999; Ryan & Deci, 2001; Sheldon, 2004), yet few well-being researchers have theorized happiness as a motivational factor. The consequences of happiness summarized above indicate that happiness has a motivational element, moving people to successful outcomes. However, the why and how are not yet well articulated.

In this regard, emotion theories are instructive because they have long taken into account the functional aspects of emotion. For instance, Frijda (1988) predicted a connection between each emotion state and subsequent action (e.g., fear and freezing). Schwarz and Clore (1988) postulated the evolutionary function of mood, such that positive mood signals that everything is fine, whereas negative mood signals that something is wrong. Extending these theories, Fredrickson

(2001) proposed the broaden-and-build theory: Positive emotions broaden people's momentary thought–action repertoires, which in turn serves to build their personal resources (physical and psychological), which in turn serves to maintain and increase well-being. Fredrickson's theory is an upward spiral model, in that positive emotions build attentional, cognitive, and social resources, which help generate even more positive emotions. Similar to Schwarz and Clore (1988), Carver (2003) focuses on the feedback loop in which positive emotion signals that things are going well. However, instead of continuing the thing that they have been doing, Carver argues that individuals may relax and move on to a new task when they experience positive emotions. More generally, many emotion theorists associate PA with an approach orientation and NA with an avoidance orientation (e.g., Cacioppo, Gardner, & Berntson, 1999). It is plausible, then, to assume that satisfied individuals later make more money, attain higher degrees, and have stabler romantic relationships than less satisfied individuals because of an open and outgoing attitude, and physical and social resources resulting from general happiness.

Although these theories provide a general account for the positive benefits of happiness, the effects of positive emotions are not differentiated across diverse domains. In addition, these theories so far implicitly assumed the linear relation between positive emotions and outcomes, namely, the more positive emotions, the better the outcomes are. In contrast, our findings were nonlinear in case of income, education, and political engagement. Thus, it is difficult to explain the current findings on different optimal levels of happiness purely based on the existing functional theories of emotion.

It is then important to differentiate different outcome domains. Our outcome variables could be divided into two classes: (1) achievement domains (e.g., income, education), and (2) relationship domains. Achievement domains have very clear objective criteria, either in the form of monetary value, degree, or skill levels. Improvement motivation (e.g., self-criticism, self-improvement) serves well in the achievement domains because this mindset makes clear what needs to be done to improve skills and performance. In contrast, self-complacency and positive illusions prevent one from clearly seeing one's weakness and working on them. Indeed, self-complacency and self-enhancement are *not* associated with better performance in job or academics (Baumeister, Campbell, Krueger, & Vohs, 2003). The diametric opposite of self-complacency, Tiger Woods spent long hours practicing to improve his already-amazing shot after winning his first Masters. Similarly, Larry Bird was known to have spent hours and hours after team practice improving his shooting, even though he was already one of the best shooters in the NBA. Although we have not yet examined the optimal level of happiness for health and longevity, it is likely that this optimal level is not the highest possible level of happiness. This is because health maintenance behaviors require patience and persistence, akin to achievement domains. For example,

Lance Armstrong was diagnosed with testicular cancer when he was 22 years old. His cancer was so advanced that one doctor estimated that Armstrong had a less than 3% chance of survival. With his headstrong determination, not only did he overcome cancer, but he trained hard enough to win the Tour de France, a 23-day race that covers over 2, 000 miles! If Armstrong were perfectly happy with just recovering from the cancer, he might have not even tried to run the race. With infinite desire to improve, he was able to accomplish the feat no athlete has ever achieved before: winning the Tour de France seven times in a row.

This type of perfectionism and self-improvement is often rewarded handsomely in terms of performance, income, status, and fame. The same type of motivation applied to an intimate relationship, however, does not work as well. This motivation might lead to a realization that the current partner is less than ideal, and that a better partner is somewhere out there. Indeed, in a romantic relationship, idealization of the partner is known to be associated with higher relationship satisfaction and stabler relationship (e.g., Murray, Holmes, & Griffin, 2003). In other words, positive illusion and self-enhancement motives serve well in romantic relationships, in which one might not want to pay too much attention to his or her partner's weaknesses. In the 1959 film *Some Like It Hot*, the millionaire Osgood Fielding III (played by Joe E. Brown) fell in love with Daphne (played by Jack Lemmon). In the memorable ending, Daphne confessed that she was actually a man. In response, Osgood famously said "Well, nobody's perfect!" In short, we argue that the highest possible level of happiness is associated with idealization of the partner and positive illusion about the relationship itself, which in turn results in relationship stability. In an area in which nobody can be perfect, improvement motives can be a poison.

Epilogue

We started this chapter with Ed Diener's lasting legacy in subjective well-being research. He successfully answered three key questions in the literature: "What is happiness?" "Who is happy?" and "What makes people happy?" Our investigation into two new questions (What are the consequences of happiness? What are the optimal levels of happiness?) revealed an interesting divergence between achievement and relationship domains. The divergent optimal levels of happiness for achievement and relationship domains indicate that it is generally difficult to simultaneously have an extremely high level of overall happiness, intimate relationships, *and* achievements. It is not surprising that epitomes of improvement motivation—Lance Armstrong, Martha Stewart, Tom Cruise, Michael Jordan, Donald Trump—all had marital problems, while achieving unprecedented success in their respective fields. As is the case with any rule, however, there are some exceptions. The success of Warren Buffet, Katie Couric, Bill Gates, Paul

Newman, Neil Young, and Ed Diener, among others, at work *and* love gives us hope that it is possible to have it all, if you have talent in your chosen field, are passionate about it, and can switch your motivational strategies between work and love. Of course, as Aristotle himself discovered, being lucky can't hurt either (Nussbaum, 2000).

References

Baron, R. A. (1987). Environmentally induced positive affect: Its impact on self-efficacy, task performance, negotiation, and conflict. *Journal of Applied Social Psychology, 17,* 911–926.

Baron, R. A., Rea, M. S., & Daniels, S. G. (1992). Effects of indoor lighting (illuminance and spectral distribution) on the performance of cognitive tasks and interpersonal behaviors: The potential mediating role of positive affect. *Motivation and Emotion, 16,* 1–33.

Baumeister, R. F., Campbell, J. D., Krueger, J. I., & Vohs, K. D. (2003). Does high self-esteem cause better performance, interpersonal success, happiness, or healthier lifestyles? *Psychological Science in the Public Interest, 4,* 1–44.

Berk, L. S., Tan, S. A., Fry, W. F., Napier, B. J., Lee, J. W., Hubbard, R. W., et al. (1989). Neuroendocrine and stress hormone changes during mirthful laughter. *Alternative Therapies in Health and Medicine, 7,* 62–76.

Bryant, B. K. (1983). Context of success: Affective aroused generosity. *American Educational Research Journal, 20,* 553–562.

Cacioppo, J. T., Gardner, W. L., & Berntson, G. G. (1999). The affect system has parallel and integrative processing components: Form follows function. *Journal of Personality and Social Psychology, 76,* 839–855.

Carver, C. S. (2003). Pleasure as a sign you can attend to something else: Placing positive feelings within a general model of affect. *Cognition and Emotion, 17,* 241–261.

Cohen, S., Doyle, W. J., Turner, R. B., Alper, C. M., & Skoner, D. P. (2003). Emotional style and susceptibility to the common cold. *Psychosomatic Medicine, 65,* 652–657.

Cropanzano, R., & Wright, T. A. (1999). A 5-year study of change in the relationship between well-being and job performance. *Consulting Psychology Journal: Practice and Research, 51,* 252–265.

Csikszentmihalyi, M. (1997). *Finding flow.* New York: Basic Books.

Cunningham, M. R. (1988). Does happiness mean friendliness? Induced mood and heterosexual self-disclosure. *Personality and Social Psychology Bulletin, 14,* 283–297.

Diener, E. (1984). Subjective well-being. *Psychological Bulletin, 95,* 542–575.

Diener, E., & Diener, M. (1995). Cross-cultural correlates of life satisfaction and self-esteem. *Journal of Personality and Social Psychology, 68,* 653–663.

Diener, E., Diener, M., & Diener, C. (1995). Factors predicting the subjective well-being of nations. *Journal of Personality and Social Psychology, 69,* 851–864.

Diener, E., Emmons, R. A., Larsen, R. J., & Griffin, S. (1985). The Satisfaction with Life Scale. *Journal of Personality Assessment, 49,* 71–75.

Diener, E., & Fujita, F. (1995). Resources, personal strivings, and subjective well-being: A nomothetic and idiographic approach. *Journal of Personality and Social Psychology, 68*, 926–935.

Diener, E., & Larsen, R. J. (1984). Temporal stability and cross-situational consistency of affective, behavioral, and cognitive responses. *Journal of Personality and Social Psychology, 47*, 871–883.

Diener, E., Nickerson, C., Lucas, R. E., & Sandvik, E. (2002). Dispositional affect and job outcome. *Social Indicators Research, 59*, 229–259.

Diener, E., Sandvik, E., Pavot, W., & Fujita, F. (1992). Extraversion and subjective well-being in a U.S. national probability sample. *Journal of Research in Personality, 26*, 205–215.

Diener, E., & Seligman, M. E. P. (2002). Very happy people. *Psychological Science, 13*, 81–84.

Diener, E., Suh, E. M., Lucas, R. E., & Smith, H. (1999). Subjective well-being: Three decades of progress. *Psychological Bulletin, 125*, 276–302.

Diener, E., Suh, E. M., Smith, H., & Shao, L. (1995). National differences in reported subjective well-being: Why do they occur? *Social Indicators Research, 34*, 7–32.

Eid, M., & Diener, E. (2001). Norms for experiencing emotions in different cultures: Inter- and intranational differences. *Journal of Personality and Social Psychology, 81*, 869–885.

Emmons, R. A. (1999). *The psychology of ultimate concerns.* New York: Guilford Press.

Fisher, V. E., & Marrow, A. J. (1934). Experimental study of moods. *Character and Personality, 2*, 201–209.

Flugel, J. C. (1925). A quantitative study of feeling and emotion in everyday life. *British Journal of Psychology, 9*, 318–355.

Fredrickson, B. L. (2001). The role of positive emotions in positive psychology: The broaden-and-build theory of positive emotions. *American Psychologist, 56*, 218–226.

Frijda, N. (1988). The laws of emotion. *American Psychologist, 43*, 349–358.

Hale, W. D., & Strickland, B. R. (1976). Induction of mood states and their effect on cognitive and social behaviors. *Journal of Consulting and Clinical Psychology, 44*, 155.

Harker, L., & Keltner, D. (2001). Expressions of positive emotions in women's college yearbook pictures and their relationship to personality and life outcomes across adulthood. *Journal of Personality and Social Psychology, 80*, 112–124.

Heine, S. J., Kitayama, S., Lehman, D. R., Takata, T., Ide, E., Leung, C., et al. (2001). Divergent consequence of success and failure in Japan and North America: An investigation of self-improving motivations and malleable selves. *Journal of Personality and Social Psychology, 81*, 599–615.

Hersey, R. B. (1932). *Workers' emotions in shop and home: A study of individual workers from the psychological and physiological standpoint.* Philadelphia: University of Pennsylvania Press.

Hubert, W., & de Jong-Meyer, R. (1991). Autonomic, neuroendocrine, and subjective responses to emotion-inducing film stimuli. *International Journal of Psychophysiology, 11*, 131–140.

Isen, A. M., & Levin, P. F. (1972). The effect of mood on feeling good on helping: Cookies and kindness. *Journal of Personality and Social Psychology, 21*, 384–388.

Janoff-Bulman, R., & Marshall, G. (1982). Mortality, well-being, and control: A study of a population of institutionalized aged. *Personality and Social Psychology Bulletin, 8,* 691–698.

Johnson, W. B. (1937). Euphoric and depressed moods in normal subjects: I and II. *Character and Personality, 6,* 79–98.

Lucas, R. E., Clark, A. E., Georgellis, Y., & Diener, E. (2003). Reexamining adaptation and the set point model of happiness: Reactions to changes in marital status. *Journal of Personality and Social Psychology, 84,* 527–539.

Lyubomirsky, S., King, L., & Diener, E. (2005). The benefits of frequent positive affect: Does happiness lead to success? *Psychological Bulletin, 131,* 803–855.

Magnus, K., Diener, E., Fujita, F., & Pavot, W. (1993). Extraversion and neuroticism as predictors of objective life events: A longitudinal analysis. *Journal of Personality and Social Psychology, 65,* 1046–1053.

Marks, G. N., & Fleming, N. (1999). Influences and consequences of well-being among Australian young people: 1980–1995. *Social Indicators Research, 46,* 301–323.

Middleton, R. A., & Byrd, E. K. (1996). Psychosocial factors and hospital readmission status of older persons with cardiovascular disease. *Journal of Applied Rehabilitation Counseling, 27,* 3–10.

Murray, H. A., & Kluckhohn, C. (1948). Outline of a conception of personality. In C. Kluckhohn & H. A. Murray (Eds.), *Personality in nature, society, and culture* (pp. 3–32). New York: Knopf.

Murray, S. L., Holmes, J. G., & Griffin, D. W. (2003). Reflections on the self-fulfilling effects of positive illusions. *Psychological Inquiry, 14,* 289–295.

Myers, D. G., & Diener, E. (1995). Who is happy? *Psychological Science, 6,* 10–19.

Nussbaum, M. C. (2000). *The fragility of goodness: Luck and ethics in Greek tragedy and philosophy.* Cambridge, UK: Cambridge University Press.

Oishi, S., & Diener, E. (2003). Culture and well-being: The cycle of action, evaluation and decision. *Personality and Social Psychology Bulletin, 29,* 939–949.

Oishi, S., Diener, E., & Lucas, R. E. (in press). The optimum level of well-being: Can people be too happy? *Perspectives on Psychological Science.*

Oishi, S., Diener, E., Suh, E., & Lucas, R. E. (1999). Value as a moderator in subjective well-being. *Journal of Personality, 67,* 157–184.

Oishi, S., Wyer, R. S., Jr., & Colcombe, S. (2000). Cultural variation in the use of current life satisfaction to predict the future. *Journal of Personality and Social Psychology, 78,* 434–445.

Palmore, E., & Cleveland, W. (1976). Aging, terminal decline, and terminal drop. *Journal of Gerontology, 31,* 76–81.

Pavot, W., & Diener, E. (1993). Review of the Satisfaction with Life Scale. *Psychological Assessment, 5,* 164–172.

Pettit, J. W., Kline, J. P., Gencoz, T., Gencoz, F., & Joiner, T. E. (2001). Are happy people healthier?: The specific role of positive affect in predicting self-reported health symptoms. *Journal of Research in Personality, 35,* 521–536.

Pressman, S. D., & Cohen, S. (2005). Does positive affect influence health? *Psychological Bulletin, 131,* 925–971.

Roberts, B. W., Caspi, A., & Moffitt, T. E. (2003). Work experiences and personality development in young adulthood. *Journal of Personality and Social Psychology, 84,* 582–593.

Roberts, B. W., & Robins, R. W. (2000). Broad dispositions, broad aspirations: The intersection of personality traits and major life goals. *Personality and Social Psychology Bulletin, 26,* 1284–1296.

Ruvolo, A. P. (1998). Marital well-being and general happiness of newlywed couples: Relationships across time. *Journal of Social and Personal Relationships, 15,* 470–489.

Ryan, R. M., & Deci, E. L. (2001). On happiness and human potentials: A review of research on hedonic and eudaimonic well-being. *Annual Review of Psychology, 52,* 141–166.

Ryff, C. D., Singer, B. H., & Dienberg Love, G. (2004). Positive health: Connecting well-being with biology. *Philosophical Transactions of the Royal Society of London Series B, Biological Sciences, 359,* 1382–1394.

Scheldon, K. M. (2004). *Optimal human being: An integrated multi-level perspective.* Mahwah, NJ: Erlbaum.

Schwarz, N., & Clore, G. L. (1988). How do I feel about it? Informative functions of affective states. In K. Fiedler & J. Forgas (Eds.), *Affect, cognition, and social behavior* (pp. 44–62). Toronto: Hogrefe International.

Spanier, G. B., & Furstenberg, F. F. (1982). Remarriage after divorce: A longitudinal analysis of well-being. *Journal of Marriage and the Family, 44,* 709–720.

Staw, B. M., Sutton, R. I., & Pelled, L. H. (1994). Employee positive emotion and favorable outcomes at the workplace. *Organization Science, 5,* 51–71.

Suh, E., Diener, E., & Fujita, F. (1996). Events and subjective well-being: Only recent events matter. *Journal of Personality and Social Psychology, 70,* 1091–1102.

Sumner, L. W. (1996). *Welfare, happiness, and ethics.* New York: Oxford University Press.

Veenhoven, R. (1984). *Conditions of happiness.* Dordrecht, The Netherlands: Reidel.

Veenhoven, R. (1988). The utility of happiness. *Social Indicators Research, 20,* 333–354.

Veenhoven, R. (1989). *How harmful is happiness?: Consequences of enjoying life or not.* Rotterdam, The Netherlands: Universitaire Pers Roterdam.

Watson, D. (2000). *Mood and temperament.* New York: Guilford Press.

Wessman, A. E., & Ricks, D. T. (1966). *Mood and personality.* New York: Holt, Rinehart, & Winston.

Wilson, W. (1967). Correlates of avowed happiness. *Psychological Bulletin, 67,* 294–306.

Wright, R. J., Rodriguez, M., & Cohen, S. (1998). Review of psychosocial stress and asthma: An integrated biopsychosocial approach. *Thorax, 53,* 1066–1074.

Wright, T. A., & Staw, B. M. (1999). Affect and favorable work outcomes: Two longitudinal tests of the happy–productive worker thesis. *Journal of Organizational Behavior, 20,* 1–23.

15

Material Wealth and Subjective Well-Being

ROBERT M. BISWAS-DIENER

Throughout history the question of whether money buys happiness has captured the collective imagination. The question is a fascinating one, in part because it is so universally relevant. So important is this issue that philosophers, religious leaders, academics, and laypeople alike have all contributed opinions. In the Book of Deuteronomy, for example, Moses emphasizes the desirability of material prosperity when he reviews the divine covenant with the Hebrew people, saying, "The Lord will give you abounding prosperity in the issue of your womb, the offspring of your cattle, and the produce of your soil" (Torah, p. 590). Jesus preached on the issue, saying that it is easier for a "camel to go through the eye of a needle than for a rich man to enter into the kingdom of God" (King James Bible, p. 869). More recently, in the social landscape of modern capitalism, the notion of acquiring material wealth is often regarded as an appropriate and desirable personal goal.

In what may be the best-known modern theory of material wealth and happiness, Maslow (1954) proposed that basic physical needs, such as having adequate shelter and access to nutritious food, must be satisfied before lasting psychological fulfillment can be achieved. Indeed, Maslow's theory highlights several intriguing issues surrounding the relation between material wealth and happiness. First, Maslow's theory begs the question, how basic are basic needs?

Will a shanty with a tin roof suffice for shelter, or do people need larger, more durable homes? Do so-called luxury items contribute nothing to happiness, or might Maslow have overlooked their possible importance? Second, although Maslow's theory has intuitive appeal when applied to individuals, it does not speak directly to the well-being of whole societies. For instance, are quality hospitals—arguably products of material wealth at the societal level—basic needs?

Psychologists and other social science researchers have attended to questions such as these for half a century. In early work on subjective well-being (a term I use interchangeably with *happiness* in this chapter) researchers were interested in broad correlates of happiness, including wealth (e.g., Wilson, 1967). The topic of material wealth as it relates to happiness has been the subject of economic theories (e.g., Sen, 1999), sociological theories (e.g., Veenhoven, 1991), and psychological theories (e.g., Ryff, 1989). Subjective well-being researchers, in particular, have attended to the nuances of this topic (e.g., Diener & Biswas-Diener, 2002). A link between subjective well-being and material wealth is plausible for several reasons. Because subjective well-being contains emotional components such as joy and pride, the hedonic appeal of physical pleasures associated with wealth could contribute to increased happiness. People with greater access to high-quality food, stimulating recreational opportunities, and comfortable home furnishings, for instance, might benefit from the positive rewards that their material prosperity brings. In addition, subjective well-being also contains a cognitive (life satisfaction) component, which could be enhanced through the sense of autonomy, purpose, and progress toward personally valued goals that additional material resources can make possible (Diener, 1984).

Given the amount of scientific attention that has been given to the issue of money and happiness, it is interesting to consider what researchers have found. In a review of the literature on income and subjective well-being Diener and Biswas-Diener (2002) report finding a trend toward a significant, yet modest, correlation between these two variables. The authors reported on surveys from a variety of demographic groups and nations showing significant positive correlations between income and life satisfaction. This finding is consistent with a broad trend in data from nationally representative samples showing a positive correlation between income and happiness (e.g., Cummins, 2002; Diener & Oishi, 2000). Thus, it appears that income, as a means of assessing material wealth, contributes to subjective well-being, but is, perhaps, not the most important factor in the attainment of happiness.

There is also some agreement among scholars in this field about the curvilinear nature of the relation between income and subjective well-being. In many cases, researchers have found that income correlates with subjective well-being more strongly at the lower incomes levels, and that the strength of the relationship between these two variables diminishes as income raises (e.g., Cummins, 2002; Diener & Oishi, 2000; Inglehart, 1997; Diener, Sandvik, Seidlitz, &

Diener, 1993). This diminishing marginal utility, in which the psychological effects of additional income decrease at the higher economic levels, is consistent with Maslow's (1954) basic needs theory. It should be noted, however, that there is some uncertainty about the extent to which diminishing marginal utility of income exists (e.g., Easterlin, 2005; Oswald, 2005).

Despite the preponderance of evidence pointing to the conclusion that income correlates with subjective well-being, scholarly opinions vary about the precise nature of the relation between these two variables. For instance, work by Wachtel (1989) and Schor (1999) suggests that affluence is associated with certain psychological downsides, including, but not limited to, increased feelings of anxiety and higher rates of divorce. Similarly, Kasser (2003, 2004) argues that the attitudes of materialism that can accompany increasing wealth, both at the individual and national level, can be toxic to personal psychological health and environmental sustainability.

In this chapter I examine the relation of material wealth and subjective well-being based on a trajectory of material accumulation. At the beginning of this developmental course is the acquisition of Maslow's basic needs, in which research and theory address considerations of the most fundamental kind, such as food and housing. I term this level the "simple life scenario" and consider results from studies of people living a materially simple lifestyle. Next, I review research from groups living a more affluent lifestyle, which I term the "abundance scenario." Finally, I discuss major theories explaining the relation between material wealth and subjective well-being.

The question of whether money, or material wealth in any form, buys happiness is more than a topic of idle curiosity or academic interest. The answer to this question has direct implications for policy. If increased wealth, whether at the individual or national level, translates to higher subjective well-being, than research and theory on this topic are important resources to direct the development of social programs, social policies, and psychological interventions. On the other hand, to the extent that material wealth is toxic to personal fulfillment or environmental sustainability, these cautions would suggest important policy considerations and recommendations for consumer behaviors as well.

Basic Needs and the Simple Life Scenario

In his classic theory Maslow (1954) proposed a hierarchy of needs that rested on the foundation of meeting basic requirements for the physical nourishing of life. Maslow hypothesized that it would be difficult to develop "higher" social and psychological pursuits, such as altruism, meaning, and aesthetic appreciation, if one were contending daily with starvation or similar threats to physical health. Maslow's theory has, in fact, received support from research on income and subjective well-being. Large international studies show that people living in nations with relatively low per capita income report lower happiness, on average, than do their counterparts in wealthier countries, even controlling for purchasing power and cost of living (e.g., Diener & Biswas-Diener, 2002; Diener & Oishi, 2000; Diener, Suh, Lucas, & Smith, 1999; Diener & Diener, 1995).

And yet, even among nonindustrialized groups living a traditional lifestyle we see the development of art, ritual, sophisticated social organization, and meaningful personal bonds. Ethnographies of tribal groups living a technologically primitive lifestyle show that even at the hunter–gatherer level of existence basic needs appear to be met sufficiently to allow for "higher-order" social and psychological development (e.g., Turnbull, 1987; Chagnon, 1972; Malinowski, 1922/1984). How, then, are we to identify basic needs and learn about the role they play in happiness? One way for us to evaluate the merits of Maslow's theory is to identify groups who do not sufficiently meet their basic needs. Of those unfortunate people living in extreme poverty, the most visible are the homeless.

Poverty is a problem that affects all societies, and homelessness is pandemic. Studies have shown that homelessness is associated with strained family relationships (Nyamathi, Wenzel, Keenan, Leake, & Gelberg, 1999), higher exposure to trauma (Buhrich, Hodder, & Teesson, 2000), increased anger and depression (Marshall, Burnam, Koegel, Sullivan, & Benjamin, 1996), and the negative psychological impact of social stigma (Lankenau, 1999). Perhaps because of the many social and psychological ills associated with homelessness, most of the research in this area has focused on psychopathology, social discord, and health problems. Only a handful of studies have examined the subjective well-being of the homeless.

In a study looking at the relative strengths and resources of extremely poor and homeless individuals in Calcutta, India, Biswas-Diener and Diener (2001) found unexpectedly high levels of life satisfaction. People from all three groups studied—slum dwellers (those in impoverished neighborhoods), pavement dwellers (homeless), and sex workers (prostitutes)—reported, on average, positive levels of satisfaction regarding variables associated with basic needs such as food, housing, and income. Despite this surprising trend, the authors found significantly lower levels of material satisfaction, as well as the overall life satisfaction, between the pavement dwellers and the other two groups. Because the pavement dwellers live at the basic needs level—most own only a handful of possessions, are forced to beg or forage for food, and are dramatically affected by the weather due to inadequate housing—this study lends support to Maslow's basic needs theory.

In a follow-up study comparing another homeless sample in India with two such groups in the United States, Biswas-Diener and Diener (2006) found that homelessness was associated with relatively low levels of subjective well-being. Although homeless individuals in Calcutta reported positive levels of overall life satisfaction, their counterparts in Fresno (California) and Portland (Oregon) reported negative satisfaction with life. Members of all three groups reported negative satisfaction with material resources, income, housing, and health. When compared with the relatively high scores of university students and other more affluent individuals from other studies using the same measures, this finding appears to lend further support to Maslow's hypothesis. Interestingly, however, satisfaction with food was high for members of all three groups, raising questions about how this variable is subjectively evaluated.

Taken together, the two studies of the subjective well-being of the homeless described above (as well as the larger body of research on the negative psychological impact of homelessness) appear to support Maslow's conclusions regarding basic needs, at the level of extreme deprivation. Inadequate food, insecure income, and substandard shelter appear to have a deleterious effect on subjective well-being. Consistent with Maslow's theory, physical and health problems associated with poor living conditions likely factor into the equation, but so might social concerns such as the stigma attached to poverty (Biswas-Diener & Diener, 2001) and estranged family relationships (Diener & Seligman, 2002) common among those who are homeless.

But, what about the case of those who do not live in poverty but still engage in a lifestyle that is relatively free of material luxuries? How might their material wealth affect their happiness? For those who champion the simple life, material luxury is often seen as synonymous with environmental devastation and spiritual emptiness. But the "simple life scenario" is not only a political position that endorses the benefits of limiting material acquisitions, it is an empirical question. There is a relatively small research literature on individuals living above the poverty level but still maintaining a materially simple lifestyle, perhaps because of methodological difficulties associated with studying these groups. Groups representing the "simple life scenario" include tribal groups utilizing preindustrial technologies, religious orders that eschew materialism for spiritual reasons, and individuals who voluntarily simplify their lives.

In one such study Yamamoto (2005) conducted 480 interviews with tribal Amazonians, rural people, and urban folk living in Peru. He asked them to rate the importance of various types of goals, such as those related to achievement, basic physical needs, and social harmony. Yamamoto found sharing and support were valued in preindustrial groups, as opposed to an emphasis on accumulation of material goods that he found in urban areas. These findings might indicate that the relatively modest material resources of the tribal Amazonians influence their overall happiness by structuring their personal aspirations and values. Yamamoto concluded that the high goal–resource coherence found among his tribal sample leads to relatively high levels of life satisfaction. This conclusion is consistent with research by Diener and Fujita (1995), in which the relevance of resources to personal strivings predicts subjective well-being.

Research with other tribal groups living a materially simple life has shown similar results. In a study of samples from three materially simple societies Biswas-Diener, Vitterso, and Diener (2005) found that, on average, members of each group were happy. The researchers collected data from diverse cultural and geographic samples, including tribal Maasai (Kenya) living a traditional pastoralist lifestyle, Inughuit people (Greenland) who still employ traditional hunting practices, and Amish people (United States), who eschew the use of many modern conveniences and technologies. Members of each group reported positive levels of life satisfaction, as well as positive levels of satisfaction with domains related to basic needs such as housing, food, income, and health. Thus, those who live a simple life appear, at least in these specific but diverse instances, to be satisfied not only with their material needs but with their lives, in general. These findings are consistent with other research on the Amish, such as mean scores for a single life satisfaction item reported by Diener and Seligman (2004), in which the Amish were found to be in the positive range.

One demographic subset of the simple life scenario is comprised of individuals who voluntarily choose a materially simple lifestyle, usually for spiritual or ecological reasons. Among those who engage in the simple life for environmental sustainability there is relatively little data. In one such study, however, Jacob and Brinkerhoff (1999) assessed a group of 565 individuals who moved away from cities to practice "environmentally friendly" lifestyles. Although these individuals reported high levels of satisfaction on many domains, zero-order correlations between income and life satisfaction were nonsignificant, suggesting that mediating factors such as living "mindfully" or living a values-congruent lifestyle might account for their relatively high psychological quality of life. In another study, Brown and Kasser (2005) evaluated hundreds of people engaged in "voluntary simplicity" (VS) against a matched sample of nonsimplicity Americans. The VS participants consumed less and repaired and reused more of their material possessions than their sample counterparts. The researchers found that the VS sample reported significantly higher life satisfaction as well as more positive affect balance.

In the end, the simple life scenario suggests that material luxuries are not a necessary precondition for happiness. The high levels of happiness found among diverse groups living a materially simple lifestyle could be due to a variety of reasons, ranging from a feeling of living in accord with one's own values to benefiting from high resource–aspiration consonance to a slower pace of life. The crucial issue, where the simple life scenario is concerned, is the degree of simplicity. At some point a threshold is reached at which material simplicity is better described as deprivation, as in the case of homeless people. Although this threshold is not clearly defined and likely depends on a number of complicated factors (see Diener & Biswas-Diener, 2002, for further discussion), research on homelessness appears to converge on the conclusion that material deprivation generally takes a heavy psychological toll on people.

The Abundance Scenario

Beyond living a simple life, is there happiness to be gained through the additional acquisition and consumption of material goods? Do luxuries such as air conditioning and opportunities to travel for leisure lead to more happiness? In fact, higher income has been shown to be related to a variety of widely valued variables, including increased longevity (Wilkenson, 1996), better health (Salovey, Rothman, Detweiler, & Steward, 2000), and greater life satisfaction (Diener, Horowitz, & Emmons, 1985). Greater income at individual and societal levels could, at least theoretically, translate to greater feelings of security, autonomy, civil peace, access to enjoyable leisure activities, and other benefits that enhance happiness. Studies investigating the subjective well-being of relatively affluent individuals, and those from wealthy nations, can help us understand the link between material wealth and subjective well-being above the level of basic needs or the simple life.

At the individual level of analysis there is research to support the idea that increased material wealth is associated with higher subjective well-being, even at levels well above basic needs. In a unique study, Diener and colleagues (1985) assessed the relative happiness of the very wealthy. In this study, the researchers received reports of happiness from 49 individuals from the Forbes list of the wealthiest Americans (those with a net worth of $125 million [U.S. dollars] or more), and compared these scores against a matched sample from the same geographic areas. The rich respondents in the study reported significantly higher life satisfaction, being happier a greater percentage of the time, and lower feelings of NA. The factors that account for the high happiness of the super-rich are unclear but may be explained by the status, privilege, or feelings of security and power associated with extreme wealth. In addition, personality factors may play a role, such that the highly selected individuals in this study were predisposed to happiness.

Data from a variety of sources further support the idea that living a materially abundant life is, indeed, associated with increased happiness. In a review of data from the World Values Survey II, Diener and Biswas-Diener (2002) found within-nation differences in happiness between high-income individuals (typically representing "middle-class" and "upper-middle-class" people) and their low-income counterparts. Similarly, Diener and Oishi (2000), again in an analysis of data from the World Values Survey II, found small but significant within-nation differences between the top and penultimate income groups, even controlling for satisfaction differences between nations and for financial satisfaction. This finding suggests that, although income explains a relatively small portion of the overall variance in most subjective well-being, the relation between these two variables is not confined to the lowest economic levels.

Further evidence for the happiness benefits of the abundant life can be seen in comparisons of analyses of international data. Data from international surveys show that respondents from richer countries generally score higher on measures of subjective well-being than do their counterparts in poor countries. In a survey of 55 countries, for example, Diener, Diener, and Diener (1995) found a general trend in which respondents from more affluent nations reported higher subjective well-being. In their analysis, for instance, respondents from countries such as Iceland, the United States, and Canada showed higher levels of happiness compared to samples from nations such as China, India, and Cameroon, which showed somewhat negative levels of happiness. Interestingly, data suggest that even poor people living in rich countries fare better than their counterparts in poor countries (Diener & Biswas-Diener, 2002), suggesting that these individuals might benefit from the material wealth of the larger society in the form of high-quality infrastructure, civil peace, or social welfare benefits. This finding is consistent with research on national wealth by Diener and Diener (1995), who investigated indices of quality of life such as social justice, happiness, homicide and suicide rates, income equality, and Nobel prizes per capita, and found that national wealth correlated significantly with 26 of 32 outcome measures. In his "livability theories" Veenhoven (1995) suggests that a large amount of societal variance in subjective well-being can be attributed to differences in objective conditions such as education nutrition, and equality, which are often related to national wealth. Table 15.1 summarizes the life satisfaction ratings across the material spectrum.

It appears that Maslow (1954) was correct in that needs, at their most basic, must be fulfilled before people can prosper psychologically. Research on the deleterious effects of severe poverty helps confirm this idea (e.g., Biswas-Diener &

TABLE 15.1. Life Satisfaction across the Material Spectrum

Group	Score
Forbes richest Americans	5.8
Traditional Maasai	5.4
Amish (Pennsylvania)	5.1
Illinois college students	4.7
Calcutta slum dwellers	4.4
Uganda college students	3.2
Calcutta homeless	3.2
California homeless	2.8

Note. Scores shown are on a 1–7 scale, where 4 is neutral. Scores are based on an average of the five items on the Satisfaction with Life Scale, and a single satisfaction item for the Forbes sample. Adapted from Diener and Biswas-Diener (2005). Copyright 2005 by Ed Diener and Robert Biswas-Diener. Adapted by permission.

Diener, 2006). Research from people living the simple life, however, suggests that the threshold for what constitutes "basic" may be quite low (e.g., Brown & Kasser, 2005). Studies of the subjective well-being of preindustrial tribal groups, for instance, show that humans can flourish emotionally, even at the materially simple nomadic pastoral level (e.g., Biswas-Diener et al., 2005). It may be that social and other non-material needs are more basic than Maslow thought and that, together, material, social, and autonomy needs form a constellation of universal basic needs (Sheldon, Elliot, Kim, & Kasser, 2001). In addition, the fact that income and subjective well-being are correlated even at higher income levels suggests that basic needs theory, in itself, is inadequate to explain individual and societal differences in happiness.

Alternative Explanatory Theories

Material wealth, often operationalized in research as income, correlates significantly and positively with subjective well-being. Even above the materially simple life, income appears to correlate with subjective well-being, although the size of the relationship diminishes some as wealth increases. Certainly, the meeting of basic physical needs cannot account for the variability found in happiness at higher income levels. Several accounts have been proposed to explain the relation between material wealth and subjective well-being, and I discuss two that have received substantial attention in the research literature: (1) goals and values, and (2) relative standards.

Goals and Values

Goals have been shown to be personally important to individuals and an important contributing factor in happiness (Emmons, 1986, 1999). To the extent that material wealth is a resource that can be used in the service of pursuing goals, it makes sense—at least theoretically—that goal theory might explain some of the relation between income and subjective well-being, even at the higher income levels. Research by Diener and Fujita (1995) illustrates that goals and personal resources (including material wealth) must be consonant to result in happiness. This finding suggests that certain goals, such as those that are too lofty materially, may actually be counterproductive to happiness.

Emmons (1999) proposed that goals are the behavioral units by which we enact and measure our personal values. Research shows that not all values contribute equally well to personal fulfillment. Although research supports the conclusion that income is positively associated with subjective well-being, it is less clear that desiring wealth contributes to personal happiness. Studies on materialism—that is, on the value an individual places on accumulating income and wealth—suggest that actively wanting money might actually be toxic to happiness. Research by Solberg, Diener, and Robinson (2004), for instance, suggests that materialism is negatively correlated with measures of subjective well-being, and that people who value money above other pursuits, such as love, are generally less satisfied with their lives. This finding is consistent with theory by Kasser (in press) that thrifty behaviors may be related to higher subjective well-being, especially when they are consonant with personal values. Other explanations exist as well, such as the possibility that those who highly value material acquisition also undervalue social relations or other aspects of life that contribute to subjective well-being (Van Boven, 2005).

Another way to examine the role of materialism, as it relates to subjective well-being, is to consider the ways in which people spend their money and how this behavior affects them psychologically. Van Boven and Gilovich (2003) conducted a set of studies in which they investigated the way in which people spent money and evaluated the happiness produced by various types of purchases. In their studies, the researchers distinguished between experiential purchases aimed at gaining life experience, such as a family vacation, and material purchases aimed at acquiring a physical object, such as a new automobile. Across three studies, using large samples and multiple methods, the researchers were able to replicate findings suggesting that experiential purchases contributed to happiness more than did material purchases, in part, because experience is more open to personal (and positive) interpretation.

Thus, although having material wealth appears to be related to subjective well-being, especially at the lower economic levels, actually wanting wealth seems to work counter to happiness. Excessive materialism is associated with lower subjective well-being, and the acquisition of material objects generally does not create lasting happiness (Kasser, 2003). It may be that materialists have a tendency to overlook other important aspects of life or that adaptation (discussed below) works against them in their pursuit of happiness.

Relative Standards

Relative standards is the term given to models that are based on the idea that people make comparison judgments and consult other internal standards for evaluating their subjective well-being (Diener & Lucas, 2000). These standards may include comparisons with others (Festinger, 1954), comparisons with past performance or future expectations (Michalos, 1985), and can be made upward or downward (Helgeson & Taylor, 1993). Relative standards have been hypothesized to influence income satisfaction (Easterlin, 1974) as well as comparisons with prior financial status (Parducci, 1995), and they have been found to affect job satisfaction (Clark & Oswald, 1996)—all of which are variables that moderate subjective well-being (Diener & Biswas-Diener, 2002). Similarly, Clark (1999) found that unemployed people who live in areas of high unemployment are more satisfied than their peers who live in more job-secure areas.

As the case of unemployment illustrates, income is generally not static, and changes in material wealth can be associated with various evaluations of relative standards. Parducci (1995) suggested that adaptation to new material circumstances may play an important role in how people make subjective evaluations of the quality of their lives. Over time natural psychological adaptation to income change may heavily influence satisfaction judgments and, in turn, subjective well-being. There is a large research literature on the homeostatic nature of emotion, in general, and subjective well-being, in particular (e.g., Lucas, in press; Heady & Wearing, 1992). According to scholars, humans (on average) have an evolutionarily determined relatively narrow, mildly positive emotional setpoint, wherein the positivity facilitates approach behaviors necessary for individual and societal functioning (Ito & Cacioppo, 1999; Fredrickson, 2001). As people interact with the environment, various pleasant and unpleasant circumstances raise and lower moods from the baseline; but then people tend to adapt back to their personal setpoint (for a more in-depth discussion, see Frederick & Lowenstein, 1999).

The process of psychological adaptation has particular bearing on the case of material wealth and subjective well-being. Brickman and Campbell (1971) proposed the idea of a "hedonic treadmill," in which individuals adjust to new circumstances and are required to increase their resources, aspirations, and opportunities for positive hedonic experiences in order to maintain an inflated level of subjective well-being. In an early study on this topic, Brickman, Coates, and Janoff-Bulman (1978) reported that individuals who won large sums of money in lotteries experienced a spike in happiness but adapted back to "normal" levels of happiness over time. This finding has been replicated in later studies showing that, although people might derive initial satisfaction from a pay raise (Parducci, 1995) or new purchase (Van Boven & Gilovich, 2003), the emotional effects are either small or short-lived.

Further support for and explanation of this position is provided by Easterlin's (1974) research. In analyses of international income data, Easterlin showed that rapid economic growth at the national level is not associated with similar gains in happiness. Other researchers have produced similar findings (e.g., Diener & Oishi, 2000; Oswald, 1997; Duncan, 1975). This so-called "Easterlin paradox" is explained, in part, by the increases in personal aspirations that normally accompany increased material wealth that occurs over the lifespan (Easterlin, 2002). The concept of adaptation in the context of Easterlin's theory may partly explain why highly materialistic goals do not typically translate to increased happiness.

Relative standards likely play an important role in the relationship between material wealth and subjective well-being. Economic status, at both the individual and societal levels, is subject to change, and change affects how people evaluate not only their financial satisfaction but their happiness in general. Further, natural psychological adaptation appears to influence how people make subjective evaluations of their objective life circumstances and overall subjective well-being.

Conclusion

The overall picture of the relation between material wealth and subjective well-being is a complex one. Research with a wide range of groups and large international samples points to the conclusion that material wealth correlates modestly and positively with subjective well-being. Further, researchers tend to agree that the nature of this correlation is curvilinear, such that money appears to correlate with subjective well-being more strongly at the lower economic levels. This set of findings offers support for basic needs theory and suggests that attention to issues of poverty and geographic displacement are important for improving the subjective well-being of the extremely poor. Preliminary research also shows that social and other psychological needs may be as "basic" as physical needs (e.g., Biswas-Diener & Diener, 2001), and Sheldon and colleagues suggest that a reexamination of the primacy of physical needs is in order (Sheldon et al., 2001). Further research is needed to determine both the threshold for basic physical needs and the ways in which social and personal needs interact with physical needs to enhance subjective well-being.

Although there appear to be diminishing returns for subjective well-being at the higher economic levels, researchers still report significant correlations between income and subjective well-being among relatively high wage earners, as well as between relatively affluent nations (e.g., Diener & Oishi, 2000). These findings suggest that explanations beyond those offered by basic needs theories are required to better understand this phenomenon. Using income as a resource to fulfill personal strivings is one such explanation (see Emmons, 1999, for further discussion of this issue). Additional income may also translate to greater feelings of autonomy and opportunities for mastery (Ryff, 1989). According to Cummins (2002), higher income allows individual increased control of their environments and helps buffer them from unpleasant events. Other explanations for societal differences in subjective well-being are also possible, including cultural differences in norms for emotions (see Kitiyama & Markus, 1994, for a more in-depth discussion of these issues).

Interestingly, although *having* material wealth appears to be related to happiness, *strongly desiring* wealth may be toxic to it. A growing body of research shows that attitudes of excessive materialism are associated with lower levels of subjective well-being, even among those who are relatively affluent. The reasons for this are not entirely clear but may be related to hedonic adaptation (Lucas, Clark, Georgellis, & Diener, 2004) or the ways in which people make subjective appraisals (Van Boven, 2005). Further research is needed to explore the relation between materialism, material and income satisfaction, and subjective well-being.

In the end, income and happiness are linked, although this relation is small in comparison to other factors that contribute to subjective well-being (see other chapters, this volume, for discussion of those factors). Material wealth appears to be most important for the subjective well-being of those living in impoverished conditions, although the threshold for these circumstances is not well-established. Interestingly, income and subjective well-being are correlated, albeit modestly, even at higher economic levels. Goals theory, relative standards models, and cultural factors all likely play a role in explaining national differences in subjective well-being, even those between relatively affluent societies. Although significant, the relative weakness of this relation is potentially instructive for individuals living in more affluent societies, because it cautions against putting too much stock in material aspirations.

References

Biswas-Diener, R., & Diener, E. (2001). Making the best of a bad situation: Satisfaction in the slums of Calcutta. *Social Indicators Research, 55*, 329–352.

Biswas-Diener, R., & Diener, E. (2006). Subjective well-being of the homeless, and related lessons for happiness. *Social Indicators Research, 76*, 185–205.

Biswas-Diener, R., Vitterso, J., & Diener, E. (2005). Most people are pretty happy, but there is cultural variation: The Inughuit, the Amish, and the Maasai. *Journal of Happiness Studies, 6*, 205–226.

Brickman, P., & Campbell, D. T. (1971). Hedonic relativism and planning the good society. In M. H. Appley (Ed.), *Adaptation level theory: A symposium* (pp. 287–304). New York: Academic Press.

Brickman, P., Coates, D., & Janoff-Bulman, R. (1978). Lottery winners and accident victims: Is happiness relative? *Journal of Personality and Social Psychology, 36*, 917–927.

Brown, K. W., & Kasser, T. (2005). Are psychological and ecological well-being compatible? The role of values, mindfulness, and lifestyle. *Social Indicators Research, 74*, 349–368.

Buhrich, N., Hodder, T., & Teesson, M. (2000). Lifetime prevalence of trauma among homeless people in Sydney. *Australian and New Zealand Journal of Psychiatry, 34*, 963–966.

Clark, A. E. (1999). Are wages habit forming? Evidence from micro-data. *Journal of Economic Behavior and Organization, 39*, 179–200.

Clark, A. E., & Oswald, A. J. (1996). Satisfaction and comparison income. *Journal of Public Economics, 61*, 359–381.

Chagnon, N. (1972). *Yanomamo: The fierce people*. New York: Holt, Rinehart & Winston.

Cummins, R. (2002). Subjective well-being from rich and poor. In W. Glatzer (Ed.),

Rich and poor: Disparities, perceptions, concomitants (pp. 137–156). Dordrecht, The Netherlands: Kluwer.

Diener, E. (1984). Subjective well-being. *Psychological Bulletin, 95,* 542–575.

Diener, E., & Biswas-Diener, R. (2002). Will money increase subjective well-being?: A literature review and guide to needed research. *Social Indicators Research, 57,* 119–169.

Diener, E., & Biswas-Diener, R. (2005). Psychological empowerment and subjective well-being. In D. Narayan (Ed.), *Measuring empowerment: Cross-disciplinary perspectives* (pp. 125–140). Washington, DC: World Bank.

Diener, E., & Diener, C. (1995). The wealth of nations, revisited: Income and quality of life. *Social Indicators Research, 36,* 275–286.

Diener, E., Diener, M., & Diener, C. (1995). Factors predicting the subjective well-being of nations. *Journal of Personality and Social Psychology, 69,* 851–864.

Diener, E., & Fujita, F. (1995). Resources, personal strivings, and subjective well-being: A nomothetic and idiographic approach. *Journal of Personality and Social Psychology, 68,* 926–935.

Diener, E., Horowitz, J., & Emmons, R. (1985). Happiness of the very wealthy. *Journal of Personality Assessment, 49,* 71–75.

Diener, E., & Lucas, R. E. (2000). Explaining differences in societal levels of happiness: Relative standards, need fulfillment, culture, and evaluation theory. *Journal of Happiness Studies, 1,* 41–78.

Diener, E., & Oishi, S. (2000). Money and happiness: Income and subjective well-being across nations. In E. Diener & E. M. Suh (Eds.), *Culture and subjective well-being* (pp. 185–218). Cambridge, MA: MIT Press.

Diener, E., Sandvik, E., Seidlitz, L., & Diener, M. (1993). The relationship between income and subjective well-being: Relative or absolute? *Social Indicators Research, 28,* 195–223.

Diener, E., & Seligman, M. E. P. (2002). Very happy people. *Psychological Science, 13,* 81–84.

Diener, E., & Seligman, M. E. P. (2004). Beyond money: Toward an economy of well-being. *Psychological Science in the Public Interest, 5,* 1–31.

Diener, E., Suh, E. M., Lucas, R. E., & Smith, H. E. (1999). Subjective well-being: Three decades of progress. *Psychological Bulletin, 125,* 276–302.

Duncan, O. (1975). Does money buy satisfaction? *Social Indicators Research, 2,* 267–274.

Easterlin, R. A. (1974). Does economic growth improve the human lot? In P. A. David & M. W. Reder (Eds.), *Nations and households in economic growth: Essays in honor of Moses Abramovitz.* New York: Academic Press.

Easterlin, R. A. (2002). The income–happiness relationship. In W. Glatzer (Ed.), *Rich and poor: Disparities, perceptions, concomitants* (pp. 157–175). Dordrecht, The Netherlands: Kluwer.

Easterlin, R. A. (2005). Diminishing marginal utility of income? Caveat Emptor. *Social Indicators Research, 70,* 243–255.

Emmons, R. A. (1986). Personal strivings: An approach to personality and subjective well-being. *Journal of Personality and Social Psychology, 51,* 1058–1068.

Emmons, R. A. (1999). *The psychology of ultimate concerns: Motivation and spirituality in personality.* New York: Guilford Press.

Festinger, L. (1954). A theory of social comparison processes. *Human Relations*, 7, 117–140.

Frederick, S., & Loewenstein, G. (1999). Hedonic adaptation. In D. Kahneman, E. Diener, & N. Schwarz (Eds.), *Well-being: The foundations of hedonic psychology* (pp. 302–329). New York: Sage.

Fredrickson, B. (2001). The role of positive emotions in positive psychology: The broaden-and-build theory of positive emotions. *American Psychologist*, 56, 218–226.

Headey, B., & Wearing, A. (1992). *Understanding happiness: A theory of subjective well-being*. Melbourne: Lonman Cheshire.

Helgeson, V., & Taylor, S. E. (1993). Social comparisons and adjustment among cardiac patients. *Journal of Applied Social Psychology*, 23, 1171–1195.

Inglehart, R. (1997). *Modernization and post-modernization*. Princeton, NJ: Princeton University Press.

Ito, T. A., & Cacioppo, J. T. (1999). The psychophysiology of utility appraisals. In D. Kahneman, E. Diener, & N. Schwartz (Eds.), *Well-being: The foundations of hedonic psychology* (pp. 470–488). New York: Sage.

Ito, T. A., Cacioppo, J. T., & Lang, P. J. (1998). Eliciting affect using the International Affective Picture System: Trajectories through evaluative space. *Personality and Social Psychology Bulletin*, 24, 855–879.

Jacob, J. C., & Brinkerhoff, M. B. (1999). Mindfulness and subjective well-being in the sustainability movement: A further elaboration of multiple discrepancies theory. *Social Indicators research*, 46, 341–368.

Kasser, T. (2003). *The high price of materialism*. Cambridge, MA: MIT Press.

Kasser, T. (2004). The good life or the goods life? Positive psychology and personal well-being in the culture of consumption. In P. A. Linley & S. Joseph (Eds.), *Positive psychology in practice* (pp. 55–67). Hoboken, NJ: Wiley.

Kasser, T. (2005). *Can thrift bring happiness?* Manuscript submitted for publication.

King James Bible. (1991). New York: Ivy Books.

Kitiyama, S., & Markus, H. (1994). *Emotion and culture: Empirical studies of mutual influence*. Washington, DC: American Psychological Association.

Lankenau, S. E. (1999). Stronger than dirt: Public humiliation and status enhancement among panhandlers. *Journal of Contemporary Ethnography*, 28, 288–318.

Lucas, R. E. (2005). Time does not heal all wounds: A longitudinal study of reaction and adaptation to divorce. *Psychological Science*, 16, 945–950.

Lucas, R. E., Clark, A. E., Georgellis, Y., & Diener, E. (2004). Unemployment alters the set point for life satisfaction. *Psychological Science*, 15, 8–13.

Malinowski, B. (1984/1922). *Argonauts of the Western Pacific*. Long Grove, IL: Waveland Press. (Original work published 1922)

Marshall, G. N., Burnam, M. A., Koegel, P., Sullivan, G., & Benjamin, B. (1996). Objective life circumstances and life satisfaction: Results from the Course of Homelessness Study. *Journal of Health and Behavior*, 37, 44–58.

Maslow, A. H. (1954). *Motivation and personality*. New York: Harper & Row.

Michalos, A. C. (1985). Multiple discrepancies theory: MDT. *Social Indicators Research*, 16, 347–413.

Nyamathi, A., Wenzel, S., Keenan, C., Leake, B., & Gelberg, L. (1999). Associations between homeless women's intimate relationships and their health and well-being. *Research in Nursing and Health*, 22, 486–495.

Oswald, A. J. (1997). Happiness and economic performance. *Economic Journal, 107*, 1815–1831.

Oswald, A. J. (2005). *On the common claim that happiness equations demonstrate the diminishing marginal utility of income.* Discussion Paper No. 1781. Institute for the Study of Labor (IZA). Bonn, Germany.

Parducci, A. (1995). *Happiness, pleasure, and judgment: The contextual theory and its applications.* Mahwah, NJ: Erlbaum.

Ryff, C. (1989). Happiness is everything, or is it? Explorations on the meaning of psychological well-being. *Journal of Personality and Social Psychology, 57*, 1069–1081.

Salovey, P., Rothman, A. J., Detweiler, J. B., & Steward, W. T. (2000). Emotional states and physical health. *American Psychologist, 55*, 110–121.

Schor, J. B. (1999). *The overspent American: Why we want what we don't need.* New York: Harper.

Sen, A. (1999). *Development as freedom.* New York: Random House.

Sheldon, K. M., Elliot, A. J., Kim, Y., & Kasser, T. (2001). What is so satisfying about satisfying events? Testing 10 candidate psychological needs. *Journal of Personality and Social Psychology, 80*, 325–339.

Solberg, E. C., Diener, E., & Robinson, M. D. (2004). Why are materialists less satisfied? In T. Kasser & A. D. Kanner (Eds.), *Psychology and consumer culture: The struggle for a good life in a materialistic world* (pp. 29–48). Washington, DC: American Psychological Association.

Torah: The Five Books of Moses (3rd ed.). (1999). New York: Jewish Publication Society.

Turnbull, C. (1987). *The forest people.* Camichael, CA: Touchstone Books.

Van Boven, L. (2005). Experientialism, materialism, and the pursuit of happiness. *Review of General Psychology, 9*, 132–142.

Van Boven, L., & Gilovich, T. (2003). To do or to have? That is the question. *Journal of Personality and Social Psychology, 85*, 1193–1202.

Veenhoven, R. (1991). Is happiness relative? *Social Indicators Research, 24*, 1–34.

Veenhoven, R. (1994). *World database of happiness: Correlates of happiness: 7,837 findings from 603 studies in 69 nations 1911–1994, Vols. 1–3.* Rotterdam, The Netherlands: Erasmus University Rotterdam.

Veenhoven, R. (1995). Test of predictions implied in three theories of happiness: The cross-national pattern of happiness. *Social Indicators Research, 34*, 33–68.

Wachtel, P. L. (1989). *The poverty of affluence: A psychological portrait of the American way of life.* Philadelphia: New Society.

Wilkenson, R. G. (1996). *Unhealthy societies: The affliction of inequality.* London: Routledge.

Wilson, W. (1967). Correlates of avowed happiness. *Psychological Bulletin, 67*, 294–306.

Yamamoto, J. (2005, October). *Happiness, adaptation, and evolution: Lessons from remote Andean and Amazonian villages.* Paper presented at the 7th International Positive Psychology Summit, Washington, DC.

16

Religion and Human Flourishing

DAVID G. MYERS

I am honored to add my tribute to the person I have often described as "the Jedi Master of happiness research." Many people, including many contributors to this volume, have made signal contributions to the emerging scientific understanding of positive well-being. But more than anyone else it was Ed Diener whose work in the mid to late 1980s first caught my eye and inspired my effort to give the field away, through *The Pursuit of Happiness* (Myers, 1992) and subsequent articles, including essays we coauthored for *Scientific American, Psychological Science,* and the *Harvard Mental Health Letter.* For me, Ed Diener exemplifies psychological science at its rigorous yet humanly significant best (not to mention his also being such an articulate, committed, and compassionate human being). How fitting that his grateful admirers should honor him with this volume.

Although I have been mostly a cub reporter and publicist for the field, not a pioneering contributor, I have paid especially close attention to explorations of wealth and well-being, and to what I report on here: explorations of religion and well-being.

Let us first acknowledge what is self-evident: Mirth and misery, mischief and morality, cruelty and compassion are exhibited by people of all faiths as well as no faith. Thus theologian Langdon Gilkey (1966) could see the human religious dimension as "not only the ground of its only hope but the source of life's deepest perversion." Religion has been associated with ecstatic joy and with what Richard Dawkins (2001) called the "insane courage" that enabled the horror of 9/11. No wonder Stephen Jay Gould (1999) could observe that much of his "fascination" with religion "lies in the stunning historical paradox that organized religion has fostered, throughout western history, both the most unspeakable horrors and the most heartrending examples of human goodness."

Let us acknowledge, second, that explorations of religion's associations with happiness, coping, health, character, and compassion, and with intolerance and aggression, have no bearing on the truth claims made by the various religions. Are spiritual people pursuing an illusion, perhaps a mental opiate, or are they apprehending a deep truth? What follows in this chapter will not answer that question. And for seekers and doubters it is truth that matters: If religious claims were known to be true, but were discomfiting, what honest person would want to disbelieve? If known to be untrue, though comforting, what honest person would want to believe?

Science can, however, help us assess the contrasting hypotheses—that religion breeds joy ("Joy is the serious business of heaven," offered C. S. Lewis in *The Four Loves*), and that religion is an "obsessional neurosis" (Freud, 1928/1964, p. 71) that breeds sexually repressed, guilt-laden unhappiness.

Religion and Individual Well-Being

In North America and Western Europe, where most of the pertinent research has been done, what are the associations of religiousness with individual and communal well-being, and with health?

Happiness

In survey after survey, actively religious people have reported markedly greater happiness and somewhat greater life satisfaction than their irreligious counterparts (Ciarrochi & Deneke, 2005; Francis & Kaldor, 2002; Francis & Katz, 2002; Hadaway, 1978; Pollner, 1989; Poloma & Pendleton, 1990; Willits & Crider, 1988; Witter, Stock, Okun, & Haring, 1985).

Some examples:

• The Gallup Organization's (1984) "Religion in America" surveys revealed that those highest in "spiritual commitment" (i.e., those who consistently agreed with statements such as "God loves me even though I may not always please him" and "My religious faith is the most important influence in my life") were twice as likely as those least spiritually committed to report being "very happy."

• National Opinion Research Center (NORC) surveys (National Opinion Research Center, 2006) reveal higher self-reported happiness among Americans who feel "extremely close to God" (40% "very happy") rather than "not very close" (21%) or "not close at all" (24%). (There are no marked differences by religion; about one in three Protestants, Catholics, and Jews has reported being very happy.)

• The NORC surveys also reveal a marked correlation between frequency of religious attendance and self-reported happiness, as shown in Figure 16.1. A comparable result was obtained by a new Pew (2006) study of happiness in the United States, with 43% of weekly or more attenders and 26% of seldom or never attenders reporting themselves "very happy."

• The Gallup Organization (Winseman, 2002) extended this association to life satisfaction with their finding that 55% of "engaged" congregational members reported being "completely satisfied with the conditions of my life," as did 25% of those "actively disengaged."

• A slew of studies in the 1980s focused on the association between religiousness and well-being among older adults (Hunsberger, 1985; Koenig, Kvale, & Ferrel, 1988; Levin & Markides, 1988; Markides, Levin, & Ray, 1987; Poloma & Pendleton, 1990; Stock, Okun, Haring, & Witter, 1983). In their meta-analysis, Okun and Stock (1987) found that the two best predictors of well-being among older persons were health and religiousness. Elderly people tend to be happier and more satisfied with life if religiously committed and engaged.

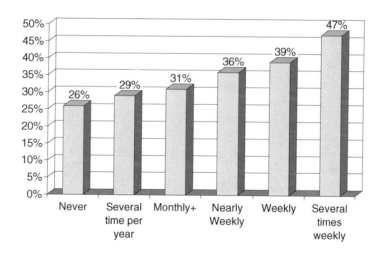

FIGURE 16.1. Percent very happy, by religious attendance (n = 42,845, NORC, 1972–2004). From National Opinion Research Center (2006).

Coping with Loss

Other studies have explored the connection between religious faith and coping with crises. Compared to religiously inactive new widows, recently wid- owed women who worship regularly have reported more joy in their lives (Harvey, Barnes, & Greenwood, 1987; McGloshen & O'Bryant, 1988; Siegel & Kuykendall, 1990). Among mothers of developmentally challenged children, those with a deep religious faith are less vulnerable to depression (Friedrich, Cohen, & Wilturner, 1988). People of faith also tend to retain or recover greater happiness after suffering divorce, unemployment, serious illness, or bereavement (Ellison, 1991; McIntosh, Silver, & Wortman, 1993). Not surprisingly, then, a meta-analysis of more than 200 studies revealed that high religiousness predicts a mildly lower risk of depression, especially for those undergoing stress (Smith, McCullough, & Poll, 2003). Actively religious North Americans have also been much less likely than those irreligious to become delinquent, abuse drugs and alcohol, and commit suicide (Batson, Schoenrade, & Ventis, 1993; Colasanto & Shriver, 1989).

Explaining the Religion–Happiness Correlation

An active religious faith hardly precludes stress or suffering (as the biblical story of Job reminds people of the Abrahamic faiths). Yet religiousness does correlate with expressed happiness, and it may help buffer stress. Seeking to explain the correlation, researchers have entertained several possibilities.

Social Support: "Where Two or Three Are Gathered"

If Martin Seligman (1988) was right that "rampant individualism" has contrib- uted to today's elevated depression rates, and if humans indeed have a fundamen- tal "need to belong" (Baumeister & Leary, 1995), then one factor is surely the social support provided by North America's estimated 350,000 faith communi- ties (Ellison, Gay, & Glass, 1989). People usually practice their religion commu- nally, through "the fellowship of kindred spirits," "the bearing of one another's burdens," "the ties of love that bind." As John Winthrop (1630/1965, p. 92) explained to one of the first groups of Puritans before disembarking to their new world, "We must delight in each other, make others' conditions our own, rejoice together, mourn together, labor and suffer together, always having before our eyes our community as members of the same body." Pennsylvania's commu- nal old-order Amish are known not only for their agrarian, pacifistic culture, but also their low rates of major depression (Egeland & Hostetter, 1983; Egeland, Hostetter, & Eshelman, 1983).

Meaning and Purpose: "Something Worth Living and Dying For"

After controlling for the greater social activity and support experienced by actively religious folk, some correlation between religiousness and well-being remains (Ellison et al., 1989). The 19th-century Polish poet Cyprian Norwid (1850) offered a clue to another possible factor: "To be what is called happy, one should have 1) something to live on, 2) something to live for, 3) something to die for. The lack of one of these results in drama. The lack of two results in tragedy."

Studies confirm that a sense of life's meaning and purpose enhances well-being, and that many people find both through their religious faith (Paloutzian, 1981; Zika & Chamberlain, 1987). Seligman (1988) has argued that a loss of meaning underlies today's high depression rate, and that finding meaning requires

> an attachment to something larger than the lonely self. To the extent that young people now find it hard to take seriously their relationship with God, to care about their relationship with the country or to be part of a large and abiding family, they will find it very difficult to find meaning in life. To put it another way, the self is a very poor site for finding meaning.

For Rabbi Harold Kushner (1987), religion satisfies "the most fundamental human need of all. That is the need to know that somehow we matter, that our lives mean something, count as something more than just a momentary blip in the universe." In the Nazi death camps Viktor Frankl (1962) similarly observed a lowered apathy and death rate among fellow inmates who retained a sense of meaning—a purpose for which to live, or even be willing to die for. Many of these, he reported, were devout Jews, who found in their faith the strength to live and to resist their oppressors.

Durable Self-Esteem: "Accepting One's Acceptance"

Baumeister, Campbell, Krueger, and Vohs (2005) have persuasively argued that self-esteem is not an all-purpose armor that protects and sustains us. Moreover, when inflated self-images are punctured, people may respond with aggression. But self-esteem does predict happiness. Paul Tillich (1988) and other theologians have argued that the religious message that God loves you—just as you are—can form a psychological basis for a durable and nondefensive self-worth. No longer is there any need to define one's self-worth by achievements, material well-being, or social approval. To find self-acceptance, said Tillich, "Do not seek for anything; do not perform anything; do not intend anything. *Simply accept the fact that you are accepted!* . . . If that happens to us, we experience grace. After such an experience we may not be better than before, and we may not believe more than before. But everything is transformed."

People who have this idea of God's "grace"—who see God as redemptively loving, accepting, and caring—not only enjoy greater self-esteem but also warmer marriages (Greeley, 1991). There is a seeming interplay between our God-concept and our self-concept.

Terror Management: An "Eternal Perspective"

Writing from a college whose symbol is the "Anchor of Hope," I cannot resist noting what our late colleague C. R. Snyder so often reminded us: of the psychological significance of hope. "Hope is itself a species of happiness, and, perhaps, the chief happiness which this world affords," wrote Samuel Johnson. Many religious worldviews not only propose answers to some of life's deepest questions, they also encourage an ultimate hope, especially when confronting what Solomon, Greenberg, and Pyszczynski (1991) call "the terror resulting from our awareness of vulnerability and death." Different faiths offer different paths, but most offer its adherents a sense that they, or something meaningful they are part of, will survive their death. Aware of the great enemies, suffering, and death, they offer a hope that in the end, the very end, "all shall be well and all shall be well and all manner of things shall be well" (Julian of Norwich). And that hope may help people cope with whatever punctuates life between now and death.

In the best of circumstances it also may provide vision and courage for the present. If human life and identity are believed to have value that make them worth preserving, and if one foresees a utopian afterlife marked by peace, justice, and love, then one has a back-to-the-present vision for life on earth. Thus Martin Luther King, Jr. could declare "I have a dream" of a future reality without oppression and suffering. With a dream worth dying for and a hope that even death could not kill it, he declared that "If physical death is the price I must pay to free my white brothers and sisters from a permanent death of the spirit, then nothing can be more redemptive" (1964, p. 10). As Alves (1972, p. 195), put it, "Hope is hearing the melody of the future. Faith is to dance to it."

Promoting Positive Virtues: Humility, Forgiveness, Gratitude, and Compassionate "Losing One's Life" for Others

Fundamentalist views often feed ingroup bias and hostility toward infidels; the circle that defines "us" also defines "them." Yet most religions also advocate many of the human virtues identified in Peterson and Seligman's (2004) *Character Strengths and Virtues* and in Snyder and Lopez's (2007) *Handbook of Positive Psychology*. And, note Peterson and Seligman, "religiousness, broadly speaking, also has been empirically linked to a range of human virtues, including forgiveness, kindness, and compassion."

Humility is intrinsic to theism, which assumes that (1) there is a God, and (2) it's not you or me. Humans, the theist assumes, are finite, fallible creatures—with dignity but not deity. Therein lies the religious foundation for open-minded skepticism of all human ideas, including one's own untested assumptions, and for free-spirited scientific inquiry. "It's all God's truth," so let's have at it. "To be humble," notes Emmons (1999), "is not to have a low opinion of oneself, it is to have an accurate opinion of oneself. It is the ability to keep one's talents and accomplishments in perspective" and to understand one's imperfections, free of both arrogance and self-deprecation. From such humility, adds Tangney (2002), comes an "openness to new ideas, contradictory information, and advice." By contrast, adds Tangney, "researchers have shown that narcissistic individuals are sensitive to interpersonal slights, quick to anger, and less inclined to forgive."

Forgiveness, or a concept close to it, is a shared feature of Judaism, Christianity, Islam, Buddhism, and Hinduism, note Peterson and Seligman (2004). Psychological researchers engaged in the recent wave of forgiveness studies agree that forgiveness is not denying, minimizing, excusing, condoning, or forgetting. Rather, forgiveness cultivates positive, prosocial responses such as compassion, which supplant hurtful and bitter thoughts, motivations, emotions, and behaviors (McCullough & Witvliet, 2002). Although not always possible or wise—as in cases of abuse or neglect—forgiveness can lead to reconciliation—the restoration of a fractured relationship. In both laboratory and clinical intervention studies, forgiveness also is associated with improved emotional and physical well-being (McCullough & Witvliet, 2002).

Gratitude "is a felt sense of wonder, thankfulness, and appreciation for life," say Emmons and Shelton (2002). And it is, they add, another "highly prized human disposition in Jewish, Christian, Muslim, Buddhist, and Hindu thought," and is found in their texts, prayers, and teachings. Indeed, an attitude of gratitude is linked with religiousness. "Those who regularly attend religious services and engage in religious activities such as prayer or reading religious material are more likely to be grateful," note Peterson and Seligman (2004).

Much as rumination prolongs and intensifies depression, so counting one's blessings enhances well-being. Students asked to keep a weekly log of things for which they are grateful come to "feel better about their lives as a whole," report Emmons and Shelton (2002). Ditto for those who, in their follow-up study, kept daily gratitude logs.

Compassion and its associated "kindness, generosity, nurturance, care . . . and altruistic love" are positive character traits that orient "the self toward the other" (Peterson & Seligman, 2004). Schwartz and Huismans (1995) explored such norms among Jews in Israel, Catholics in Spain, Calvinists in The Netherlands, the Orthodox in Greece, and Lutherans and Catholics in West Germany, and consistently observed that highly religious people tended to be less hedonistic and self-oriented: "Religions encourage people to seek meaning beyond everyday existence . . . [and] exhort people to pursue causes greater than their personal desires. The opposed orientation, self-indulgent materialism, seeks happiness in the pursuit and consumption of material goods."

In the U.S. General Social Survey data confirm that "volunteering some time to community service" is felt to be an "important obligation" by 19% of those attending religious services less than once a year and by 40% of those attending every week or more (National Opinion Research Center, 2006). And those who feel this "important obligation" are also more likely to report themselves "very happy" (39%) than are those who don't (27%).

Mother Teresa observed that "Nothing makes you happier than when you really reach out in mercy to someone who is badly hurt" (Teresa, 1968). Putting this idea to the test, Rimland (1982) asked 216 students to list the initials of the 10 people they knew best, yielding a grand list of some 2,000 names. Then he asked them to indicate whether each person seemed happy or not, and, finally, whether each seemed more selfish (devoted mostly to his or her own welfare) or unselfish (willing to be inconvenienced for others). The striking result: 70% of those judged unselfish seemed happy, and 95% of those judged selfish seemed *un*happy. Paradoxically, those who sought first their own happiness found less of it.

So, if compassionate values are espoused by religions and by religious people, and if compassionate people are happier, can we close the circle by linking religiousness with altruistic behavior?

Religion, Altruism, and Communal Well-Being

Religion has been associated with both love and hate. History offers us Bible-thumping slave owners, Ku Klux Klanners, apartheid defenders, and gay bashers. It also offers us the clergy who helped lead the abolitionist, civil rights, and anti-apartheid movements, and the founding of hospitals, orphanages, and universities worldwide. The horrors and heroes aside, what does the evidence show?

Religion and Prejudice

A mid 20th-century cluster of religion–prejudice studies painted a mixed picture (Myers, 2005): On the one hand, U.S. church members expressed more racial prejudice than nonmembers, and those with conservative Christian beliefs expressed more racial prejudice than those less conservative. For many people, religion seems a cultural habit—something not so much practiced as professed by those who adhere to their community's attitudes and traditions. On the other hand, faithful church attenders expressed less prejudice than nominal members. Moreover, clergy were more supportive of civil rights efforts than laypeople. And those for whom religion was an intrinsic end ("My religious beliefs are what really lie behind my whole approach to life") were less prejudiced than those who used religion as an extrinsic means ("A primary reason for my interest in religion is that my church is a congenial social activity"). Ergo, among the churched, the devout were consistently less prejudiced than were those who gave religion lip service. As Jonathan Swift (1727) observed, "We have just enough religion to make us hate, but not enough to make us love one another." "The role of religion is paradoxical," said Gordon Allport (1958, p. 413). "It makes prejudice and it unmakes prejudice."

Religion and Altruism

Some have enough religion to motivate self-sacrificial love, as memorably illustrated by the World War II Protestant, Catholic, and Jewish "Four Chaplains." As their *SS Dorchester* was sinking into icy waters after being torpedoed, they each gave away their life jackets and were last seen on the deck, with arms linked, saying their final prayers (fourchaplains.org). But does religion actually promote selflessness?

Volunteerism

In studies of college students and the general public, religiously committed individuals have (compared to those religiously uncommitted) reported volunteering more hours, for example, as relief workers, tutors, and campaigners for social justice (Benson et al., 1980; Hansen, Vandenberg, & Patterson, 1995; Penner, 2002). Among the 12% of Americans whom Gallup (1984) labeled "highly spiritually committed," 46% reported presently working among the infirm, the poor, or the elderly—double the 22% among those "highly uncommitted." In a follow-up Gallup survey, charitable and social service volunteering was reported by 28% of those who rated religion "not very important" in their lives and by 50% of those who rated it "very important" (Colasanto, 1989). And 37% of those attending religious services yearly or less, and 76% of those attending weekly, reported thinking at least a "fair amount" about "responsibility to the poor" (Wuthnow, 1994).

Do the religious links with volunteerism extend to other communal organizations? Putnam (2000) analyzed national survey data from 22 types of organizations, including hobby clubs, professional associations, self-help groups, and service clubs, concluding: "It was membership in religious groups that was most closely associated with other forms of civic involvement, like voting, jury service, community projects, talking with neighbors, and giving to charity" (p. 67).

Charitable Giving

The anonymous jest—"When it comes to giving, some people stop at nothing"— is seldom true of church and synagogue members. In a Gallup survey, Americans who said they never attended church or synagogue reported giving away 1.1% of their incomes (Hodgkinson, Weitzman, & Kirsch, 1990). Weekly attenders were two and a half times as generous. This 24% of the population gave 48% of all charitable contributions. The other three-quarters of Americans gave the remaining half. Follow-up 1990 and 1992 Gallup surveys and a 2001 Independent Sector survey confirmed the faith and philanthropy correlation (Hodgkinson & Weitzman, 1992; Hodgkinson et al., 1990).

An analysis by *Fortune* (Bollinger, 1997) magazine of America's top philanthropists found that most are "religious: Jewish, Mormon, Protestant, and Catholic. And most attribute their philanthropic urges at least in part to their religious backgrounds" (p. 96). According to the *Nonprofit Times* (2002), the seven financially largest, publicly supported U.S. philanthropies (YMCA, Red Cross, Catholic Charities, Salvation Army, Goodwill, United Jewish Communities, Boys and Girls Clubs) share one thing in common: They all have religiously motivated foundings. "Religion is the mother of philanthropy," observed Andrews (1953, p. 85).

Moral Behaviors

Other moral behaviors also correlate with religiousness. In a U.S. Values Survey, frequent worship attendance predicted lower scores on a dishonesty scale that assessed, for example, self-serving lies, tax cheating, and failing to report damaging a parked car (Marini, 1990). Moreover, cities with high church-going rates tend to be cities with low crime rates (Myers, 2000). After examining 40 religion–delinquency studies, Johnson and his colleagues (Johnson, Li, Larsen, & McCullough, 2000) concluded that "most delinquent acts were committed by juveniles who had low levels of religious commitment." To be sure, many are good without God, and many believers go to sleep behind bars each night. Yet even when controlling for other factors, such as socioeconomic level, neighborhood, and peer influences, kids who went to church rarely were delinquent.

Caveats

So, religion has been implicated in ingroup bias and intolerance, yet religiousness also correlates with happiness and altruistic ideals and behaviors. None of this research indicates the truth or falsity of religious claims. Even skeptics such as

Shermer (2000, 2004) acknowledge (in fact, contend) that religion exists because it contributes to evolutionary fitness, such as by encouraging within-group solidarity and by inhibiting antisocial behaviors. Although similarly skeptical of religion, biologist E. O. Wilson (1998, p. 244) likewise acknowledges that "religious conviction is largely beneficent. Religion . . . nourishes love, devotion, and above all, hope." Ditto the 18th-century skeptic Voltaire, who regarded religion as "infamy," but nevertheless regarded it as useful among the masses. "I want my attorney, my tailor, my servants, even my wife to believe in God. . . . Then I shall be robbed and cuckolded less often" (quoted by Wilson, 1993, p. 219). He once silenced a discussion about atheism until he had dismissed the servants, lest in losing their faith they lose their morality.

A second caveat: Like so many predictor variables in the subjective well-being literature, religion is confounded with other predictors. Religion is like political party affiliation—which a recent Pew (2006) survey shows is also predictive of happiness. Republicans (45%) more often than Democrats (30%) say they are "very happy." Republicans are also more likely to be married, to have high income, and to be religious, each of which, to varying extents, predicts happiness. So is it the essential "Republicanness" or these other associated variables that are decisive?

Religion encompasses social support, a purpose for living, devotion to a reality beyond self, an ultimate source of self-acceptance, hope for the timeless future, and the promotion of positive virtues. If we were to control for such facets, would there be anything left of "the religion factor"? Might this be rather like a hurricane analyst asking whether, after controlling for the effects of the wind, tidal surge, and rain, there is any effect of a hurricane? The hurricane factor, and the religion factor, are package variables. Religion, for example, entails social support—because religion, unlike New Age spirituality, is intrinsically communal. The word root *religion* means "to bind together." It is something you believe and practice in community.

Still, we may wonder about the extent to which a social support variable, such as marriage, helps explain the religion–happiness correlation. Consider:

- Married people (more than never-married people) report being "very happy" (40% versus 23% among those surveyed by the National Opinion Research Center between 1972 and 2004; National Opinion Research Center, 1996).
- Religiously active people (more than religiously inactive people) also report being "very happy" (see Figure 16.1).
- Religiously active people (more than religiously inactive people) report being married. (Sixty-three percent of adults who attend religious services weekly or more report being married, as do 46% of those never attending.)

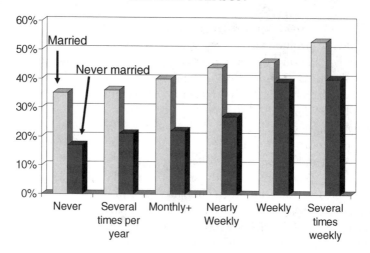

FIGURE 16.2. Percent very happy, by marital status and religious attendance (n = 42,845, NORC, 1972–2004). From National Opinion Research Center (1996).

We might wonder whether, after controlling for religious activity, marriage still correlates with happiness. (Is marriage just a proxy for religion?) Or we might wonder whether, after controlling for marital status, religious activity still correlates with happiness. (Is religion just a proxy for marriage?) Given that most religions encourage marriage, either question is reasonable. Thus Figure 16.2 recasts Figure 16.1, but with the religion–happiness association depicted separately for those married and never married. Although controlling for marital status leaves the religion–happiness correlation largely intact, we could surely, by extracting additional subcomponents of the religion factor, reduce its apparent impact (much as we could eliminate the residual effects of a hurricane after extracting the influence of its associations). Doing so would neither debunk nor validate the religious factor; it would simply illuminate its makeup.

Religion and Physical Well-Being[1]

As humans suffered ills and sought healing throughout history, two healing traditions—religion and medicine—have joined hands in caring for them. Often those hands belonged to the same person—the spiritual leader was also the healer. Maimonides was a 12th-century rabbi and a renowned physician. Hospi-

---

[1] This section is adapted, with permission, from Myers (2007). Copyright 2007 by Worth Publishers. Adapted by permission.

tals, which were first established in monasteries and then spread by missionaries, often carry the names of saints or faith communities.

As medical science matured, healing and religion diverged. Rather than asking God to spare their children from smallpox, people were able to vaccinate them. Rather than seeking a spiritual healer when burning with bacterial fever, they were able to use antibiotics. Recently, however, religion and healing are converging once again:

- Of the 135 medical schools in the United States, 101 offered spirituality and health courses in 2005, up from 5 in 1992 (Koenig, 2002, personal communication; Puchalski, 2005, personal communication).
- Duke University has established a Center for Spirituality, Theology, and Health.
- A Yankelovich survey (1997) found 94% of U.S. health maintenance organization (HMO) professionals and 99% of family physicians agreeing that "personal prayer, meditation, or other spiritual and religious practices" can enhance medical treatment.
- Booksellers are featuring such titles as *The Healing Power of Faith* (Koenig, 1999), *Handbook of Religion and Health* (Koenig, McCullough, & Larson, 2000), and *Faith, Medicine, and Science* (Levin & Koenig, 2005).

Is there fire underneath all this smoke? More than a thousand studies have sought to correlate "the faith factor" with health and healing. For example, Kark and his colleagues (1996) compared the death rates for 3,900 Israelis either in one of 11 religiously orthodox or in one of 11 matched, nonreligious collective settlements (kibbutz communities). The researchers reported that over a 16-year period, "belonging to a religious collective was associated with a strong protective effect" not explained by age or economic differences. In every age group, religious community members were about half as likely to have died as were their nonreligious counterparts. This finding is roughly comparable to the gender difference in mortality.

In response to such findings, Sloan and his skeptical colleagues remind us that mere correlations can leave many factors uncontrolled. Consider one obvious possibility: Women are more religiously active than men, and women outlive men. So perhaps religious involvement is merely an expression of the gender effect on longevity (Sloan, 2005; Sloan & Bagiella, 2002; Sloan, Bagiella, & Powell, 1999; Sloan, Bagiella, VandeCreek, & Poulos, 2000).

However, several new studies find the religiosity–longevity correlation among men alone, and even more strongly among women (McCullough, Hoyt, Larson, Koenig, & Thoresen 2000; McCullough & Laurenceau, 2005). One study that followed 5,286 Californians over 28 years found that, after controlling for age, gender, ethnicity, and education, frequent religious attendees were 36% less likely to have died in any year (Figure 16.3).

A U.S. National Health Interview Survey (Hummer, Rogers, Nam, & Ellison, 1999) followed 21,204 people over 8 years. After controlling for age, sex, race, and region, researchers found that nonattenders were 1.87 times more likely to have died than were those attending church services more than weekly. This translated into a life expectancy at age 20 of 83 years for frequent attenders and 75 years for infrequent attenders (Figure 16.4).

These correlational findings do not indicate that nonattenders who start attending services and change nothing else will live 8 years longer. But they do indicate that as a *predictor* of health and longevity, religious involvement rivals nonsmoking and exercise effects. Such findings demand explanation. What intervening variables might account for the correlation?

First, religiously active people have healthier lifestyles; for example, they smoke and drink less (Lyons, 2002; Strawbridge, Shema, Cohen, & Kaplan, 2001). Health-oriented, vegetarian Seventh Day Adventists have a longer-than-usual life expectancy (Berkel & de Waard, 1983). Religiously orthodox Israelis eat less fat than do their nonreligious compatriots. But such differences are not great enough to explain the dramatically reduced mortality in the religious kib-

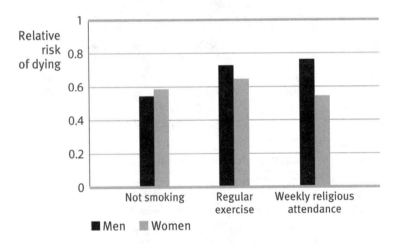

FIGURE 16.3. Predictors of mortality: not smoking, frequent exercise, and regular religious attendance. Epidemiologist William Strawbridge and his coworkers (Strawbridge, 1999; Strawbridge, Cohen, & Shema, 1997; Oman, Kurata, Strawbridge, & Cohen, 2002) followed 5,286 Alameda, California, adults over 28 years. After adjusting for age and education, the researchers found that not smoking, regular exercise, and religious attendance all predicted a lowered risk of death in any given year. Women attending weekly religious services, for example, were only 54% as likely to die in a typical study year as were nonattenders.

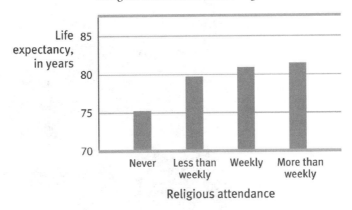

FIGURE 16.4. Religious attendance and life expectancy. In a national health survey financed by the U.S. Centers for Disease Control and Prevention, religiously active people had longer life expectancies. Data from Hummer and others (1999).

butzim (Kark, Shemi, Friedlander, Martin, Manor, & Blondheim, 1996). In the recent U.S. studies, too, about 75% of the longevity difference remains after controlling for unhealthy behaviors such as inactivity and smoking (Musick, Herzog, & House, 1999).

For health, as for happiness, social support is another variable that helps explain the "faith factor" (George, Ellison, & Larson, 2002). Moreover, as noted earlier, religion encourages another predictor of health and longevity—marriage. In the religious kibbutzim, for example, divorce has been almost nonexistent.

But even after controlling for gender, unhealthy behaviors, social ties, and preexisting health problems, the studies report that much of the mortality reduction remains (George, Larson, Koenig, & McCullough, 2000; Powell, Schahabi, & Thoresen, 2003). Researchers therefore speculate that a third set of intervening variables is the stress protection and enhanced well-being associated with a coherent worldview, a sense of hope for the long-term future, feelings of ultimate acceptance, and the relaxed meditation of prayer or Sabbath observance (Figure 16.5). These variables might also help to explain other recent findings among the religiously active, such as healthier immune functioning and fewer hospital admissions, and, for AIDS patients, fewer stress hormones and longer survival (Ironson et al., 2002; Koenig & Larson, 1998; Lutgendorf, Russell, Ullrich, Harris, & Wallace, 2004).

Although the religion–health correlation is yet to be fully explained, Harold Pincus (1997), deputy medical director of the American Psychiatric Association, believes that these findings "have made clear that anyone involved in providing health care services . . . cannot ignore . . . the important connections between spirituality, religion, and health."

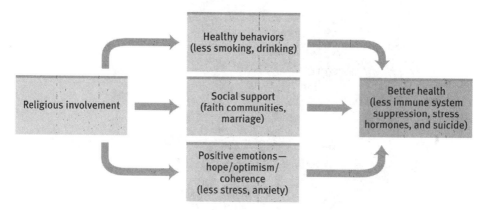

FIGURE 16.5. Possible explanations for the correlation between religious involvement and health/longevity.

Conclusions

Religious affiliation has sometimes fostered the opposite of the love, peace, and justice that the major religions so often profess. Extrinsically motivated religion has fostered ingroup bias, antipathy to ethnic and sexual minorities, and self-justification for oppression. Expressed religiosity in the Western world does, nevertheless, exhibit positive correlations with happiness, coping with loss, character virtues, volunteerism, charitable giving, and health. Religion is a package variable that, psychologically speaking, encompasses social support, meaning, existential terror management, and health-promoting behaviors.

References

Allport, G. W. (1958). *The nature of prejudice* (abridged). Garden City, NY: Anchor Books.

Alves, R. (1972). *Tomorrow's child: Imagination, creativity, and the rebirth of culture.* New York: Harper & Row.

Andrews, F. M. (1953). *Attitudes toward giving.* New York: Bureau of Social Research.

Batson, C. D., Schoenrade, P. A., & Ventis, W. L. (1993). *Religion and the individual: A social-psychological perspective.* New York: Oxford University Press.

Baumeister, R. F., Campbell, J. D., Krueger, J. I., & Vohs, K. D. (2005, January). Exploding the self-esteem myth. *Scientific American,* 84–91.

Baumeister, R. F., & Leary, M. R. (1995). The need to belong: Desire for interpersonal attachment as a fundamental human motivation. *Psychological Bulletin, 117,* 497–529.

Benson, P. L., Dehority, J., Garman, L., Hanson, E., Hochschwender, M., Lebold, C., et al. (1980). Intrapersonal correlates of nonspontaneous helping behavior. *Journal of Social Psychology*, *110*, 87–95.

Berkel, J., & de Waard, F. (1983). Mortality pattern and life expectancy of Seventh Day Adventists in the Netherlands. *International Journal of Epidemiology*, *12*, 455–459.

Bollinger, C. (1997). America's Most Generous—Which of the nation's tycoons are putting their fortunes to good use? *Fortune*, *135*(1), 96–102.

Ciarrochi, J. W., & Deneke, E. (2005). Happiness and the varieties of religious experience: Religious support, practices, and spirituality as predictors of well-being. *Research in the Social Scientific Study of Religion*, *15*, 209–223.

Colasanto, D. (1989). Americans show commitment to helping those in need. *Gallup Report*, (290), 17–24.

Colasanto, D., & Shriver, J. (1989). Mirror of America: Middle-aged face marital crisis. *Gallup Report*, (284), 34–38.

Dawkins, L. (2001, September 15). Discussion: That's religion for you. *The Guardian*.

Egeland, J. A., & Hostetter, A. M. (1983). Amish study: I. Affective disorders among the Amish, 1976–1980. *American Journal of Psychiatry*, *140*, 56–61.

Egeland, J. A., Hostetter, A. M., & Eshleman, S. K. (1983). Amish study: III. The impact of cultural factors on diagnosis of bipolar illness. *American Journal of Psychiatry*, *140*, 67–71.

Ellison, C. G. (1991). Religious involvement and subjective well-being. *Journal of Health and Social Behavior*, *32*, 80–99.

Ellison, C. G., Gay, D. A., & Glass, T. A. (1989). Does religious commitment contribute to individual life satisfaction? *Social Forces*, *68*, 100–123.

Emmons, R. A. (1999). *The psychology of ultimate concerns: Motivation and spirituality in personality*. New York: Guilford Press.

Emmons, R. A., & Shelton, C. M. (2002). Gratitude and the science of positive psychology. In C. R. Snyder & S. J. Lopez (Eds.), *Handbook of positive psychology*. New York: Oxford University Press.

Francis, L. J., & Kaldor, P. (2002). The relationship between psychological well-being and Christian faith and practice in an Australian population sample. *Journal for the Scientific Study of Religion*, *49*, 179–184.

Francis, L. J., & Katz, Y. J. (2002). Religiosity and happiness: A study among Israeli female undergraduates. *Research in the Social Scientific Study of Religion*, *13*, 75–86.

Frankl, V. E. (1962). *Man's search for meaning: An introduction to logotherapy*. Boston: Beacon Press.

Freud, S. (1964). *The future of an illusion*. Garden City, NY: Doubleday. (Original work published 1928)

Friedrich, W. N., Cohen, D. S., & Wilturner, L. T. (1988). Specific beliefs as moderator variables in maternal coping with mental retardation. *Children's Health Care*, *17*, 40–44.

Gallup, G., Jr. (1984). Religion in America. *The Gallup Report*, (222).

George, L. K., Ellison, C. G., & Larson, D. B. (2002). Explaining the relationships between religious involvement and health. *Psychological Inquiry*, *13*, 190–200.

George, L. K., Larson, D. B., Koenig, H. G., & McCullough, M. E. (2000). Spirituality and health: What we know, what we need to know. *Journal of Social and Clinical Psychology*, *19*, 102–116.

Gilkey, L. (1966). *The Shantung compound: The story of men and women under pressure.* New York: Harper & Row.

Gould, S. J. (1999). *Rocks of ages.* New York: Ballantine.

Greeley, A. M. (1991). *Faithful attraction.* New York: Tor Books.

Hadaway, C. K. (1978). Life satisfaction and religion: A reanalysis. *Social Forces, 57,* 636–643.

Hansen, D. E., Vandenberg, B., & Patterson, M. L. (1995). The effects of religious orientation on spontaneous and nonspontaneous helping behaviors. *Personality and Individual Differences, 19,* 101–104.

Harvey, C. D., Barnes, G. E., & Greenwood, L. (1987). Correlates of morale among Canadian widowed persons. *Social Psychiatry, 22,* 65–72.

Hodgkinson, V. A., & Weitzman, M. S. (1992). *Giving and volunteering in the United States.* Washington, DC: Independent Sector.

Hodgkinson, V. A., Weitzman, M. S., & Kirsch, A. D. (1990). From commitment to action: How religious involvement affects giving and volunteering. In R. Wuthnow, V. A. Hodgkinson, & Associates (Eds.), *Faith and philanthropy in America: Exploring the role of religion in America's voluntary sector.* San Francisco: Jossey-Bass.

Hummer, R. A., Rogers, R. G., Nam, C. B., & Ellison, C. G. (1999). Religious involvement and U.S. adult mortality. *Demography, 36,* 273–285.

Hunsberger, B. (1985). Religion, age, life satisfaction, and perceived sources of religiousness: A study of older persons. *Journal of Gerontology, 40,* 615–630.

Inglehart, R. (1990). *Culture shift in advanced industrial society.* Princeton, NJ: Princeton University Press.

Ironson, G., Solomon, G. F., Balbin, E. G., O'Cleirigh, C., George, A., Kumar, M., et al. (2002). The Ironson–Woods spiritual/religiousness index is associated with long survival, health behaviors, less distress, and low cortisol in people with HIV/AIDS. *Annals of Behavioral Medicine, 24,* 34–48.

Johnson, B. R., Li, S. D., Larson, D., & McCullough, M. (2000). A systematic review of the religiosity and delinquency literature: A research note. *Journal of Contemporary Criminal Justice, 16,* 32–52.

Johnson, S. (1791). From J. Boswell *The life of Samuel Johnson.*

Julian of Norwich. (1368). *Showing of love, Part I.* Westminster Cathedral manuscript.

Kark, J. D., Shemi, G., Friedlander, Y., Martin, O., Manor, O., & Blondheim, S. H. (1996). Does religious observance promote health? Mortality in secular vs. religious kibbutzim in Israel. *American Journal of Public Health, 86,* 341–346.

King, M. L., Jr. (1964, June 6). I have a dream. *New York Times,* p. 10.

Koenig, H. G. (1999). *The healing power of faith.* New York: Simon & Schuster.

Koenig, H. G., Kvale, J. N., & Ferrel, C. (1988). Religion and well-being in later life. *Gerontologist, 28,* 18–28.

Koenig, H. G., & Larson, D. B. (1998). Use of hospital services, religious attendance, and religious affiliation. *Southern Medical Journal, 91,* 925–932.

Koenig, H. G., McCullough, M. E., & Larson, D. B. (2000). *Handbook of religion and health.* New York: Oxford University Press.

Kushner, H. (1987). You've got to believe in something. *Redbook, 12,* 92–94.

Levin, J., & Koenig, H. G. (2005). *Faith, medicine, and science.* Binghamton, NY: Haworth Pastoral Press.

Levin, J. S., & Markides, K. S. (1988). Religious attendance and psychological well-being in middle-aged and older Mexican Americans. *Sociological Analysis*, *49*, 66–72.

Lutgendorf, S. K., Russell, D., Ullrich, P., Harris, T. B., & Wallace, R. (2004). Religious participation, interleukin-6, and mortality in older adults. *Health Psychology*, *23*, 465–475.

Lyons, L. (2002, June 25). Are spiritual teens healthier? *Gallup Tuesday Briefing*, Gallup Organization. Available at *www.gallup.com/poll/tb/religValue/20020625b.asp*.

Marini, M. M. (1990). *The rise of individualism in advanced industrial societies*. Paper presented at the Population Association of America annual meeting, Toronto.

Markides, K. S., Levin, J. S., & Ray, L. A. (1987). Religion, aging, and life satisfaction: An eight-year, three-wave longitudinal study. *Gerontologist*, *27*, 660–665.

McCullough, M. E., Hoyt, W. T., Larson, D. B., Koenig, H. G., & Thoresen, C. (2000). Religious involvement and mortality: A meta-analytic review. *Health Psychology*, *19*, 211–222.

McCullough, M. E., & Laurenceau, J.-P. (2005). Religiousness and the trajectory of self-rated health across adulthood. *Personality and Social Psychology Bulletin*, *31*, 560–573.

McCullough, M. E., & Witvliet, C. V. (2002). The psychology of forgiveness. In C. R. Snyder & S. J. Lopez (Eds.), *Handbook of positive psychology*. New York: Oxford University Press.

McGloshen, T. H., & O'Bryant, S. L. (1988). The psychological well-being of older, recent widows. *Psychology of Women Quarterly*, *12*, 99–116.

McIntosh, D. N., Silver, R. C., & Wortman, C. B. (1993). Religion's role in adjustment to a negative life event: Coping with the loss of a child. *Journal of Personality and Social Psychology*, *65*, 812–821.

Mother Teresa. (1968). In an interview with Malcolm Muggeridge for the BBC.

Musick, M. A., Herzog, A. R., & House, J. S. (1999). Volunteering and mortality among older adults: Findings from a national sample. *Journal of Gerontology*, *54B*, 173–180.

Myers, D. G. (1992). *The pursuit of happiness: Who is happy and why*. New York: William Morrow.

Myers, D. G. (2000). *The American paradox*. New Haven, CT: Yale University Press.

Myers, D. G. (2005). *Social psychology* (7th ed.). New York: McGraw-Hill.

Myers, D. G. (2007). *Psychology* (8th ed.). New York: Worth.

National Opinion Research Center. (2006). General social survey archive. Available at *www.sda.berkeley.edu*.

Nonprofit Times (2002). Cited by M. Guillen, *Can a smart person believe in God?* Nashville : Thomas Nelson.

Okun, M. A., & Stock, M. J. (1987). Correlates and components of subjective well-being among the elderly. *Journal of Applied Gerontology*, *6*, 95–112.

Oman, D., Kurata, J. H., Strawbridge, W. J., & Cohen, R. D. (2002). Religious attendance and cause of death over 31 years. *International Journal of Psychiatry in Medicine*, *32*, 69–89.

Paloutzian, R. F. (1981). Purpose in life and value changes following conversion. *Journal of Personality and Social Psychology*, *41*, 1153–1160.

Penner, L. A. (2002). Dispositional and organizational influences on sustained volunteerism: An interactionist perspective. *Journal of Social Issues*, *58*, 447–467.

Peterson, C., & Seligman, M. E. P. (2004). *Character strengths and virtues: A handbook and classification*. New York: Oxford University Press.

Pew Research Center. (2006, February 13). Are we happy yet? Available at *www.pewresearch.org*.

Pincus, H. A. (1997). Commentary: Spirituality, religion, and health: Expanding and using the knowledge base. *Mind/Body Medicine, 2*, 49.

Pollner, M. (1989). Divine relations, social relations, and well-being. *Journal of Health and Social Behavior, 30*, 92–104.

Poloma, M. M., & Pendleton, B. F. (1990). Religious domains and general well-being. *Social Indicators Research, 22*, 255–276.

Powell, L. H., Schahabi, L., & Thoresen, C. E. (2003). Religion and spirituality: Linkages to physical health. *American Psychologist, 58*, 36–52.

Putnam, R. (2000). *Bowling alone*. New York: Simon & Schuster.

Rimland, B. B. (1982). The altruism paradox. *Southern Psychologist, 2*(1), 1–9.

Schwartz, S. H., & Huismans, S. (1995). Value priorities and religiosity in four Western religions. *Social Psychology Quarterly, 58*, 88–107.

Seligman, M. (1988, October). Boomer blues. *Psychology Today*, 50–55.

Shermer, M. (2000). *How we believe: Science, skepticism, and the search for God*. New York: Holt.

Shermer, M. (2004). *The science of good and evil*. New York: Holt.

Siegel, J. M., & Kuykendall, D. H. (1990). Loss, widowhood, and psychological distress among the elderly. *Journal of Consulting and Clinical Psychology, 58*, 519–524.

Sloan, R. P. (2005). Field analysis of the literature on religion, spirituality, and health. Available at *www.metanexus.net/tarp*.

Sloan, R. P., & Bagiella, E. (2002). Claims about religious involvement and health outcomes. *Annals of Behavioral Medicine, 24*, 14–21.

Sloan, R. P., Bagiella, E., & Powell, T. (1999). Religion, spirituality, and medicine. *Lancet, 353*, 664–667.

Sloan, R. P., Bagiella, E., VandeCreek, L., & Poulos, P. (2000). Should physicians prescribe religious activities? *New England Journal of Medicine, 342*, 1913–1917.

Smith, T. B., McCullough, M. E., & Poll, J. (2003). Religiousness and depression: Evidence for a main effect and the moderating influence of stressful life events. *Psychological Bulletin, 129*, 614–636.

Snyder, C. R., & Lopez, S. (Eds.). (2007). *Handbook of positive psychology*. New York: Oxford University Press.

Solomon, S., Greenberg, J., & Pyszczynski, T. (1991). A terror management theory of social behavior: The psychological functions of self-esteem and cultural worldviews. *Advances in Experimental Social Psychology, 24*, 93–159.

Stock, W. A., Okun, M. A., Haring, M. J., & Witter, R. A. (1983). Age and subjective well-being: A meta-analysis. In R. J. Light (Ed.), *Evaluation studies: Review Annual* (Vol. 8). Beverly Hills: Sage.

Strawbridge, W. J. (1999). *Mortality and religious involvement: A review and critique of the results, the methods, and the measures*. Paper presented at a Harvard University conference on religion and health, sponsored by the National Institute for Healthcare Research and the John Templeton Foundation, Boston.

Strawbridge, W. J., Cohen, R. D., & Shema, S. J. (1997). Frequent attendance at religious services and mortality over 28 years. *American Journal of Public Health, 87*, 957–961.

Strawbridge, W. J., Shema, S. J., Cohen, R. D., & Kaplan, G. A. (2001). Religious attendance increases survival by improving and maintaining good health behaviors, mental health, and social relationships. *Annals of Behavioral Medicine, 23*, 68–74.

Swift, J. (1727). *Thoughts on various subjects.*

Tangney, J. P. (2002). Humility. In C. R. Snyder & S. J. Lopez (Eds.), *Handbook of positive psychology.* New York: Oxford University Press.

Teresa, M. (1985). Quoted by Malcolm Muggeridge in a BBC interview and reported by R. Schuller, *The be-happy attitudes: Eight positive attitudes that can transform your life!* Waco, TX: Word Books.

Tillich, P. (1988). *Shaking the foundations.* Gloucester, MA: Smith Publishers.

Willits, F. K., & Crider, D. M. (1988). Religion and well-being: Men and women in the middle years. *Review of Religious Research, 29*, 281–294.

Wilson, E. O. (1998). *Consilience.* New York: Knopf.

Wilson, J. Q. (1993). *The moral sense.* New York: Free Press.

Winseman, A. L. (2002, February 26). Congregational engagement index: Life satisfaction and giving. *The Gallup Poll.* Available at *www.poll.gallup.com.*

Winthrop, J. (1965). A model of Christian charity. In E. S. Morgan (Ed.), *Puritan political ideas, 1558–1794.* Indianapolis: Bobbs-Merrill. (Original work published 1630)

Witter, R. A., Stock, W. A., Okun, M. J., & Haring, M. J. (1985). Religion and subjective well-being in adulthood: A quantitative synthesis. *Review of Religious Research, 26*, 332–342.

Wuthnow, R. (1994). *God and mammon in America.* New York: Free Press.

Yankelovich Partners. (1997, December 15). *Ability of spirituality to help people who are sick* [Press release]. Chapel Hill, NC: Authors.

Zika, S., & Chamberlain, K. (1987). Relation of hassles and personality to subjective well-being. *Journal of Personality and Social Psychology, 53*, 155–162.

IV

SUBJECTIVE WELL-BEING
IN THE INTERPERSONAL DOMAIN

17

What Makes People Happy?

A Developmental Approach to the Literature on Family Relationships and Well-Being

MARISSA L. DIENER
and MARY BETH DIENER MCGAVRAN

Subjective well-being (SWB) is a broad category that includes positive emotional responses, such as joy, elation, happiness, and contentment, as well as long-term moods and cognitive dimensions (Diener, Suh, Lucas, & Smith, 1999). It also reflects the balance of positive emotions relative to negative emotions, such as guilt and shame, sadness, anger, anxiety and negative moods, and a cognitive evaluation of one's life and of particular domains in that life, such as self, work, family, and health.

Early research on subjective well-being identified its correlates (see Diener et al., 1999), and recent research has also identified processes that underlie subjective well-being. One important process appears to be the progression toward certain types of goals (Kasser & Ryan, 1996). Although working toward a variety of goals may provide satisfaction, affiliation goals appear to be particularly rewarding. In fact, the "need to belong" has been proposed as a fundamental, intrinsic motivation (Baumeister & Leary, 1995). Theorists have suggested that social relationships are fundamental to human development (e.g., Bowlby, 1969), psychological well-being (Myers, 2004; Ryff, 1995), and human flourishing (Maslow, 1954). Indeed, it has been argued that human beings have evolved to establish and maintain social networks (Bowlby, 1969). Not only are social relationships an important source of subjective well-being (Reis & Gable, 2003), they are often considered an important component, in and of themselves, of psychological well-being (Keyes, 1998; Ryff, 1995).

Researchers interested in the correlates of subjective well-being have examined social relationships as one predictor of it. For example, Myers's (2000) review concluded that social relationships can both support and damage psychological well-being. Support from social relationships is seen as beneficial for subjective well-being (Diener, 1984); those with close relationships cope better with stresses. For example, Landau and Litwin (2001) found, in a sample of Jewish Israelis over the age of 75 years, that social network supportiveness significantly predicted life satisfaction, even after controlling for demographic factors, locus of control, and physical capacity. Conversely, those who prefer high incomes and occupational success to the detriment of close friendships and marriage are more likely to describe themselves as unhappy (Perkins, 1991). Similarly, Emmons (2003) examined the differential correlates of intimacy strivings, which reflect a concern for establishing close interpersonal relationships, and power strivings, which reflect a concern for influencing and impacting other people. He reported that people who emphasize intimacy strivings over power strivings tend to have greater levels of subjective well-being. Likewise, Reis, Sheldon, Gable, Roscoe, and Ryan (2000) showed that satisfaction with the intrinsic need of relatedness was significantly associated with daily fluctuations in positive affect. As individuals' satisfaction with relatedness increased, so too did positive affect.

Social relationships seem necessary but not sufficient for high happiness (Diener & Seligman, 2002). A classic study conducted by Campbell, Converse, and Rodgers (1976) showed that the most important domains for life satisfaction as a whole were those involving social relationships: family life, marriage, and friendship. Diener and Seligman's (2002) findings on very happy individuals indicate that these individuals have satisfying social relationships and spend little time alone, compared to people who are closer to the average in happiness. In fact, people report feeling happier when they are with others (Pavot, Diener, & Fujita, 1990). Biswas-Diener and Diener (2001) examined life satisfaction and domain satisfaction among prostitutes, homeless individuals, and those living in slums in Calcutta. They found that these extremely poor individuals were fairly satisfied with their social relationships, and that greater satisfaction with friends, family, and romantic relationships all predicted greater life satisfaction among these disadvantaged groups. In contrast, homeless people in the United States frequently report extreme social isolation, lack of social support, and lower levels of subjective well-being (Biswas-Diener & Diener, 2001). The researchers concluded that the strong social support provided by family and friends in the Calcutta sample buffered the negative effects of extreme poverty.

Relationships are not always positive, and just as our greatest joys arise from relationships, so, too may our greatest conflicts and sorrows. Social relationships of poor quality or characterized by conflict are associated with greater stress and anxiety and may actually lower subjective well-being (Antonucci, Akiyama, & Lansford, 1998; Rook, 1992). Likewise, divorce, death of a child or spouse, or the end of a relationship produces an increase in negative affect and a decrease in positive affect (e.g., Booth & Amato, 1991; Lehman, Wortman, & Williams, 1987). Similarly, relationships characterized by negative interactions are associated with more negative moods, stress, and depression (Finch, Okun, Barrera, Zautra, & Reich, 1989; Pagel, Erdly, & Becker, 1987; see Rook, 1992 for review). For example, Antonucci et al. (1998) found that for men, feeling that people in their social network were too demanding was associated with lower levels of happiness, and for women, having people in their social network that "got on their nerves" predicted less happiness.

Clearly, social relationships are an important piece of the subjective well-being mosaic. Social relationships occur in many different areas of people's lives and take many forms. The present review focuses on the links between close family relationships and subjective well-being. Several types of family relationships, including parent–child relationships, sibling relationships, and marital and romantic relationships, are examined. Although friendships are also important, due to space constraints, only family relationships are considered here.

Family relationships appear to be consistent correlates of subjective well-being. For example, Diener and Diener (1995) showed that satisfaction with family was related to life satisfaction across 31 nations. Campbell et al.'s (1976) classic study demonstrated that the most important domains for life satisfaction were family life and marriage. Much of the research on family life and subjective well-being has been correlational, and consequently, the potential causal mechanisms underlying the associations remain unclear. Potential mechanisms by which family relationships and subjective well-being are related are discussed where evidence is available. This review addresses well-being across the lifespan, including research examining infants, children, and adults. The research on children's well-being has tended to examine less direct indicators of psychological well-being, such as the absence of externalizing and internalizing behaviors or other types of behavior problems, rather than direct subjective assessments of well-being. Nonetheless, this body of research is included here as a step toward bridging the developmental literature on close relationships with the adult literature on subjective well-being.

Parent–Child Relationships and Well-Being

Parent–child relationships are often the primary relationships in infants' and young children's lives. As such, they are often considered critical to children's well-being. However, little research has examined the correlates of subjective well-being per se (especially life satisfaction) in young children. Of course, young children may be unable to provide verbal global assessments of their life. Many of the studies reviewed here examine indirect indicators of well-being, such as the absence of internalizing and externalizing behaviors, but should not be considered measures of subjective well-being per se. Some of the research, however, includes indicators, often observationally assessed, of some components of subjective well-being—specifically, positive and negative affect.

The most prominent theory in the study of early socioemotional development is that of attachment theory (Thompson, 2000), and this theory can be used to understand individual differences in positive and negative affect in children. Attachment theory is an ethological formulation that postulates that attachment relationships evolved because they increased the likelihood of child–caregiver proximity and thus maximized survival (Bowlby, 1969). According to attachment theory, infants are biologically predisposed to form these relationships. However, the nature and quality of these relationships differ, of course, from one dyad to another. Bowlby theorized that, on the basis of repeated parent–child interactions, the child forms a cognitive model of the availability and supportiveness of the caregiver that affects his or her psychological well-being. That is, early experiences with sensitive or insensitive care shape individuals' "internal working models"—their expectations of future relationships, self-appraisals, and behavior toward others. The child uses the internal working model to filter information selectively, evoke responses from other people, select niches, and appraise experience (Belsky & Cassidy, 1994). These internal working models become self-perpetuating both because of the confirmation biases inherent in them and because the child elicits responses consistent with them (see Thompson, 1999, for further discussion).

According to Bowlby (1969) and Ainsworth (1979; Ainsworth, Blehar, Waters, & Wall, 1978) an early, enduring, warm relationship (a secure relationship) with a caregiver promotes psychological well-being. A securely attached child comes to expect that his or her emotional signals will be addressed. A secure attachment is the beginning of a parent–child relationship characterized by mutual cooperation: The parent is sensitive to the child's needs, and the child is receptive to the caregiver's socialization. This mutual cooperation may promote both positive affect and more optimal functioning as the child develops. The securely attached child brings a secure internal working model to other relationships; he or she seeks and expects supportive, satisfying relationships with other people and acts in a way to elicit such support (Thompson, 1999). In contrast, insensitive or rejecting care, a lack of availability, or maltreatment will promote an insecure attachment. An insecurely attached child develops an expectation that his or her emotional signals will be met only selectively. These expectations are internalized and affect conscious and unconscious rules for organizing and accessing information about experiences, emotions, and relationships (Belsky & Cassidy, 1994). Insecurely attached children bring distrust to new and old relationships and expect less support from others. These children are expected to be at greater risk for depression, anxiety, anger, and interpersonal difficulties later. Thus, the internal working model acts as an unconscious filter through which relationships are interpreted and self-understanding is developed.

Because these outcomes are multiply determined, however, insecure attachment is just one risk factor for later development. Theorists differ in their estimations of the effects of attachment relationships on later outcomes. In a narrow view of attachment, early attachment relationships should affect the child's later trust and confidence in the parent and possibly other close partners (Thompson, 1999). In a broad view of attachment, early attachment relationships affect emergent personality characteristics (Thompson, 1999), which may subsequently affect subjective well-being.

Quality of Parent–Child Relationships during Infancy and Later Well-Being

Early studies on attachment security during infancy indicated that patterns of affective behavior differentiated securely and insecurely attached infants. For example, infants classified as securely attached to their mothers showed more smiling and enthusiasm playing with their mothers 6 months later (Waters, Wippman, & Sroufe, 1979). Similarly, infants classified as securely attached at 18 months were more enthusiastic and positive in a problem-solving task at 28 months (Matas, Arend, & Sroufe, 1978). Securely attached infants were more likely to show patterns of increased smiling in interaction with the mother over the first year, whereas the majority of insecurely attached infants showed a pattern of decreased smiling over the first year of life (Malatesta, Culver, Tesman, & Shepard, 1989). Not only is infant affect associated with the quality of relationship with the mother, it is also associated with father–infant relationships. For example, infants in secure father–infant relationships showed greater positive affect than infants in insecure father–infant relationships (Diener, Mangelsdorf, McHale, & Frosch, 2002). In contrast, infants in insecure-resistant attachment relationships exhibited higher levels of distress with both mothers and fathers in a competing demands situation than did securely attached infants (Diener et al., 2002). Other studies have also found that insecure resistant infants exhibit more fear or distress than secure infants (e.g., Calkins & Fox, 1992). These studies of parent–child relationships during infancy suggest that infants in secure attachment relationships exhibit greater positive affect and less negative affect than children in insecure relationships.

There are a number of longitudinal studies examining attachment security in the early years of life and later child well-being. These studies have produced mixed results. Some studies, especially those from the Minnesota research group, have demonstrated that early attachment security predicts later child well-being (e.g., Arend, Gove, & Sroufe, 1978; Erickson, Sroufe, & Egeland, 1985; Urban, Carlson, Egeland, & Sroufe, 1991). For example, Bohlin, Hagekull, and Rydell (2000) found that both early attachment and concurrent attachment was associated with more positive social behavior at age 8 years. Preschool attachment security predicted more positive perceptions of maternal support at age 8 years (Booth, Rubin, & Rose-Krasnor, 1998). In contrast, Lewis, Feiring, and Rosenthal (2000) failed to find an association between attachment security at 1 year and maladjustment in adolescence. However, they found concurrent associations between attachment representations and adolescent maladjustment at both 13 and 18 years. Furthermore, they found that children from divorced families had less positive representations of attachment relationships during adolescence and showed greater maladjustment than did children from married-parent families, suggesting that disruption of close family relationships is associated with lower well-being. There are a number of reasons to expect lawful discontinuity in attachment security and later outcomes (see Thompson, 1999), including change in parenting behavior over time, other attachment relationships, and mediating factors, such as emotion regulation strategies. Thus, it is not surprising that some studies fail to find an association between early attachment and later well-being. Research has moved toward understanding the conditions in which early attachment relationships will and will not predict later well-being.

The National Institute of Child Health and Human Development (NICHD) Study of Early Child Care is unique in its sample size ($n = 1,030$ at first grade), its inclusion of multiple child outcomes measured via multiple informants, and its longitudinal design (National Institute of Child Health and Human Development, 2006). Families were recruited from 10 sites around the United States at birth. Attachment security was assessed at 15 months, and mothers and their children were seen in the laboratory or in their homes repeatedly until the child was in first grade. Early attachment relationships predicted either mothers' or teachers' ratings of social competence, internalizing behaviors, and externalizing behaviors in first grade. However, the authors showed that continuity in parenting quality accounted for the link between attachment quality during infancy and later child outcomes. More specifically, positive parenting assessed through observations and interviews between 15 and 54 months, rather than early attachment classifications, predicted social competence, externalizing, and teacher-rated internalizing scores. This finding provides evidence for the continuity in care mechanism, which is discussed in more detail below (National Institute of Child Health and Human Development, 2006). Moreover, children's early attachment relationships predicted how they responded to changes in parenting quality. Children who were classified as securely attached at 15 months did not show increased externalizing behavior in the classroom when parenting quality declined, as did insecurely attached children. The securely attached children seemed to be somewhat protected from declines in positive parenting. It may be that the securely attached children are able to approach social situations with positive views of themselves and positive expectations from others, even when their mothers show decreased sensitivity. For insecurely attached children, a decline in maternal sensitivity may confirm their more negative sense of self and others.

In addition to being associated with affect and internalizing and externalizing behaviors, parent–child relationships may be associated with the ability to form other social relationships. A meta-analysis of 63 studies that examined the associations between attachment security and peer relations demonstrated that attachment security with the mother was significantly related to peer relations (effect size = .20; Schneider, Atkinson, & Tardif, 2001). Attachment security was more strongly related to children's close friendships than to more distal peer relations, and was more strongly related to older children's relations than younger children's peer relations. For example, Kerns (1994) found that securely attached children at age 4 years had more positive interactions with a friend 1 year later than did insecurely attached children.

The causal mechanism underlying early attachment relationships and later child well-being is still unclear. There are a number of potential mechanisms: temperamental effects, continuity in the quality of the caregiving environment, emotion regulation styles, and the effects of attachment security via the internal working model (see Thompson, 1999). These processes are not mutually exclusive, and research, discussed below, supports each of them.

There has been considerable debate about the extent to which certain temperamental affective characteristics promote secure or insecure attachment (see Goldsmith & Harman, 1994 for a review). A meta-analysis of infant negative affect and attachment security found little evidence for an association between temperamental distress and later attachment security (Goldsmith & Alansky, 1987). Nonetheless, some studies have demonstrated a connection between specific temperamental characteristics and later attachment security. For example, Mangelsdorf, McHale, Diener, Goldstein, and Lehn (2001) showed that securely attached infants were higher on positive affect and lower on fearfulness than were insecurely attached infants. It may be that certain temperamental characteristics promote secure attachment and later well-being, especially given that personality is one of the strongest and most consistent predictors of subjective well-being (Diener et al., 1999). To the extent that temperament is a precursor to later personality, temperament may be associated with both attachment security and later subjective well-being.

There is also evidence that continuity in caregiving contributes to both attachment security and later child outcomes (see Thompson, 1998, for discussion). In this view, the sensitive caregiving that initially promoted a secure attachment also contributes, if it continues, to greater emotional well-being as the child develops. Thus, it is not necessarily the quality of the attachment relationship during infancy that promotes later child well-being but, rather, the fact that the same parent or caregivers who sensitively responded to their child's needs during infancy also provide high-quality care that meets their child's needs during later childhood. When parents meet their children's needs, their children experience greater well-being and better relationships with their parents.

Another potential mechanism that accounts for the relation between parent–child and peer relationships is emotion regulation styles. Emotion regulation is one of the functions of the parent–child attachment relationship (Bowlby, 1969). Thompson (1998) states that one of the important lessons learned in the parent–child relationship is how to interpret, express, and cope with the intense emotions experienced in intimate relationships. Attachment theory hypothesizes that the patterns of emotion regulation within the parent–child relationship become internalized by the child and are shown in other contexts as well (Cassidy, 1994). Contreras, Kerns, Weimer, Gentzler, and Tomich (2000) examined concurrent associations among parent–child attachment security, emotion regulation, and teacher-rated peer competence. They demonstrated that effective emotion regulation mediated the relation between attachment security and peer competence. Diener et al. (2002) demonstrated that infants' emotion regulation styles were significantly associated with their attachment relationships with fathers. Securely attached infants showed more effective emotion regulation styles. These findings suggest that attachment security may be related to more effective emotion regulation strategies, and these strategies may partially account for the associations between attachment security and later well-being. More research is clearly needed to examine how emotion regulation styles might mediate the association between attachment security and later well-being.

Although less research has examined the internal working model mechanism proposed by Bowlby (1969), Laible and Thompson (1998) examined concurrent associations between attachment security and emotional understanding in preschoolers. They found that securely attached children had better understanding of negative emotions than did insecurely attached children. Two longitudinal studies have demonstrated that children process affective information differently based upon their attachment relationship histories during infancy. These studies provide preliminary support for the idea that early attachment relationships may affect social information processing. Belsky, Spritz, and Crnic (1996) assessed attachment security with mothers at 12 months. Two years later they examined children's memory for positive and negative events with a laboratory puppet show. After controlling for verbal intelligence, they found that children with secure attachment histories remembered positive events during the puppet show more accurately than negative events. In contrast, children with insecure attachment histories remembered the negative events during the puppet show more accurately than the positive events. It is important to note that 12-month emotionality was not related to memory for the events, so differences in emotionality do not appear to account for differences in memory.

If children process information in real life as they did in the laboratory, these provocative findings suggest that children may experience the same events very differently. Ziv, Oppenheim, and Sagi-Schwartz (2004) examined attachment security at 12 months and social information processing at 7 or 8 years of age. They found that secure children differed from insecure children in their evaluations of responses to peers in videotaped vignettes. More specifically, securely attached children were more likely to believe that competent responses would produce positive outcomes with peers than were insecurely attached children. Additionally, the securely attached children were able to differentiate between situations in which positive behavior would, or would not, be effective with peers, whereas insecurely attached children were not. These findings provide preliminary support for the idea that attachment relationships may influence children's information processing in such as way as to ultimately affect their subjective well-being.

Parent–Adolescent Child Relationships and Subjective Well-Being

Unlike research with younger children, research on older children and adolescents has examined the correlations of parent–child relationships with specific components of subjective well-being, likely because older children are better able to provide self-reports of subjective well-being. This literature suggests that parent–child relationships continue to be a predictor of subjective well-being in adolescents. For example, in a study specifically designed to measure life satisfaction in children ranging from 10 to 13 years of age, Huebner (1991) examined the associations among global life satisfaction and satisfaction with specific domains. Satisfaction with family life was more strongly associated with global life satisfaction than was satisfaction with friends. Moreover, recent school grades, parents' occupational status, and other demographic characteristics were not significantly associated with global life satisfaction. Thus, these findings underscore the importance of close family relationships for children's life satisfaction.

Although research with younger children has tended to emphasize the role of mothers over fathers, research indicates that both are important for adolescents' subjective well-being. In Israel, a sample of 121 adolescents and their parents showed that adolescent–father relationship quality, as reported by both parents and the adolescent, was related to the concurrently assessed subjective well-being of adolescents (Ben-Zur, 2003). Mastery and optimism were also related to adolescent subjective well-being. Ducharme, Doyle, and Markiewicz (2002) showed that adolescents' perceptions of attachment security with their parents were associated with their diary reports of the quality of interaction with their parents. More specifically, adolescents who perceived themselves to be securely attached to one or both parents reported significantly more positive and fewer negatively toned interactions with their parents than did adolescents insecurely attached to both parents. It is unclear from these data whether there were objective differences in the emotional quality of interactions, or whether these were differences in perceptions of the relationships.

Demo and Acock (1996) used data from the National Survey of Households, a nationally representative sample, to examine how family structure, demographic factors, marital quality, maternal reports of adolescent adjustment and mother–adolescent relationship quality were associated. They found that the strongest and most consistent predictor of adolescent well-being was mother–adolescent disagreement, which predicted lower well-being. Although they relied on maternal reports, their findings are consistent with research with younger children showing that concurrent assessments of parent–child relationship quality are associated with child well-being. Emotional involvement with both mothers and fathers predicted both self-esteem and life satisfaction in longitudinal data from the National Survey of Children (Wenk, Hardesty, Morgan, & Blair, 1994). Similarly, Amato (1994) showed, in a national sample of young adults, that closeness to both fathers and mothers made unique, independent contributions to happiness, life satisfaction, and psychological distress. Thus, regardless of the quality of the mother–child relationship, greater closeness to fathers predicted greater happiness, more satisfaction, and less distress. In a recent review of children's perceived quality of life, Huebner, Suldo, Smith, and McKnight (2004) concluded that family relationships were consistent predictors of children's perceived quality of life.

As with the literature on parent–child relationships with younger children, the causal mechanisms are unclear, and directionality of effects is an issue. For example, Allen, McElhaney, Kuperminc, and Jodl (2004) conducted a longitudinal study from age 16 years to 18 years. They found that adolescents' reported levels of depression at age 16 years predicted declines in attachment security from ages 16 to 18 years, even after controlling for the baseline effects of security at age 16. It may be that personality factors, such as extraversion, contribute to both positive parent–child relationships and adolescents' subjective well-being. Or the direction of effects may be from subjective well-being to parent–child relationships, such that happy, satisfied adolescents are easier to get along with and have better relationships with their parents.

In summary, correlational data indicate that parent–child relationship quality is associated with subjective well-being for both younger and older children. Overall, effect sizes tend to be small to moderate, and of course, other influences are also important for child well-being. Temperamental influences and demographic factors are often also related to subjective well-being. Although most studies have examined relationships with mothers, it is likely that relationships with multiple caregivers are important—mothers, fathers, and extrafamilial caregivers. In fact, Diener, Isabella, Behunin, and Wong (in press) found that children who reported higher levels of attachment security with both parents perceived themselves, and were rated by teachers, as more competent than children who were securely attached to only one parent. In addition, more research is needed to elucidate the processes underlying the associations between parent–child relationships and subjective well-being, and the factors that moderate these relationships. It is important to note that most of these studies do not include traditional self-report measures of subjective well-being. Instead, they tend to rely on observational measures of affect or teacher or parent report of children's behavior. Thus, they are not really assessing subjective experience, except insofar as the observational measures may reflect subjective experience.

Parent–Adult Child Relationships and Subjective Well-Being

The literature on parent–adult child relationships and subjective well-being has focused on two main issues: first, whether adults with children experience greater subjective well-being than those without any or with fewer children, and second, how adult–child relationship quality is associated with subjective well-being. The gerontological literature has suggested that adult children are important for providing social and instrumental support for older people. Thus, it might be expected that childless elders would be at risk for lower subjective well-being than elders with children. Furthermore, the majority of people around the world become parents. Thus, being a parent may be viewed by most as an expected event. Whether people remain childless voluntarily or due to other factors likely has an impact on their well-being.

Connidis and McMullin (1993) examined whether childless people chose to remain childless or perceived childlessness to be a matter of circumstance. They found that people who were childless by choice were not significantly different in subjective well-being (happiness, depression, and satisfaction with life) than parents who were close with their children. However, those childless by circumstance and those with distant relationships with their children were significantly less happy, less satisfied with life, and more depressed than parents who were emotionally close to their children. Similarly, Koropeckyj-Cox (2002) examined depression and loneliness for individuals ages 50–84 years old, with and without children, using the National Survey of Families and Households. Her findings indicate that childless women who desired children reported greater loneliness and depression than childless women who thought it was acceptable to be childless and women with children with high-quality relationships. For men, fathers with good parent–child relationships reported lower levels of loneliness and depression than men without children and men with poor-quality parent–child relationships. Poorer-quality parent–child relationships were significantly predictive of greater loneliness and depression for both men and women. In contrast,

Somers (1993) examined the life satisfaction of voluntarily child-free adults and parents and found that there were no significant differences in life satisfaction between the two groups when she controlled for age and income. It is likely that being voluntarily childless is quite a different experience from expecting and desiring to have children but failing to do so.

These findings on the benefits of children, especially for those who desire children, appear across many countries. Diener and Suh (1998) showed, across 43 diverse nations and 60,000 respondents, a slight but significant tendency for people with more children to have higher life satisfaction. This effect did not differ by age. It was unclear whether happier people had more offspring or whether offspring made people happier. Also, they were unable to differentiate whether individuals were childless by choice or experienced infertility.

In contrast, parents who have lost children, especially unexpectedly, show dramatic declines in subjective well-being and prolonged periods of intense grief (Dyregrov, 1990; Lehman et al., 1987). Losing a child is often described as one of the most difficult and painful losses one may experience. This loss may be especially difficult because it is an unexpected event. The majority (80%) of children's deaths are due to accidents, suicides, or homicides (U.S. National Center for Health Statistics, 2000); in other words, most children do not suffer from an illness that might forewarn the parents of their child's impending death. Children usually outlive their parents, and thus, in most cases, parents do not anticipate that they will experience their own child's death. Research on anticipatory grieving indicates that forewarning of the death often improves affect and functioning later (Frederick & Loewenstein, 1999). Even when a child's death is anticipated, however, experiencing the death of a child is often associated with permanent and dramatic declines in subjective well-being.

Clearly, losing a child can be negatively related to subjective well-being; on the flip side, a high-quality relationship with a child can be positively related to subjective well-being. In fact, relationship quality with one's children may be a better predictor of subjective well-being than status as a parent per se. A meta-analysis of 286 studies on the associations between social networks and subjective well-being in later life showed that higher-quality relations with adult children were significantly associated with greater life satisfaction, and these effects were stronger for women than for men (Pinquart & Sorensen, 2000). High-quality relationships with adult children were more strongly related to subjective well-being than was quantity of contact. These results show that just having children does not protect against loneliness or depression, but rather, the benefits of children are conditional on having a good-quality relationship with them. It appears that having a close, emotionally supportive relationship with adult children is associated with greater subjective well-being.

Sibling Relationships and Subjective Well-Being

Sibling relationships are unique in that they are often the longest lasting relationships that individuals have, continuing from the birth of the younger sibling until the death of one of them. Siblings can serve as sources of support (e.g., Dunn, 1996) as well as sources of conflict and negativity (e.g., De Hart, 1999). Furthermore, sibling relationships are important sources of socialization in many children's lives (Dunn, 1996), and children may learn to negotiate conflict and competition (Volling, 2003), as well as experience companionship and warmth, with their brothers and sisters. For example, Cicirelli (1980) found that college women perceived as much emotional support from their closest sibling as they did from their mothers. Despite the salience of sibling relationships for many individuals, the majority of research on close relationships in childhood has focused on parent–child relationships and peer relationships. However, researchers are increasingly recognizing the importance of sibling relationships and designing studies to examine their influences on development. Most research has focused on the association between sibling relationships and outcomes such as externalizing and internalizing symptoms, perspective taking, and cognitive skills. Little research on sibling relationships during childhood has focused on subjective well-being per se, although research on adult-sibling relationships has examined subjective well-being.

Research on Only Children

Similar to the literature on parent–child relationships, one issue in the literature on siblings is whether the presence of siblings, by itself, is associated with greater subjective well-being. The stereotype of only children is that they are lonely and isolated. One might expect, then, that they would have lower levels of subjective well-being. However, research does not support this view. Studies of only children tend to show no differences in emotional well-being, or they show differences that favor only children. For example, in a sample of Dutch adolescents, Veenhoven and Verkuyten (1989) found that only children did not differ from children with siblings in terms of life satisfaction or mood. A meta-analysis of 141 studies (Polit & Falbo, 1987) showed that only children were better adjusted than individuals who were middle-born. Adjustment included a variety of categories, including measures of anxiety and self-esteem, teachers' ratings of negative affect and contentment, and the studies included a wide range of ages (mean age 17 years). Thus, it appears that individuals are not disadvantaged emotionally by being only children. They likely form other close relationships that provide support, and they are not subject to the conflict and rivalry that can lower subjective well-being in sibling relationships.

Sibling Relationship Quality and Subjective Well-Being

A second issue is how sibling relationship quality is associated with subjective well-being. Evidence of a positive relationship between sibling and greater subjective well-being is mixed. Sibling relationships, at least in childhood, tend to be marked by greater conflict and negativity than relationships with peers (e.g., Volling, Youngblade, & Belsky, 1997). There are notable individual differences in the emotional qualities of sibling relationships (see Volling, 2003, for a review). Some sibling relationships are characterized by intimacy and support, whereas others are marked by hostility, aggression, and rivalry. The degree to which sibling relationships predict outcomes seems to depend on their level of warmth and conflict. The next section reviews research on the associations among socioemotional development and sibling relationships, organized by age.

Sibling Relationships during Childhood

Sibling relationships during childhood are associated with children's individual adjustment (see Brody, 1998, for a review). Findings converge to suggest that high hostility in sibling relationships, especially in combination with low warmth, is associated with poor socioemotional adjustment. For example, Hetherington (1988) showed that brothers in relationships characterized by high conflict and low warmth showed less positive peer relations and more externalizing problems than brothers in high-conflict but high-warmth relationships. Similarly, Stormshak, Bellanti, and Bierman (1996) demonstrated that children in sibling relationships involving moderate levels of conflict and warmth showed better adjustment than did children in sibling relationships characterized by high conflict and low warmth. Pike, Coldwell, and Dunn (2005) examined 101 families with two children between the ages of 4 and 8 years. They found that sibling relationship quality was associated with the older siblings' adjustment, even after controlling for the quality of the relationship with parents (that is, they controlled for the "spillover" effect). Positive (but not negative) sibling behavior was associated with greater prosocial behavior and better adjustment (i.e., fewer emotional symptoms, conduct problems, and peer problems). Other research has demonstrated that sibling behavior during the preschool period is associated with adjustment 7 years later, during middle childhood. More specifically, more negative and less positive relationships with a sibling during preschool were correlated with greater externalizing and internalizing behavior later (Dunn, Slomkowski, Beardsall, & Rende, 1994). Deater-Deckard, Dunn, and Lussier (2002) examined the associations among 5-year-olds' relationships with siblings and their socioemotional adjustment within different family types (i.e., single mother, married parents, and stepfamilies). They found that sibling negativity was related to greater internalizing and externalizing behavior for children with married parents, but not for children in stepparent or single-mother families. The data comparing sibling relationships in various family constellations are cross-sectional, so it is unclear what accounts for this pattern of findings. However, there seems to be some evidence that older siblings can buffer younger siblings in situations of high parental conflict and divorce (Jenkins, 1992).

In summary, the quality of sibling relationships seems to be related to children's well-being, as defined in terms of emotional adjustment and externalizing behavior. However, little research has examined subjective well-being directly in relation to sibling relations.

Adolescent-Sibling Relationships and Well-Being

Although sibling relationships become less emotionally intense in adolescence (Dunn, Deater-Deckard, Pickering, & Golding,1999), ratings of intimacy, affection, and admiration among siblings remain relatively high. Furthermore, adolescents still spend about 13% of their time with their siblings (Kleiber, Larson, & Csikszentmihalyi, 1986). Thus, they likely remain important relationships that may be associated with adolescent subjective well-being. Seginer (1998) examined adolescents' relationships with peers, parents, and older siblings and found that positive sibling relationships were associated with satisfaction with social support, independent of perceived support. Furthermore, adolescents who experienced low peer acceptance but high sibling warmth and closeness were just as satisfied with their emotional support as adolescents experiencing high peer acceptance. Thus, sibling relationships seemed to compensate for poor peer acceptance. In a longitudinal study examining sibling relationships and problematic behaviors, Branje, van Lieshout, van Aken, and Haselager (2004) found that greater sibling support was associated concurrently with fewer externalizing problems. Sibling problem behavior was related to greater internalizing behavior, regardless of whether the sibling was older or younger. Moser and Jacob (2002) found that conflict in sibling relationships significantly predicted adolescent internalizing behavior, even after controlling for parenting behavior. Although these sibling studies did not address subjective well-being directly, they provide some insight into the association between sibling relationships and emotional well-being.

Having a sibling sets up the possibility that parents will treat their children differently. Children use the parents' behavior as a barometer indicating the extent to which they feel loved or rejected by their parents (Brody, 2004). Children in the same family make social comparisons between their own and their siblings' treatment by their parents. Children and adolescents who believe they unfairly receive less warmth or more negativity from their parents, relative to their siblings, show poorer emotional functioning (e.g., Kowal, Kramer, Krull, & Crick, 2002; Reiss, Neiderhiser, Hetherington, & Plomin, 2000). For example, children who reported receiving equal affection also reported greater self-worth and greater satisfaction with their parent–child relationships when compared to those who reported receiving differential affection (McHale, Crouter, McGuire, & Updegraff, 1995). Thus, another way that siblings may affect children is by the perception of unfair or unjustified differential treatment, which children use as evidence that they are not valued or worthy of love (Brody, 2004). This sense of rejection may be associated with lower levels of emotional well-being and higher levels of negative affect. For example, in a large, multimethod, multimeasure longitudinal study of adolescents, greater negativity and less warmth directed to a child, relative to the sibling, predicted greater depressive symptoms, even after accounting for the absolute levels of hostility and warmth directed at the child (Feinberg & Hetherington, 2001). Furthermore, the effects of differential treatment seemed to be most pronounced for children experiencing greater absolute levels of negativity or low levels of warmth. In addition, perceived favoritism predicts negative outcomes in the sibling who is not favored. For example, experiencing perceived disfavoritism has been associated with greater anxiety and fear in children with a sibling with cancer (Cairns, Clark, Smith, & Lansky, 1979); anxiety and depression in children with a disabled sibling (McHale & Gamble, 1989); depression and anger in adolescents (Harris & Howard, 1984); and more frequent shame and more intense fear in undergraduates (Brody, Copeland, Sutton, Richardson, & Guyer, 1998).

Although the data about differential treatment or perceived differential treatment and associated negative outcomes are substantial, most studies have used correlational designs, and the direction of causality cannot be determined. It may that child characteristics evoke certain kinds of treatment from parents. For example, depressed children may evoke higher levels of negativity and less warmth from their parents. Moreover, advances in understanding social comparisons may shed greater light on how differences in perceptions and upward and downward comparisons with siblings may be associated with children's and adolescents' subjective well-being. This area, as with several mentioned above, deserves further research.

Adult-Sibling Relationships and Well-Being

Sibling relationships remain important in adulthood. Circirelli (1989) found that closeness with sisters was related to less depression in both men and women (mean age of respondents, 72 years); in addition, closeness with brothers was related to less depression for men (but not for women). Women's perceptions of conflict in their relationships with sisters was related to greater depression (Circirelli, 1989). Taken together, these findings suggest that close sibling relationships are related to better mental health, and conflict with siblings is related to more problems with well-being, although there is some evidence that close relationships with sisters are more beneficial to well-being than close relationships with brothers (Cicirelli, 1989; McGhee, 1985).

Some studies show that frequency of interaction with siblings is unrelated to well-being in old age (Lee & Ihinger-Tallman, 1980). However, other studies show that siblings are associated with greater well-being in older adults (see Cicirelli, 1991, for review). O'Bryant (1988) found that widows' interaction with their married sisters was associated with greater positive affect. Shortt and Gottman (1997) demonstrated in a laboratory setting, that close sibling relationships during young adulthood are associated with greater positive affect. Moreover, close siblings showed greater emotion regulation in terms of lower levels of physiological reactivity in a conflictual discussion than did distant siblings, suggesting that close sibling relationships may buffer individuals from the effects of stress and negative affect.

Romantic Relationships and Subjective Well-Being

The majority of the people worldwide develop a close relationship with a spouse in marriage, and it is well-documented that marriage is related to greater subjective well-being (Diener et al., 1999). Most research shows that married people are happier than never-married, divorced, separated, or widowed individuals (e.g., Argyle, 2001; Glenn & Weaver, 1979; Gove, Style, & Hughes, 1990; Myers, 1992; Diener & Seligman, 2002). Furthermore, many of these studies include large, representative samples. A 1985 meta-analysis concluded that marriage was modestly and positively related to subjective well-being (Haring-Hidore, Stock, Okun, & Witter, 1985). Data from the World Values Survey II showed that across most nations examined ($n = 43$), married people experienced greater life satisfaction, more positive emotions and fewer negative emotions than divorced people (Diener, Gohm, Suh, & Oishi, 2000). Furthermore, the ending of a romantic relationship in the form of a divorce has a well-documented effect of distress (Johnson & Wu, 2002; Hope, Rodgers, & Power, 1999). In a cross-sectional study Kamp Dush and Amato (2005) showed that being in a romantic relationship (either with a spouse, a cohabiting partner, or a steady dating partner) was associated with greater subjective well-being, compared to single individuals not dating or individuals dating multiple people. Moreover, the greater the commitment in the relationship, the greater the association between the romantic relationship and subjective well-being. Even after controlling for relationship quality, married individuals still had the highest levels of subjective well-being.

A number of explanations have been proposed for the association between marriage and subjective well-being, and these explanations are not mutually exclusive. The first is that there is a selection effect. The idea here is that people have certain psychological characteristics that predispose them to experience marital events; thus, subjective well-being may, in part, cause certain marital events, such as entering a marriage or divorcing. That is, happy people are more likely to successfully attract and retain a mate, whereas unhappy people may be less likely to find a mate, and if they do find a mate, they may be more likely to subsequently divorce. The second explanation is a social role one. An unmarried status is associated with different types of hardships, such as decreased sources of social support and financial troubles. Married people may have greater practical and emotional support than divorced people, and divorced people are less likely than married people to have strong social support networks and are more likely to experience financial strain. Spouses provide material support, social support, and a source of shared enjoyable activities (Argyle & Martin, 1991). Furthermore, marriage receives a great deal of support from the wider community, for example, from religious institutions, the government, the legal system, etc. The third explanations is the crisis or event explanation, which involves the proposal that marital transitions may cause short-term changes in subjective well-being, but these changes should dissipate when time since the event (e.g., the marriage or the divorce) has been accounted for. According to this explanation, people eventually adapt to their current life circumstances, and their subjective well-being returns to initial levels. As can be seen from these differing explanations, the direction of causality between subjective well-being and marital status is still under debate (Diener et al., 1999). Support for each of these explanations is discussed below.

Longitudinal evidence suggests that selection effects do occur—happier people are more likely to marry and stay married (e.g., Mastekaasa, 1992). However, it is likely that marriage also has protective effects against stress and thereby generates positive well-being (Kessler & Essex, 1982). Thus, bidirectional effects are likely among subjective well-being and marital status.

Support for all three explanations for the association between subjective well-being and marital status can be found in a recent longitudinal study of a nationally representative sample of 30,000 Germans (Lucas, 2005). He showed that lower levels of happiness found during a baseline period of marriage predicted marriages that divorced later. Moreover, people who got married and stayed married were more satisfied with life even well before the marriage occurred. These findings are evidence for selection effects. He also found positive effects of marriage beyond selection effects. Long-term levels of satisfaction after divorce were lower than long-term levels of satisfaction before divorce, indicating that satisfaction did not return to baseline levels following divorce. Some adaptation occurred, but it was not complete. Thus, the relationship between divorce and life satisfaction appears to be due to both preexisting differences and lasting changes following divorce.

The findings on divorce point to the downside of romantic relationships: When they end, there is often an accompanying decrease in subjective well-being. For example, widowhood is associated with lower subjective well-being, and this effect is largest in recent widows (Mastekaasa, 1994). Mastekaasa argues that lower levels of subjective well-being found in recent widows is a temporary effect, and that 3 years or more after the death of a spouse, widows are just as high on subjective well-being as married individuals. However, Mastekaasa's data are cross-sectional, and longitudinal data do not support these conclusions. The Lucas (2005) study, reviewed above, indicates that adaptation to divorce is not complete. This study is strong because it is a longitudinal study, so it can control for preexisting differences in subjective well-being between those who divorced and those who did not. Although people in that study did adapt to divorce somewhat, after about 5 years that adaptation leveled off and did not reach levels of satisfaction that were as high as those during marriage. Similarly, Lucas, Clark, Georgellis, and Diener (2003) found that adaptation to widowhood occurred very gradually over a period of 8 years (a substantial period of time) and never returned to initial baseline levels. They demonstrated that there were large individual differences in the extent to which marital transitions affected an individual's subjective well-being. The most satisfied people reacted most negatively to divorce and widowhood and least positively to marriage.

Moderators of the Associations between Marriage and Subjective Well-Being

Although the relationship between subjective well-being and marriage is well established, the effect sizes are small. These effect sizes may appear small because other factors may moderate the relationship between marriage and subjective well-being. One of these factors is culture (Diener et al., 2000). There are cross-national differences in the extent to which marriage is associated with subjective well-being (Lucas & Dyrenforth, 2005). Both the World Values Survey and the General Social Survey indicate that in the United States, marriage is positively associated with subjective well-being. Effect sizes are modest, rs around .20. However, results from the World Values Survey also indicate that the association between marriage and subjective well-being differs by nation. For example, in other countries (e.g., Latvia in 1995) marriage was negatively associated with subjective well-being (Lucas & Dyrenforth, 2005). The benefit of being married over divorced was smaller in collectivist countries than in individualist nations (Diener et al., 2000).

Timing theories suggest that the timing of life events is also an important moderator of the relationship with subjective well-being. If events such as widowhood occur at a usual time, they may have less of an effect on subjective well-being than if they occur at an unusual time (Hagestad, 1986). In fact, Diener and

Suh (1998) showed that social expectations played a role in the association between marriage and life satisfaction. They found, consistent with other research (George, Okun, & Landerman, 1985), that widowhood was more strongly associated with lower life satisfaction in younger people than in older people. Thus, the effects of marriage on life satisfaction may vary on the basis of one's social expectations. Older women may expect to outlive their husbands, whereas younger women may expect their husbands to share their future. When marital transitions violate expectations, they may have more of a negative impact on subjective well-being.

There is also some evidence that marriage impacts subjective well-being differently for men and women. Women may benefit less from marriage than men (Argyle & Martin, 1991; Diener et al., 1999), although this issue is still open to debate. Some studies show that the relations between marital status and subjective well-being are similar for men and women (e.g., Mastekaasa, 1994). Other studies show that men may benefit more (e.g., Gove et al., 1990). If men do benefit more, this may be because women serve as better confidants than do men (Argyle & Martin, 1991). In conclusion, one probable reason that effect sizes are modest is that other factors, such as timing, culture, age, and marital quality, moderate the association between marriage and subjective well-being.

Family Relationships in Old Age

Although social interaction declines over old age, it appears that social relationships become increasingly satisfying, and that older adults are less lonely than young and middle-age adults (Lang & Carstensen, 1994). According to socioemotional selectivity theory, individuals emphasize different functions of social relationships over the life course. One function of relationships is emotion regulation and affective rewards, another is information gain, and a third function is the potential for future contact (Fredrickson & Carstensen, 1990). Goals surrounding information gain and future social contact seem to be most salient for adolescents, whereas elderly people emphasize affective rewards to a greater extent than information gain and future social contact. That is, as individuals become knowledgeable about the world over their lifespan, they have less need to seek information from social partners and increasingly focus on deriving emotional meaning from them. As such, older adults seek interactions with fewer close partners, as opposed to a wider range of mere acquaintances, who are less likely to provide the emotionally meaningful relationships that older adults desire (Carstensen, 1992).

Empirical research provides support for this theory about the changing nature of relationships over the life course. For example, both European American and African American older people have social networks composed of many emotionally close relationships, such as spouses and children, and fewer distal relationships, such as acquaintances, than do younger adults (Fung, Carstensen, & Lang, 2001). In a longitudinal study using interviews with participants when they were 18, 30, 40, and 52 years, patterns of interaction frequency, emotional closeness, and satisfaction were rated for various relationships (Carstensen, 1992). Satisfaction, emotional closeness, and frequency of interaction for sibling relationships increased from age 30 to 40 years. Similarly, interaction frequency, emotional closeness, and satisfaction with parents increased from age 18 to 50 years. In contrast, significant decreases were observed in interaction and satisfaction with acquaintances over time. In a sample of older adults, ages 70–104 years old, people with nuclear family members felt more socially embedded than individuals who did not have nuclear family members (i.e., a spouse or children; Lang & Carstensen, 1994). These findings suggest that individuals' social partners become increasingly selected, that these social partners become more satisfying and emotionally close over the adult life course, and that these close relationships are often with family members (Carstensen, 1992). As adults age, they appear to invest more in close relationships that provide affective gains, and they reduce interactions with casual acquaintances who provide fewer affective rewards.

Conclusion

Our review of the research suggests that close family relationships are associated with direct measures of subjective well-being and with less direct indicators throughout the lifespan. The type of familial relationship that is central to well-being depends upon the need at various developmental levels, such that parent–child relationships are central in infancy and early childhood, and over the lifespan, other relationships, such as romantic relationships, become important.

Despite the research reviewed here, which indicates that close family relationships tend to be a correlate of subjective well-being, family relationships provide only one window to subjective well-being, which is multiply determined. Most of the research we have discussed, with a few exceptions, is correlational, and the direction of causality cannot be determined. It is tempting to draw conclusions such as "close relationships affect individuals' subjective well-being," but it is also likely that individuals' levels of subjective well-being impact their relationships with others. For example, it may be that it is more difficult to establish a secure attachment relationship with an infant who is very irritable (van den Boom, 1994), and it may be more difficult to be happily married if an individual is neurotic and disagreeable. Thus, effects are likely bidirectional. Furthermore, relatively little research has examined the mechanisms by which relationships and subjective well-being are associated. More research is needed to elucidate these processes. Understanding the process by which relationships affect subjective well-being is important for creating appropriate interventions.

In order to thoroughly explicate the processes by which close family relationships and subjective well-being are related, more research is needed on the moderating influence of other factors. Temperament, emotion regulation strategies, age, and gender all may moderate the effects of these relationships on well-being. Moreover, subjective well-being may itself be a moderator of other outcomes. For example, Suldo and Huebner (2004) showed that authoritative parenting predicted adolescents' perceived quality of life, but also that perceived quality of life mediated the link between parenting practices and adolescents' internalizing and externalizing behaviors. Not only is subjective well-being important as an outcome variable, but it may also be important as a pathway through which social relationships predict other behavioral outcomes (Huebner et al., 2004).

The bulk of the research reviewed here is cross-sectional in nature and largely based upon self-report measures. The direction of causality is unknown, and it may be that in the case of family relationships, the same characteristics that promote positive relationship qualities also promote well-being, and these characteristics may have a genetic basis. Thus, future research should include more longitudinal studies, as well considering how genetic and relationship factors interact to produce well-being. Finally, given the reliance on self-report measures, research using multimethod measurement using latent variables is needed in order to determine the effects that method variance may have on the results described here.

References

Allen, J. P., McElhaney, K. B., Kuperminc, G. P., & Jodl, K. M. (2004). Stability and change in attachment security across adolescence. *Child Development, 75,* 1792–1805.

Ainsworth, M. S. (1979). Infant–mother attachment. *America Psychologist, 34,* 932–937.

Ainsworth, M. S., Blehar, M. C., Waters, E., & Wall, S. (1978). *Patterns of attachment: A psychological study of the strange situation.* Oxford, UK: Erlbaum.

Amato, P. R. (1994). Father–child relations, mother–child relations, and offspring psychological well-being in early adulthood. *Journal of Marriage and the Family, 56,* 1031–1042.

Antonucci, T. C., Akiyama, H., & Lansford, J. E. (1998). Negative effects of close social relationships. *Family Relations, 47,* 379–384.

Arend, R., Gove, F., & Sroufe, L. A. (1979). Continuity of individual adaptation from infancy to kindergarten: A predictive study of ego-resiliency and curiosity in preschoolers. *Child Development, 50,* 950–960.

Argyle, M. (1991). *The psychology of happiness* (2nd ed.). New York: Routledge.

Argyle, M., & Martin, M. (1991). The psychological causes of happiness. In F. Strack, M. Argyle, & N. Schwarz (Eds.), *Subjective well-being: An interdisciplinary perspective* (pp. 77–100). Elmsford, NY: Pergamon Press.

Baumeister, R., & Leary, M. R. (1995). The need to belong: Desire for interpersonal attachments as a fundamental human motivation. *Psychological Bulletin, 117,* 497–529.

Belsky, J., & Cassidy, J. (1994). Attachment: Theory and evidence. In M. Rutter & D. Hay (Eds.), *Development through life* (pp. 373–402). Oxford, UK: Blackwell.

Belsky, J., Spritz, B., & Crnic, K. (1996). Infant attachment security and affective–cognitive information processing at age 3. *Psychological Science, 7,* 111–114.

Ben-Zur, H. (2003). Happy adolescents: The link between subjective well-being, internal resources, and parental factors. *Journal of Youth and Adolescence, 32,* 67–79.

Biswas-Diener, R., & Diener, E. (2001). Making the best of a bad situation: Satisfaction in the slums of Calcutta. *Social Indicators Research, 55,* 329–352.

Bohlin, G., Hagekull, B., & Rydell, A. M. (2000). Attachment and social functioning: A longitudinal study from infancy to middle childhood. *Social Development, 9,* 24–39.

Booth, A., & Amato, P. (1991). Divorce and psychological stress. *Journal of Health and Social Behavior, 32,* 396–407.

Booth, C. L., Rubin, K. H., & Rose-Krasnor, L. (1998). Perceptions of emotional support from mother and friend in middle childhood: Links with social–emotional adaptation and preschool attachment security. *Child Development, 69,* 427–442.

Bowlby, J. (1969). *Attachment and loss: Vol. 1. Attachment.* New York: Basic Books.

Branje, S. J. T., van Lieshout, C. F. M., van Aken, M. A. G., & Haselager, G. J. T. (2004). Perceived support in sibling relationships and adolescent adjustment. *Journal of Child Psychology and Psychiatry, 45,* 1385–1396.

Brody, G. H. (1998). Sibling relationship quality: Its causes and consequences. *Annual Review of Psychology, 49,* 1–24.

Brody, G. H. (2004). Siblings' direct and indirect contributions to child development. *Current Directions in Psychological Science, 13,* 124–126.

Brody, L. R., Copeland, A. P., Sutton, L. S., Richardson, D. R., & Guyer, M. (1998). Mommy and Daddy like you best: Perceived family favouritism in relation to affect, adjustment, and family process. *Journal of Family Therapy, 20,* 269–291.

Cairns, N. U., Clark, G. M., Smith, S. D., & Lansky, S. B. (1979). Adaptation of siblings to childhood malignancy. *Journal of Pediatrics, 95,* 484–487.

Calkins, S., & Fox, N. A. (1992). The relations among infant temperament, security of attachment and behavioral inhibition at 24 months. *Child Development, 63,* 1456–1472.

Campbell, A., Converse, P. E., & Rodgers, W. L. (1976). *The quality of American life.* New York: Sage.

Carstensen, L. L. (1992). Social and emotional patterns in adulthood: Support for socioemotional selectivity theory. *Psychology and Aging, 7,* 331–338.

Cassidy, J. (1994). Emotion regulation: Influences of attachment relationships. In N. A. Fox (Ed.), The development of emotion regulation: Biological and behavioral considerations. *Monographs of the Society for Research in Child Development, 59*(240), 228–249.

Cicirelli, V. G. (1980). A comparison of college women's feelings toward their siblings and parents. *Journal of Marriage and the Family, 42,* 111–118.

Cicirelli, V. G. (1989). Feelings of attachment to siblings and well-being in later life. *Psychology and Aging, 4,* 211–216.

Cicirelli, V. G. (1991). Sibling relationships in adulthood. *Marriage and Family Review, 16,* 291–310.

Connidis, I. A., & McMullin, J. A. (1993). To have or have not: Parent status and the subjective well-being of older men and women. *Gerontologist, 33,* 630–636.

Contreras, J. M., Kerns, K. A., Weimer, B. L., Gentzler, A. L., & Tomich, P. L. (2000). Emotion regulation as a mediator of associations between mother–child attachment and peer relationships in middle childhood. *Journal of Family Psychology, 14,* 111–124.

Deater-Deckard, K., Dunn, J., & Lussier, G. (2002). Sibling relationships and socioemotional adjustment in different family contexts. *Social Development, 11,* 571–590.

De Hart, G. B. (1999). Conflict and averted conflict in preschoolers' interactions with siblings and friends. In W. A. Collins & B. Laursen (Eds.), *Relationships as developmental contexts; The Minnesota symposia on child psychology* (Vol. 30, pp. 281–303). Mahwah, NJ: Erlbaum.

Demo, D. H., & Acock, A. C. (1996). Family structure, family process, and adolescent well-being. *Journal of Research on Adolescence, 6,* 457–488.

Diener, E. (1984). Subjective well-being. *Psychological Bulletin, 95,* 542–575.

Diener, E., & Diener, M. L. (1995). Cross-cultural correlates of life satisfaction. *Journal of Personality and Social Psychology, 68,* 653–663.

Diener, E., Gohm, C. L., Suh, E., & Oishi, S. (2000). Similarity of the relations between marital status and subjective well-being across cultures. *Journal of Cross-Cultural Psychology, 31,* 419–436.

Diener, E., & Seligman, M. E. P. (2002). Very happy people. *Psychological Science, 13,* 81–84.

Diener, E., & Suh, E. M. (1998). Subjective well-being and age: An international analysis. In K. W. Schaie & M. P. Lawton (Eds.), *Annual review of gerontology and geriatrics: Vol. 17. Focus on emotion and adult development* (pp. 304–324). New York: Spring.

Diener, E., Suh, E. M., Lucas, R. E., & Smith, H. L. (1999). Subjective well-being: Three decades of progress. *Psychological Bulletin, 125,* 276–302.

Diener, M. L., Isabella, R. A., Behunin, M., & Wong, M. S. (in press). Attachment to mothers and fathers during middle childhood: Associations with child gender, grade, and competence. *Social Development.*

Diener, M. L., Mangelsdorf, S. C., McHale, J. L., & Frosch, C. (2002). Infants' behavioral strategies for emotion regulation with mothers and fathers: Associations with emotional expressions and attachment quality. *Infancy, 5,* 151–172.

Ducharme, J., Doyle, A. B., & Markiewicz, D. (2002). Attachment security with mother and father: Associations with adolescents' reports of interpersonal behavior with parents and peers. *Journal of Social and Personal Relationships, 19,* 203–231.

Dunn, J. (1996). Brothers and sisters in middle childhood and adolescence: Continuity and change in individual differences. In G. Brody (Ed.), *Sibling relationships: Their causes and consequences* (pp. 31–46). Norwood, NJ: Ablex.

Dunn, J., Deater-Deckard, K., Pickering, K., & Golding, J. (1999). Siblings, parents, and partners: Family relationships with in a longitudinal community study. *Journal of Child Psychology and Psychiatry, 40*, 1025–1037.

Dunn, J., Slomkowski, C., Beardsall, L., & Rende, R. (1994). Adjustment in middle childhood and early adolescence: Links with earlier and contemporary sibling relationships. *Journal of Child Psychology and Psychiatry, 35*, 491–504.

Dyregrov, A. (1990). Parental reactions to the loss of an infant child: A review. *Scandinavian Journal of Psychology, 31*, 266–280.

Emmons, R. A. (2003). Personal goals, life meaning, and virtue: Wellsprings of a positive life. In C. L. M. Keyes & J. Haidt (Eds.), *Flourishing: Positive psychology and the life well-lived* (pp. 105–128). Washington, DC: American Psychological Association.

Erickson, M., Sroufe, L. A., & Egeland, B. (1985). The relationship between quality of attachment and behavior problems in preschool in a high-risk sample. *Monographs of the Society for Research in Child Development, 50*(1–2, Serial No. 209), 147–166.

Feinberg, M., & Hetherington, E. M. (2001). Differential parenting as a within-family variable. *Journal of Family Psychology, 15*, 22–37.

Finch, J. F., Okun, M. A., Barrera, M., Zautra, A. J., & Reich, J. W. (1989). Positive and negative social ties among older adults: Measurement models and the prediction of psychological distress and well-being. *American Journal of Community Psychology, 17*, 585–605.

Frederick, S., & Loewenstein, G. (1999). Hedonic adaptation. In D. Kahneman, E. Diener, & N. Schwarz (Eds.), *Well-being: The foundations of hedonic psychology* (pp. 302–329). New York: Sage.

Fredrickson, B. L. (2002). Positive emotions. In C. R. Synder & S. L. Lopez (Eds.), *Handbook of positive psychology* (pp. 120–134). New York: Oxford University Press.

Fredrickson, B. L., & Carstensen, L. L. (1990). Choosing social partners: How old age and anticipated endings make people more selective. *Psychology and Aging, 5*, 335–347.

Fung, H. H., Carstensen, L. L., & Lang, F. R. (2001). Age-related patterns in social networks among European Americans and African Americans: Implications for socioemotional selectivity across the life span. *International Journal of Aging and Human Development, 52*, 185–206.

Glenn, N. D., & Weaver, C. N. (1988). The changing relationship of marital status to reported happiness. *Journal of Marriage and the Family, 50*, 317–324.

Goldsmith, H. H., & Alansky, J. A. (1987). Maternal and infant temperamental predictors of attachment: A meta-analytic review. *Journal of Consulting and Clinical Psychology, 55*, 805–816.

Goldsmith, H. H., & Harman, C. (1994). Temperament and attachment: Individuals and relationships. *Current Directions in Psychological Science, 3*, 53–57.

Gove, W. R., Hughes, M., & Style, C. B. (1983). Does marriage have positive effects on the psychological well-being of the individual? *Journal of Health and Social Behavior, 24*, 122–131.

Gove, W. R., Style, C. B., & Hughes, M. (1990). The effect of marriage on the well-being of adults: A theoretical analysis. *Journal of Family Issues, 11*, 4–35.

Hagestad, G. O. (1986). Dimensions of time and the family. *American Behavioral Scientist, 29*, 679–694.

Haring-Hidore, M., Stock, W. A., Okun, M. A., & Witter, R. A. (1985). Marital status and subjective well-being: A research synthesis. *Journal of Marriage and Family, 47,* 947–953.

Harris, I. D., & Howard, K. I. (1984). Correlates of perceived parental favoritism. *Journal of Genetic Psychology, 146,* 45–56.

Hetherington, E. M. (1988). Coping with family transitions: Winners, losers, and survivors. *Child Development, 60,* 1–14.

Hope, S., Rodgers, B., & Power, C. (1999). Marital status transitions and psychological distress: Longitudinal evidence from a national population sample. *Psychological Medicine, 29,* 381–389.

Huebner, E. S. (1991). Correlates of life satisfaction in children. *School Psychology Quarterly, 6,* 103–111.

Huebner, E. S., Suldo, S. M., Smith, L. C., & McKnight, C. G. (2004). Life satisfaction in children and youth: Empirical foundations and implications for school psychologists. *Psychology in the Schools, 41,* 81–93.

Jenkins, J. (1992). Sibling relationships in disharmonious homes: Potential difficulties and protective effects. In F. Boer & J. Dunn (Eds.), *Children's sibling relationships: Developmental and clinical issues* (pp. 125–138). Hillsdale, NJ: Erlbaum.

Johnson, D. R., & Wu, J. (2002). An empirical test of crisis, social selection, and role explanations of the relationship between marital disruption and psychological distress: A pooled time-series analysis of four-wave panel data. *Journal of Marriage and the Family, 63,* 211–224.

Kamp Dush, C. M., & Amato, P. R. (2005). Consequences of relationships status and quality for subjective well-being. *Journal of Social and Personal Relationships, 22,* 607–627.

Kasser, T., & Ryan, R. M. (1996). Further examining the American dream: Differential correlates of intrinsic and extrinsic goals. *Personality and Social Psychology Bulletin, 22,* 80–87.

Kerns, K. A. (1994). A longitudinal examination of links between mother–child attachment and children's friendships in early childhood. *Journal of Social and Personal Relationships, 11,* 379–381.

Kessler, R. C., & Essex, M. (1982). Marital status and depression: The importance of coping resources. *Social Forces, 61,* 484–507.

Keyes, C. L. M. (1998). Social well-being. *Social Psychology Quarterly, 61,* 121–140.

Kleiber, D., Larson, R., & Csikszentmihalyi, M. (1986). The experience of leisure in adolescence. *Journal of Leisure Research, 18,* 169–176.

Koropeckyj-Cox, T. (2002). Beyond parental status: Psychological well-being in middle and old age. *Journal of Marriage and Family, 64,* 957–971.

Kowal, A., Kramer, L., Krull, J. L., & Crick, N. R. (2002). Children's perceptions of the fairness of parental preferential treatment and their socioemotional well-being. *Journal of Family Psychology, 16,* 297–306.

Laible, D. J., & Thompson, R. A. (1998). Attachment and emotional understanding in preschool children. *Developmental Psychology, 34,* 1038–1045.

Landau, R., & Litwin, H. (2001). Subjective well-being among the old-old: The role of health, personality, and social support. *International Journal of Aging and Human Development, 52,* 265–280.

Lang, F. R., & Carstensen, L. L. (1994). Close emotional relationships in later life: Further support for proactive aging in the social domain. *Psychology and Aging, 9,* 315–324.

Lang, F. R., & Schutze, Y. (2002). Adult children's supportive behaviors and older parents' subjective well-being: A developmental perspective on intergenerational relationships. *Journal of Social Issues, 58,* 661–680.

Lee, G. R., & Ihinger-Tallman, M. (1980). Sibling interaction and morale: The effects of family relations on older people. *Research on Aging, 2,* 367–391.

Lehman, D. R., Wortman, C. B., & Williams, A. F. (1987). Long-term effects of losing a spouse or child in a motor vehicle crash. *Journal of Personality and Social Psychology, 52,* 218–231.

Lewis, M., Feiring, C., & Rosenthal, S. (2000). Attachment over time. *Child Development, 71,* 707–720.

Lucas, R. E. (2005). Time does not heal all wounds: A longitudinal study of reaction and adaptation to divorce. *Psychological Science, 16,* 945–950.

Lucas, R. E., Clark, A. E., Georgellis, Y., & Diener, E. (2003). Reexamining adaptation and the set point model of happiness: Reactions to change in marital status. *Journal of Personality and Social Psychology, 84,* 527–539.

Lucas, R. E., & Dyrenforth, P. S. (2005). The myth of marital bliss? *Psychological Inquiry, 16,* 111–115.

Malatesta, C. Z., Culver, C., Tesman, J. R., & Shepard, B. (1989). The development of emotion expression during the first two years of life. *Monographs of the Society for Research in Child Development, 54*(Serial No. 219).

Mangelsdorf, S. C., McHale, J. L., Diener, M. L., Goldstein, L. H., & Lehn, L. (2000). Infant attachment: Contributions of infant temperament and maternal characteristics. *Infant Behavior and Development, 23,* 175–196.

Maslow, A. H. (1954). *Motivation and personality.* Oxford, UK: Harper.

Mastekaasa, A. (1992). Marriage and psychological well-being: Some evidence on selection into marriage. *Journal of Marriage and the Family, 54,* 901–911.

Mastekaasa, A. (1994). The subjective well-being of the previously married: The importance of unmarried cohabitation and time since widowhood or divorce. *Social Forces, 73,* 665–692.

Matas, L., Arend, R. A., & Sroufe, L. A. (1978). Continuity in adaptation: Quality of attachment and later competence. *Child Development, 49,* 547–556.

McGhee, J. L. (1985). The effects of siblings on the life satisfaction of the rural elderly. *Journal of Marriage and the Family, 47,* 85–91.

McHale, S. M., Crouter, A. C., McGuire, S. A., & Updegraff, K. A. (1995). Congruence between mothers' and fathers' differential treatment of siblings: Links with family relations and children's well-being. *Child Development, 66,* 116–128.

McHale, S. M., & Gamble, W. C. (1989). Sibling relationships of children with disabled and nondisabled brothers and sisters. *Developmental Psychology, 25,* 421–429.

Moser, R. P., & Jacob, T. (2002). Parental and sibling effects in adolescent outcomes. *Psychological Reports, 91,* 463–479.

Myers, D. G. (1992). *The pursuit of happiness: Who is happy and why.* New York: Morrow.

Myers, D. G. (2000). The funds, friends, and faith of happy people. *American Psychologist, 55,* 56–67.

Myers, D. G. (2004). Human connections and the good life: Balancing individuality and community in public policy. In P. A. Linley & S. Joseph (Eds.), *Positive psychology in practice* (pp. 641–657). Hoboken, NJ: Wiley.

National Institute of Child Health and Human Development, Early Child Care Research Network. (2006). Infant–mother attachment classification: Risk and protection in relation to changing maternal caregiving quality. *Developmental Psychology, 42,* 38–58.

O'Bryant, S. L. (1988). Sibling support and older widows' well-being. *Journal of Marriage and Family, 50,* 173–183.

Pagel, M. D., Erdly, W. W., & Becker, J. (1987). Social networks: We get by with (and in spite of) a little help from our friends. *Journal of Personality and Social Psychology, 53,* 793–804.

Pavot, W., Diener, E., & Fujita, F. (1990). Extraversion and happiness. *Personality and Individual Differences, 11,* 1299–1306.

Perkins, H. W. (1991). Religious commitment, yuppie values, and well-being in post-collegiate life. *Review of Religious Research, 32,* 244–251.

Pike, A., Coldwell, J., & Dunn, J. F. (2005). Sibling relationships in early/middle childhood: Links with individual adjustment. *Journal of Family Psychology, 19,* 523–532.

Pinquart, M., & Sorensen, S. (2000). Influences of socioeconomic status, social network, and competence on subjective well-being in later life: A meta-analysis. *Psychology and Aging, 15,* 187–224.

Polit, D. F., & Falbo, T. (1987). Only children and personality development: A quantitative review. *Journal of Marriage and Family, 49,* 309–325.

Reis, H. T., & Gable, S. L. (2003). Toward a positive psychology of relationships. In C. L. Keyes & J. Haidt (Eds.), *Flourishing: Positive psychology and the life well-lived* (pp. 129–159). Washington, DC: American Psychological Association.

Reis, H. T., Sheldon, K. M., Gable, S. L., Roscoe, J., & Ryan, R. M. (2000). Daily well-being: The role of autonomy, competence, and relatedness. *Personality and Social Psychology Bulletin, 26,* 419–435.

Reiss, D., Neiderhiser, J. M., Hetherington, E. M., & Plomin, R. (2000). *The relationship code: Deciphering genetic and social influences on adolescent development.* Cambridge, MA: Harvard University Press.

Rook, K. S. (1992). Detrimental aspects of social relationships: Taking stock of an emerging literature. In H. O. F. Viel & U. Baumann (Eds.), *The meaning and measurement of social support* (pp. 157–169). New York: Hemisphere.

Ryff, C. D. (1995). Psychological well-being in adult life. *Current Directions in Psychological Science, 32,* 119–128.

Schneider, B. H., Atkinson, L., & Tardif, C. (2001). Child–parent attachment and children's peer relations: A quantitative review. *Developmental Psychology, 37,* 86–100.

Seginer, R. (1998). Adolescents' perceptions of relationships with older siblings in the context of other close relationships. *Journal of Research on Adolescence, 8,* 287–308.

Shortt, J. W., & Gottman, J. M. (1997). Closeness in young adult sibling relationships: Affective and physiological processes. *Social Development, 6,* 142–164.

Somers, M. D. (1993). A comparison of voluntarily child-free adults and parents. *Journal of Marriage and the Family, 55,* 643–650.

Stormshak, E. A., Bellanti, C., Bierman, K. L., & Conduct Problems Prevention Research Group. (1996). The quality of sibling relationships and the development of social competence and behavioral control in aggressive children. *Developmental Psychology, 32,* 79–89.

Suldo, S. M., & Huebner, E. S. (2004). The role of life satisfaction in the relationship between parenting styles and adolescent problem behavior. *Social Indicators Research, 66,* 165–195.

Thompson, R. A. (1998). Early sociopersonality development. In W. Damon & N. Eisenberg (Eds.), *Handbook of child psychology: Social, emotional, and personality development* (5th ed., Vol. 3, pp. 25–104). Hoboken, NJ: Wiley.

Thompson, R. A. (1999). Early attachment and later development. In J. Cassidy & P. R. Shaver (Eds.), *Handbook of attachment* (pp. 265–286). New York: Guilford Press.

Thompson, R. A. (2000). The legacy of early attachments. *Child Development, 71,* 145–152.

Urban, J., Carlson, E., Egeland, B., & Sroufe, L. A. (1991). Patterns of individual adaptation across childhood. *Development and Psychopathology, 3,* 445–460.

U.S. National Center for Health Statistics. (2000). *Deaths and death rates for the 10 leading causes of death in specified age groups, by race and sex: United States, 1998.* Washington, DC: U.S. Government Printing Office.

van den Boom, D. C. (1994). The influence of temperament and mothering on attachment and exploration: An experimental manipulation of sensitive responsiveness among lower-class mothers with irritable infants. *Child Development, 65,* 1457–1477.

Vennhoven, R., & Verkuyten, M. (1989). The well-being of only children. *Adolescence, 24,* 155–166.

Volling, B. L. (2003). Sibling relationships. In M. H. Bornstein, L. Davidson, C. L. M. Keyes, & K. A. Moore (Eds.), *Well-being: Positive development across the life course* (pp. 205–219). Mahwah, NJ: Erlbaum.

Volling, B. L., Youngblade, L. M., & Belsky, J. (1997). Young children's social relationships with siblings and friends. *American Journal of Orthopsychiatry, 67,* 102–111.

Waters, E., Wippman, J., & Sroufe, L. A. (1979). Attachment, positive affect, and competence in the peer group: Two studies in construct validation. *Child Development, 50,* 821–829.

Wenk, D., Hardesty, C. L., Morgan, C. S., & Blair, S. L. (1994). The influence of parental involvement on the well-being of sons and daughters. *Journal of Marriage and Family, 56,* 229–234.

Ziv, Y., Oppenheim, D., & Sagi-Schwartz, A. (2004). Social information processing in middle childhood: Relations to infant–mother attachment. *Attachment and Human Development, 6,* 327–348.

18

Research on Life Satisfaction of Children and Youth

Implications for the Delivery of School-Related Services

E. Scott Huebner and Carol Diener

Major school reform efforts have been undertaken in U.S. public schools during the last several decades. These efforts have emphasized academic outcomes, to the relative negative of emotional well-being and/or quality-of-life concerns (Baker, Dilly, Aupperlee, & Patil, 2003; Schalock & Alonso, 2002). As early as 1976, Epstein and McPartland argued that the evaluation of schooling should include quality-of-life variables, including life satisfaction and satisfaction with school experiences, in addition to academic performance variables (e.g., standardized achievement test scores). More recently, Rutter and Maughan's (2002) analysis of the school effectiveness literature led them to conclude that "much more attention needs to be paid to the characteristics of schools that matter most for noncognitive outcomes" (p. 469). Although the association between emotional well-being and academic outcomes is robust (Roeser, 2001), the promotion of emotionally healthy students is important in its own right (Hegarty, 1994).

The study of individual differences in students' affective reactions to schooling fits well within the general framework of subjective well-being research. *Subjective well-being* has been defined as a person's cognitive and affective evaluations of his or her life (Diener, 2000). In the Diener model, these evaluations include judgments of life satisfaction as well as emotional reactions, including frequent positive affect (e.g., joyful, alert) and infrequent negative affect (anxious, sad). The scientific study of the subjective well-being of adults has grown rapidly. In the mid-1980s, Diener (1984) reviewed the relatively substantial body of research that had accumulated to that point in time. The subsequent review of Diener, Suh, Lucas, and Smith (1999) reflected the continuing explosion of research in the area. Much progress has been made in understanding the antecedents and consequences of individual differences in adult subjective well-being.

In contrast to the study of adults, research on the subjective well-being of children and youth has lagged behind. Although there have been numerous studies of negative affect (e.g., depression) in children for many years, studies of life satisfaction and positive affect have only recently been undertaken. Although the reasons for this gap are unclear, one possibility involves the relatively later development of psychometrically sound measures of positive emotional well-being appropriate for children.

Measurement of Life Satisfaction in Children

Few measures of positive affect appropriate for children and youth have been developed, although there are some notable exceptions (e.g., Positive and Negative Affect Scale for Children [PANAS-C]: Laurent et al., 1999). Child-oriented measures of life satisfaction have been more abundant, although still limited. Gilman and Huebner (2000) reviewed the extant literature on measures of life satisfaction and concluded that although the various measures would benefit from further research, several measures were acceptable for research purposes with children and youth, beyond approximately the third grade. Overall, self-reports of global and domain-specific life satisfaction show adequate internal consistency reliability among children and youth. Life satisfaction reports also demonstrate reasonable test–retest reliability across several time frames, up to 1 year. Thus they do not likely vary from moment to moment or day to day, as do affective experiences such as moods. However, life satisfaction reports of children and youth are influenced by changes in life experiences and systematic psychosocial interventions (Farrell, Valois, & Meyer, 2003; Gilman & Handwerk, 2001).

Life satisfaction reports also show evidence of validity. They relate significantly to the reports of significant others, such as parents or teachers (Huebner, Brantley, Nagle, & Valois, 2002), as well as theoretically related constructs (see Huebner, 2004, for a review). They are weakly related to social desirability responding (Huebner, 1991). Also, self-reports of life satisfaction show acceptable psychometric properties for children and youth with mild disabilities, including emotional and learning disabilities (Griffin & Huebner, 2000; McCullough & Huebner, 2003).

Existing measures of life satisfaction have used primarily unidimensional or multidimensional models of life satisfaction. Based upon the work of Diener, Emmons, Larsen, and Griffin (1985), Huebner (1991) developed the Students' Life Satisfaction Scale (SLSS). The unidimensional SLSS is composed exclusively of context-free life satisfaction items (e.g., "I have a good life"), which allow children to use their own criteria for determining their satisfaction with life as a whole. In contrast, Huebner (1994) also developed a multidimensional life satisfaction scale for children and youth, the Multidimensional Students' Life Satisfaction Scale (MSLSS). The MSLSS assesses satisfaction with five specific life domains—family, friends, self, school, and living environment—all of which are deemed important by children from ages 8 to 18 (Seligson, Huebner, & Valois, 2003, 2005). Analogous to the domain-free measures, the school satisfaction subscale of the MSLSS is comprised of items that tap *global* perceptions of their school experiences (e.g., "I look forward to going to school"). Thus, students can utilize their own criteria (e.g., interpersonal relationships, academic content, physical characteristics of the school) to formulate their overall appraisals of their quality of school life.

Additional multidimensional measures have been developed, including the Quality of Student Life Questionnaire (Keith & Schalock, 1995), Comprehensive Quality of Life Scale—Student Version (Cummins, 1997), and Perceived Life Satisfaction Scale (Adelman, Taylor, & Nelson, 1989). Unidimensional and multidimensional life satisfaction scales offer unique information, with multidimensional measures displaying incremental concurrent and predictive validity (Haranin, Huebner, & Suldo, 2007). Multidimensional scales offer potentially important information (e.g., profiles of needs and assets) for intervention programs for enhancing life satisfaction in clinical contexts, including school-related contexts (Huebner, Gilman, & Suldo, 2007).

Importance of Global Life Satisfaction of Children

Like adults (Diener & Diener, 1996), most children and youth are satisfied with their overall lives and with important domains of their lives (e.g., family, friends, school). Although most children report satisfaction above the neutral point, few report the highest levels of life satisfaction. Adolescents who do report that they are very happy show generally positive functioning across intrapersonal, interpersonal, and school-related domains (Gilman & Huebner, 2006; Suldo & Huebner, 2006). Children who are very unhappy with their lives demonstrate pervasive difficulties, including problems with aggressive behavior, internalizing behaviors, suicidal thinking, sexual risk taking, alcohol and drug use, eating and physical health problems, and physical inactivity (see Huebner, Gilman, & Suldo, 2006, for a review). They are also more likely to be subject to victimization experiences, both physical and relational in nature (Martin & Huebner, 2007).

Research on Global Life Satisfaction of Children

Similar to studies with adults, demographic variables account for little variance in global life satisfaction reports of children and youth (see Gilman & Huebner, 2003, for a review). Global life satisfaction reports of children, above the age of 8, do not appear to differ significantly as a function of age. Life satisfaction reports do not reflect gender differences as well. Boys and girls appear equally satisfied with their lives as a whole.

The effects of socioeconomic status (SES) and ethnicity have been equivocal, with some studies suggesting that children from low-income minority backgrounds have somewhat lower life satisfaction (e.g., Huebner, Drane, & Valois, 2000; Huebner, Valois, Paxton, & Drane, 2005); however, some studies show no effects (e.g., Huebner, 1991). In a related vein, differences in neighborhoods relate to global life satisfaction. Children who live in commercial areas of cities report greater dissatisfaction than those who live in residential areas (Homel & Burns, 1989). Thus, overall, demographic variables may play a modest role in individual differences in overall life satisfaction, at least once the basic needs of children have been met.

As is the case with adults, research findings suggest that environmental experiences influence life satisfaction but do not tell the complete story. For example, McCullough, Huebner, and Laughlin (2000), in a sample of high school students, found the following correlations between life satisfaction and (1) positive daily events: .39; (2) negative daily events: −.34; (3) positive major events: .30; and (4) negative major events: −.22. Similar results have been reported in Ash and Huebner (2001). Thus, life experiences contribute moderate amounts of variance to the life satisfaction reports of children and youth; other variables appear to be necessary for a complete explanation.

Not surprisingly, the quality of children's interpersonal relationships is an important correlate of their life satisfaction. The perceived positivity of their relationships with their family is crucial from ages 8 to 18. Similarly, relationships with peers and teachers are also important for children in this age range. In a study of students in grades 4–8, trust was identified as the most salient attachment variable related to life satisfaction for both parent and peer relationships (Nickerson & Nagle, 2004). In a study of parenting behavior, adolescents indicated that perceived emotional support was a stronger predictor of life satisfaction than supervision and autonomy granting, although all three behaviors were important for early, middle, and late adolescents (Suldo & Huebner, 2004b).

Several individual difference variables are strongly associated with children's life satisfaction. Children who have a high self-esteem, internal locus of control, and emotionally stable temperaments appear to have the highest life satisfaction (Dew & Huebner, 1994; Rigby & Huebner, 2004). Interestingly, in one study, children's perceptions of internal versus external control mediated the relationships between life experiences and life satisfaction judgments (Ash & Huebner,

2001). The attribution styles of children, incorporating positive and negative attributions, also significantly predicted life satisfaction (Rigby & Huebner, 2004). Life satisfaction reports of adolescents do not relate to IQ test scores, however (Huebner & Alderman, 1993).

Finally, although there is a paucity of research on cultural effects, such factors must be considered. The multidimensionality of life satisfaction reports among children and youth in the United States shows comparability across children and youth from several other countries (e.g., Spain, South Korea). Nevertheless, some research suggests that the correlates of global life satisfaction may differ across cultures. For example, Park and Huebner (2005) found that school satisfaction was more strongly related to global life satisfaction among Korean students versus U.S. students. On the other hand, satisfaction with family experiences was equally important across the U.S. and Korean students. Grob, Little, Warner, Wearing, and Euronet (1996) found that problem-oriented coping was more strongly related to adolescents' subjective well-being for students in Western countries than for those in Eastern countries.

Much additional research is needed to explain the interrelationships among environmental circumstances, temperament, and cognitive variables, as is the case for adults (Diener et al., 1999). A variety of "ingredients" likely comprises the determinants of a given child's life satisfaction (cf. Diener & Seligman, 2002). The interactions are probably complex and accentuated by developmental differences from childhood through adolescence. Unfortunately, little attention has been paid to developmental issues in children's life satisfaction research to date.

Importance of Children's School Satisfaction

Most students report positive levels of *global* life satisfaction, as well as satisfaction with family, friends, self, school, and living environment (Huebner et al., 2000; Huebner et al., 2005). However, there is variability in satisfaction ratings across the five domains, with adolescents reporting most dissatisfaction with their school experiences. For example, in the Huebner et al. (2000) study of high school students, nearly one-quarter of the students reported dissatisfaction, with 9% describing their school experiences as "terrible."

Like children who are very dissatisfied with their lives overall, children who are very unhappy with their school experiences display pervasive adaptive difficulties across multiple life domains. Children who report that they dislike school are more likely to show a variety of disturbances, such as externalizing and internalizing behavior problems (DeSantis-King, Huebner, Suldo, & Valois, in press; Huebner & Gilman, 2006; Suldo & Huebner, 2002), including suicidal ideation (Locke & Newcomb, 2004), psychosomatic symptoms (Katja, Paivi, Marja-Terttu, & Pekka, 2002), substance use (Stevens, Freeman, Mott, Youells, & Linsey, 1993), and depression (Eamon, 2002). Students who dislike school also show differences in academic behavior and functioning, including lower grades (Epstein & McPartland, 1976; Huebner & Gilman, 2006), lower standardized test scores (Cock & Halvari, 1999), and less participation in extracurricular activities (Gilman, 2001; Huebner & Gilman, 2006). Using a longitudinal design, Ladd, Buhs, and Seid (2000) demonstrated that kindergarten students' school dissatisfaction preceded school disengagement behaviors, which in turn reduced their school achievement. This study thus addressed the directionality of the effects of school satisfaction, suggesting that it is low subjective well-being that determines a student's level of engagement, and not the reverse. Such a finding underscores the importance of students' affective reactions to schooling in relation to their academic success. Such a finding is also not inconsistent with theories of the differential functions of positive and negative emotions, such as Frederickson's (2001) broaden and build theory.

School satisfaction is related to life satisfaction, but generally in the range of .30–.40 for U.S. students (Huebner, Laughlin, Ash, & Gilman, 1998; Seligson et al., 2003). It is often the weakest correlate of the five domains, thus suggesting a degree of separability of the constructs. For this reason, studies of global or domain-free life satisfaction, in general, and school satisfaction, in particular, are reviewed separately.

Research on Children's School Satisfaction

Compared to the study of children's global life satisfaction, studies of children's school satisfaction are meager. Nevertheless, a number of important personal and environmental factors has been identified.

Similar to findings with general life satisfaction, studies of the demographic correlates of school satisfaction have revealed weak associations for most variables. Exceptions may include age/grade and gender effects. Some studies suggest that females report higher school satisfaction, although the effect sizes are modest (Huebner et al., 2000; Huebner et al., 2005). More substantial age/grade effects are suggested in studies, with significant decreases occurring between grades 1 and 8 (Chapman & McAlpine, 1988; Hirsch & Rabkin, 1987; Ito & Smith, 2005; Karatzias, Power, Flemming, Lennan, & Swanson, 2002; Okun, Braver, & Weir, 1990).

The relationship between school satisfaction and personality and/or temperament variables has received little attention. One study (Karatzias et al., 2002) showed a significant relationship between school satisfaction and positive and negative trait affect. Another study showed significant positive relationships between school engagement (i.e., absences) and openness to experience, emotional stability, and conscientiousness, and a negative relationship with agreeableness (Lounsbury, Steel, Loveland, & Gibson, 2004). School satisfaction has also been linked with locus of control (Huebner, Ash, & Laughlin, 2001), and academic and social self-esteem (Verkuyten & Thijs, 2002). The link between school satisfaction and academic self-efficacy was positive in a study involving primarily affluent, white private high school students (Huebner & McCullough, 2000), whereas it was negative in a study involving primarily low-income, black public elementary school students (Baker, 1998). Thus, this relationship may be moderated by the school environment.

A few studies of environmental correlates have also been reported. The role of interpersonal experiences in school seems crucial. Perceived quality of teacher support has been a strong correlate of school satisfaction in several studies, as has been perceived quality of classmate support (Baker, 1998; Gest, Welsh, & Domitrovich, 2005; Ito & Smith, 2005). Student–parent relationships are also associated with school satisfaction (DeSantis-King et al., in press; Rosenfeld, Richman, & Bowen, 2000).

The contribution of teacher social support may differ for students with different needs, however. For example, Leone, Luttig, Zlotlow, and Trickett (1990) found that students with behavior disorders who were placed in regular classes showed a nonsignificant relationship between their school satisfaction and teacher supportiveness, whereas students with behavior disorders who were placed in special education classes showed a significant, positive relationship.

The nature of the classroom environment has received little attention to date. One exception is a study by Felner et al. (1993), who reported increased school satisfaction among students who were paired with the same teacher and student cohort for multiple school years. Other exceptions include Baker's (1998, 1999) studies that demonstrated the importance of school climate, including classroom structure, rules, and teacher behavior. For example, Baker (1999) found relationships between school satisfaction and differences in teacher behavior. Specifically, she found that dissatisfied students received more positive teacher comments when they approached their teachers with questions about their school work. However, the dissatisfied students also received more verbal reprimands for misbehavior than their satisfied counterparts.

Characteristics of the instructional environment that influence the emotional well-being of students have also been the focus of work by Csikszentmihalyi and colleagues (e.g., Csikszentmihalyi & Schneider, 2000). Conceptually distinguishable from school satisfaction, Csikszentmihalyi's work has focused on the related concept of flow. *Flow states* are experienced when the difficulty level of a task is matched to the individual's skills so that the individual is maximally engaged in the task, rather than bored or anxious. Frequent flow states are associated with classroom activities that actively engage the learners, are relatively structured, and are perceived as meaningful and voluntary (Maton, 1990; Shernoff, Csikszentmihalyi, Schneider, & Shernoff, 2003). Although flow states are considered nonemotional at the time of occurrence, they are often described as satisfying afterward and are related to life satisfaction in adults (Peterson, Park, & Seligman, 2005). Presumably, such circumstances may apply to children as well. Notably, Wong and Csikszentmihalyi (1991) found that flow states did not influence shorter-term academic outcomes, such as grades, but did influence the difficulty level of the courses in which students enrolled during their high school years.

Although the literature is sparse, students' nonschool experiences also appear to contribute to their school satisfaction. Huebner and McCullough (2000) found that nonschool experiences (e.g., family relations, recreational activities, physical appearance concerns) were more strongly related to adolescent's school satisfaction than were school-related experiences (e.g., good grades). School satisfaction is likely affected by a variety of more distal environmental variables yet to be studied.

Taken together, the studies suggest that school satisfaction, like global life satisfaction, is a meaningful variable for children and has a wide ranging network of important life correlates. Life satisfaction appears to be meaningful to children, even as young as kindergarten, in the case of school satisfaction.

Functional Roles of Life and School Satisfaction

It is important to highlight the functional role that life satisfaction plays in adolescent behavior problems. Cross-sectional studies suggest that life satisfaction mediates the relationship between stressful life events and internalizing behavior problems of adolescents (McKnight, Huebner, & Suldo, 2002). Using a more rigorous design, the aforementioned longitudinal study of Ladd et al. (2000) supported a functional role for school satisfaction in the development of school disengagement behaviors. Furthermore, additional longitudinal research showed that adolescents who were low in life satisfaction were more likely to report symptoms of externalizing behavior problems in the future (Suldo & Huebner, 2004a). Thus, life and school satisfaction judgments are more than an epiphenomenon, they affect important outcomes.

Implications for Further Research

Research in children's school and life satisfaction is in its infancy. There are many avenues of investigation needed to advance the respective knowledge bases of these two areas. This discussion focuses on three major *overarching* needs to advance research in both areas. First, both the children's global life satisfaction and school satisfaction literatures are limited by a lack of theory-guided work.

Subsequent research efforts would benefit from attempts to situate the research in appropriate theoretical frameworks. For example, research in school satisfaction parallels that of job satisfaction and may benefit from attempts to link the two areas (Epstein & McPartland, 1976). The divergent purposes of jobs and schools necessitate recognition of the important distinctions between the contexts. Investigations of the nature of the relationships between school satisfaction and life satisfaction, within and across cultures, would be informative in their own right.

Second, research efforts in both school and life satisfaction have largely lacked a developmental focus. Much of the research highlights similarities in the determinants and consequences of life satisfaction among children and adults, failing to reflect the distinctiveness between adults and children of different ages. Developmental differences in cognitive abilities, social–emotional needs, interests, physical maturation, and so forth, suggest possible important developmental considerations. Longitudinal research would be particularly beneficial, providing the opportunity to monitor the course and development of life satisfaction determinants and sequalae and determine the directionality of relationships. For example, enhanced understanding of the interactions of temperament, acute and ongoing environmental circumstances, and cognitive processes across time could facilitate the development of systematic interventions to promote satisfying lives for all children and youth as well as help redirect the development of those students with unsatisfying lives.

Third, cross-cultural efforts are needed to assess the generalizability of findings. Research with adults has demonstrated many meaningful differences in the nature, correlates, and consequences of individual differences in life satisfaction and related well-being variables across nations and cultures (Diener & Suh, 2000). Research with children has been sparse, although some notable exceptions exist. As previously mentioned, Park and Huebner (2005) found significant differences in the life satisfaction–school satisfaction link between Korean and American students, underscoring the separability of the dimensions as well as a potentially meaningful contextual difference in the importance and effects of schooling across the two nations.

Implications for Practice

Professionals who work with children and youth, particularly in school settings, are often asked to evaluate children's development, especially for purposes of determining whether they have special needs. Unfortunately, "special needs" is often limited to the notion of a handicapping condition or a disability that requires "special" or "remedial" attention. In practice, the job of school psychologists and related professionals is considered complete by some when they have made determinations of whether or not a child qualifies for special education services under one of several diagnostic categories (e.g., learning disability, emotional disability). In some cases, school psychologists use more refined diagnostic systems (e.g., DSM-IV) to further specify the nature of the psychopathological condition (e.g., attention-deficit/hyperactivity disorder [ADHD], anxiety disorder). Traditionally, many psychological tests have been designed to aid in the determination of the specific disability, with items that focus on assessing the presence of psychopathological symptoms (e.g., short attention span, aggressive behaviors, sleep disruptions). Whatever the case, when the differential diagnosis is determined, then intervention efforts focused on the disorder or disability are undertaken. Interestingly, seldom does the diagnostic and intervention process include recognition of special strengths or assets that are relevant to a child's educational functioning (Epstein et al., 2003; Jimerson, Sharkey, Nyborg, & Furlong, 2004).

My (ESH) experiences in training school psychologists to conduct "comprehensive" psychological assessments of children and youth led to an early understanding of the shortcoming of this traditional model of mental health, which defines positive mental health as the absence of psychopathological symptoms. Upon sending out trainees to practice assessment skills with "normal" children, it was discovered that the trainees were bewildered as to what to report about students who had no "problems." With few or no symptoms to report, the traditional conceptualization of mental health in association with the typical assessment devices provided little information to convey beyond something akin to "the child shows normal functioning." When psychopathological problems were present, the models and methods again provided a lack of means to describe a person as more than his or her disability.

The development of measures of positive psychological constructs, such as life satisfaction, enables differentiation of responses above a "neutral" point, assessing the full range of well-being from "very dissatisfied" through neutral through "very satisfied." Including measures of other positive psychology constructs, such as hope, self-efficacy, and emotional competence (see Peterson & Seligman, 2004, for a taxonomy of human strengths), in their assessment procedures, school psychologists can be armed with the ability to describe positive levels of functioning, beyond simply enumerating the presence or absence of psychological symptoms.

Children's life satisfaction research also has implications for the delivery of psychologically healthy environments for children, including the school environment. Several recommendations for promoting healthy schools can be gleaned from the school satisfaction literature. These implications include monitoring school and life satisfaction, individualizing experiences for students, providing supportive interpersonal relationships, and increasing the active engagement of students.

First, healthy schools appreciate the reciprocal interaction between students' emotional well-being (e.g., life satisfaction) and their academic performance. Healthy schools thus recognize that they must be inhabited by emotionally healthy students. Healthy schools thus would monitor their students' life satisfaction, especially their school satisfaction. Given that school dissatisfaction appears to operate, at the least, as a "marker," if not a determinant, of a variety of academic and behavioral problems, then knowledge of the levels and fluctuations in students' school satisfaction, at the individual and group levels, should provide useful information for school personnel as they attempt to design, monitor, and evaluate the "psychological health" of their schools. Students who show decreasing trajectories of school satisfaction should be targeted for group or individual interventions to determine the nature of their dissatisfaction and develop strategies to improve their emotional well-being. Healthy schools also recognize that by maintaining students' life satisfaction, they are supporting an important buffer against the development of behavior problems in their students.

Second, healthy schools capitalize upon individual differences in temperament, abilities, and interests to maximize the goodness of fit between the school experience and students' needs. This focus includes attention to a student's unique personal strengths and environmental assets as well as his or her deficits. This approach applies not only to "normal" students but also to students with special needs and those at risk. In the latter cases, the articulation of personal strengths and environmental supports can balance the identification of "pathology," so that such students can be perceived and educated in a more holistic manner. Students are more likely to be satisfied with their school experiences and report overall life satisfaction if they are perceived and treated as persons with strengths, self-efficacy, respect, and so forth.

Third, healthy schools recognize the importance of supportive teacher and peer relationships. Furthermore, they intentionally design behavioral settings in the school to maximize the occurrence of positive interactions among the participants. For example, schoolwide positive behavior support programs have been implemented, that promote positive behaviors by providing a facilitative framework to guide teacher–student and student–student interactions (Lewis, Sugai, & Colvin, 1998).

Fourth, healthy schools emphasize instructional tasks that maintain student involvement through the provision of appropriately challenging, interesting, and voluntary activities to the maximum extent possible. Csikszentmihalyi and Schneider (2000) provide a variety of useful recommendations pertinent to educational policy for secondary schools.

The final implication of life satisfaction research relates to program planning and evaluation efforts. Students are the recipients of a wide variety of psychosocial, educational, and medical "programs" as individuals and as part of groups. Life satisfaction research, coupled with the quality-of-life literature, underscores the importance of monitoring the effects of universal interventions (e.g., public school programs) as well as selected interventions (e.g., individualized education program for a student with special needs, medication treatment for children with

ADHD). In all cases, programs should be evaluated from the minimum ethical perspective of "doing no harm" to the longer-term quality of life of the children they serve (Huebner & Gilman, 2005). The development of a life satisfaction research base and measures appropriate for children of a wide age and ability range opens the doors to the evaluation of many programs with respect to their impact upon recipients' subjective quality of life. Life satisfaction research can thus provide additional means to ensure that programs support the healthy development of children in both school and nonschool settings.

References

Adelman, H., Taylor, L., & Nelson, P. (1989). Minors' dissatisfaction with their life circumstances. *Child Psychiatry and Human Development, 20,* 135–147.

Ash, C., & Huebner, E. S. (2001). Environmental events and life satisfaction reports of adolescents: A test of cognitive mediation. *School Psychology International, 22,* 320–336.

Baker, J. A. (1998). The social context of school satisfaction among urban, low income, African-American students. *School Psychology Quarterly, 13,* 25–44.

Baker, J. A. (1999). Teacher–student interaction in urban at-risk classrooms: Differential behavior, relational quality, and student satisfaction with school. *Elementary School Journal, 100,* 57–70.

Baker, J. A., Dilly, L. J., Aupperlee, J. L., & Patil, S. A. (2003). The development of school satisfaction: Schools as psychologically healthy environments. *School Psychology Quarterly, 18,* 206–221.

Chapman, J. W., & McAlpine, D. D. (1988). Students' perceptions of ability. *Gifted Child Quarterly, 31,* 222–225.

Cock, D., & Halvari, H. (1999). Relations among achievement motives, autonomy, performance in mathematics, and satisfaction of pupils in elementary school. *Psychological Reports, 84,* 983–997.

Csikszentmihalyi, M., & Schneider, B. (2000). *Becoming adult: How teenagers prepare for the world of work.* New York: Basic Books.

Cummins, R. A. (1997). *Manual for the Comprehensive Quality of Life Scale—Student (Grades 7–12)* (5th ed.). Melbourne, Australia: Deakin University, School of Psychology.

DeSantis-King, A., Huebner, E. S., Suldo, S. M., & Valois, R. F. (in press). An ecological view of school satisfaction in adolescence: Linkages between social support and behavior problem. *Applied Research in Quality of Life.*

Dew, T., & Huebner, E. S. (1994). Adolescents' perceived quality of life: An exploratory investigation. *Journal of School Psychology, 33*(2), 185–199.

Diener, E. (1984). Subjective well-being. *Psychological Bulletin, 95,* 542–575.

Diener, E. (2000). Subjective well-being: The science of happiness and a proposal for a national index. *American Psychologist, 55,* 34–43.

Diener, E., & Diener, C. (1996). Most people are happy. *Psychological Science, 7,* 181–185.

Diener, E., Emmons, R. A., Larsen, R. J., & Griffin, S. (1985). The Satisfaction with Life Scale. *Journal of Personality Assessment, 49*, 71–75.

Diener, E., & Seligman, M. E. P. (2002). Very happy people. *Psychological Science, 31*, 81–84.

Diener, E., & Suh, E. M. (2000). *Culture and subjective well-being.* Cambridge, MA: MIT Press.

Diener, E., Suh, E. M., Lucas, R. E., & Smith, H. L. (1999). Subjective well-being: Three decades of progress. *Psychological Bulletin, 125*, 276–302.

Eamon, M. K. (2002). Influences and mediators of the effect of poverty on young adolescent depressive symptoms. *Journal of Youth and Adolescence, 31*, 231–242.

Epstein, J. L. (1981). Patterns of classroom participation, student attitudes, and achievements. In J. L. Epstein (Ed.), *Quality of school life* (pp. 81–116). Lexington, MA: Heath.

Epstein, J. L., & McPartland, J. M. (1976). The concept and measurement of the quality of school life. *American Educational Research Journal, 13*, 15–30.

Epstein, M. H., Harniss, M. K., Robbins, V., Wheeler, L., Cyrulik, S., Kriz, M., et al. (2003). Strengths-based approaches to assessment in schools. In M. D. Weist, S. W. Evans, & N. A. Lever (Eds.), *Handbook of school mental health: Advancing practice and research* (pp. 285–299). New York: Kluwer.

Farrell, A., Valois, R. F., & Meyer, A. L. (2003). Impact of the RIPP violence prevention program on rural middle school students. *Journal of Primary Prevention, 24*, 143–167.

Felner, R. D., Brand, S., Adan, A. M., Murshall, P. F., Flowers, N., Sartain, B., et al. (1993). Restructuring the ecology of the school as an approach to prevention during school transitions: Longitudinal follow-ups and extensions of the school Transitional Environment Project (STEP). *Prevention in Human Services, 10*, 103–136.

Frederickson, B. L. (2001). The role of positive emotions in positive psychology: The broaden-and-build theory of positive emotions. *American Psychologist, 56*, 218–226.

Gest, S. D., Welsh, J. A., & Domitrovich, C. E. (2005). Behavioral predictors of changes in social relatedness and liking school in elementary school. *Journal of School Psychology, 43*, 281–301.

Gilman, R. (2001). The relationship between life satisfaction, social interest, and frequency of extracurricular activities among adolescent students. *Journal of Youth and Adolescence, 30*, 749–767.

Gilman, R., & Handwerk, M. L. (2001). Changes in life satisfaction as a function of stay in a residential setting. *Residential Treatment for Children and Youth, 18*, 47–65.

Gilman, R., & Huebner, E. S. (2000). Review of life satisfaction measures for adolescents. *Behaviour Change, 17*, 178–195.

Gilman, R., & Huebner, E. S. (2003). A review of life satisfaction research with children and adolescents. *School Psychology Review, 18*, 192–205.

Gilman, R., & Huebner, E. S. (2006). Characteristics of adolescents who report very high life satisfaction. *Journal of Youth and Adolescence, 35*, 311–319.

Gilman, R., Meyers, J., & Perez, L. (2004). Structured extracurricular activities among adolescents: Findings and implications for school psychologists. *Psychology in the Schools, 41*, 31–42.

Griffin, M., & Huebner, E. S. (2000). Multidimensional life satisfaction reports of students with emotional disturbance. *Journal of Psychoeducational Assessment, 18,* 111–124.

Grob, A. T., Little, T. D., Warner, B., Wearing, A. J., & Euronet. (1996). Adolescent well-being and perceived control across fourteen sociocultural contexts. *Journal of Personality and Social Psychology, 71,* 785–795.

Haranin, E., Huebner, E. S., & Suldo, S. M. (2007). Predictive and incremental validity of global and domain-based adolescent life satisfaction reports. *Journal of Psychoeducational Assessment, 25,* 127–138.

Hegarty, S. (1994). Quality of life at school. In D. Goode (Ed.), *Quality of life for persons with disabilities: International perspectives and issues* (pp. 241–249). Cambridge, MA: Brookline.

Hirsch, B. J., & Rabkin, B. D. (1987). The transition to junior high school: A longitudinal study of self-esteem, psychological symptomatology, school life, and social support. *Child Development, 58,* 1235–1243.

Homel, R., & Burns, A. (1989). Environmental quality and the well-being of children. *Social Indicators Research, 21,* 133–158.

Huebner, E. S. (1991). Initial development of the Students' Life Satisfaction Scale, *School Psychology International, 6,* 103–111.

Huebner, E. S. (1994). Preliminary development and validation of a multidimensional life satisfaction scale for children. *Psychological Assessment, 6,* 149–158.

Huebner, E. S. (2004). Research on assessment of life satisfaction of children and adolescents. *Social Indicators Research, 66,* 3–33.

Huebner, E. S., & Alderman, G. L. (1993). Convergent and discriminant validation of a children's life satisfaction scale: Its relationship to self- and teacher-reported psychological problems and school functioning. *Social Indicators Research, 30,* 71–82.

Huebner, E. S., Ash, C., & Laughlin, J. E. (2001). Life experiences, locus of control, and school satisfaction in adolescence. *Social Indicators Research, 55,* 167–183.

Huebner, E. S., Brantley, A., Nagle, R. J., & Valois, R. F. (2002). Correspondence between parent and adolescent ratings of life satisfaction for adolescents with and without mental disabilities. *Journal of Psychoeducational Assessment, 16,* 118–134.

Huebner, E. S., Drane, W., & Valois, R. F. (2000). Levels and demographic correlates of adolescent life satisfaction reports. *School Psychology International, 21,* 281–292.

Huebner, E. S., & Gilman, R. (2004). Perceived quality of life: A neglected component of assessment and intervention plans for students in school settings. *California School Psychologist, 9,* 127–134.

Huebner, E. S., & Gilman, R. (2006). Children who like and dislike school. *Applied Research in Quality of Life, 1,* 139–150.

Huebner, E. S., Gilman, R., & Suldo, S. M. (2007). Assessing perceived quality of life in children and youth. In S. Smith & L. Handler (Eds.), *The clinical assessment of children and adolescents: A practitioner's guide* (pp. 349–366). Mahwah, NJ: Erlbaum.

Huebner, E. S., Laughlin, J. E., Ash, C., & Gilman, R. (1998). Further validation of the Multidimensional Students' Life Satisfaction Scale. *Journal of Psychoeducational Assessment, 16,* 118–134.

Huebner, E. S., & McCullough, G. (2000). Correlates of school satisfaction among adolescents. *Journal of Educational Research, 93,* 331–335.

Huebner, E. S., Suldo, S. M., & Gilman, R. (2006). Life satisfaction. In G. Bear & K. Minke (Eds.), *Children's needs–III* (pp. 357–368). Washington, DC: National Association of School Psychologists.

Huebner, E. S., Suldo, S. M., Smith, L. C., & McKnight, C. (2004). Life satisfaction in children and youth: Empirical foundations and implications for school psychologists. *Psychology in the Schools, 41*, 81–93.

Huebner, E. S., Valois, R. F., Paxton, R., & Drane, W. (2005). Middle school students' perceptions of quality of life. *Journal of Happiness Studies, 6*, 15–24.

Ito, A., & Smith, D. C. (2005). Predictors of school satisfaction among Japanese and U.S. youth. *Community Psychologist, 12*, 19–21.

Jimerson, S. R., Sharkey, J. D., Nyborg, V., & Furlong, M. J. (2004). Strengths-based assessment and school psychology: A summary and synthesis. *California School Psychologist, 9*, 9–20.

Karatzias, A., Power, K. G., Flemming, J., Lennan, F., & Swanson, V. (2002). The role of demographics, personality variables, and school stress on predicting school satisfaction/dissatisfaction: Review of the literature and research findings. *Educational Psychology, 22*, 33–50.

Katja, R., Paivi, A., Marja-Terttu, T., & Pekka, L. (2002). Relationships among adolescent subjective well-being, health behavior, and school satisfaction. *Journal of School Health, 72*, 243–249.

Keith, K. D., & Schalock, R. L. (1995). *Quality of Student Life Questionnaire.* Worthington, OH: IDS.

Ladd, G. W., Buhs, E. S., & Seid, M. (2000). Children's initial sentiments about kindergarten: Is school liking an antecedent of early classroom participation and achievement? *Merrill–Palmer Quarterly, 46*, 255–278.

Laurent, J., Cantanzaro, J. S., Thomas, J. E., Rudolph, D. K., Potter, K. I., Lambert, S., et al. (1999). A measure of positive and negative affect for children: Scale development and preliminary validation. *Psychological Assessment, 11*, 141–169.

Leone, P. E., Luttig, P. G., Zlotlow, S., & Trickett, E. J. (1990). Understanding the social ecology of classrooms for adolescents with behavioral disorders: A preliminary study of differences in perceived environments. *Behavioral Disorders, 16*, 55–56.

Lewis, T. J., Sugai, G., & Colvin, G. (1998). Reducing problem behavior through a schoolwide system of effective behavioral support: Investigation of a schoolwide social skills training program and contextual interventions. *School Psychology Review, 27*, 446–459.

Locke, T. F., & Newcomb, M. D. (2004). Adolescent predictors of young adult and adult alcohol involvement and dysphoria in a prospective community sample of women. *Prevention Science, 5*, 151–167.

Lounsbury, J. W., Steel, R. P., Loveland, J. M., & Gibson, L. W. (2004). An investigation of personality traits in relation to adolescent school absenteeism. *Journal of Youth and Adolescence, 33*, 457–466.

Martin, K. M., & Huebner, E. S. (2007). Peer victimization and prosocial experiences and subjective well-being in middle school students. *Psychology in the Schools, 44*, 199–208.

Maton, K. I. (1990). Meaningful involvement in instrumental activity and well-being:

Studies of older adolescents and at-risk teenagers. *Journal of Community Psychology, 18,* 297–320.

McCullough, G., & Huebner, E. S. (2003). Life satisfaction reports of adolescents with learning disabilities and normally achieving adolescents. *Journal of Psychoeducational Assessment, 21,* 311–324.

McCullough, G., Huebner, E. S., & Laughlin, J. E. (2000). Life events, self-concept, and adolescent positive subjective well-being. *Psychology in the Schools, 37,* 281–290.

McKnight, C. G., Huebner, E. S., & Suldo, S. M. (2002). Relationships among stressful life events, temperament, problem behavior, and global life satisfaction in adolescents. *Psychology in the Schools, 39*(6), 677–687.

Nickerson, A., & Nagle, R. J. (2004). The influence of parent and peer attachments on life satisfaction in middle childhood and early adolescence. *Social Indicators Research, 66,* 35–60.

Okun, M., Braver, M. W., & Weir, R. M. (1990). Grade level differences in school satisfaction. *Social Indicators Research, 22,* 419–427.

Park, N., & Huebner, E. S. (2005). A cross-cultural study of the levels and correlates of life satisfaction among children and adolescents. *Journal of Cross-Cultural Research, 36,* 444–456.

Peterson, C., Park, N., & Seligman, M. E. P. (2005). Orientations to happiness and life satisfaction: The full life versus the empty life. *Journal of Happiness Studies, 6,* 25–41.

Peterson, C., & Seligman, M. E. P. (2004). *Character strengths and virtues: A handbook and classification.* New York: Oxford University Press.

Rigby, B., & Huebner, E. S. (2004). Do causal attributions mediate the relationship between personality and life satisfaction in adolescence? *Psychology in the Schools, 41,* 91–99.

Roeser, R. W. (2001). To cultivate the positive: Introduction to the special issue on schooling and mental health issues. *Journal of School Psychology, 39,* 99–110.

Rosenfeld, L. B., Richman, J. M., & Bowen, G. L. (2000). Social support networks and school outcomes: The centrality of the teacher. *Child and Adolescent Social Work Journal, 17,* 205–226.

Rutter, M., & Maughan, B. (2002). School effectiveness findings, 1979–2002. *Journal of School Psychology, 40,* 451–475.

Schalock, R., & Alonson, M. A. V. (2002). *Handbook on quality of life for human service providers.* Washington, DC: American Association of Mental Retardation.

Seligson, J. L., Huebner, E. S., & Valois, R. F. (2003). Preliminary validation of the Brief Multidimensional Students' Life Satisfaction Scale (BMSLSS). *Social Indicators Research, 61,* 121–145.

Seligson, J. L., Huebner, E. S., & Valois, R. F. (2005). An investigation of a brief life satisfaction scale with elementary students. *Social Indicators Research, 73,* 355–374.

Shernoff, D. J., Csikszentmihalyi, M., Schneider, B., & Shernoff, E. S. (2003). Student engagement in high school classrooms from the perspective of flow theory. *School Psychology Quarterly, 18,* 158–176.

Stevens, M. M., Freeman, D. H., Jr., Mott, L. A., Youells, F. E., & Linsey, S. C. (1993). Smokeless tobacco use among children: The New Hampshire Study. *American Journal of Preventative Medicine, 9*(3), 160–167.

Suldo, S. M., & Huebner, E. S. (2002, March). *Influence of parenting styles on adolescent school satisfaction and problem behavior.* Paper presented at the National Association of School Psychologists, Chicago.

Suldo, S. M., & Huebner, E. S. (2004a). Does life satisfaction moderate the effects of stressful life events on psychopathological behavior in adolescence? *School Psychology Quarterly, 19,* 93–105.

Suldo, S. M., & Huebner, E. S. (2004b). The role of life satisfaction in the relationship between authoritative parenting dimensions and adolescent problem behavior. *Social Indicators Research, 66,* 165–195.

Suldo, S. M., & Huebner, E. S. (2006). Characteristics of very happy youth. *Social Indicators Research, 78,* 179–203.

Verkuyten, M., & Thijs, J. (2002). School satisfaction of elementary school children: The role of performance, peer relations, ethnicity, and gender. *Social Indicators Research, 59,* 203–228.

Wong, M. M., & Csikszentmihalyi, M. (1991). Motivation and academic achievement: The effects of personality traits and the quality of experience. *Journal of Personality, 59,* 539–574.

19

Job Satisfaction
Subjective Well-Being at Work

TIMOTHY A. JUDGE and RYAN KLINGER

Work is central to most people's identities. When asked a general question, "What do you do"?, most people respond with their job title. Moreover, across many languages, a significant number of people's surnames are based on occupations (e.g., in English, just to name a few: *abbot, archer, baker, barber, barker, brewer, carpenter, carter, clark, collier, cook, cooper, farmer, fisher, fowler, goldsmith, hooper, mason, miller, porter, roper, sawyer, smith, taylor, thatcher, turner, weaver, wright*). Furthermore, more than half of the nonretired adult population spends most of its waking hours at work. Thus, no research on subjective well-being can be complete without considering subjective well-being at work.

Beyond their centrality to identities, job attitudes are important to consider for other reasons. First, the most widely investigated job attitude—job satisfaction—may be the most extensively researched topic in the history of industrial/organizational psychology (Judge & Church, 2000). Second, in the organizational sciences, job satisfaction occupies a central role in many theories and models of individual attitudes and behaviors. Finally, as we note later, job satisfaction research has practical applications for the enhancement of individual lives as well as organizational effectiveness.

In this chapter we provide a review of significant theoretical and empirical contributions to the job satisfaction literature, emphasizing several current conceptual and methodological issues. We begin with a discussion of the definition of job satisfaction, noting several features of the definition that make job satisfaction an inherently complex social attitude. Next we discuss the measurement of job satisfaction, bridging definitional/conceptual issues and practical considerations. Then we discuss several prominent theories of the antecedents of job satisfaction followed by an overview of empirical support for various significant outcomes of job satisfaction. Finally, we mention some areas of research that we believe are particularly deserving of future exploration.

Definitional Issues

The concept of job satisfaction has been defined in many ways. However, the most-used definition of job satisfaction in organizational research is that of Locke (1976), who described job satisfaction as "a pleasurable or positive emotional state resulting from the appraisal of one's job or job experiences" (p. 1304). Building on this conceptualization, Hulin and Judge (2003) noted that job satisfaction includes multidimensional psychological responses to one's job, and that such responses have cognitive (evaluative), affective (or emotional), and behavioral components. This tripartite conceptualization of job satisfaction fits well with typical conceptualizations of social attitudes (Eagley & Chaiken, 1993). However, there are two apparent difficulties with this viewpoint.

First, as noted by Hulin and Judge (2003), social attitudes are generally weak predictors of specific behaviors (Eagley & Chaiken, 1993; Fishbein, 1980; Wicker, 1969), yet job attitudes are generally reliably and moderately strongly related to relevant job behaviors. If job satisfaction is a social attitude, then how might we resolve this apparent inconsistency? Although we have more to say about this issue when discussing the outcomes of job satisfaction, one possible reason for the apparent contradiction is that job attitudes may be more salient and accessible for workers than the social attitudes typically assessed in social attitude research. For instance, cognitive and affective outcomes of job dissatisfaction are likely to permeate and influence an individual's thoughts from the moment he or she wakes to the moment the individual returns home from work (and possibly spill over into nonwork domains as well). Attitudes toward a political party or a marketing campaign are likely considerably less salient for the average individual.

Second, although most researchers include affect in their definitions of job satisfaction, such as provided by measures of life satisfaction, instruments used to evaluate job satisfaction tend to assess cognitive more than affective aspects. This bias has led some to conclude that the missing affective component sufficiently impairs extant measures, and thus to recommend entirely new measures of job satisfaction (Brief & Weiss, 2002; Weiss, 2002). We consider this topic further in our discussion of measurement issues.

Measurement of Job Satisfaction

Most researchers recognize that job satisfaction is a global concept that is comprised of, or indicated by, various facets. The most typical categorization (Smith, Kendall, & Hulin, 1969) considers five facets of job satisfaction: pay, promotions, coworkers, supervision, and the work itself. Locke (1976) adds a few other facets: recognition, working conditions, and company and management. Furthermore, it is common for researchers to separate job satisfaction into intrinsic and extrinsic elements whereby pay and promotions are considered extrinsic factors and coworkers, supervision, and the work itself are considered intrinsic factors.

The astute reader will notice a rather casual use of measurement terms ("comprised of," "indicated by") that, in the measurement literature, generally indicates very different conceptualizations of a concept. This looseness is intentional. Particularly, use of the term *comprised of* generally denotes treatment of a concept as a manifest or aggregate or formative variable, wherein specific facets or items cause the concept. Conversely, use of the term *indicated by* generally connotes a latent or reflective concept, where the subscales or items indicate a higher-order concept. Although clarity in thinking about concepts is often recommended in this literature (Law, Wong, & Mobley, 1998), we think considerable confusion can be created by making false choices. Specifically, in this case, concepts can be either manifest or latent, depending on how the researcher wishes to treat them. Clearly, when considering the facets of job satisfaction, it is a manifest variable in that overall job satisfaction is comprised of more specific satisfactions in different domains. Just as clearly, though, job satisfaction is also a latent variable in that it is likely that people's overall attitude toward their job or work causes specific satisfactions to be positively correlated. Thus, we do not think that conceptualizations or measures of job satisfaction are advanced by forcing false dichotomies into the literature.

With that caveat in mind, two further issues warrant discussion. First, we wish to reprise our earlier discussion of the (missing) role of affect in job satisfaction measures, and its implications for research on, and measurement of, job satisfaction. Second, there is the practical issue of how to measure job satisfaction for research purposes. We address each in turn.

As we noted earlier, affect is central to any definition of job satisfaction, or job attitudes more generally. However, this acknowledgment of the role of affect creates problems for researchers. As noted by Brief and Weiss (2002) and Hulin and Judge (2003) in the job satisfaction literature, and Diener and Larson (1984) in the subjective well-being literature, affective reactions are likely to be fleeting and episodic—state variables rather than consistent chronic, trait-like variables. Measurement of affect should reflect its state-like, episodic nature. Otherwise we become enmeshed in a methodological stalemate (Larson & Csikszentmihalyi, 1983) in which researchers attempt to study propositions of newly developed theories with methods and analyses appropriate only to the needs of an older generation of theoretical models.

To some degree, we are discussing a research design issue. This problem has been addressed, and partially solved, by event signal methods (ESM), or momentary ecological assessments, and multilevel statistical analyses that combine within- and between-person effects (Bryk & Raudenbush, 1992). ESM designs show that when job satisfaction is measured on an experience-sampled basis, roughly one-third to one-half of the variation in job satisfaction is within-individual. Thus, typical "one-shot" between-person research designs miss a considerable portion of the variance in job satisfaction by treating within-individual variation as transient error.

However, another, perhaps more, controversial issue is whether extant measures of job satisfaction are poorly suited to assess the affective nature of job satisfaction. This is a complex issue, and space allows only a few cursory thoughts here. First, it is very difficult, perhaps insurmountably so, to separate measures of cognition and affect. Isen and colleagues (e.g., Ashby, Isen, & Turken, 1999; Isen, 2002, 2003) have made this point repeatedly in reference to positive affect. Indeed, there is some discussion that even neuroimaging techniques such as magnetic resonance imaging (MRI), functional magnetic resonance imaging (fMRI), and positron emission tomography (PET) scans are not sufficiently sensitive to separate cognitive and affective processes. If we cannot make such separations in neuroimaging, it seems inconceivable that survey measures will be *more* sensitive. A second and related point is to express dubious regard toward efforts to develop measures of "job affects" as distinct from measures of "job cognitions." For example, Brief (1998) and Brief and Roberson (1989) have argued that job affect should be assessed separately from job satisfaction, owing to the overly cognitive focus of the latter measures. However, the Brief and Roberson's measure of job cognitions correlated as strongly with affect as did their measure of job satisfaction. Another study showed that cognition and affect each contributes (roughly equally) to job satisfaction (Weiss, Nicholas, & Daus, 1999). Perhaps the best advice that can be offered here is that research on discrete moods and emotions should continue, alongside research on job satisfaction. Including separate measures of moods (such as positive and negative affect) or specific emotions with job satisfaction certainly seems advisable without posing any potentially false dualities between cognition and affect.

To be clear, we are not suggesting that the dual roles of affect and cognition should *not* be studied in the context of job satisfaction. What we are objecting to is (1) the characterization of measures of job satisfaction as either cognitive or affective; and (2) the need to develop new, affectively laden measures of job satisfaction or to replace measures of job satisfaction with "work affect" measures. Cognition and affect concepts can help us better understand the nature of job satisfaction, but they are not substitutes for job satisfaction any more than the accumulated body parts of a cadaver substitute for a living human.

Turning to practical issues in measuring job satisfaction, in the literature the two most extensively validated employee attitude survey measures are the Job Descriptive Index (JDI; Smith et al., 1969) and the Minnesota Satisfaction Questionnaire (MSQ; Weiss, Dawis, England, & Lofquist, 1967). The JDI assesses satisfaction with five different job areas: pay, promotion, coworkers, supervision, and the work itself. This index is reliable and has an impressive array of validation evidence. The MSQ has the advantage of versatility—long and short forms are available, as well as faceted and overall measures.

As for overall measures of job satisfaction, Brayfield and Rothe's (1951) job satisfaction scale is commonly used. In some of our research (e.g., Judge, Bono, & Locke, 2000) we have used a reliable (i.e., internal consistencies [α] at .80 or above) five-item version of this scale. The five items are:

1. I feel fairly satisfied with my present job.
2. Most days I am enthusiastic about my work.
3. Each day at work seems like it will never end.
4. I find real enjoyment in my work.
5. I consider my job to be rather unpleasant.

Two additional issues concerning the measurement of job satisfaction are worth consideration. First, some measures, such as the JDI, are faceted, whereas others are global. If a measure is facet-based, overall job satisfaction is typically defined as a sum of the facets. Scarpello and Campbell (1983) found that individual questions about various aspects of the job did not correlate well with a global measure of overall job satisfaction. Based on these results, the authors argued that faceted and global measures do not measure the same construct. In other words, the whole is not the same as the sum of the parts. Scarpello and Campbell concluded, "The results of the present study argue against the common practice of using the sum of facet satisfaction as the measure of overall job satisfaction" (p. 595). This conclusion is probably premature. Individual items generally do not correlate highly with independent measures of the same construct. If one uses job satisfaction *facets* (as opposed to individual job satisfaction *items*) to predict an independent measure of overall job satisfaction, the correlation is considerably higher. For example, using data I (T.A.J.) collected, and using the JDI facets to predict a measure of overall job satisfaction, the combined multiple correlation is $r = .87$. If this correlation were corrected for unreliability, it would be very close to unity. As has been noted elsewhere (e.g., Judge & Hulin, 1993), the job satisfaction facets are correlated highly enough to suggest that they indicate a common construct. Thus, there may be little difference between measuring general job satisfaction with an overall measure and measuring it by summing facet scores.

Second, although most job satisfaction researchers have assumed that single-item measures are unreliable and therefore should not be used, this view has not gone unchallenged. Wanous, Reichers, and Hudy (1997) found that the reliability of single-item measures of job satisfaction is .67. In addition, for the G. M. Faces scale, another single item measure of job satisfaction that asks individuals to check one of five facets that best describes their overall satisfaction (Kunin, 1955), the reliability was estimated to be .66. Though these are respectable levels of reliability, it is important to keep in mind that these levels are lower than most multiple-item measures of job satisfaction. For example, Judge, Boudreau, and Bretz (1994) used a three-item measure of job satisfaction with an interitem reliability of $\alpha = .85$. The items in this measure were:

1. All things considered, are you satisfied with your present job (circle one)? YES NO

2. How satisfied are you with your job in general (circle one)?

1	2	3	4	5
Very Dissatisfied	Somewhat Dissatisfied	Neutral	Somewhat Satisfied	Very Satisfied

3. Below, please write down your best estimates on the percent of time you feel satisfied, dissatisfied, and neutral about your present job on average. The three figures should add up to equal 100%. ON THE AVERAGE:

The percent of time I feel satisfied with my present job _____%
(*note*: only this response is scored)

The percent of time I feel dissatisfied with my present job _____%

The percent of time I feel neutral about my present job _____%

TOTAL _____%

When used in practice, these items need to be standardized before summing. Although this measure is no substitute for the richness of detail provided in a faceted measure of job satisfaction, we do believe it is a reasonably valid measure of overall job satisfaction and more reliable than a single-item measure.

Theories of Antecedents of Job Satisfaction

Several theories concerning causes of job satisfaction have been proposed in the organizational literature. These theories can be loosely classified into one of three categories:

1. Situational theories, which hypothesize that job satisfaction results from the nature of one's job or other aspects of the environment.

2. Dispositional approaches, which assume that job satisfaction is rooted in the personological makeup of the individual.

3. Interactive theories, which propose that job satisfaction results from the interplay of situational and personological factors.

As with all areas of psychology, some theories are never really seriously investigated (e.g., Salancik & Pfeffer's [1977, 1978] social information processing approach), some take off and then are either discredited (e.g., Herzberg's [1967] two-factor theory) or broadly supported (though we have difficulty finding any job satisfaction theory to fit in this category), and still others lie dormant for years, only to be investigated at a later time (e.g., Landy's [1978] opponent process theory, which recently was reappraised [Bowling, Beehr, Wagner, & Libkuman, 2005]). We now turn our focus to several theories that have garnered a considerable portion of the attention and/or support of job satisfaction researchers.

Job Characteristics Model

The job characteristics model (JCM) argues that jobs that contain intrinsically motivating characteristics will lead to higher levels of job satisfaction (Hackman & Oldham, 1976). Five core job characteristics define an intrinsically motivating job: (1) *task identity*—degree to which one can see one's work from beginning to end; (2) *task significance*—degree to which one's work is seen as important and significant; (3) *skill variety*—extent to which job allows one to do different tasks; (4) *autonomy*—degree to which one has control and discretion over how to conduct one's job; and (5) *feedback*—degree to which the work itself provides feedback for how one is performing the job. According to the theory, jobs that are enriched to provide these core characteristics are likely to be more satisfying and motivating than jobs that do not provide these characteristics. More specifically, it is proposed that the core job characteristics lead to three critical psychological states—experienced meaningfulness of the work, responsibility for outcomes, and knowledge of results—which, in turn, lead to outcomes such as job satisfaction.

There is both indirect and direct support for the validity of the model's basic proposition that core job characteristics lead to more satisfying work. In terms of indirect evidence, research studies across many years, organizations, and types of jobs show that when employees are asked to evaluate different facets of their job, such as supervision, pay, promotion opportunities, coworkers, and so forth, the nature of the work itself generally emerges as the most important job facet (Judge & Church, 2000; Jurgensen, 1978). In addition, of the major job satisfaction facets—pay, promotion opportunities, coworkers, supervision, and the work itself—satisfaction with the work itself is almost always the facet most strongly correlated with overall job satisfaction, as well as with important outcomes such as employee retention (e.g., Frye, 1996; Parisi & Weiner, 1999; Rentsch & Steel, 1992; Weiner, 2000). Research directly testing the relationship between workers' reports of job characteristics and job satisfaction has produced consistently positive results. For instance, Frye (1996) reported a true score correlation of .50 between job characteristics and job satisfaction.

Initially a purely situational model, the JCM was modified by Hackman and Oldham (1976) to account for the fact that two employees may have the same job, experience the same job characteristics, and yet have different levels of job satisfaction. The concept of growth need strength (GNS)—an employee's desire for personal development—was added as a moderator of the relationship between intrinsic job characteristics and job satisfaction. According to this interactional form of the model, intrinsic job characteristics are especially satisfying for individuals who score high on GNS. Empirical evidence supports this position: The relationship between work characteristics and job satisfaction is stronger for high-GNS employees (average $r = .68$) than for low-GNS employees (average $r = .38$) (Frye, 1996). However, it should be noted that task characteristics are related to job satisfaction even for those who score low on GNS.

Value-Percept Theory

Locke (1976) argued that individuals' values would determine what satisfied them on the job. Only the unfulfilled job values that were important to the individual would be dissatisfying. According to Locke's value-percept model, job satisfaction can be modeled by the formula

$$S = (V_c - P) \times V_i$$

or

Satisfaction = (want − have) × importance

where S is satisfaction, V_c is value content (amount wanted), P is the perceived amount of the value provided by the job, and V_i is the importance of the value to the individual. Thus, value-percept theory predicts that discrepancies between what is desired and what is received are dissatisfying only if the job facet is important to the individual. Because individuals consider multiple facets when evaluating their job satisfaction, the cognitive calculus is repeated for each job facet. Overall satisfaction is estimated by aggregating across all contents of a job, weighted by their importance to the individual.

The value-percept model expresses job satisfaction in terms of employees' values and job outcomes. A particular strength of the model is that it highlights the role of individual differences in values and job outcomes. However, one potential problem with the value-percept theory is that what one desires (V_c or want) and what one considers important (V_i or importance) are likely to be highly correlated. In addition, the use of weighting may be inappropriate unless weighting variables are measured with very high reliability. The model also ignores influences from exogenous factors, such as costs of holding a job, or current and past social, economic, or organizational conditions external to the individual/job nexus.

Dispositional Approaches

Over the past 20 years, research on job satisfaction antecedents has been dominated by dispositional approaches As reviewed by Judge and Larsen (2001), these studies have been both indirect—inferring a dispositional source of job satisfaction without measuring personality—and direct. We provide a brief review each of these types of studies.

Indirect Studies

Staw and Ross (1985) exploited the National Longitudinal Surveys (NLS) database and found that measures of job satisfaction were reasonably stable over time (over 2 years, $r = .42$; over 3 years, $r = .32$; over 5 years, $r = .29$). They also found that job satisfaction showed modest stability even when individuals changed both employers and occupations over a 5-year period of time ($r = .19$, $p < .01$). Finally, the authors found that prior job satisfaction was a stronger predictor of current satisfaction ($b = .27$, $t = 14.07$, $p < .01$) than changes in pay ($b = .01$, $t = 2.56$, $p < .01$) or changes in status ($b = .00$). In a separate line of research, Arvey, Bouchard, Segal, and Abraham (1989) found significant consistency in job satisfaction levels between 34 pairs of monozygotic twins reared apart from early childhood. The intraclass correlation (ICC) of the general job satisfaction scores of the twin pairs was .31 ($p < .05$). As Judge and Larsen (2001) and others (Gerhart, 2005) have noted, the problem with indirect studies is that alternative explanations are obvious. For example, correlations of satisfaction levels across time and jobs may reflect relative consistency in jobs as much as it does stable individual dispositions; those who are able to secure a good, high-quality job at one time are likely to secure an equivalent job at a later time, and thus situational explanations for job satisfaction consistency are not ruled out, even if individuals change jobs (Hulin & Judge, 2003).

Direct Studies

More recent studies have linked direct measures of personality traits to job satisfaction. Most of the studies in this area have focused on one of four typologies: (1) positive and negative affectivity; (2) the five-factor model of personality; (3) core self-evaluations; (4) other measures of affective disposition. Probably the heir to the throne of indirect studies were studies that related positive affectivity and negative affectivity (trait PA and trait NA) to job satisfaction. Counter to the theory that PA is more strongly related to positive outcomes than NA, Thoresen et al.'s (Thoresen, Kaplan, Barsky, Warren, & de Chermont, 2003) meta-analysis revealed that trait NA was somewhat more strongly related to job satisfaction than was trait PA ($\rho = -.37$ and $\rho = .33$, respectively). As for the five-factor model, Judge, Heller, and Mount (2002) found that three Big Five traits— neuroticism, extraversion, and conscientiousness—each displayed moderate, nonzero relationships with job satisfaction: neuroticism, $\rho = -.29$; extraversion, $\rho = .25$; conscientiousness, $\rho = .26$.

Judge, Locke, and Durham (1997) introduced the construct of core self-evaluations. According to these authors, core self-evaluations are fundamental premises that individuals hold about themselves and their functioning in the world. Judge et al. argued that core self-evaluation is a broad personality construct comprised of several more specific traits: (1) self-esteem; (2) generalized self-efficacy; (3) locus of control; and (4) neuroticism or emotional stability. Judge and Bono (2001) completed a meta-analysis of 169 independent correlations (combined $N = 59,871$) between each of the four core traits and job satisfaction. When the four meta-analyses where combined into a single composite measure, the overall core trait correlates .37 with job satisfaction. Judge, Locke, Durham, and Kluger (1998) found that one of the primary causal mechanisms was through the perception of intrinsic job characteristics, a finding that has also generalized to objective measures of job complexity (Judge, Bono, & Locke, 2000).

Finally, in terms of other measures of affective disposition, in order to gauge relative job satisfaction more accurately, Weitz (1952) developed a "gripe index" that takes into account individuals' tendencies to feel negatively or positively about many aspects of their lives. Judge and Hulin (1993) found that employees' responses to neutral objects were correlated with job satisfaction, a finding replicated by Judge and Locke (1993). However, Judge et al. (1998) and Piccolo, Judge, Takahashi, Watanabe, and Locke (2005) found that, compared to core self-evaluations, affective disposition explained less variance in job satisfaction.

Cornell Model

Hulin, Roznowski, and Hachiya (1985) and Hulin (1991) provide a model of job satisfaction that attempts to integrate previous theories of attitude formation. The model proposes that job satisfaction is a function of the balance between role inputs—what the individual puts into the work role (e.g., training, experience, time, and effort)—and role outcomes—what is received by the individual (pay, status, working conditions, and intrinsic factors). All else equal, the more outcomes received relative to inputs invested, the higher work role satisfaction will be. Furthermore, according to the Cornell model, an individual's opportunity costs affect the value the individual places on inputs. In periods of labor oversupply (i.e., high unemployment), individuals will perceive their inputs as less valuable due to the high competition for few alternative positions, and the opportunity cost of their work role declines (i.e., work role membership is less costly relative to other opportunities). Therefore, as unemployment (particularly in one's local or occupational labor market) rises, the subjective utility of inputs falls—making perceived value of inputs less, relative to outcomes—thus increasing satisfaction. Finally, the model proposes that an individual's frames of reference, which represent past experiences with outcomes, influence how he or she perceives current outcomes received. This concept of frames of reference, as generated and modified by individuals' experience, accounts, in part, for differences in job satisfactions of individuals with objectively identical jobs. However, direct tests of the model are lacking.

Summary

Of the job satisfaction theories that have been put forth, it appears that three have garnered the most research support: Locke's value-percept theory, the job characteristics model, and the dispositional approach. It is interesting to note that one of these theories is, essentially, a situational theory (job characteristics model), another is a person theory (dispositional approach), and another is a person–situation interactional theory (value-percept model). Although this outcome may lead one to assume that these theories are competing or incompatible explanations of job satisfaction, this is not necessarily the case. Judge et al. (1997), in seeking to explain how core self-evaluations would be related to job satisfaction, proposed that intrinsic job characteristics would mediate this relationship. Indeed, Judge et al. (1998) showed that individuals with positive core self-evaluations perceived more intrinsic value in their work, and Judge, Bono, and Locke (2000) showed that the link between core self-evaluations and intrinsic job characteristics was not solely a perceptual process—core self-evaluations was related to the actual attainment of complex jobs. Because job complexity is synonymous with intrinsic job characteristics, this result shows that part of the reason individuals with positive core self-evaluations perceived more challenging jobs and reported higher levels of job satisfaction is that they actually have obtained more complex (and thus challenging and intrinsically enriching) jobs. The work of Judge and colleagues thus shows that dispositional approaches and the job characteristics model are quite compatible with one another.

Outcomes of Job Satisfaction

Evidence indicates that job satisfaction is strongly and consistently related to subjective well-being. All studies that we reviewed found significant relationships between job satisfaction and life satisfaction (reported correlations ranged from .19 to .49). Researchers have speculated that there are three possible forms of this relationship: (1) *spillover*, wherein job experiences spill over onto life experiences, and vice versa; (2) *segmentation*, wherein job and life experiences are balkanized and have little to do with one another; and (3) *compensation*, wherein an individual seeks to compensate for a dissatisfying job by seeking fulfillment and happiness in his or her nonwork life, and vice versa. Judge and Watanabe (1994) argued that these different models may exist for different individuals and that individuals can be classified into the three groups. On the basis of a national stratified random sample of workers, they found that 68% of workers could be classified as falling into the spillover group, 20% fell into the segmentation group, and 12% fell into the compensation group. Thus, the spillover model, whereby job satisfaction spills into life satisfaction, and vice versa, appears to characterize most U.S. employees. Consistent with the spillover model, a quantitative review of the literature indicated that job and life satisfaction are moderately strongly correlated—a meta-analysis revealed the average "true score" correlation of +.44 (Tait, Padgett, & Baldwin, 1989).

Given that a job is a significant part of one's life, the correlation between job and life satisfaction makes sense—one's job experiences spill over into nonwork life. However, it also seems possible that the causality could go the other way—a happy nonwork life spills over into job experiences and evaluations. In fact, research suggests that the relationship between job and life satisfaction is reciprocal—job satisfaction does affect life satisfaction, but life satisfaction also affects job satisfaction (Judge & Watanabe, 1993).

Job satisfaction is also related to an impressive array of workplace behaviors. These include (1) attendance at work (Smith, 1977; Scott & Taylor, 1985); (2) turnover decisions (Carsten & Spector, 1987; Hom, Katerberg, & Hulin, 1979; Hom, 2001; Hulin, 1966, 1968; Mobley, Horner, & Hollingsworth, 1978; Miller, Katerberg, & Hulin, 1979); (3) decisions to retire (Hanisch & Hulin, 1990, 1991; Schmitt & McCune, 1981); (4) psychological withdrawal behaviors (Roznowski, Miller, & Rosse, 1992); (5) prosocial and organizational citizenship behaviors (Bateman & Organ, 1983; Farrell, 1983; Roznowski et al., 1992); (6) pro-union representation votes (Getman, Goldberg, & Herman, 1976; Schriesheim, 1978; Zalesny, 1985); (7) prevote unionization activity (Hamner & Smith, 1978); (8) job performance (Judge, Thoresen, Bono, & Patton, 2001); and (9) workplace incivility (Mount, Ilies, & Johnson, 2006).

Although job satisfaction is related to an impressive array of behaviors, the correlations are not large, typically in the .15–.35 range. As Fishbein and Ajzen (1974) have noted, much mischief has been created in the attitude–behavior literature by failing to achieve correspondence between attitudes and behaviors. One means of achieving attitude–behavior correspondence is to use specific attitudes to predict specific behaviors, as has been the course of action pursued in Fishbein and Ajzen's research. For example, we might use a specific behavioral intention (e.g., intent to quit smoking) to predict a specific behavior (e.g., quitting smoking) within a relatively delimited time period. However, another approach is to use a general attitude to predict a general behavior. Because job attitudes are general concepts, we may expect the relationship between job satisfaction and behavior to increase if we broaden the conceptualization of the relevant behavioral set. For instance, Harrison, Newman, and Roth (2006) found that the relationship between general job attitude (comprised of job satisfaction and organizational commitment) and individual effectiveness (a construct comprised of a broad set of workplace behaviors, including focal performance, contextual performance, lateness, absenteeism, and turnover) was much stronger ($r = .59$) than those typically reported in the job attitude literature.

Future of Job Satisfaction Research

Based on our review of the job satisfaction literature, we now suggest several fruitful directions for future job satisfaction research. First, as might be gathered from this review, and has been noted in the subjective well-being literature more broadly (Diener, 1984), there is no consensus on the roles of cognition and affect in job satisfaction research. Although we have made our position known in the section on measurement, we do not mean to imply that this is "settled law"—there is more to be learned about how cognition and affect are intertwined in job satisfaction research. Rather than focusing on measurement properties, our preference is for future research to look at more substantive issues in cognitive processing and to focus on moods and emotions. For example, despite the considerable impact of affective events theory (Weiss & Cropanzano, 1996) on job attitudes research, we still have a very poor idea of what affective events are most salient to individuals, how individuals process this information, and what the cognitive, affective, and behavioral implications of these events might be.

Another area for future research is the role of goals in job satisfaction. As Diener (1984) noted in his review, the telic perspective has been an important one in conceptualizations of subjective well-being. However, the role of goals in well-being is not perfectly clear. Some have argued that the explicit goal of happiness is likely to make the realization of this goal elusive (Gilbert, 2006). Research by Mento, Locke, and Klein (1992) suggests that goals, although improving performance, are likely to breed dissatisfaction because they involve holding oneself to a high standard. On the other hand, the self-concordance model suggests that the type of goal matters—goals pursued for intrinsic reasons are more likely to bring happiness than those pursued for extrinsic reasons; there is support for this position in both the subjective well-being (Sheldon & Elliot, 1999) and job satisfaction (Judge, Bono, Erez, & Locke, 2005) literatures. Thus, more work on goals and job satisfaction is needed, conceptually and empirically.

A third area for research concerns the issue of stability and change. In the personality literature we have come to understand that stability and change coexist (Roberts, Walton, & Viechtbauer, 2006). There is considerable rank-order consistency in personality, though, naturally, consistency declines over time (Srivastava, John, & Gosling, 2003). However, there are also forces of change—personality does change over time, and time does not do the same thing to each trait. For example, there is evidence that individuals become more conscientious but less open over time (Srivastava et al., 2003). Within the subjective well-being literature, there are similar dialogues and debates. Clearly, there is a genetic basis to life satisfaction, no doubt operating through genetic effects on personality traits, abilities, physical characteristics, and so forth. The genetic basis is so strong that some have argued that life satisfaction is defined by a "setpoint" from which individuals rarely deviate (Headey & Wearing, 1989; Lykken & Tellegen, 1996). However, other research suggests that whereas some events do little to change one's characteristic level of life satisfaction, other events can have profound effects on happiness. For example, although it appears that there is adaptation to marriage such that, over time, individuals return to their setpoint before courtship began (see Lucas & Dyrenforth, 2005), adaptation is partial but less complete in the other direction—when marriage results in divorce (Lucas, 2005b). Our point here is that this debate on the dominance of a setpoint and the importance of events in changing life satisfaction has seemingly been lost on job satisfaction research. Many of the concepts, arguments, and methods could be incorporated into studies on job satisfaction, and we can see no reason why this should not take place.

Fourth and related, Brickman and Campbell's (1971) "hedonic treadmill" concept suggests that although individuals do react rather strongly to good and bad events, over time they then tend to adapt to these events and return to their original level of happiness. As noted by Diener (2000), one of the explanations for this adaptation effect is that individuals constantly change their expectancies and goals in response to new information. If an individual receives a pay raise at work, he or she quickly adjusts aspirations and mentally "spends" the reward. However, whereas adaptation effects are not uncommon, it is clear that people do not completely habituate to all conditions. As reported in Diener, Lucas, and Scollon (2006), using data from two large longitudinal studies, Lucas (2005a) found that individuals whose well-being was measured, on average, 7 years before and 7 years after onset of a disability reported substantial drops in life satisfaction and little evidence of adaptation (returning to predisability life satisfaction levels) over time. As Diener et al. (2006) conclude in examining the evidence on adaptation to positive and negative events, "Adaptation may proceed slowly over a period of years, and in some cases the process is never complete" (p. 311). Although some subjective well-being research has considered work events such as job loss, very little of this line of research has made its way into organizational psychology. Clearly, it is not a long bridge to build.

Fifth, as Judge and Church (2000) noted, the extent to which organizations have adopted the term *job satisfaction* and institutionalized interventions based on job-satisfaction-related theory and research is mixed, at best. Job satisfaction, for example, is rarely included as part of an organization's key values, basic beliefs, core competencies, or guiding principles, nor is the topic given much direct exposure in popular business books. Judge and Church (2000) conducted a survey of practitioners (most of whom were employed in the human resource area) regarding their organization's general perception of job satisfaction, its relative importance, and the use of the term in their organizations. Roughly half of the practitioners indicated that job satisfaction as a term and singular construct was rarely, if ever, mentioned or considered in their organizations. When asked next about the utilization of current theory and research on job satisfaction, the results were even less optimistic. Most practitioners indicated that research was rarely, if ever, consulted or valued in their organizations. There is a real gap between how job satisfaction is viewed by researchers and organizations, and given the centrality of work to individual's well-being, we think most researchers are hampered by a somewhat Panglossian belief that because we believe organizations *should* value job satisfaction and the well-being of their employees, they *do* so. But the values of organizational managers and subjective well-being researchers are not necessarily the same.

Finally, increasingly we see the chasm between psychology and economics being bridged. Some economists, for example, are using neuroscience to determine how brain activity is related to economic decision making (Camerer, Loewenstein, & Prelec, 2005). Kahneman and Krueger (2006) have applied economic concepts to the study of well-being. Outside of work on how labor market conditions can affect the degree to which individuals will leave dissatisfying jobs (Iverson & Currivan, 2003), however, little job satisfaction research has made use of economic concepts. Although the Cornell model (reviewed earlier) is an interesting blend of economic and psychological concepts, we are not aware of any direct tests of the model, in whole or in part. Such tests would prove worthwhile.

Conclusion

In summary, job satisfaction is a salient and perhaps inveterate attitude, permeating cognitive, affective, and behavioral aspects of peoples' work and nonwork lives. These features accentuate the importance of job satisfaction as a construct worthy of attention in the organizational sciences as well as subjective well-being research more generally. The reciprocal nature of job attitudes and subjective well-being highlights the fact that a sound understanding of one domain is incomplete without due consideration of the other.

References

Arvey, R. D., Bouchard, T. J., Segal, N. L., & Abraham, L. M. (1989). Job satisfaction: Environmental and genetic components. *Journal of Applied Psychology, 74,* 187–192.

Ashby, F. G., Isen, A. M., & Turken, U. (1999). A neuropsychological theory of positive affect and its influence on cognition. *Psychological Review, 106,* 529–550.

Bateman, T. S., & Organ, D. W. (1983). Job satisfaction and the good soldier: The relationship between affect and employee "citizenship." *Academy of Management Journal, 26,* 587–595.

Bowling, N. A., Beehr, T. A., Wagner, S. H., & Libkuman, T. M. (2005). Adaptation level theory, opponent process theory, and dispositions: An integrated approach to the stability of job satisfaction. *Journal of Applied Psychology, 90,* 1044–1053.

Brayfield, A. H., & Rothe, H. F. (1951). An index of job satisfaction. *Journal of Applied Psychology, 35,* 307–311.

Brickman, P., & Campbell, D. T. (1971). Hedonic relativism and planning the good society. In M. H. Appley (Ed.), *Adaptation level theory: A symposium* (pp. 287–302). New York: Academic Press.

Brief, A. P. (1998). *Attitudes in and around organizations.* Thousand Oaks, CA: Sage.

Brief, A. P., & Roberson, L. (1989). Job attitude organization: An exploratory study. *Journal of Applied Social Psychology, 19,* 717–727.

Brief, A. P., & Weiss, H. M. (2002). Organizational behavior: Affect at work. *Annual Review of Psychology, 53,* 279–307.

Byrk, A. S., & Raudenbush, S. W. (1992). *Hierarchical linear models: Applications and data analysis methods.* Newbury Park, CA: Sage.

Camerer, C. F., Loewenstein, G. F., & Prelec, D. (2005). Neuroeconomics: How neuroscience can inform economics. *Journal of Economic Literature, 43,* 9–64.

Carsten, J. M., & Spector, P. W. (1987). Unemployment, job satisfaction, and employee turnover: A meta-analytic test of the Muchinsky model. *Journal of Applied Psychology, 72,* 374–381.

Diener, E. (1984). Subjective well-being. *Psychological Bulletin, 95,* 542–575.

Diener, E. (2000). Subjective well-being: The science of happiness and a proposal for a national index. *American Psychologist, 55,* 34–43.

Diener, E., & Larsen, R. (1984). Temporal stability and cross-situational consistency of affective, behavioral, and cognitive responses. *Journal of Personality and Social Psychology, 47,* 871–883.

Diener, E., Lucas, R. E., & Scollon, C. N. (2006). Beyond the hedonic treadmill: Revising the adaptation theory of well-being. *American Psychologist, 61,* 305–314.

Eagley, A. H., & Chaiken, S. (1993). *The psychology of attitudes.* New York: Harcourt.

Farrell, D. (1983). Exit, voice, loyalty, and neglect as responses to job dissatisfaction: A multidimensional scaling study. *Academy of Management Journal, 26,* 596–607.

Fishbein, M. (1980). A theory of reasoned action: Some applications and implications. In H. Howe & M. M. Page (Eds.), *Nebraska symposium on motivation: Beliefs, attitudes, and values* (pp. 65–116). Lincoln: University of Nebraska Press.

Fishbein, M., & Ajzen, I. (1974). Attitudes towards objects as predictors of single and multiple behavioral criteria. *Psychological Review, 81,* 59–74.

Frye, C. M. (1996). *New evidence for the job characteristics model: A meta-analysis of the job characteristics–job satisfaction relationship using composite correlations.* Paper presented at the 11th annual meeting of the Society for Industrial and Organizational Psychology, San Diego, CA.

Gerhart, B. (2005). The (affective) dispositional approach to job satisfaction: Sorting out the policy implications. *Journal of Organizational Behavior, 26,* 79–97.

Getman, J. G., Goldberg, S. B., & Herman, J. B. (1976). *Union representation elections: Law and reality.* New York: Sage.

Gilbert, D. (2006). *Stumbling on happiness.* New York: Knopf.

Hackman, J. R., & Oldham, G. R. (1976). Motivation through the design of work: Test of a theory. *Organizational Behavior and Human Performance, 16,* 250–279.

Hamner, W., & Smith, F. J. (1978). Work attitudes as predictors of unionization activity. *Journal of Applied Psychology, 63,* 415–421.

Hanisch, K. A., & Hulin, C. L. (1990). Retirement as a voluntary organizational withdrawal behavior. *Journal of Vocational Behavior, 37,* 60–78.

Hanisch, K. A., & Hulin, C. L. (1991). General attitudes and organizational withdrawal: An evaluation of a causal model. *Journal of Vocational Behavior, 39,* 110–128.

Harrison, D. A., Newman, D. A., & Roth, P. L. (2006). How important are job attitudes? Meta-analytic comparisons of integrative behavioral outcomes and time sequences. *Academy of Management Journal, 49,* 305–325.

Headey, B., & Wearing, A. (1989). Personality, life events, and subjective well-being: Toward a dynamic equilibrium model. *Journal of Personality and Social Psychology, 57,* 731–739.

Herzberg, F. (1967). *Work and the nature of man.* Cleveland, OH: World Book.

Hom, P. W. (2001). The legacy of Hulin's work on turnover thinking and research. In F. D. Drasgow & J. M. Brett (Eds.), *Psychology of work: Theoretically based empirical research* (pp. 169–187). Mahwah, NJ: Erlbaum.

Hom, P. W., Katerberg, R., & Hulin, C. L. (1979). A comparative examination of three approaches to the prediction of turnover. *Journal of Applied Psychology, 64,* 280–290.

Hulin, C. L. (1966). Job satisfaction and turnover in a female clerical population. *Journal of Applied Psychology, 50,* 280–285.

Hulin, C. L. (1968). The effects of changes in job satisfaction levels on turnover. *Journal of Applied Psychology, 52,* 122–126.

Hulin, C. L. (1991). Adaptation, persistence, commitment in organizations. In M. Dunnette & L. Hough (Eds.), *Handbook of industrial and organizational psychology* (2nd ed., pp. 445–507). Palo Alto, CA: Consulting Psychologists Press.

Hulin, C. L., & Judge, T. A. (2003). Job attitudes. In W. C. Borman, D. R. Ilgen, & R. J. Klimoski (Eds.), *Handbook of psychology: Industrial and organizational psychology* (pp. 255–276). Hoboken, NJ: Wiley.

Hulin, C. L., Roznowski, M., & Hachiya, D. (1985). Alternative opportunities and withdrawal decisions: Empirical and theoretical discrepancies and an integration. *Psychological Bulletin, 97,* 233–250.

Isen, A. M. (2002). Missing in action in the AIM: Positive affect's facilitation of cognitive flexibility, innovation, and problem solving. *Psychological Inquiry, 13,* 57–65.

Isen, A. M. (2003). Positive affect as a source of human strength. In L. G. Aspinwall & U.

M. Staudinger (Eds.), *A psychology of human strengths: Fundamental questions and future directions for a positive psychology* (pp. 179–195). Washington, DC: American Psychological Association.

Iverson, R. D., & Currivan, D. B. (2003). Union participation, job satisfaction, and employee turnover: An event-history analysis of the exit-voice hypothesis. *Industrial Relations, 42,* 101–105.

Judge, T. A., & Bono, J. E. (2001). Relationship of core self-evaluations traits—self-esteem, generalized self-efficacy, locus of control, and emotional stability—with job satisfaction and job performance: A meta-analysis. *Journal of Applied Psychology, 86,* 80–92.

Judge, T. A., Bono, J. E., Erez, A., & Locke, E. A. (2005). Core self-evaluations and job and life satisfaction: The role of self-concordance and goal attainment. *Journal of Applied Psychology, 90,* 257–268.

Judge, T. A., Bono, J. E., & Locke, E. A. (2000). Personality and job satisfaction: The mediating role of job characteristics. *Journal of Applied Psychology, 85,* 237–249.

Judge, T. A., Boudreau, J. W., & Bretz, R. D. (1994). Job and life attitudes of male executives. *Journal of Applied Psychology, 79,* 767–782.

Judge, T. A., & Church, A. H. (2000). Job satisfaction: Research and practice. In C. L. Cooper & E. A. Locke (Eds.), *Industrial and organizational psychology: Linking theory with practice* (pp. 166–198). Oxford, UK: Blackwell.

Judge, T. A., Heller, D., & Mount, M. K. (2002). Five-factor model of personality and job satisfaction: A meta-analysis. *Journal of Applied Psychology, 87,* 530–541.

Judge, T. A., & Hulin, C. L. (1993). Job satisfaction as a reflection of disposition: A multiple-source causal analysis. *Organizational Behavior and Human Decision Processes, 56,* 388–421.

Judge, T. A., & Larsen, R. J. (2001). Dispositional affect and job satisfaction: A review and theoretical extension. *Organizational Behavior and Human Decision Processes, 86,* 67–98.

Judge, T. A., & Locke, E. A. (1993). Effect of dysfunctional thought processes on subjective well-being and job satisfaction. *Journal of Applied Psychology, 78,* 475–490.

Judge, T. A., Locke, E. A., & Durham, C. C. (1997). The dispositional causes of job satisfaction: A core evaluations approach. *Research in Organizational Behavior, 19,* 151–188.

Judge, T. A., Locke, E. A., Durham, C. C., & Kluger, A. N. (1998). Dispositional effects on job and life satisfaction: The role of core evaluations. *Journal of Applied Psychology, 83,* 17–34.

Judge, T. A., Thoresen, C. J., Bono, J. E., & Patton, G. K. (2000). The job satisfaction–job performance relationship: A qualitative and quantitative review. *Psychological Bulletin, 127,* 376–407.

Judge, T. A., & Watanabe, S. (1993). Another look at the job satisfaction–life satisfaction relationship. *Journal of Applied Psychology, 78,* 939–948.

Judge, T. A., & Watanabe, S. (1994). Individual differences in the nature of the relationship between job and life satisfaction. *Journal of Occupational and Organizational Psychology, 67,* 101–107.

Jurgensen, C. E. (1978). Job preferences (What makes a job good or bad?). *Journal of Applied Psychology, 50,* 479–487.

Kahneman, D., & Krueger, A. (2006). Developments in the measurement of subjective well-being. *Journal of Economic Perspectives, 20,* 3–24.

Kunin, T. (1955). The construction of a new type of attitude measure. *Personnel Psychology, 8,* 65–77.

Landy, F. J. (1978). An opponent process theory of job satisfaction. *Journal of Applied Psychology, 63,* 533–547.

Larson, R., & Csikszentmihalyi, M. (1983). The experience sampling method. In H. T. Reis (Ed.), *Naturalistic approaches to studying social interaction* (pp. 41–56). San Francisco: Jossey-Bass.

Law, K. S., Wong, C. S., & Mobley, W. H. (1998). Towards a taxonomy of multidimensional constructs. *Academy of Management Review, 23,* 741–755.

Locke, E. A. (1976). The nature and causes of job satisfaction. In M. D. Dunnette (Ed.), *Handbook of industrial and organizational psychology* (pp. 1297–1343). Chicago: Rand McNally.

Lucas, R. E. (2005a). *Happiness can change: A longitudinal study of adaptation to disability.* Manuscript submitted for publication.

Lucas, R. E. (2005b). Time does not heal all wounds: A longitudinal study of reaction and adaptation to divorce. *Psychological Science, 16,* 945–950.

Lucas, R. E., & Dyrenforth, P. S. (2005). The myth of marital bliss? *Psychological Inquiry, 16,* 111–115.

Lykken, D., & Tellegen, A. (1996). Happiness is a stochastic phenomenon. *Psychological Science, 7,* 186–189.

Mento, A. J., Locke, E. A., & Klein, H. J. (1992). Relationship of goal level to valence and instrumentality. *Journal of Applied Psychology, 77,* 395–405.

Miller, H. E., Katerberg, R., & Hulin, C. L. (1979). Evaluation of the Mobley, Horner, and Hollingsworth model of employee turnover. *Journal of Applied Psychology, 64,* 509–517.

Mobley, W. H., Horner, S. O., & Hollingsworth, A. T. (1978). An evaluation of precursors of hospital employee turnover. *Journal of Applied Psychology, 63,* 408–414.

Mount, M., Ilies, R., & Johnson, E. (2006). Relationship of personality traits and counterproductive work behaviors: The mediating effects of job satisfaction. *Personnel Psychology, 59,* 591–622.

Parisi, A. G., & Weiner, S. P. (1999, April). *Retention of employees: Country-specific analyses in a multinational organization.* Poster presented at the 14th annual conference of the Society for Industrial and Organizational Psychology, Atlanta, GA.

Piccolo, R. F., Judge, T. A., Takahashi, K., Watanabe, N., & Locke, E. A. (2005). Core self-evaluations in Japan: Relative effects on job satisfaction, life satisfaction and happiness. *Journal of Organizational Behavior, 26,* 965–984.

Rentsch, J. R., & Steel, R. P. (1992). Construct and concurrent validation of the Andrews and Withey Job Satisfaction Questionnaire. *Educational and Psychological Measurement, 52,* 357–367.

Roberts, B. W., Walton, K. E., & Viechtbauer, W. (2006). Patterns of mean-level change in personality traits across the life course: A meta-analysis of longitudinal studies. *Psychological Bulletin, 132,* 1–25.

Roznowski, M., Miller, H. E., & Rosse, J. G. (1992, August). *On the utility of broad-band measures of employee behavior: The case for employee adaptation and citizenship.* Paper presented at the annual meeting of the Academy of Management, Las Vegas.

Salancik, G. R., & Pfeffer, J. (1977). An examination of need–satisfaction models of job attitudes. *Administrative Science Quarterly, 22,* 427–456.

Salancik, G. R., & Pfeffer, J. (1978). A social information processing approach to job attitudes and task design. *Administrative Science Quarterly, 23,* 224–253.

Scarpello, V., & Campbell, J. P. (1983). Job satisfaction: Are all the parts there? *Personnel Psychology, 36,* 577–600.

Schmitt, N., & McCune, J. T. (1981). The relationship between job attitudes and the decision to retire. *Academy of Management Journal, 24,* 795–802.

Schriesheim, C. (1978). Job satisfaction, attitudes toward unions, and voting in a union representation election. *Journal of Applied Psychology, 63,* 548–552.

Scott, K. D., & Taylor, G. S. (1985). An examination of conflicting findings on the relationship between job satisfaction and absenteeism: A meta-analysis. *Academy of Management Journal, 28,* 599–612.

Sheldon, K. M., & Elliot, A. J. (1999). Goal striving, need satisfaction, and longitudinal well-being: The self-concordance model. *Journal of Personality and Social Psychology, 76,* 482–497.

Smith, F. J. (1977). Work attitudes as predictors of attendance on a specific day. *Journal of Applied Psychology, 62,* 16–19.

Smith, P. C., Kendall, L. M., & Hulin, C. L. (1969). *The measurement of satisfaction in work and retirement.* Chicago: Rand McNally.

Srivastava, S., John, O. P., & Gosling, S. D. (2003). Development of personality in early and middle adulthood: Set like plaster or persistent change? *Journal of Personality and Social Psychology, 84,* 1041–1053.

Staw, B. M., & Ross, J. (1985). Stability in the midst of change: A dispositional approach to job attitudes. *Journal of Applied Psychology, 70,* 469–480.

Tait, M., Padgett, M. Y., & Baldwin, T. T. (1989). Job and life satisfaction: A reevaluation of the strength of the relationship and gender effects as a function of the date of the study. *Journal of Applied Psychology, 74,* 502–507.

Thoresen, C. J., Kaplan, S. A., Barsky, A. P., Warren, C. R., & de Chermont, K. (2003). The affective underpinnings of job perceptions and attitudes: A meta-analytic review and integration. *Psychological Bulletin, 129,* 914–945.

Wanous, J. P., Reichers, A. E., & Hudy, M. J. (1997). Overall job satisfaction: How good are single-item measures? *Journal of Applied Psychology, 82,* 247–252.

Weiner, S. P. (2000, April). Worldwide technical recruiting in IBM: Research and action. In P. D. Bachiochi (Chair), *Attracting and keeping top talent in the high-tech industry.* Practitioner forum at the 15th annual conference of the Society for Industrial and Organizational Psychology, New Orleans, LA.

Weiss, D. J., Dawis, R. V., England, G. W., & Lofquist, L. H. (1967). *Manual for the Minnesota Satisfaction Questionnaire.* Minneapolis: Industrial Relations Center, University of Minnesota.

Weiss, H. M. (2002). Deconstructing job satisfaction: Separating evaluations, beliefs and affective experiences. *Human Resource Management Review, 12,* 173–194.

Weiss, H. M., & Cropanzano, R. (1996). Affective events theory: A theoretical discussion of the structure, causes, and consequences of affective experiences at work. *Research in Organizational Behavior, 18*, 1–74.

Weiss, H. M., Nicholas, J. P., & Daus, C. S. (1999). An examination of the joint effects of affective experiences and job beliefs on job satisfaction and variations in affective experiences over time. *Organizational Behavior and Human Decision Processes, 78*, 1–24.

Weitz, J. (1952). A neglected concept in the study of job satisfaction. *Personnel Psychology, 5*, 201–205.

Wicker, A. W. (1969). Attitudes versus actions: The relationship of verbal and overt behavioral responses to attitude objects. *Journal of Social Issues, 25*, 41–78.

Zalesny, M. D. (1985). Comparison of economic and noneconomic factors in predicting faculty vote preference in a union representation election. *Journal of Applied Psychology, 70*, 243–256.

20

Comparing Subjective Well-Being across Cultures and Nations

The *"What"* and *"Why"* Questions

EUNKOOK M. SUH and JAYOUNG KOO

Diener's (1984) landmark review paper published in *Psychological Bulletin* sparked numerous lines of research activities under the heading of *subjective well-being*. One research area that started to create its own niche in the early 1990s was the field of culture and subjective well-being. This period overlapped with the publication of prominent articles on culture (Markus & Kitayama, 1991; Triandis, 1989), and also with the growing recognition that subjective well-being should be understood as an individual-level as well as a collective-level phenomenon.

A number of early articles set the stage for this field and challenged some of the prevalent opinions of the time. In particular, three papers are noteworthy. Diener, Diener, and Diener (1995) found that one of the strongest predictors of national differences in subjective well-being was the degree of collectivism–individualism (even after controlling for national income level). This was a very important finding because at the time economic factors were deemed most critical for the occurrence of national differences in subjective well-being. An article by Diener and Diener (1995) also drew attention because it suggested that self-esteem, a psychological factor traditionally deemed indispensable for mental health in the West, seemed far less crucial in determining subjective well-being in other cultures. Finally, Diener, Suh, Smith, and Shao (1995) demonstrated that several methodological artifacts that may plague cross-cultural research (e.g., response bias, translation) do not completely explain the subjective well-being differences between cultures. The reasons underlying cultural differences in subjective well-being levels seemed to be substantial ones (e.g., difference in emotion norms) rather than methodological errors.

Prompted by these initial research issues, the field of culture and subjective well-being has grown rapidly in a short span of time. Figure 20.1 shows the number of publications (journal articles, books, dissertations) found by PsycINFO using the combined keywords of *culture* and *well-being* from 1991 to 2005. In a single decade (from 97 during 1991–1995 to 481 during 2001–2005), there has been roughly a fivefold increase in the sheer number of publications on this topic! Along with the quantitative increase, a special issue published by the *Journal of Happiness Studies* (Suh & Oishi, 2004), an *Annual Review of Psychology* chapter (Diener, Oishi, & Lucas, 2003), and an edited volume (Diener & Suh, 2000) has been recently devoted to the topic of culture and subjective well-being.

Given the highly vibrant research activities during the past decade, it seems like an opportune time to evaluate and digest the major findings from this productive period and to target the set of issues that warrants more concentrated research attention in the upcoming years. Although a wide array of questions has been investigated during the decade, many of those were serial efforts prompted by the two large questions set up by the early papers. *What* are the key components of subjective well-being across cultures (Diener & Diener, 1995)? *Why* do national/cultural differences in mean levels of subjective well-being occur (Diener, Diener, & Diener, 1995; Diener et al., 1995)?

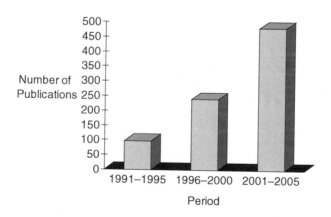

FIGURE 20.1. Total number of publications on *culture* and *well-being* from 1991 to 2005. Data from PsycINFO.

It is not the goal of this chapter to offer an exhaustive review of the latest research. Rather, attention is selectively centered on a few lines of findings that have been particularly influential in informing us of the interplay between culture and subjective well-being. Also, because the vast majority of empirical data come from East Asian (e.g., Japan, Korea, China) and U.S. samples, discussions focus most often on these two cultural regions.

What Makes Up Happiness across Cultures?

Virtually all human beings—from Nigerians to Peruvians to French-Canadians—think happiness is a desirable state. The precise affective experiences, the recommended means, and the conceptualizations surrounding this ultimate human desire, however, seem to show cultural variations.

An analogy is provided by humor: Everyone across the globe enjoys humor, but each cultural group is drawn to particular types of humor and has different ways of telling a joke. This analogy naturally raises two questions. First, what are the most popular types of jokes in each culture and how are they delivered? This is akin to asking what the culture-specific contents of happiness are. The second (and tougher) question is whether the jokes in some cultures are intrinsically more hilarious than those of others, and if so, why (i.e., why are some cultures happier than others?). A decade of research offers some insights on these two questions. Let's begin with the relatively easier one—what makes up happiness in different cultures?

To begin, there seem to be some cultural differences in the definitional accounts of happiness. Although this idea is hardly surprising, empirical investigation on this topic has been scarce, in part because of the practical and methodological difficulties posed by qualitative data. However, Lu and Gilmour (2004) recently asked Chinese and U.S. students to write essays on "What Is Happiness?" Although both groups agreed that happiness is a positive, desirable state of the mind, the Chinese emphasized spiritual cultivation and transcendence of the present, whereas the Americans' account of happiness was comparably more uplifting, elated, and emphasized the enjoyment of present life. Also importantly, the Asian respondents expressed the desire for a balanced emotional life and underlined the importance of fulfilling social expectations in their overall sense of happiness. The Americans, in contrast, asserted the importance of personal agency over social restrictions and believed that the pursuit of personal happiness cannot be compromised in any way.

Recent empirical findings (for review, see Diener et al., 2003; Uchida, Norasakkunkit, & Kitayama, 2004) strike a similar cord with the open-ended responses documented by Lu and Gilmour (2004). Generally speaking, the critical predictors of happiness among Western cultural members are comprised of elements that promote, signify, and maintain a highly independent and agentic mode of being. Important predictors of happiness in the East, on the other hand, seem to affirm the fundamental interconnectedness between the self and significant others (Kitayama & Markus, 2000). Among the wide array of specific affective, cognitive, and motivational phenomena that support this general picture, several findings stand out.

First, the role of emotion in people's judgment and experience of subjective well-being seems to vary. Compared to individualistic cultural members, collectivists are less inclined to equate an emotionally "happy life" with a "good, satisfying life." The correlation between affect balance (relative frequency of pleasant minus unpleasant emotions) and overall life satisfaction is much weaker in collectivist than in individualistic nations (Schimmack, Radhakrishna, Oishi, Dzokoto, & Ahadi, 2002; Suh, Diener, Oishi, & Triandis, 1998). The relatively idiosyncratic and unique nature of emotional experience may embody less significance compared to social cues, such as the opinions held by others in one's life (cf. Potter, 1988). In direct support of this idea, when the social connectedness of self-identity is primed, individuals pay greater attention to how their life is appraised by significant others than to their inner emotions in their life satisfaction judgment process (Suh, Diener, & Updegraff, in press).

Another interesting finding in the affect and subjective well-being area is that pleasant emotional experience, such as happiness, explicitly requires a social component in East Asian cultures. According to Kitayama, Markus, and Kurokawa (2000), happiness is associated more strongly with interpersonally engaging emotions (e.g., friendly feelings) in Japan, whereas it is more closely related with interpersonally disengaging emotions (e.g., pride) in the United States. In a related line, Park, Choi, and Suh (2006) recently found that the amount of pleasantness reported by Koreans while engaging in a task varied significantly between interpersonal conditions—whether they collaborated with a friend or a stranger. This discriminative emotional experience pattern was especially prominent among individuals with a strong interdependent self. In other words, the "with whom" factor seems to loom large in determining the experience of pleasant emotions of those with a strongly relation-oriented identity.

Research on motives and goals is another piece in the *what* puzzle. Given the centrality of others in conceptualizations of self-identity, the happiness of Asian Americans, more so than European Americans, is elevated after fulfilling goals that are directed to please or receive approval from significant others (Iyengar & Lepper, 1999; Oishi & Diener, 2001; Oishi & Sullivan, 2005). On surface, these findings may seem inconsistent with recent claims that, regardless of culture, self-directed goals are more conducive to subjective well-being than externally imposed goals (e.g., Chirkov, Ryan, & Willness, 2005; Sheldon et al., 2004).

How should we reconcile this latest controversy on goals and subjective well-being? The key seems to be the degree of internalization of the culturally sanctioned values. Even among East Asians, not all derive greater pleasure from fulfilling parental expectations than from engaging in personally rewarding activities. It depends on whether the person following the parent's desires feels coerced and obligated or is acting spontaneously with sincere pleasure. The cultural difference is that the *probability* of encountering a person who genuinely prefers to satisfy his or her parents' wishes before his or her own is higher in the East than West. Regardless of the content of the behavior, it seems reasonable to conclude that humans, by design, have a greater chance of experiencing positive experiences when they do "what they enjoy and believe in" (Sheldon et al., 2004, p. 220). Much of the cultural variations documented in this area seems to be about the "what" part; the "enjoy and believe in" part seems universal.

Finally, several dispositional qualities that were traditionally believed to be essential for mental health are being reevaluated in a cross-cultural context. For instance, recent findings suggest that psychologists might have overestimated the importance of having a strong sense of personal control (Morling, Kitayama, & Miyamoto, 2003), high self-esteem (Diener et al., 1995; Chen, Cheung, Bond, & Leung, 2006), and a consistent self-identity (Suh, 2002) in the achievement of mental health. These are important findings that highlight the power of cultural influence. At the same time, however, it is important not to overinterpret the data. At an intracultural level, even in Eastern cultures, individuals with high self-esteem and a more consistent self-identity are happier than those who score low on these dimensions. These constructs seem less critical in predicting the person's subjective well-being in the East only in an intercultural sense (compared to the West). To date, no psychological quality has been found that strongly and consistently correlates with subjective well-being in *opposite* directions between cultures.

Returning to our humor analogy, the types of jokes that are most popular in one culture may not be the most enjoyed ones in another. That is, a great deal of cultural nuance exists in the conceptualization of, and in the shades of experiences related with happiness. However, are these differences simply a matter of different cultural tastes, or do they partly explain why some cultures are happier than others? With this key question in mind, we move on to the next section.

Why Are Some Cultures Happier Than Others?

Arguably one of the most solid findings from the cross-cultural/national research on subjective well-being is that individualistic nations are happier than collectivistic countries (Diener et al., 1995; Diener & Suh, 1999; Veenhoven, 1999). The mean-level difference between individualistic and collectivistic cultures, to some extent, arises from societal and political factors confounded with individualism (e.g., income level, Diener et al., 1995; democracy, Inglehart & Klinge-mann, 2000; political empowerment, Frey & Stutzer, 2002).

However, a decade of research makes it clear that these socioeconomic con-ditions alone are insufficient for explaining why individualistic nations consis-tently report higher levels of happiness than collectivistic nations. Besides income level or political structure, cultures also vary along a wide spectrum of psycho-logical habits and characteristics that are related to the experience and expressions of happiness. For instance, emotion norms (Eid & Diener, 2001), socialization of emotions (Diener & Lucas, 2004), and cognitive biases (Diener, Lucas, Oishi, & Suh, 2002; Oishi, 2002) associated with happiness vary considerably across cul-tures.

A recent study by Rice and Steele (2004) further implies that cultural differ-ences in subjective well-being may reflect something more than the objective conditions of life. They found that the relative ranking of the subjective well-being levels of Americans with ancestors from 20 different nations is quite similar to the subjective well-being levels obtained from the citizens of the correspond-ing nations. By surveying U.S. residents only, this study controls for many of the confounding social-condition factors between cultures/nations. The findings by Rice and Steele suggest that the cultural agents that influence subjective well-being might be quite amorphous and stubborn, and this might partly explain why national differences in subjective well-being are temporally so stable (Inglehart & Klingemann, 2000; Veenhoven, 1999).

One key reason for examining mean differences in subjective well-being between nations/cultures is to gain insights about the collective conditions that enhance or suppress human happiness. At first brush, individualism and collectiv-ism neither seems to have a clear edge in producing higher subjective well-being (cf. Diener & Suh, 1999). Different cultural members may prefer different activi-ties and experiences in their pursuit of happiness, but one might think that the different paths are equally potent means for reaching the destination. If this is the case, should we expect the "perfect Japanese" to be every bit as happy as a "per-fect American"? Many of the current investigators in this field may answer "yes" to this question; however, it is quite plausible that the answer is "no."

A strong version of cultural relativism (i.e., different cultural strategies for achieving happiness are equally viable; they are merely different in content) would find it difficult to explain why the difference in subjective well-being level between individualistic and collectivistic societies remains so robust. All cultures are evolved to efficiently resolve pressing human needs, such as reproduction or safety needs. However, ecological opportunities and restrictions configure the nuts and bolts that sustain each cultural system, including its norms, values, prac-tices, and central ideologies (Triandis & Suh, 2002). Among the various meta-assumptions held by cultures, particularly significant is the one concerning the re-lation between the individual and the society. Certain cultures are built around the premise that the individual exists for the larger collective unit; in other cultures, the opposite is assumed. Crudely speaking, collectivism is prototypical of the former type of culture, and individualism is a prime example of the latter.

Most important to our discussion, these two contrasting cultural schemes may *not* be designed to produce the same type of cultural capital (see Ahuvia, 2002). Collectivism has its ultimate sight on social order and harmony, and hence the system constantly reinforces and idealizes the type of self that is able to keep its desires in check for the greater goods of the family, group, and community. Self-regulation is sanctioned over self-expression, and fulfillment of social obligations comes before discussions of personal rights and preferences. In contrast, individualism believes in the irrevocable value, power, and capabilities of, literally, the individual. The normative cultural expectation is that each person should be self-directive and self-sufficient, and find, consolidate, and uplift the best within the self. *Self-actualization*, the key word in the discussion of ideal living in the West, encapsulates these beliefs. In the East, in contrast, people are encouraged to perfect the inner attributes of the self for a social reason—to be used appropriately *for* the service of the larger society (Cho, 2006).

Between the two cultural systems, which one has an edge in producing "happy individuals"? This chapter suggests two general possibilities for why individualistic cultures may have the advantage. First, greater sacrifice of instinctive needs and desires is required to live an "appropriate" collectivist than an individualist life. As Freud (1930/1961) claimed in *Civilization and Its Discontents*, conflict and friction between individual desires and social constraints is the rule rather than an exception. In the continuous bargain between the self and society, the individual gives up his or her instinctive impulses in exchange for social rewards. One of the biggest social awards is social acceptance by others (Baumeister, DeWall, Ciarocco, & Twenge, 2005), which is more crucial for the functioning of a collectivistic than an individualistic pattern of life. As a result, by necessity, collectivist cultural members are more likely than individualists to curb their instinctive, self-gratifying desires (often including personal happiness) in their bargain for social approval.

One might argue that the social gains (e.g., social approval, respect) may fully make up for the negatives of giving up personal desires in collectivistic cultures. This would be a valid argument only if one unit of social reward translated to an exactly equivalent amount of personal happiness in Eastern cultures. This idea seems rather unrealistic. Although it is true that social rewards constitute a very important part of the collectivist's sense of personal happiness, incommensurable differences still remain between the two. Social rewards are strongly related to happiness in the East, but still, it is *not* happiness itself.

In fact, several scholars have argued that even in collectivistic cultures, people who adopt individualistic values report higher levels of subjective well-being and self-esteem than the more collective-minded ones (Heine, Lehman, Markus,

& Kitayama, 1999). Preliminary findings from Korean university samples indicate that subjective well-being is related positively with independent self-construal and negatively with the interdependent self-view (Koo & Suh, 2006). Similarly, from mainland Chinese and Taiwanese samples, Lu and Gilmour (2006) found that the frequency of experiencing positive emotions is related more closely with the independent than the interdependent self.

The above findings have an important implication. They seem to go against the idea that those who enjoy high levels of happiness are people who have psychological dispositions that fit into the cultural template (e.g., being interdependent in collectivistic cultures). Rather, these latest findings imply that, regardless of the cultural context, the independent styles of thinking and behaving may have a more direct connection to personal happiness than the collectivistic approach. However, the individualistic strategies will meet a "tipping point" where the personal costs incurred by ignoring collective demands start to outweigh the positive payoffs. Collectivist cultural members confront this tipping point more often, and in more domains of life, than individualist cultural members.

Secondly, collectivism may nurture various dispositional qualities that unintentionally create potholes in the road to happiness. It seems that the East Asian self-system is optimized for maintaining social connections with others. However, a self that is preoccupied with social concerns may acquire a wide range of psychological characteristics—motivational, cognitive, emotional, and behavioral—that create friction in the pursuit of personal happiness (see Suh, in press, for a detailed discussion). For instance, at a cognitive level, the highly socially oriented self construes and evaluates itself more often by concrete and specific social criteria (e.g., gaining admission to a top college) than by idiosyncratic terms. Many findings demonstrate that chronic reliance on explicit external criteria, such as social comparison information, is related with lower levels of subjective well-being (Lyubomirsky & Ross, 1997; White & Lehman, 2005). This is because external social standards allow less latitude in interpretation and therefore are more difficult to tailor to the advantage of the self than idiosyncratically defined standards (e.g., Dunning & McElwee, 1995).

Other disadvantages could occur at the motivational and behavioral levels for the highly collectively oriented East Asians. When the focal concern is fulfilling social obligations and living up to the expectations of others (as in Japan), failing to meet these standards has a bigger blow than the rewards for surpassing them (Heine et al., 2001). In the long run, individuals in such cultures find themselves framing goals more in prevention-oriented than in promotion-oriented terms (Elliot, Chirkov, Kim, & Sheldon, 2001). This is unfortunate because a large body of evidence indicates that positive emotions and subjective well-being are inherently related to approach-oriented behaviors, thoughts, and neurological processes (e.g., Elliot & Thrash, 2002; Lee, Aaker, & Gardner,

2000; Updegraff, Gable, & Taylor, 2004; Urry et al., 2004). Finally, at the level of emotion, the experience and expression of positive affect are not as much idealized in Eastern cultures as in the West (Eid & Diener, 2001; Diener & Lucas, 2004; Diener & Suh, 1999). This is probably because East Asians believe that strong positive emotions (pride, happiness) have a potential to disrupt interpersonal harmony or lead to negligent behaviors. Such beliefs may have a cost. They could discourage individuals from engaging in various behavioral and cognitive practices that are found to enhance or prolong subjective well-being (see Larsen & Prizmic, Chapter 13, this volume), such as capitalizing on positive life events (Gable, Reis, Impett, & Asher, 2004).

In conclusion, it is worth questioning whether the ultimate blueprint of all cultures is to enhance happiness at a personal level. Some cultures, such as East Asian collectivistic societies, might have arrived at the present form because it maximized the chances of maintaining collective harmony and order. Believing that happiness is meant to be the goal of life could be a view most representative of contemporary Western cultures.

For the Future

Merely a decade ago, the terms *subjective well-being* and *culture* were rarely paired together in the research agendas of psychologists. In a relatively short span of time, however, the almost nonexistent field has become a highly active research area of subjective well-being. Much research has accumulated during the past decade, thanks to innovative studies, bold ideas, and improvements in measurements and data analyses strategies. In short, the past decade has been an extremely fruitful one. Following are a few research agendas that might make the upcoming decade an even more productive one.

First, it is hoped that the methodological arsenals in this field continue to develop and expand in the upcoming years. Various developments have occurred in the areas of measurement (e.g., Kim, 2004; Scollon, Diener, Oishi, & Biswas-Diener, 2004; Suh & Sung, 2006) and statistical methods (e.g., Eid & Diener, 2001). Particularly promising is the finding by Scollon et al. that different measurements render similar conclusions about the relative position of the subjective well-being of different cultural groups. Hopefully, future studies will include two types of powerful data that are currently missing in the field: longitudinal and brain imaging techniques.

At the conceptual level, two questions seem particularly worthy of future investigation. First, what are the consequences of happiness in different cultures? Lyubomirsky, King, and Diener (2005) offered compelling evidence that positive affect, at least in the United States, is a cause of many desirable life outcomes. Does this finding hold true in cultures that express somewhat ambivalent attitudes about happiness? It seems extremely unlikely that happiness is a personal liability in any culture. However, the particular life domains in which the happy person benefits the most and the magnitude of this outcome need to be determined empirically, especially through longitudinal data.

Another highly promising research candidate is the study of lay theories about happiness. One important reason for why various aspects of subjective well-being differ across cultures is because different cultural members have different ideas about the genesis, attainability, desirability, and outcomes of happiness. Whether such lay beliefs are really true is not the point; what is important is the fact that the way happiness is represented in people's mind (even if incorrectly) affects virtually every decisions and judgments made about happiness.

To illustrate, unlike Western cultural members, East Asians take a more dialectic perspective on the relation between happiness and unhappiness (Kitayama & Markus, 1999; Suh, 2000). One outcome of such belief is the prediction of future happiness. For instance, the happiness that has linearly increased since the past is expected to reverse its future trajectory by Chinese, whereas Americans believe that the trend will continue (Ji, Nisbett, & Su, 2001). Prediction of happiness is related to another type of lay belief. In an ongoing line of research (Koo & Suh, 2006), we are examining people's belief about whether a fixed or an unlimited amount of happiness exists in their personal lives and in the world. As expected, the "finite amount" theory holders were reluctant to capitalize on positive events (probably fearing that happiness would vanish), predicted that future fortune would reverse the current trend, and perceived overly happy people as being naïve and immature. Understanding the lay beliefs about happiness will offer refreshing insights about why, when, and how people feel happy in different cultures.

In Closing

There is limited scientific value in merely describing cultural differences in subjective well-being. Such descriptive efforts, however, are necessary for understanding the various *why* questions that arise in the study of culture and subjective well-being. One question that has occupied the minds of many researchers is why happy people are more easily found in individualistic than in collectivistic cultures. In search for the answer, the possibility that cultures are not equally enthusiastic about the idea of promoting individual happiness needs full consideration. This line of thinking does not imply that certain cultures are intrinsically better than others; it simply means that different cultures might have different opinions about what is most worth the pursuit. The opinion may change over time. But, very slowly.

References

Ahuvia, A. (2002). Individualism/collectivism and cultures of happiness: A theoretical conjecture on the relationship between consumption, culture and subjective well-being at the national level. *Journal of Happiness Studies, 3*, 23–36.

Baumeister, R. F., DeWall, C. N., Ciarocco, N. J., & Twenge, J. M. (2005). Social exclusion impairs self-regulation. *Journal of Personality and Social Psychology, 88*, 589–604.

Chen, S. X., Cheung, F. M., Bond, M. H., & Leung, J. (2006). Going beyond self-esteem to predict life satisfaction: The Chinese case. *Asian Journal of Social Psychology, 9*, 24–35.

Chirkov, V., Ryan, R., & Willness, C. (2005). Cultural context and psychological needs in Canada and Brazil: Testing a self-determination approach to the internalization of cultural practices, identity, and well-being. *Journal of Cross-Cultural Psychology, 36*, 423–443.

Cho, G. (2006). *The ideal personhood: East versus West.* Seoul: Jishiksanup-sa.

Diener, E. (1984). Subjective well-being. *Psychological Bulletin, 95*, 542–575.

Diener, E., & Diener, M. (1995). Cross-cultural correlates of life satisfaction and self-esteem. *Journal of Personality and Social Psychology, 68*, 653–663.

Diener, E., Diener, M., & Diener, C. (1995). Factors predicting the subjective well-being of nations. *Journal of Personality and Social Psychology, 69*, 851–864.

Diener, E., Lucas, R., Oishi, S., & Suh, E. M. (2002). Looking up and looking down: Weighting good and bad information in life satisfaction judgments. *Personality and Social Psychology Bulletin, 28*, 437–445.

Diener, E., Oishi, S., & Lucas, R. (2003). Personality, culture, and subjective well-being: Emotional and cognitive evaluations of life. *Annual Review of Psychology, 54*, 403–425.

Diener, E., & Suh, E. M. (1999). National differences in subjective well-being. In D. Kahneman, E. Diener, & N. Schwarz (Eds.), *Well-being: The foundations of hedonic psychology* (pp. 434–450). New York: Sage.

Diener, E., & Suh, E. M. (2000). *Culture and subjective well-being.* Cambridge, MA: MIT Press.

Diener, E., Suh, E., Smith, H., & Shao, L. (1995). National differences in subjective well-being: Why do they occur? *Social Indicators Research, 34*, 7–32.

Diener, M., & Lucas, R. E. (2004). Adults' desires for children's emotions across 48 countries: Associations with individual and national characteristics. *Journal of Cross-Cultural Psychology, 35*, 525–547.

Dunning, D., & McElwee, R. O. (1995). Idiosyncratic trait definitions: Implications for self-description and social judgment. *Journal of Personality and Social Psychology, 68*, 936–946.

Eid, M., & Diener, E. (2001). Norms for experiencing emotions in different cultures: Inter- and intranational differences. *Journal of Personality and Social Psychology, 81*, 869–885.

Elliot, A. J., Chirkov, V. I., Kim, Y., & Sheldon, K. M. (2001). A cross-cultural analysis of avoidance (relative to approach) personal goals. *Psychological Science, 12*, 505–510.

Elliot, A. J., & Thrash, T. M. (2002). Approach–avoidance motivation in personality: Approach and avoidance temperaments and goals. *Journal of Personality and Social Psychology, 82,* 804–818.

Freud, S. (1961). *Civilization and its discontents.* New York: Norton. (Original work published 1930)

Frey, B. S., & Stutzer, A. (2002). *Happiness and economics.* Princeton, NJ: Princeton University Press.

Gable, S. L., Reis, H. T., Impett, E., & Asher, E. (2004). What do you do when things go right? The intrapersonal and interpersonal benefits of sharing positive events. *Journal of Personality and Social Psychology, 87,* 228–245.

Heine, S., Kitayama, S., Lehman, D. R., Takata, T., Ide, E., Leung, C., et al. (2001). Divergent consequences of success and failure in Japan and North America: An investigation of self-improving motivations and malleable selves. *Journal of Personality and Social Psychology, 81,* 599–615.

Heine, S., Lehman, D., Markus, H., & Kitayama, S. (1999). Is there a universal need for positive self-regard? *Psychological Review, 106,* 766–794.

Inglehart, R., & Klingemann, H. (2000). Genes, culture, democracy, and happiness. In E. Diener & E. M. Suh (Eds.), *Culture and subjective well-being* (pp. 165–184). Cambridge, MA: MIT Press.

Iyengar, S., & Lepper, M. (1999). Rethinking the value of choice: A cultural perspective on intrinsic motivation. *Journal of Personality and Social Psychology, 76,* 349–366.

Ji, L., Nisbett, R., & Su, Y. (2001). Culture, change, and prediction. *Psychological Science, 12,* 450–456.

Kim, D. Y. (2004). The implicit life satisfaction measure. *Asian Journal of Social Psychology, 7,* 236–261.

Kitayama, S., & Markus, H. (1999). The yin and yang of the Japanese self: The cultural psychology of personality coherence. In D. Cervone & Y. Shoda (Eds.), *The coherence of personality: Social cognitive bases of personality consistency, variability, and organization* (pp. 242–302). New York: Guilford Press.

Kitayama, S., & Markus, H. R. (2000). The pursuit of happiness and the realization of sympathy: Cultural patterns of self, social relations, and well-being. In E. Diener & E. M. Suh (Eds.), *Culture and subjective well-being.* Cambridge, MA: MIT Press.

Kitayama, S., Markus, H. R., & Kurokawa, M. (2000). Culture, emotion and well-being: Good feelings in Japan and in the United States. *Cognition and Emotion, 14,* 93–124.

Koo, J., & Suh, E. M. (2006). [Belief in fixed amount of happiness (BIFAH) and subjective well-being.] Unpublished raw data, Yonsei University, Korea.

Lee, A. Y., Aaker, J. L., & Gardner, W. L. (2000). The pleasure and pains of distinct self-construals: The role of interdependence in regulatory focus. *Journal of Personality and Social Psychology, 78,* 1122–1134.

Lu, L., & Gilmour, R. (2004). Culture and conceptions of happiness: Individual oriented and social oriented SWB. *Journal of Happiness Studies, 5,* 269–291.

Lu, L., & Gilmour, R. (2006). Individual-oriented and socially oriented cultural conceptions of subjective well-being: Conceptual analysis and scale development. *Asian Journal of Social Psychology, 9,* 36–49.

Lyubomirsky, S., King, L., & Diener, E. (2005). The benefits of frequent positive affect: Does happiness lead to success? *Psychological Bulletin, 131,* 803–855.

Lyubomirsky, S., & Ross, L. (1997). Hedonic consequences of social comparison: A contrast of happy and unhappy people. *Journal of Personality and Social Psychology, 73,* 1141–1157.

Markus, H., & Kitayama, S. (1991). Culture and the self: Implications for cognition, emotion, and motivation. *Psychological Review, 98,* 224–253.

Morling, B., Kitayama, S., & Miyamoto, Y. (2003). American and Japanese women use different coping strategies during normal pregnancy. *Personality and Social Psychology Bulletin, 29,* 1533–1546.

Oishi, S. (2002). The experiencing and remembering of well-being: A cross-cultural analysis. *Personality and Social Psychology Bulletin, 28,* 1398–1406.

Oishi, S., & Diener, E. (2001). Goals, culture, and subjective well-being. *Personality and Social Psychology Bulletin, 27,* 1674–1682.

Oishi, S., & Sullivan, H. (2005). The mediating role of parental expectations in culture and well-being. *Journal of Personality, 73,* 1267–1294.

Park, J., Choi, I., & Suh, E. M. (2006). *The "whom" versus "what" in the Korean's equation of happiness.* Manuscript in preparation.

Potter, S. H. (1988). The cultural construction of emotion in rural Chinese social life. *Ethos, 16,* 181–208.

Rice, T. W., & Steele, B. J. (2004). Subjective well-being and culture across time and space. *Journal of Cross-Cultural Psychology, 35,* 633–647.

Schimmack, U., Radhakrishnan, P., Oishi, S., Dzokoto, V., & Ahadi, S. (2002). Culture, personality, and subjective well-being: Integrating process models of life satisfaction. *Journal of Personality and Social Psychology, 82,* 582–593.

Scollon, C. N., Diener, E., Oishi, S., & Biswas-Diener, R. (2004). Emotions across cultures and methods. *Journal of Cross-Cultural Psychology, 35,* 304–326.

Sheldon, K., Elliot, A., Rtan, R., Chirkov, V., Kim, Y., Wu, C., et al. (2004). Self-concordance and subjective well-being in four cultures. *Journal of Cross-Cultural Psychology, 35,* 209–223.

Suh, E. M. (2000). Self, the hyphen between culture and subjective well-being. In E. Diener & E. M. Suh (Eds.), *Culture and subjective well-being* (pp. 63–86). Cambridge, MA: MIT Press.

Suh, E. M. (2002). Culture, identity consistency, and subjective well-being. *Journal of Personality and Social Psychology, 83,* 1378–1391.

Suh, E. M. (in press). Downsides of an *overly* context-sensitive self: Implications from the culture and subjective well-being research. *Journal of Personality.*

Suh, E. M., & Diener, E. (2006). *Stereotypes of a "happy person": Cultural variations.* Manuscript in preparation, Yonsei University, Seoul, South Korea.

Suh, E. M., Diener, E., Oishi, S., & Triandis, H. C. (1998). The shifting basis of life satisfaction judgments across cultures: Emotions versus norms. *Journal of Personality and Social Psychology, 74,* 482–493.

Suh, E. M., Diener, E., & Updegraff, J. (in press). From culture to priming conditions: How self-construal influences life satisfaction judgments. *Journal of Cross-Cultural Psychology.*

Suh, E. M., & Oishi, S. (2004). Culture and subjective well-being: Introduction to the special issue. *Journal of Happiness Studies, 5,* 219–222.

Suh, E. M., & Sung, M. (2006, August). *Affective experience patterns across interpersonal con-*

texts: Findings from the day reconstruction method (DRM). Paper presented at the annual Korean Psychological Association Conference, Seoul, Korea.

Triandis, H. C. (1989). The self and social behavior in differing cultural contexts. *Psychological Review, 96*, 506–520.

Triandis, H. C., & Suh, E. M. (2002). Cultural influences on personality. *Annual Review of Psychology, 53*, 133–160.

Uchida, Y., Norasakkunkit, V., & Kitayama, S. (2004). Cultural constructions of happiness: Theory and empirical evidence. *Journal of Happiness Studies, 5*, 223–239.

Updegraff, J. A., Gable, S. L., & Taylor, S. E. (2004). What makes experience satisfying? The interaction of approach–avoidance motivations and emotions in well-being. *Journal of Personality and Social Psychology, 86*, 496–504.

Urry, H., Nitschke, J., Dolski, I., Jackson, D., Kim, D., Mueller, C., et al. (2004). Making a life worth living: Neural correlates of well-being. *Psychological Science, 15*, 367–372.

Veenhoven, R. (1999). Quality-of-life in individualistic society. *Social Indicators Research, 48*, 159–188.

White, K., & Lehman, D. R. (2005). Culture and social comparison seeking: The role of self-motives. *Personality and Social Psychology Bulletin, 31*, 232–242.

MAKING PEOPLE HAPPIER

21

Interventions for Enhancing Subjective Well-Being
Can We Make People Happier, and Should We?

LAURA A. KING

Those who have been fortunate enough to hear Ed Diener give a talk have probably heard an anecdote about the first time he informed a former graduate advisor of his interest in studying subjective well-being. An established researcher in the social psychology of deindividuation, aggression, and the like, Ed was looking for a new, more positive horizon. There it was: the little studied but important field of happiness. The response was less than enthusiastic: Who would care about such a topic? Certainly, the years since have demonstrated that his instincts were spot on. It is clear that subjective well-being has become not only a vital area of scholarly activity but also important to everyday people. Enormous amounts of scholarship have been dedicated to subjective well-being —its definition, measurement, structure, correlates, and predictors. It is fair to say (witness the present volume) that we know (and are continuing to learn) a lot about subjective well-being. My purpose in the present chapter is to consider the next step. If we know what subjective well-being is and have established that it is a good thing to have, how might we enhance subjective well-being in people's lives?

Before considering this central question, two important issues warrant attention. First, *should* we seek to enhance subjective well-being? And second, if we
should, is it possible? In reviewing some the issues in subjective well-being
research and the challenges involved in trying to make real changes in subjective
well-being, I hope to demonstrate that one of the key ways that subjective well-
being can be changed (if, indeed, it should be changed) is to engage in a rich
emotional life—to be engaged in the many facets of life—the good and the bad.
It may be that engagement in life via goals allows an individual to enjoy subjective well-being in a way that is relatively free from the dangers of the hedonic
treadmill (more on this later). Finally, in considering goal change and life transitions, I argue that the pursuit of happiness may be viewed as a powerful motivator of personality development. Before addressing these provocative notions, let's
consider the first of our key questions.

Should We Enhance Subjective Well-Being?

I begin with what might seem an odd question—really, who would not want to
be happy or happier? Certainly, a happy life is a desirable life (King & Napa,
1998; Scollon & King, 2005). Indeed, when we have invited people to make
three wishes for "anything at all," happiness is a very common wish (King &
Broyles, 1997). One of the few wholly psychological aspects of the Declaration
of Independence is its recognition of the right to "pursue happiness." People
want to be happy. But should they?

Eudaimonia and Hedonism: A Tale of Two "Happinesses"?

Within the broad context of research on human well-being, two approaches
have been identified and labeled after Aristotle's (350 B.C.E./1998 C.E.) classical
distinction between eudaimonia and hedonism. Within psychology, eudaimonia
has typically been defined as the fulfillment (including positive feelings) that
comes from engagement in meaningful activity and the actualization of one's
potential (e.g., Deci & Ryan, 2000). Research in this tradition responds to what
has been seen by some (e.g., Ryff, 1989) as an overemphasis on happiness to the
detriment of our knowledge about other important aspects of the good life (e.g.,
Ryff & Singer, 1998). Hedonism, in contrast, is viewed as focusing on positive
feelings, per se. Within this tradition, subjective well-being is typically defined as
high levels of life satisfaction (LS) and positive affect (PA) and lower levels of
negative affect (NA) (e.g., Diener, 1984, 1994). Ryan and Deci (2001) proposed
that research on well-being is rightly divided into these two camps, with work by
themselves, Ryff (e.g., 1989) and others identified as eudaimonic, whereas work
by Diener (e.g., Diener, Lucas, & Scollon, 2006) and others is seen as contribut-

ing to our knowledge of hedonism or, perhaps less alarmingly, "hedonics" (Kahneman, 1999).

Viewed in this way, the eudaimonia versus hedonism division takes on an almost moral character. After all, the Marquis de Sade is the most salient and oft-cited example of what happens when a person focuses solely on the attainment of pleasure. Aristotle is typically presented as laying the foundation for eudaimonic work, whereas the little-read, much-maligned, and generally not-quite-so bright Aristippes is the philosophical founder of hedonism (Ryan & Deci, 2001). Thus, eudaimonic research may be thought of as an interest in something that is some-how better than just being happy. Indeed, by definition, subjective well-being research has largely focused on how people feel about their lives—how happy they are, how unhappy, and how they feel about that.

Importantly, this distinction between eudaimonia and hedonics is arguably quite artificial and potentially unnecessary. Aristotle, himself, saw pleasure as an integral part of eudaimonic living. In his discussion of eudaimonia, in the *Nicomachean Ethics*, he noted, "Happiness . . . is the best, noblest, *most pleasant* thing in the world, and *these attributes are not severed*" (Aristotle, 350 B.C.E./1998 C.E., p. 17, emphasis added). The research literature is rife with examples of how eudaimonia and hedonics intertwine. Intrinsic motivation, perhaps a hallmark of eudaimonic activity, is often measured by enjoyment (Ryan, Koestner, & Deci, 1991). The organismic needs of relatedness, autonomy, and competence (Ryan & Deci, 2001; Sheldon, 2002) gain validity through their relations to measures of subjective well-being (happiness; e.g., Kasser & Ryan, 1996; Sheldon, 2002). Indeed, many aspects of the good life (e.g., warm relations with others, personal mastery, a purpose in life) do relate strongly to subjective well-being. It is diffi-cult to imagine that such relationships would be taken as anything but a sign of the vital importance of these eudaimonic variables to the good life. Certainly, happiness is not everything, but perhaps in the right context, it is something. Pairing pleasurable emotion with adaptive activities is evolution's way of ensur-ing that we engage in the behaviors necessary to our survival (de Waal, 1996).

Perhaps the distinction between eudaimonia and hedonism is not so much about being happy versus not, but concern over identifying the roots of that hap-piness. If eudaimonia can be boiled down to feeling happy for the right reasons (e.g., "I volunteered as a literacy tutor") versus the wrong ones (e.g., "I just got a new sports car"), then once again, we can see from the empirical evidence that the dichotomy has been drawn too sharply. Research has shown that intrinsically motivated activity contributes to subjective well-being *more strongly* than extrinsi-cally motivated activity. It is actually quite remarkable that, apparently, subjective well-being is sensitive to the dynamics of eudaimonics—the better we live, the better we feel. Finally, happy feelings can be seen as precursors or concomitants of higher-level constructs such as flow (Csikszentmihalyi, 1990), generosity and religious faith (Myers, 2000), kindness (e.g., Magen & Aharoni, 1991), creativity

(Estrada, Isen, & Young, 1994), enthusiastic pursuit of goals (Emmons, 1986), approach coping (Carver, Scheier, & Pozo, 1992), and meaning in life (King, Hicks, Krull, & Del Gaiso, 2006).

The search for something superior to plain old "feeling good about one's life" is unnecessary. As Aristotle might have predicted, research on the goods of life often shows that these are associated with feeling better about one's life. One is reminded, here, of William James's (1902) declaration that "All Goods are disguised by the vulgarity of their concomitants, in this work-a-day world; but woe to him who can only recognize them when he thinks them in their pure and abstract form!" (p. 125). As we consider enhancing subjective well-being, it is important to keep in mind that we are not discussing a program of action that derives from de Sade. Despite its rather modest trappings in transparent self-report measures, subjective well-being may be our best means of tracking the good life as it is lived every day.

Leaving the debate of the importance of subjective well-being to notions of "the good life," if subjective well-being represents happiness as it is experienced in "this work-a-day world," are there reasons beyond its pleasantness and its role as an outcome of eudaimonia that indicate we ought to enhance it? Increasingly, research has shown that subjective well-being is not only a consequence of the goods of life but is also a predictor of these positive outcomes. A recent meta-analysis by Lyubomirsky, King, and Diener (2005) surveyed a broad array of studies in support of the notion that happiness might not only be viewed as an outcome of life success but also a correlate, predictor, and possible cause of such success. Moving from the considerable cross-sectional literature on the correlates of subjective well-being, these authors present compelling evidence from longitudinal research demonstrating that PA as well as other measures of well-being relate prospectively to altruism, sociability, activity, self-esteem, other esteem, conflict resolution, physical health, and immune function (see Lyubomirsky et al., 2005). It seems likely that if someone were to make a prescription for happiness, he or she might list the following: a good marriage, satisfying work, warm friendships, and a long, healthy life. Importantly, the results of the review by Lyubomirsky et al. suggest that happiness is not simply an outcome of these experiences but that happiness may *foster* them. Happiness is a precursor to a broad array of goods, including satisfying relationships (Lyubomirsky, Sheldon, & Schkade, 2005), career success, superior coping, and even physical health, and survival (Lyubomirsky et al., 2005). Drawing from lab studies on mood, Lyubomirsky and colleagues (2005) contend that the types of processes (cognitive, intrapersonal, and social) that are set in motion by PA may help to explain the benefits of general subjective well-being. Thus, happiness is a potential cause of life success.

The chronically unhappy reader may be feeling a bit irked at this point. Happy people not only get to feel good much of the time (cf. Diener, Sandvik,

& Pavot, 1992; Larsen & Ketelaar, 1991), but these pleasant feelings may be associated with a variety of other goods in life. Meanwhile, the unhappy are not only miserable, they are less likely to enjoy so many of life's rewards: Where's the justice? Clearly, then, it's time to consider whether happiness can be fostered.

Can We Enhance Subjective Well-Being? And If So, How?

If we accept the tentative answer that yes, we really should be interested in enhancing subjective well-being, the obvious next question, is "Is such enhancement possible?" Looking to the literature on the correlates of subjective well-being, we can see that some aspects of life that are associated with higher levels of subjective well-being are changeable and some less so. For instance, research on the heritability of well-being has tended to show that the variance in well-being is quite heritable (with estimates ranging from .50 to .80; Lykken & Tellegen, 1996; Braungart, Plomin, DeFries, & Fulker, 1992; Tellegen et al., 1988). That is, a great deal of within-group phenotypic variance in subjective well-being might be attributable to genotypic variance. At first blush, such statistics might seem to indicate that there is little sense in trying to change subjective well-being, because it is largely genetic. Such a conclusion, however, would miss the definition of heritability, itself. Heritability is a statistic, of course, and as such it describes characteristics of a group. Heritability estimates vary across groups and over time. As a statistic, heritability cannot specify down to the single case (any more than a single case can be generalized to an entire group). Knowing that one has particularly miserable parents does not doom that person to a life of unhappiness. So, though variation in a group on subjective well-being is explained to some degree by genetic variation in the members of that group, the experience of subjective well-being by an individual may or may not reflect genetic heritage. Thus, these substantial heritability estimates do not preclude the possibility of fostering subjective well-being, one unhappy person at a time.

Personality traits also relate to subjective well-being. Particularly, extraversion and neuroticism seem most relevant to well-being (e.g., Diener & Lucas, 1999; DeNeve & Cooper, 1998; McCrae & Costa, 1990). And both of these traits have shown to remain quite stable over time (McCrae & Costa, 1990). Should introverts set a goal to enhance their subjective well-being by becoming more extraverted? Probably not. To the extent that traits are relatively unchanging, they may not be the best avenues for intervention.

Some correlates of subjective well-being are life circumstances that do change. For instance, though the effect is relatively small, income is related to enhanced subjective well-being (Diener, Lucas, & Scollon, 2006; Graham, Eggers, & Sukhtankar, 2004). Subjective well-being is also enhanced by marriage and religiosity (e.g., Diener, 1984). Notably, these life experiences are not typically performed *explicitly* in the pursuit of personal happiness. Surely, no one gets married because he or she *wants* to be miserable, but few would walk down the aisle or sit in the pew *simply* as part of a subjective well-being enhancement program. Rather, these aspects of human life carry with them the promise of fulfillment in a larger sense. Indeed, the strong relationships between these life circumstances and subjective well-being highlights one of the dilemmas of enhancing subjective well-being, to wit: The pursuit of happiness is rarely successful when done for its own sake. When happiness is the explicit goal, the pursuit is likely to backfire (Schooler, Ariely, & Loewenstein, 2003). In a sense, explicitly focusing on enhancing what is more consciously considered a byproduct of life experiences renders the pursuit itself less than fulfilling.

Another way to approach the problem of enhancing subjective well-being is to focus on its components: LS, PA, and NA. Can we change each of these? Life satisfaction is, of course, the most complex of these components, because it involves the cognitive evaluation of one's life. Certainly cognitive–behavioral interventions might come into play in this area. Such interventions might be aimed at helping a person judge his or her current circumstances in a more positive light. Alternatively (and, perhaps, more easily) we might focus interventions on the mood components of subjective well-being. The notion of changing subjective well-being by enhancing PA is one potentially fruitful avenue.

A promising approach to enhancing subjective well-being, in a way that is durable has been suggested by Lyubomirsky, Sheldon, and Schkade (2005). Acknowledging the many reasons why sustainable changes in subjective well-being might be less than easy to attain, these authors suggest that the place to begin is in intentional activities. Indeed, there are a variety of factors that are associated with enhanced PA: for example, activity, kindness, positive self-reflection, goal striving, and experiencing meaning (Lyubomirsky et al., 2005). Indeed, the fact that social psychologists have spent careers debating whether there truly is any such thing as selfless altruistic behavior (i.e., altruistic behavior without mood benefits) suggests that the strong link between altruistic behavior and PA is all but inescapable. Changing genes is impossible (at least to date) and changing traits is quite difficult. Even seeking out the larger experiences of marriage, employment, etc., are not easily incorporated into a daily "happiness" program. But these concrete intentional activities (e.g., kind acts, physical exercise) would seem to represent a way for everyone to benefit from frequent PA. Drawing from Lyubomirsky et al. (2004), then, we might suggest the following plan to an unhappy person who wants to be happy: "Do something useful for others. Stop reading self-help books and start exploring options to help others."

The effectiveness of another method for enhancing subjective well-being has been demonstrated in studies employing the Pennebaker expressive writing paradigm (e.g., Pennebaker & Chung, 2007). In a study in my lab (King, 2001a), participants were asked to write about their most traumatic life experiences, their best possible future selves, or a control topic (their plans for the day) for 20 minutes a day over 4 days. The best possible self-instructions included the following:

> Imagine your life in the future. Everything has gone as well as it possibly could have. You have worked hard and succeeded in accomplishing all of your goals. Think of this as the realization of your life dreams. (King, 2001a, p. 801).

Mood was measured before and after writing and participants completed measures of subjective well-being nearly a month later. Results demonstrated that the best possible self condition led to enhanced PA immediately after writing (in contrast to previous studies using only the trauma topic) and, more importantly, enhanced subjective well-being several weeks after writing. Expanding upon this evidence, Sheldon and Lyubomirsky (2006) initiated a program of research examining the potential for interventions to enhance subjective well-being in a way that is maintained over time. They assigned individuals to write about gratitude, their best possible selves, or a life details control condition. In accord with past research, they found that the best possible self writing condition was particularly likely to foster PA and intrinsic motivation.

Thus, writing optimistically about the future may be a promising way to increase subjective well-being, at least in the short term. It is no coincidence that these two writing studies focused on best possible selves—personalized representations of goals. Indeed, Lyubomirsky et al. (2005; see also Sheldon & Lyubomirsky, 2006) also focus wisely on the role of the pursuit of goals in subjective well-being as a potential avenue for sustainable change in subjective well-being, a possibility to which we now turn.

Goals and Subjective Well-Being

The role of goal investment in subjective well-being is certainly well established. The term *personal goals* refers to those goals that a person is typically trying to accomplish in his or her everyday behavior (Emmons, 1986). Personal goals appear on the midlevel "to-do" lists that drive everyday life (King, 2007). Working toward valued goals is an important aspect of subjective well-being (e.g., Brunstein, 1993; King, 2007; King, Richards, & Stemmerich, 1998; Pervin, 1989; Sheldon & Elliot, 1999). Indeed, research has demonstrated that simply having important, valued goals is related to subjective well-being, as is making progress on those goals. Personal goals have been shown to organize daily experience and mediate the relationship between events and daily emotional life (Diener & Fujita, 1995). Events matter to us to the extent that they affect our goals. Goal pursuit provides the glue that meaningfully links a chain of life events—providing life with beginnings, middles, and ends. To the extent that goals direct attention, draw our thoughts to them, and drive the extraction of meaning from life events, they are a kind of psychic hub in our mental lives (King, 2007).

Optimal Goal Pursuit

The considerable literature on goal investment offers a variety of ideas about the types of goals that are likely to enhance subjective well-being. To optimize the subjective well-being payoffs of goal processes, one ought to pursue goals that are important and personally valuable (Emmons, 1986; Sheldon & Elliot, 1999). These goals should be moderately challenging and should share an instrumental relationship with each other (Emmons & King, 1988). Goals should be construed in approach (rather than avoidance) terms (Elliot & Sheldon, 1997). Having daily goals that serve the function of leading us to our broader life dreams is related to enhanced subjective well-being, and progress on those goals is particularly rewarding (King et al., 1998). Optimal goal content might be defined as those goals that serve underlying needs for organismic values (e.g., Sheldon & Kasser, 1998, 1999).

One advantage of goals as an entryway to enhanced subjective well-being is that they allow us to enjoy subjective well-being without explicitly pursuing it. Personal goals may range from the trivial to the grand, but they typically include more than the goal "to be happy." Thus, goals allow us to capitalize on our implicit tie to our overall subjective well-being. That is, goals allow us to pursue happiness while we are pursuing other things. Indeed, it is notable that those who explicitly link goal progress to happiness fare quite poorly (McIntosh, Harlow, & Martin, 1995).

Goals versus Other Ways to Increase Subjective Well-Being: The Problem of Adaptation

Perhaps the biggest challenge facing any enhancement program for subjective well-being is the "hedonic treadmill" (Brickman & Campbell, 1971; Fredrick & Loewenstein, 1999). Essentially, any changes that might occur in our lives that would presumably influence subjective well-being are likely to be adapted to quite rapidly. So, winning the lottery, moving to California, or falling in love may lead to temporary gains in the experience of joy, but eventually we go back to our baseline (cf. Diener, Lucas, & Scollon, 2006). Any new thing eventually becomes routine. Variety has an incentive value (McClelland, 1980), of course, and so it makes sense that what was once fantastic might eventually become humdrum. Whether it is the switch from broadcast to cable or from dialup to DSL, what first is experienced as a monumental life-changing improvement at the very foreground of existence eventually fades to a routine (but still necessary) aspect of life, all too soon to be taken for granted.

The hedonic treadmill highlights one of the great advantages of a goal approach to enhancing subjective well-being. Goals are dynamic variables; they change and are changed by life experience. The very definition of motivation in human life is that it serves unquenchable needs—just because we have one friend, we do not lose the desire to make friends. As a result, goal pursuit may be less susceptible to adaptation over time.

Another way that goals may allow the person to maintain traction on the hedonic treadmill is by "accentuating the positive" but *not* necessarily eliminating the negative. Critics of "positive psychology" (e.g., Lazarus, 2003) have complained that the movement overemphasizes positive thinking and "happy-ology" to the detriment of our understanding of the difficulties of life. The embeddedness of goals in our everyday mood and the capacity of goals to evoke good and bad feelings make them an ideal domain for fostering not only happiness but engagement in a multifaceted life. Goals may relate to positive or negative emotional experiences, depending on how we are progressing in their pursuit. This notion is certainly in accord with models of the role of affect in self-regulation (e.g., Carver & Scheier, 2008). Goals do not simply increase subjective well-being, they might also increase momentary unhappiness—which may be a very good thing.

Sometimes goals just do not work out, however, no matter how well chosen or how doggedly pursued. Indeed, setting a goal includes not only the promise of the fulfillment but the potential for failure, humiliation, and regret. Emotionally investing in one's daily life may mean experiencing worry over whether one will succeed (Pomerantz, Saxon, & Oishi, 2000) and experiencing disappointment when things do not go well (cf. Marsh, 1995; Kernis, Paradise, Whitaker, Wheatman, & Goldman, 2000). Truly caring about what happens in one's life, from one day to the next, may well prove challenging: Memories of loss, failure, and mistakes can become a source of considerable misery (Gilovich, Medvec, & Kahneman, 1998; Niedenthal, Tangney, & Gavanski, 1994). King and Burton (2003) reviewed all the potential ways that goal pursuit might lead to NA, concluding that, "In life, some unhappiness is inevitable. Perhaps, goals simply make the 'why' of our misery more comprehensible" (p. 64). Yes, overall, goal pursuit may lead to a happier life, but it also keeps life affectively interesting. By fostering a rich, nuanced emotional life that is also coherent and comprehensible, goals keep the positive possible and interesting. The conclusion here, for those who want to enhance subjective well-being, is to strive mightily for goals that you value. You may get lucky and fail now and then, which will only make successes all the sweeter.

More generally, a rich emotional life that encompasses both positive and negative affective experiences sidesteps the trap of the hedonic treadmill. Goals are valuable as means of enhancing subjective well-being because although they have the capacity to engender PA, they do not preclude the possibility of NA. One problem in focusing on subjective well-being or happiness as an end in itself is the tendency to view any negative emotion as problematic. Thus, the experiences of distress, regret, and disappointment are often viewed as better avoided. Focus on the maximization of PA and the minimization of NA has led to a view of the happy person as a well-defended fortress, invulnerable to the vicissitudes of life (King, 2001b). At times, researchers in the area of positive psychology have referred to an "upward spiral" (e.g., Fredrickson & Joiner, 2003; Sheldon & Houser-Marko, 2001), suggesting that characteristics such as resilience or intrinsic motivation lead to enhanced PA, which leads to higher levels of these variables, which, in turn, leads to even greater PA. This upward spiral would seem to culminate in a nonstop party of orgasmic ecstasy.

Once again, it is worth noting that even the very happiest among us must occasionally experience negative feelings. Not to do so would seem quite dysfunctional, to the extent to that mood serves as feedback about reality. Embedding subjective well-being in everyday life, in events that are sometimes out of our control, in responsibilities and hassles, as well as the many good things that happen to us, suggests that to the extent that mood is simultaneously an aspect of subjective well-being and a source of feedback on performance in areas we value, the functional life must include the good and the bad. Indeed, my own research on life transitions (e.g., King, Scollon, Ramsey, & Williams, 2000) would seem to indicate that nothing makes "everything old seem new again" like the prospect of losing it all. In the context of life transitions, the small things that were previously taken for granted become precious all over again (King, 2001b). In addition to the pursuit of goals, then, the seeker of subjective well-being might dare to seek not happiness but engagement with life, itself (Cantor & Sanderson, 1999).

The Pursuit of Happiness and the Drive to Develop

Finally, I would like to suggest a potentially important, though surprising, role for the pursuit of happiness in adult personality development. Most modern approaches to adult development include the idea that the organism is an active participant in the process. In this final section I would like to pose the question, "*Why* do we develop? What motivates adults to develop?"

Here we return for a moment to the eudaimonia–hedonism distinction. Among the eudaimonic goods of life we might recognize maturity. Does maturity include happiness? Personality development is certainly a variable for which it is difficult to imagine a person scoring "high" not also being happy. One reason for this is that many of our theoretical models of development include a sense that development culminates in a scenario of "happily every after." Certainly, Erikson (e.g., 1968) did not include "happy" as a criterion for personality development, but it is not difficult to imagine that a person who has attained "trust," "autonomy," "initiative," "industry," "identity," "intimacy," "generativity," and "integrity" is going to be happier than the unfortunate soul who ended up on the other side of those psychosocial conflicts. To some extent development might well include getting happier—and research has shown that older individuals do report themselves as happier than younger ones (e.g., Sheldon & Kasser, 2001).

One approach to development that is not typically related to subjective well-being is ego development (ED), as defined by Loevinger (e.g., Hy & Loevinger, 1999). Loevinger's ego is a buffer that exists between the self and world. ED refers to the level of complexity with which the person is able to experience him- or herself and the world (e.g., Loevinger, 1976; Hy & Loevinger, 1996). According to Loevinger's theory, at the earliest stages of ED, we are dominated by impulses, lack insight, and engage in simplistic thinking. With ED comes an increasingly complex experience of ourselves and the world. We learn to control and channel impulses. We recognize that life's big questions may have a variety of valid answers. As we develop, we increasingly recognize conflict. High levels of ED involve a more complex but also more expansive view of the self and world. In Loevinger's (1976) theory, growth can occur only when the environment fails to conform to the person's expectations. Loevinger (1976) referred to "pacers" as complex interpersonal situations that might pull an individual to a higher level of ego functioning. Research has supported the notion that ED can be spurred by challenging life experiences (Bursik, 1991; Helson, 1992; Helson & Roberts, 1994; Helson & Wink, 1992; King & S. N. Smith, 2005). Unlike subjective well-being, ED is measured using a less-than-transparent measure, the sentence completion test (SCT; Hy & Loevinger, 1999). ED is a variable that resists self-report; we cannot simply look into ourselves and rate our ED.

Wisdom is another construct that is often used to characterize maturity. Baltes and Staudinger (1993) defined wisdom as expert knowledge—"the fundamental pragmatics of life permitting exceptional insight, judgment, and advice involving complex and uncertain matters of the human condition" (p. 76). Wise thinking is characterized by relativism, uncertainty, and contextualism. Importantly, wisdom is enhanced by life experiences that involve dealing with difficult and unstructured matters of life, or "wisdom facilitative experiences" (Baltes & Staudinger, 2000). Wisdom is typically measured using an interview that involves asking participants to grapple with a variety of hypothetical scenarios. Once again, wisdom is not measured using a simple self-report. We are generally not good judges of how wise we are. There are, of course, important differences between ED and wisdom, but for the purposes of this chapter, two key similarities are noted. Both of these aspects of maturity appear to be relatively unavailable to the person and both have been shown to occur in response to life difficulties.

Why do we grow from difficult life experiences? One way to think about personality development in adulthood is through the Piagetian processes of assimilation and accommodation (Block, 1982). Confronted with a difficult life experience (e.g., going through divorce, losing a loved one), we may try to come to grips with that experience using our preexisting meaning structures (assimilation), or we may come to the realization that new structures are necessary to make sense of this new experience (accommodation). My research has shown that instances of accommodation (in narratives of life change) are related to current and future levels of ED (e.g., King & Raspin, 2004; King & Smith, 2004). Accommodation can be observed in narratives that reflect an active struggle to make sense and an admission of the need for a "paradigmatic shift" in one's sources of meaning (King, Scollon, Ramsey, & Williams, 2000).

An ambiguous issue, however, is the question of what propels growth. Accommodation may well be conceived of as a process that is driven by the person—but *why* does the person bother reinventing a new approach to life? Given that indicators of maturity are relatively out of awareness, it seems unlikely that someone might conclude, "I am not thinking wisely enough" or "I am too simplistic in my thinking." Indeed, it is not at all clear that if people were asked about their goals for maturity, the idea of coming to a more complex view of the self and world would be given (King, Hicks, & Eells, 2006).

I would suggest that a key motivator in this struggle to come to terms with life's difficulties is the pursuit of happiness itself. We know when we are happy or unhappy. This assumption underlies the reliance on self-report in subjective well-being research. The absence of feeling good about one's life is a keen loss. Perhaps development in response to life change occurs as a result of an individual's need to invent a new way of living, a new life *in which he or she can be happy* (King & Hicks, 2006). When life is difficult, finding a way to be happy may be a great challenge. That search for happiness may well involve rewriting goals and revisiting priorities: Essentially, accommodation is a result of the pursuit of happiness. Lyubomirsky, Sheldon, and Schkade (2005) somewhat offhandedly refer to the "ability to be happy." This provocative notion lies at the center of the dilemma of the individual who has experienced a significant life change—how to be happy again within the new constraints of his or her new life. The desire to be happy again necessitates personality development. That is, a person cannot be happy with his or her meaning structures so at variance with the world of experience. Perhaps, the person matures to be happy (King, 2001b). This notion is given some support by research on divorce by Bursik (1991), who found that ED increased following a divorce only in those women who had recovered their previous levels of subjective well-being. Clearly, the provocative notion that the pursuit of happiness itself serves as a motivation for development remains open for future research on subjective well-being.

Conclusions

In this chapter I have argued that subjective well-being is an important by-product and predictor of many of the most valued outcomes in human life. Subjective well-being has been shown to be sensitive to the eudaimonic value of activities and goals, relieving any concerns that enhancing subjective well-being means engaging in profligate hedonism. Thus, enhancing subjective well-being is a potentially worthwhile endeavor. In addition, there is reason to believe that low levels of subjective well-being can be changed, their relative heritability and trait associations notwithstanding. Because of the problem of adaptation, however, it is important that the pursuit of happiness focus not on the attainment of happiness, per se, but on engagement in life, particularly through the pursuit of important personal goals. Those seeking to enjoy sustained changes in their levels of subjective well-being might begin by engaging in activities known to enhance PA, but in the long run change is most likely to persist if it occurs in the context of a rich emotional life. People want to be happy, but sustainable happiness requires occasional unhappiness as well. Finally, I would suggest that low subjective well-being may be an important indicator, not simply to the researcher but to the person experiencing it, of the need for life changes, goal reevaluation, and a reconsideration of life's meaning. The common human longing for happiness may well be what drives us to develop.

References

Aristotle (1998). *The Nichomacean Ethics* (J. L. Ackrill, J. O. Urmson, & D. Ross, Trans.). New York: Oxford University Press. (Original work written in 350 B.C.)

Aspinwall, L. G. (1998). Rethinking the role of positive affect in self-regulation. *Motivation and Emotion, 22,* 1–32.

Baltes, P. B., & Staudinger, U. M. (1993). The search for a psychology of wisdom. *Current Directions in Psychological Science, 2,* 75–80.

Baltes, P. B., & Staudinger, U. M. (2000). Wisdom: A metaheuristic (pragmatic) to orchestrate mind and virtue toward excellence. *American Psychologist, 55,* 122–136.

Block, J. (1982). Assimilation, accommodation, and the dynamics of personality development. *Child Development, 53,* 281–295.

Braungart, J. M., Plomin, R., DeFries, J. C., & Fulker, D. W. (1992). Genetic influence on tester-rated infant temperament as assessed by Bayley's Infant Behavior Record: Nonadoptive and adoptive siblings and twins. *Developmental Psychology, 28,* 40–47.

Brickman, P., & Campbell, D. T. (1971). Hedonic relativism and planning the good society. In M. H. Appley (Ed.), *Adaptation-level theory* (pp. 287–302). New York: Academic Press.

Brickman, P., Coates, D., & Janoff-Bulman, R. (1978). Lottery winners and accident victims: Is happiness relative? *Journal of Personality and Social Psychology, 36*, 917–927.

Brunstein, J. (1993). Personal goals and subjective well-being: A longitudinal study. *Journal of Personality and Social Psychology, 65*, 1061–1070.

Bursik, K. (1991). Adaptation to divorce and ego development in adult women. *Journal of Personality and Social Psychology, 60*, 300–306.

Cantor, N., & Sanderson, C. A. (1999). Life task participation and well-being: The importance of taking part in daily life. In D. Kahneman, E. Diener, & B. N. Schwarz (Eds.), *Well-being: The foundations of hedonic psychology* (pp. 230–243). New York: Russell Sage Foundation.

Carver, C. S., & Scheier, M. F. (1990). Origins and functions of positive and negative affect: A control-process view. *Psychological Review, 97*, 19–35.

Carver, C. S., & Scheier, M. F. (2008). Feedback processes in the simultaneous regulation of action and affect. In J. Y. Shah & W. L. Gradner (Eds.), *Handbook of motivation science* (pp. 308–324). New York: Guilford Press.

Carver, C. S., Scheier, M. F., & Pozo, C. (1992). Conceptualizing the process of coping with health problems. In H. S. Friedman (Ed.), *Hostility, coping, and health* (pp. 167–187). Washington, DC: American Psychological Association.

Costa, P. T., McCrae, R. R., & Zonderman, A. B. (1987). Environmental and dispositional influences on well-being: Longitudinal follow-up of an American national sample. *British Journal of Psychology, 78*, 299–306.

Csikszentmihalyi, M. (1990). *Flow: The psychology of optimal experience.* New York: Harper & Row.

Danner, D. D., Snowdon, D. A., & Friesen, W. V. (2001). Positive emotions in early life and longevity: Findings from the nun study. *Journal of Personality and Social Psychology, 80*, 804–813.

Deci, E. L., & Ryan, R. M. (2000). The "what" and "why" of goal pursuits: Human needs and the self-determination of behavior. *Psychological Inquiry, 4*, 227–268.

DeNeve, K. M., & Cooper, H. (1998). The happy personality: A meta-analysis of 137 personality traits and subjective well-being. *Psychological Bulletin, 124*, 197–229.

DeWaal, F. B. M. (1996). *Good natured: The origins of right and wrong in humans and other animals.* Cambridge, MA: Harvard University Press.

Diener, E. (1984). Subjective well-being. *Psychological Bulletin, 95*, 542–575.

Diener, E. (1994). Assessing subjective well-being: Progress and opportunities. *Social Indicators Research, 31*, 103–157.

Diener, E., & Biswas-Diener, R. (2002). Will money increase subjective well-being? *Social Indicators Research, 57*, 119–169.

Diener, E., & Fujita, F. (1995). Resources, personal strivings, and subjective well-being: A nomothetic and idiographic approach. *Journal of Personality and Social Psychology, 68*, 926–935.

Diener, E., Gohm, C. L., Suh, E., & Oishi, S. (2000). Similarity of the relations between marital status and subjective well-being across cultures. *Journal of Cross-Cultural Psychology, 31*, 419–436.

Diener, E., & Lucas, R. E. (1999). Personality and subjective well-being. In D. Kahneman, E. Diener, & N. Schwartz (Eds.), *Well-being: The foundations of hedonic psychology* (pp. 213–229). New York: Sage.

Diener, E., Lucas, R. E., & Scollon, C. N. (2006). Beyond the Hedonic Treadmill: Revising the Adaptation Theory of Well-Being. *American Psychologist, 61*, 305–314.

Diener, E., Sandvik, E., Pavot, W., & Fujita, F. (1992). Extraversion and subjective well-being in a U.S. national probability sample. *Journal of Research in Personality, 26*, 205–215.

Diener, E., Sandvik, E., Seidlitz, L., & Diener, M. (1993). The relationship between income and subjective well-being: Relative or absolute? *Social Indicators Research, 28*, 195–223.

Diener, E., Suh, E. M., Lucas, R. E., & Smith, H. L. (1999). Subjective well-being: Three decades of progress. *Psychological Bulletin, 125*, 276–302.

Emmons, R. A. (1986). Personal Strivings: An approach to personality and subjective well-being. *Journal of Personality and Social Psychology, 51*, 1058–1068.

Emmons, R. A., & King, L. A. (1988). Conflict among personal strivings: Immediate and long-term implications for psychological and physical well-being. *Journal of Personality and Social Psychology, 54*, 1040–1048.

Estrada, C., Isen, A. M., & Young, M. J. (1994). Positive affect influences creative problem solving and reported source of practice satisfaction in physicians. *Motivation and Emotion, 18*, 285–299.

Erikson, E. H. (1968). *Identity, youth, and crisis.* New York: Norton.

Frederick, S., & Loewenstein, G. (1999). Hedonic adaptation. In D. Kahneman, E. Diener, & N. Schwarz (Eds.), *Well-being: The foundations of hedonic psychology* (pp. 302–329). New York: Sage.

Fredrickson, B. L., & Joiner, T. (2002). Positive emotions trigger upward spirals toward emotional well-being. *Psychological Science, 13*, 172–175.

Gallup, G. G., Jr. (1984, March). Commentary on the state of religion in the U.S. today. *Religion in America: The Gallup Report*, No. 222.

Gilovich, T., Medvec, V. H., & Kahneman, D. (1998). Varieties of regret: A debate and partial resolution. *Psychological Review, 105*, 602–605.

Graham, C., Eggers, A., & Sukhtankar, S. (2004). Does happiness pay? An exploration based on panel data from Russia. *Journal of Economic Behavior and Organization, 55*, 319–342.

Headey, B., & Wearing, A. (1989). Personality, life events, and subjective well-being: Toward a dynamic equilibrium model. *Journal of Personality and Social Psychology, 57*, 731–739.

Helson, R., & Roberts, B. W. (1994). Ego development and personality change in adulthood. *Journal of Personality and Social Psychology, 66*, 911–920.

Helson, R., & Wink, P. (1987). Two conceptions of maturity examined in the findings of a longitudinal study. *Journal of Personality and Social Psychology, 53*, 531–541.

Hy, L. X., & Loevinger, J. (1996). *Measuring ego development, second edition.* Mahwah, NJ: Erlbaum.

Kahneman, D. (1999). Objective happiness. In D. Kahneman, E. Diener, & N. Schwarz (Eds.), *Well-being: The foundations of hedonic psychology* (pp. 3–25). New York: Sage.

Kasser, T., & Ryan, R. M. (1996). Further examining the American dream: Differential correlates of intrinsic and extrinsic goals. *Personality and Social Psychology Bulletin, 22,* 280–287.

Kernis, M. H., Paradise, A. W., Whitaker, D. J., Wheatman, S. R., & Goldman, B. N. (2000). Master of one's psychological domain? Not likely if one's self-esteem is unstable. *Personality and Social Psychology Bulletin, 26,* 1297–1305.

King, L. A. (2001a). The health benefits of writing about life goals. *Personality and Social Psychology Bulletin, 27,* 798–807.

King, L. A. (2001b). The hard road to the good life: The happy, mature person. *Journal of Humanistic Psychology, 41,* 51–72.

King, L. A. (2007). Personal goals and life dreams: Positive psychology and motivation in daily life. In J. Shah & W. L. Gardner (Eds.), *Handbook of motivation science.* New York: Guilford Press.

King, L. A., & Broyles, S. J. (1997). Wishes, gender, personality, and well-being. *Journal of Personality, 65,* 49–76.

King, L. A., & Burton, C. M. (2003). The hazards of goal pursuit. In E. Chang & L. Sanna (Eds.), *Virtue, vice and personality: The complexity of behavior* (pp. 53–70). Washington, DC: American Psychological Association.

King, L. A., & Hicks, J. A. (2006). Narrating the self in the past and the future: Implications for maturity. *Research in Human Development, 3,* 121–138.

King, L. A., Hicks, J. A., & Eells, J. E. (2006). *Older but wiser,* and *happier* and *nicer: Folk concepts of maturity.* Unpublished manuscript, University of Missouri, Columbia.

King, L. A., Hicks, J. A., Krull, J., & Del Gaiso, A. K. (2006). Positive affect and the experience of meaning in life. *Journal of Personality and Social Psychology, 90,* 179–196.

King, L. A., & Napa, C. (1998). What makes a life good? *Journal of Personality and Social Psychology, 75,* 156–165.

King, L. A., & Raspin, C. (2004). Lost and found possible selves, well-being and ego development in divorced women. *Journal of Personality, 72,* 603–631.

King, L. A., Richards, J. H., & Stemmerich, E. (1998). Daily goals, life goals, and worst fears: Means, ends, and subjective well-being. *Journal of Personality, 66,* 713–744.

King, L. A., Scollon, C. K., Ramsey, C. M., & Williams, T. (2000). Stories of life transition: Happy endings, subjective well-being, and ego development in parents of children with Down syndrome. *Journal of Research in Personality, 34,* 509–536.

King, L. A., & Smith, N. G. (2004). Gay and straight possible selves: Goals, identity, subjective well-being, and personality development. *Journal of Personality, 72,* 967–994.

King, L. A., & Smith, S. N. (20050. Happy, mature, and gay: Intimacy, power, and difficult times in coming out stories. *Journal of Research in Personality, 39,* 278–298.

Larsen, R. J., & Ketelaar, T. (1991). Personality and susceptibility to positive and negative emotional states. *Journal of Personality and Social Psychology, 61,* 132–140.

Lazarus, R. S. (2003). Does the Positive Psychology movement have legs? *Psychological Inquiry, 14,* 93–109.

Loevinger, J. (1976). *Ego development: Conceptions and theories.* San Francisco, CA: Jossey-Bass.

Lucas, R. E., Clark, A. E., Georgellis, Y., & Diener, E. (2003). Reexamining adaptation and the set point model of happiness: Reactions to changes in marital status. *Journal of Personality and Social Psychology, 84,* 527–539.

Lykken, D. (2000). *Happiness: The nature and nurture of joy and contentment*. New York: St. Martin's.

Lykken, D., & Tellegen, A. (1996). Happiness is a stochastic phenomenon. *Psychological Science, 7*, 186–189.

Lyubomirsky, S., King, L. A., & Diener, E. (2005). The benefits of frequent positive affect: Does happiness lead to success? *Psychological Bulletin, 131*, 803–855.

Lyubomirsky, S., Sheldon, K. M., & Schkade, D. (2005). Pursuing happiness: The architecture of sustainable change. *Review of General Psychology, 9*, 111–131.

Magen, Z., & Aharoni, R. (1991). Adolescents contributing toward others: Relationship to positive experiences and transpersonal commitment. *Journal of Humanistic Psychology, 31*, 126–143.

Marsh, H. W. (1995). A Jamesian model of self-investment and self-esteem: Comment on Pelham (1995). *Journal of Personality and Social Psychology, 69*, 1151–1160.

Mastekaasa, A. (1994). Marital status, distress, and well-being: An international comparison. *Journal of Comparative Family Studies, 25*, 183–205.

McClelland, D. C. (1980). *Human motivation*. Cambridge, UK: Cambridge University Press.

McCrae, R. R., & Costa, P. T. (1986). Personality, coping, and coping effectiveness in an adult sample. *Journal of Personality, 54*, 385–405.

McCrae, R. R., & Costa, P. T. (1990). *Personality in adulthood*. New York: Guilford Press.

McCrae, R. R., & Costa, P. T. (1994). The stability of personality: Observations and evaluations. *Current Directions in Psychological Science, 3*, 173–175.

McGregor, I., & Little, B. R. (1998). Personal projects, happiness, and meaning: On doing well and being yourself. *Journal of Personality and Social Psychology, 74*, 494–512.

Myers, D. G. (2000). The funds, friends, and faith of happy people. *American Psychologist, 55*, 56–67.

Myers, D. G., & Diener, E. (1995). Who is happy? *Psychological Science, 6*, 10–19.

Niedenthal, P. M., Tangney, J. P., & Gavanski, I. (1994). "If only I weren't" versus "If only I hadn't": Distinguishing shame and guilt in counterfactual thinking. *Journal of Personality and Social Psychology, 67*, 585–595.

Pennebaker, J. W., & Chung, C. K. (2007). Expressive writing, emotional upheavals, and health. In H. S. Friedman & R. C. Silver (Eds.), *Foundations of health psychology* (pp. 263–284). New York: Oxford University Press.

Pervin, L. A. (Ed.). (1989). *Goal concepts in personality and social psychology*. Hillsdale, NJ: Erlbaum.

Pomerantz, E. M., Saxon, J. L., & Oishi, S. (2000). The psychological trade-offs of goal investment. *Journal of Personality and Social Psychology, 79*, 617–630.

Ryan, R. M., & Deci, E. L. (2001). On happiness and human potentials: A review of research on hedonic and eudaimonic well-being. In S. Fiske (Ed.), *Annual review of psychology* (Vol. 52, pp. 141–166). Palo Alto, CA: Annual Reviews.

Ryan, R. M., Koestner, R., & Deci, E. L. (1991). Ego-involved persistence: When free-choice behavior is not intrinsically motivated. *Motivation and Emotion, 15*(3), 185–205.

Ryff, C. D. (1989). Happiness is everything, or is it? Explorations on the meaning of psychological well-being. *Journal of Personality and Social Psychology, 57*, 1069–1081.

Ryff, C. D., & Singer, B. (1998). Contours of positive human health. *Psychological Inquiry*, *9*, 1–28.

Schkade, D. A., & Kahneman, D. (1998). Does living in California make people happy?: A focusing illusion in judgments of life satisfaction. *Psychological Science*, *9*, 340–346.

Schooler, J. W., Ariely, D., & Loewenstein, G. (2003). The explicit pursuit and assessment of happiness can be self-defeating. In I. Brocas & J. Carillo (Eds.), *The psychology of economic decisions* (pp. 41–72). Oxford, UK: Oxford University Press.

Scollon, C. N., & King, L. A. (2004). Is the good life the easy life? *Social Indicators Research*, *68*, 127–162.

Sheldon, K. M. (2002). The self-concordance model of healthy goal-striving: When personal goals correctly represent the person. In E. L. Deci & R. M. Ryan (Eds.), *Handbook of self-determination research* (pp. 65–86). Rochester, NY: University of Rochester Press.

Sheldon, K. M., & Elliot, A. J. (1998). Not all personal goals are personal: Comparing autonomous and controlled reasons for goals as predictors of effort and attainment. *Personality and Social Psychology Bulletin*, *24*, 546–557.

Sheldon, K. M., & Elliot, A. J. (1999). Goal striving, need-satisfaction, and longitudinal well-being: The self-concordance model. *Journal of Personality and Social Psychology*, *76*, 482–497.

Sheldon, K. M., & Houser-Marko, L. (2001). Self-concordance, goal-attainment, and the pursuit of happiness: Can there be an upward spiral? *Journal of Personality and Social Psychology*, *80*, 152–165.

Sheldon, K. M., & Kasser, T. (1995). Coherence and congruence: Two aspects of personality integration. *Journal of Personality and Social Psychology*, *68*, 531–543.

Sheldon, K. M., & Kasser, T. (1998). Pursuing personal goals: Skills enable progress but not all progress is beneficial. *Personality and Social Psychology Bulletin*, *24*, 1319–1331.

Sheldon, K. M., & Kasser, T. (2001). Getting older, getting better? Personal strivings and psychological maturity across the life span. *Developmental Psychology*, *37*, 491–501.

Sheldon, K. M., & Lyubomirsky, S. (2006). How to increase and sustain positive emotion: The effects of expressing gratitude and visualizing best possible selves. *Journal of Positive Psychology*, *1*, 73–82.

Suh, E. M., Diener, E., & Fujita, F. (1996). Events and subjective well-being: Only recent events matter. *Journal of Personality and Social Psychology*, *70*, 1091–1102.

Tellegen, A., Lykken, D. T., Bouchard, T. J., Wilcox, K. J., Segal, N. L., & Rich, S. (1988). Personality similarity in twins reared apart and together. *Journal of Personality and Social Psychology*, *54*, 1031–1039.

Williams, J. (1902). *The principles of psychology* (Vol. 1). New York: Holt.

22

Promoting Positive Affect

Barbara L. Fredrickson

One of Ed Diener's key contributions to social science was to point out that the ratio of people's experiences of positive to negative emotions in daily life predicts their overall levels of subjective well-being (Diener, 2000). This practice of examining the ratio of people's good to bad feelings—what I term "positivity ratios"—has proven fruitful in other domains as well. In studies of people's recovery from depression, for instance, Schwartz and colleagues (2002) found that in optimal remission, clients' positivity ratios climb from less than 1-to-1 to higher than 4-to-1. In studies of marriage, Gottman (1994) found that stable and happy marriages are characterized by positivity ratios of about 5-to-1, whereas other marriages—those Gottman (1994) describes as "on a cascade toward divorce"—sport positivity ratios that are lower than 1-to-1. In studies of business teams, Losada (1999) found that profitable and well-regarded business teams have positivity ratios of over 5-to-1 during their business meetings, whereas less profitable and less highly regarded teams have ratios of less than 1-to-1. In each of these contexts, we see that high ratios of positivity to negativity—ratios near 5-to-1—are associated with doing well, whereas low positivity ratios—those lower than 1-to-1—are associated with doing poorly.

Another of Ed Diener's key contributions was to highlight that positive and negative affect are not mere opposites. Many consequential asymmetries between these good and bad experiential states exist. Although others have emphasized that "bad is stronger than good" (Baumeister, Bratslavsky, Finkenauer, & Vohs,

2001), Diener and colleagues marshaled evidence for another important asymmetry: that "most people are happy" and "most moments are good" (Diener & Diener, 1996). These two points reflect what has come to be called the "positivity offset"—that people's most frequent emotional state is mildly positive (Cacioppo, Gardner, & Berntson, 1999). This offset is thought to be an adaptive bias that motivates people to get up in the morning and approach novelty with curiosity rather than fear. Together with the negativity bias ("bad is stronger than good"), the positivity offset ("most moments are good") may help explain why the positivity ratios for doing well and doing badly keep turning up as near 5-to-1 and 1-to-1, respectively. If, measure for measure, negative states hold more sway than positive states, then although ratios near 1:1 may represent equal "air time" for opposing states, this does not translate into equal impact. Instead such ratios portend downward spirals toward doing poorly. At the same time, if positive emotions are commonplace, perhaps positivity ratios need to appreciably exceed people's typical positivity offsets to trigger upward spirals toward doing well or optimal functioning.

However intriguing these observations may be, they raise a more critical set of questions: What is so special about positive states? How and why do they—in the right ratios—forecast optimal functioning? Do positive emotions simply track and mirror personal successes? Or, as Diener and colleagues have asked more recently (Lyubomirsky, King, & Diener, 2005), might positive affect also lead to success?

My own contribution to the study of positive states is encapsulated in what I call the broaden-and-build theory of positive emotions (Fredrickson, 1998, 2001). The theory holds that, unlike negative emotions, which narrow people's ideas about possible actions in ways that aided our ancestor's survival in life-threatening circumstances (e.g., fight, flee), positive emotions broaden people's thought and action repertoires (e.g., play, explore) in ways that spurred our ancestor's development of key assets, including their physical, mental, psychological, and social resources. In time, the resources gained during positive emotional states would have better equipped our ancestors to survive the threats to life and limb that they would inevitably face.

Several key aspects of the broaden-and-build theory have been empirically tested and supported. For instance, laboratory experiments have shown that, relative to neutral and negative states, induced positive emotions widen the scope of attention (Fredrickson & Branigan, 1998; Rowe, Hirsh, & Anderson, 2007), broaden repertoires of desired actions (Fredrickson & Branigan, 1998), dismantle physiological preparation for specific actions sparked by negative emotions (Fredrickson, Mancuso, Branigan, & Tugade, 2000), and increase openness to new experiences (Isen, 1970; Kahn & Isen, 1993). At the interpersonal level, induced positive emotions, again relative to neutral and negative states, increase people's sense of "oneness" with close others (Hejmadi, Waugh, Otake, &

Fredrickson, 2007), their trust in acquaintances (Dunn & Schweitzer, 2005), and their ability to recognize cross-race faces (Johnson & Fredrickson, 2005). Prospective correlational studies have further shown that people who, for whatever reasons, experience or express positive emotions more than others cope more effectively with adversity (Fredrickson, Tugade, Waugh, & Larkin, 2003; Folkman & Moskowitz, 2000; Stein, Folkman, Trabasso, & Richards, 1997; Bonanno & Keltner, 1997), and enjoy more successes in their work (Diener, Nickerson, Lucus, & Sandvik, 2002) and in their relationships (Harker & Keltner, 2001; Waugh & Fredrickson, 2006). People with more positive emotions and outlooks have also been shown to live longer (Danner, Snowden, & Friesen, 2001; Levy, Slade, Kunkel, & Kasl, 2002; Moskowitz, 2003; Ostir, Markides, Black, & Goodwin, 2000). Moreover, as is detailed in a later section, field experiments have demonstrated that interventions that increase people's daily experiences of positive emotions serve to build their physical, social, mental, and psychological resources (Fredrickson, Cohn, Coffey, Pek, & Finkel, 2007).

The broaden-and-build theory of positive emotions, together with its growing empirical support, provides an explanation for how and why high positivity ratios might forecast optimal functioning: By broadening people's mindsets and building consequential personal resources, positive emotional states, over time, transform people for the better, enabling them to survive, thrive, and even flourish. To *flourish* means to live within an optimal range of human functioning, one that simultaneously connotes growth, goodness, generativity, and resilience.

Another of Ed Diener's key contributions to science has been to help establish and legitimize the positive psychology movement (Diener & Seligman, 2004). One of the fruits of this new movement has been to describe, define, and measure flourishing mental health (Keyes, 2002). Epidemiological studies show that fewer than 20% of U.S. adults can be classified as enjoying flourishing mental health (Keyes, 2002). About the same percentage can be classified as fitting the diagnostic criteria for a mental illness. The rest of the population—the majority—can be described either as having only moderate mental health or as languishing. Those who languish might describe themselves as being "stuck in a rut" or "yearning for more." Although not diagnosable with any clinical disorders, these people experience as many lost workdays and illnesses as those who are depressed, costing society billions of dollars each year (Keyes & Lopez, 2002). Clearly there would be much gained by the discovery of reliable pathways toward flourishing mental health. Doing so would not only lift multiple burdens from society, but also create a society of citizens who are not merely self-sufficient but also generative and resilient—citizens well poised to make the world a more livable place for future generations.

Using the diagnostic tools developed to assess flourishing mental health, my past work has shown that, relative to people who do not flourish, those who do flourish experience higher positivity ratios (Fredrickson & Losada, 2005). More-over, there appears to be a particular threshold—or tipping point—within peo-ple's positivity ratios, above which flourishing mental health and other good out-comes become much more probable. Consider the differences between ice and water. Whereas ice is solid, rigid, and immobile, water is flowing, flexible, and dynamic. Yet despite these stark differences, to change one into the other simply requires a change in temperature: As the ambient temperature rises above 0 degrees Celsius, rigid ice melts into flowing water. Water undergoes a second phase-state change at 100 degrees Celsius, changing this time from liquid to vapor. The differences between not flourishing and flourishing may show similar properties: Our recent findings suggest that as people's habitual positivity ratios rise above about 3-to-1, they may leave behind stagnant states of languishing and begin to enjoy the more complex, dynamic, generative, and resilient states of flourishing mental health (Fredrickson & Losada, 2005). Likewise, if people's habitual positivity ratios exceed about 11-to-1, they may experience diminished generativity and resilience. Above that upper bound, negative experiences may be so infrequent that people lose their credibility as connected to reality. Just as water in its liquid state exists within a range of temperatures (bounded by 0° and 100° C), so too may humans exist within a range of positivity ratios in their flourishing states (bounded by about 3:1 and 11:1; Fredrickson & Losada, 2005). Across multiple samples, I have found that individuals classified as flourishing have positivity ratios above 3-to-1 (but less than about 11:1), whereas those who are not flourishing have positivity ratios below 3-to-1 (Fredrickson & Losada, 2005). Although the upper boundary of flourishing positivity ratios has yet to be tested empirically, the wide disdain associated with the label "Pollyanna" suggests that people intuitively recognize that an upper boundary on credible positivity exists.

So, as Ed Diener has long held, people's positivity ratios appear to be inex-tricably tied to their subjective well-being. My most recent theory and evidence, detailed in the *American Psychologist* (Fredrickson & Losada, 2005), illuminates the possible nature and dynamics of this important tie.

Increasing Positivity Ratios

If increases in people's positivity ratios might help them escape languishing and attain flourishing—like rising temperatures can melt ice into water—then it behooves us to learn ways to reliably augment people's positivity ratios. The rest of this chapter is devoted to this important topic.

Changing people's emotional habits is a tall order, akin to moving a river. Although possible, it is not something done on a whim or without tremendous and continued effort. The best new research suggests that forging lasting changes in people's emotional well-being requires as much intention, effort, and lifestyle change as does losing weight or changing cholesterol levels (Lyubomirsky, Sheldon, & Schkade, 2005).

As with many change efforts, multiple paths toward the goal are possible. A core implication of conceptualizing people's well-being and prospects for flourishing in terms of a ratio of positive to negative affect is that there are three overarching possibilities by which to increase a ratio: Either increase the numerator, decrease the denominator, or both. The principle of the negativity bias ("bad is stronger than good"; Baumeister et al., 2001) assures that efforts to decrease the denominator hold great promise (Larsen, 2002). Even so, the goal should not be to reduce all forms of negativity. Negative emotions are often appropriate and useful. It is, for instance, appropriate and even adaptive to mourn following a loss (Keller & Nesse, 2006) or to resonate on anger to fight an injustice (de Rivera, Gerstmann, & Maisels, 2002). Recall, too, that positivity ratios greater than about 11-to-1 may no longer predict flourishing mental health (Fredrickson & Losada, 2005). One implication of this upper boundary is that negative affect is, in fact, a necessary component of flourishing mental health. Yet, at times, people's emotional habits can intensify or prolong aversive feelings far beyond their usefulness. Rumination, for one, is a mental habit that can prolong feelings of sadness and increase a person's odds of falling prey to depression (Nolen-Hoeksema, 2002). Fortunately, the entire toolbox of cognitive–behavioral therapy—developed over the last several decades—is available to help people reduce their experiences of negative affect. In the present chapter, I focus exclusively on the less-studied path: increasing the numerator, or increasing positive affect.

Good intentions alone will not make anyone happier. A parallel to physical pain can illustrate this point. Suppose at this instant—for whatever reason—you wanted to make your left shin sting with pain. Could you rouse the intended experience of pain simply by thinking about this limb and willing your body to feel pain there? Not likely. To carry out this intention you would need to do more than apply sheer willpower. You would have to *do something*. And this "something" would need to be quite specific: such as banging your leg against a table leg or coaxing someone to kick you. Those and related actions could be considered leverage points by which you can carry out your intention to feel pain in your shin. By this same logic, people cannot simply will themselves to feel a positive emotion. They must instead locate one of a several quite specific leverage points to boost positive feelings. A probabilistic web of causality connects certain forms of thought and action to increases in positive emotions. So just as you must "do something" to rouse a feeling of pain out of thin air, so too must people "do something" to rouse positive emotions where none previously existed. A fundamental difference between physical pain and emotions, however, is that leverage points for emotions can involve redirections of conscious thought. This means that you can "think something" in addition to "do something" to rouse positive emotions.

The close causal ties between people's patterns of thought and their subsequent emotional experiences were introduced and tested within appraisal theories of emotion and later refined and applied within cognitive-behavioral therapies for affective disorders. A core assumption within these approaches is that changing the course of people's emotions requires that they change their course of thinking. This is as true for increasing positive emotions as it is for decreasing negative emotions. For the most part, positive emotions take root when people find and enact positive meaning within their current circumstances. Although other routes to enhanced positive affective experiences exist (e.g., through diet, exercise, facial feedback), our habits of mind and action provide perhaps the most powerful leverage points for increasing positive affectivity. In the sections that follow, I detail various ways in which changes in thinking and action can leverage positive emotions to augment positivity ratios.

Find Positive Meaning

Does the local forecast predict a partly cloudy sky? Or a partly sunny sky? Is the cup or cupboard half empty? Or half full? Most circumstances in which we find ourselves are not completely, 100%, bad. So the opportunity to find the good or accentuate the inherent positive meaning is almost always present, even if it is simply to say "This too shall pass." When people reappraise or reframe bad circumstances in positive ways, they increase the odds that positive emotions, such as hope, awe, or gratitude, will follow. Granted, these "silver lining" positive emotions may at times be subtle and may not fully neutralize the aversive situation. Yet they nonetheless appear to unlock positive dynamics. For instance, people who experience positive emotions during bereavement tend to develop more long-term plans and goals. Together with positive emotions, plans and goals predict better well-being and psychological functioning 12 months following bereavement (Stein et al., 1997). Similarly, most Americans felt a combination of sadness, anger, and fear in the wake of the 9/11 terrorist attacks. Yet those who, alongside these negative emotions, also experienced positive emotions—such as love, compassion, and gratitude—were the least likely to experience depressive symptoms and the most likely to show postcrisis growth in positive traits such as optimism, tranquility, and life satisfaction (Fredrickson et al., 2003).

One path toward finding positive meaning is to reframe or reappraise a negative event in positive terms. Another path is to infuse ordinary events with positive meaning (Folkman & Moskowitz, 2001). The strategy of "counting blessings" adopts this approach by encouraging people to recast hidden or mundane aspects of daily life as "gifts" to be cherished, and as such, these aspects of life can become sources of gratitude and other positive emotions. Experimental studies have shown that people who count their blessings, relative to those who do not, report increases in their own positive affect (Emmons & McCullough, 2003; Lyubomirsky, Sheldon, & Schkade, 2005).

Be Open

The broaden-and-build theory asserts that positive emotions broaden people's attention and thinking (Fredrickson & Branigan, 2005), and we also know that broadened attention and thinking forecasts future positive emotions (Fredrickson & Joiner, 2002). Similarly, in his study of business team meetings, Losada (1999) finds bidirectional relations between positivity and two plausible indicators of openness, namely inquiry (e.g., asking questions) and other-focus. Noting the reciprocal causal links between positive emotions and broadened, open mindsets raises the possibility that another leverage point for augmenting positive feelings is to practice openness. One way to do so is to become more open to direct sensory experience. On a morning walk, for instance, rather than being lost in your ever-expanding mental "to-do" list, you might practice being open to the colors of the leaves and blooms, the call of the nearby birds, the smell of the wet grass, the feel of the cool morning air against your skin, and the pressure of the earth beneath your feet.

Focusing on the present moment and being experientially open are viewed as the two core components of mindfulness. This consensus definition of mindfulness was articulated by Western psychological scientists and was based on the emerging clinical and empirical literature on mindfulness meditation practices, which themselves emanate from Buddhist traditions (Bishop et al., 2004). The first component of mindfulness, focusing on the present moment, involves self-regulation of attention. Unpacked further, effective self-regulation of attention requires both (1) sustained attention, to maintain awareness of current experiences and a chosen focal object (often the breath), and (2) attention switching, to return attention to the focal object once an arising thought, feeling, or sensation has been acknowledged. The second component of mindfulness, being open to experience, involves cultivating an orientation of curiosity and acceptance about the arising contents of consciousness. In this manner, thoughts, feelings, and sensations that may surface are not viewed as disruptions to be suppressed in favor of the focal object, but instead acknowledged, appreciated, and allowed to pass. Mindfulness, then, characterizes a wider, more accepting perspective on present experience than is typical. Mindfulness training, through meditation and other practices, can thus be conceptualized as a skillful means of cultivating the broad-minded attentional state that is produced automatically during positive emotional states.

Would increasing openness to experience—through mindfulness training or other means—increase positive emotions? Might it not also increase negative emotions? Certainly all experiences to which people might open themselves are not pleasant. During that morning walk, for instance, you may suddenly discover animal excrement on your shoe or in your hair. Creating openness to experience will not selectively augment positive emotions. Even so, cultivating an open, accepting stance toward negative experience can diffuse emotional distress. To illustrate, consider once again that animal excrement and imagine the affective difference between thinking to yourself "Shit!" versus "Shit happens." Intentional efforts to be open to experience are hypothesized to improve people's tolerance for negative emotions and diffuse the reactivity and intensity of aversive states (Bishop et al., 2004; Hayes, Follette, & Linehan, 2004).

But let's return to positive emotions: Why might we expect increased openness to increase positivity? One key is to consider the natural topography of good and bad experiences. We know from Diener's work on the positivity offset that unpleasant experiences are relatively rare, which is part of the reason why negative events rivet our attention (Baumeister et al., 2001; Schwartz & Garamoni, 1989). As such, when people open themselves to experience, those experiences are likely to reflect this inherent positivity offset. So, depending on people's immediate circumstances and habitual positivity ratios, increasing openness to experience is highly likely to increase the experience of positive emotions and thereby increase positivity ratios.

Being open and mindful can also expand people's awareness such that they recognize features of their environment that had previously gone unnoticed. For instance, being open and mindful can increase awareness of oneness and interconnectedness, both with other people and with the natural world. Such perceived oneness can, in turn, inspire the self-transcendent positive emotions of awe (Keltner & Haidt, 2003), gratitude (McCullough, Emmons, & Tsang, 2002), and compassion (Cialdini, Brown, Lewis, Luce, & Neuberg,1997).

By intentionally cultivating openness, people can find the good even within the bad. With high openness, for instance, that animal excrement on your morning walk might be transformed into a reminder that you are just one of many creatures co-experiencing that particular stretch of earth, and begin to draw out your fascination and awe, and even your gratitude and amusement. The link between openness and the ability to discover the good within the bad can be illustrated by an often-cited Zen meditation that goes something like this: A farmer's horse ran away. His neighbors say, "Such bad luck!" The farmer says "Maybe." The next week, the farmer's horse returns with a several other horses. His neighbors say, "What wonderful luck!" The farmer says "Maybe." A few days later, the farmer's son tries to ride one of the new horses and is thrown and breaks his leg. "Ah, such bad luck!" the farmer's neighbors cry out. "Maybe" said the farmer. A short time later, the ruler of the country comes to recruit all young men to join his army for battle. The son, with his broken leg, is left at home. "What good luck that your son was not forced into battle!" celebrated the neighbors. The farmer said "Maybe." Whereas this parable might imply that every bad experience is matched by a good one (and vice versa), we know empirically—again from Diener's work on the positivity offset—that most events and experiences are, in fact, at least mildly pleasant. So, in the end, as people increase their openness, positivity is likely to accrue in greater abundance than negativity.

Is the logic of this link between openness and positivity born out empirically? The evidence to date is scant but nonetheless suggestive. One study, for example, used an experience sampling technique to compare two groups of mindfulness meditators (Easterlin & Cardena, 1998). The groups were defined by their level of meditation experience. Advanced meditators ($n = 24$) had practiced Vipassana for 3 years or more, with at least 10 days of formal retreat experience each year, and showed advanced skill level on a self-report measure of meditation experience. Beginning meditators ($n = 19$) had less experience (on average, about 1 year) and lower skill levels. The two groups carried electronic pagers for 5 days, which signaled them at random between two and five times a day. When signaled, they completed a specially designed Experience Sampling Form (Csikszentmihalyi & Larson, 1987). Comparing the culled experiences of these two groups revealed that the advanced meditators—those more skilled in mindful, open attention—reported experiencing more positive affect, more active affect, as well as more self-awareness and acceptance (Easterlin & Cardena, 1998). Did greater openness directly account for this difference? These data do not answer that question. Although it is possible that practicing mindful attention created an openness to greater positive experiences, it is also possible that the advanced meditators perceived more success and delight in their meditation practice, and that these greater positive emotions reduced their threshold to experience further positive emotions. Plus, it is important to note that the two groups were not randomly assigned, and so the direction of causality cannot be determined. It may be, for instance, that people prone to experience more frequent positive emotions are especially likely to become effective meditators. Even so, the association between skillful practice of mindful, open attention and enhanced positivity is intriguing.

Another line of evidence regarding the effects of mindfulness meditation on emotion experience can support causal claims. The research program of Kabat-Zinn and colleagues is representative (for a review, see Kabat-Zinn, 2003). In a program of research that spans more than 25 years, Kabat-Zinn has documented the salutary effects of mindfulness training on stress, anxiety, pain, and various illnesses. More recently, Kabat-Zinn and colleagues (Davidson, Kabat-Zinn, Schumacher, et al., 2003) examined the affective, brain, and immunological effects of mindfulness practice. A sample of volunteers for a workplace study on the effects of meditation was randomly assigned either to a waitlist control group ($n = 16$) or to an 8-week mindfulness-based stress reduction workshop ($n = 25$), which required a daily practice of guided mindfulness meditation lasting about an hour. At the start of the study, immediately after the 8-week training period, and again 4 months later, the researchers assessed brain electrical activity (i.e., by an electroencephalogram [EEG]). At the end of the 8-week training period, all participants were vaccinated with influenza vaccine, and blood draws at about 4 and 8 weeks later were examined for antibody titers in response to the vaccine. As in past studies, Kabat-Zinn et al. found that trait anxiety was significantly reduced in the meditation group. More strikingly, results also showed that individuals practicing mindfulness show greater left-sided anterior activation at rest, and also during both positive and negative emotion inductions. This pattern is striking because Davidson's past work (2000) has linked it decisively to greater positive affectivity. The meditation group also showed greater increases in antibody titers to the influenza vaccine, and this salutary immune response was correlated with the magnitude of left-sided anterior brain activation. So even though self-reports of positive affect did not change as a result of the mindfulness intervention, asymmetric brain activation and immune function changed in a manner indicative of increased positivity.

A third approach to testing the connection between openness and increased positivity is illustrated by a recent study from my laboratory (Fredrickson, Cohn, Coffey, Pek, & Finkel, 2001). The aim of this study was to test the build hypothesis—derived from the broaden-and-build theory—which states that as positive emotions accumulate and compound, people show a positive trajectory of growth in which they augment or build a range of personal resources that better equip them to handle future adversity. The resources so gained may be physical (e.g., health, sleep quality), psychological (e.g., resilience, optimism), social (e.g., closeness, support given/received), and/or mental (e.g., mindfulness, savoring). To test this hypothesis, we sought an intervention that would selectively increase people's positive emotions over the course of several weeks. We chose to test the effects of a loving-kindness meditation practice, a "cousin" to mindfulness meditation.

Like mindfulness meditation, loving-kindness meditation emanates from ancient Buddhist mind-training practices. Each practice involves quiet contemplation in a seated posture, often with eyes closed and an initial focus on the breath. Yet whereas mindfulness meditation aims to train a person's attention toward the present moment, loving-kindness meditation aims to train a person's emotions toward warm, tender, and compassionate feelings. The practice, as we studied it, is akin to guided emotional imagery. Individuals are first asked to focus on their breath and their heart region and to contemplate a person for whom they already feel warm, tender, and compassionate feelings (e.g., their child or a close loved one). They are then asked to extend these warm feelings to themselves. As the practice continues, they are also asked to radiate these warm, tender, and compassionate feelings to others, first to a few people they know well, then to all their friends and family, then to all people with whom they have a connection, and finally to all people and creatures of the earth. By radiating warm feelings to an ever-widening circle of others, the practice of loving-kindness meditation cultivates not only positive emotions but also openness, or broad-minded, attention. According to the broaden-and-build theory, these two experiential consequences go hand in hand.

To test the effects of loving-kindness mediation on positive emotions and positive trajectories of growth, we recruited a sample of about 200 working adults to participate in a workplace wellness program described as a workshop on "stress-relieving meditation." We randomly assigned participants to either a wait-list control group or a 6-week meditation workshop. Before the workshop began, we assessed participants' mental health and personal resources. Mental health was conceptualized as degrees of flourishing, using Keyes's (2002) measures. Personal resources included physical (e.g., sleep quality), psychological (e.g., trait resilience), social (e.g., self–other overlap), and mental (e.g., mindfulness) domains. Over the next 8 weeks, while those assigned to the meditation group attended the workshop and initiated a daily practice of meditation, all participants (including those in the waitlist group) reported their emotion experiences daily. We assessed 10 distinct positive emotions (i.e., amusement, awe, contentment, compassion, joy, gratitude, hope, interest, love, and pride) and 8 distinct negative emotions (i.e., anger, contempt, disgust, embarrassment, fear, guilt, sadness, and shame). At the close of the study (approximately 10 days after the last workshop session), we again assessed participants' mental health and personal resources.

Analysis of the daily emotion reports revealed that, beginning in week 3 and persisting through the end of the study, participants in the meditation group, compared to those in the waitlist control group, reported more intense experiences of a wide range of positive emotions. No significant group differences emerged for the experience of negative emotions. These data document that loving-kindness meditation practice succeeds at selectively increasing positivity and therefore provides a critical manipulation check in this study.

What happened when we augmented people's daily experiences of positive emotions in this manner? The build hypothesis states that as positive emotions increase, people accrue and build personal resources, which in turn enhances their overall mental health. This hypothesis not only predicts group differences in improved resources and mental health favoring those in the meditation workshop, but it also predicts that increments in people's resources account for (i.e., mediate) the association between their increased positive emotions and their enhanced mental health. We found support for each of these predictions. First, significant group differences emerged across a wide range of resources, including one physical resource (sleep quality, Buysse, Reynolds, Monk, Berman, & Kupfer, 1989) one psychological resource (i.e., trait resilience, Block & Kremen, 1996; Fredrickson et al., 2003), two social resources (i.e., self–other overlap,

Aron, Aron, & Smollan, 1992; and social support given, Spanier, 1976), and three mental resources (mindfulness, Brown & Ryan, 2003; the ability to savor the future, Bryant, 2003; and implicit incremental theories, Hong, Chiu, Dweck, Lin, & Wan, 1999). Each significant effect reflected greater gains in the targeted resource within the meditation group. Second, group differences emerged on our index of increased flourishing, with those in the meditation group showing significantly larger gains. Finally, a test of mediation, following the Kenny et al. (1998) guidelines, confirmed that an aggregate measure that reflected all evident resource gains mediated the association between increased positive emotions and enhanced mental health. In other words, practicing loving-kindness meditation reliably augmented people's daily experiences of positive emotions, and those increases in positive emotions, in turn, accounted for gains in a wide range of personal resources, ranging from sleep quality to resilience and mindfulness. These resource gains, in turn, elevated signs of flourishing mental health. These data provide the first experimental evidence for the build hypothesis. They not only tell how to augment positivity but also underscore the consequential down-stream effects of doing so.

The design of this initial study on the effects of loving-kindness meditation does not allow us to pinpoint the active ingredients within this particular medita-tion practice. Further studies are needed to do so. The active ingredient may be the pleasantness of the emotions induced. Alternatively, it could be the greater openness inspired by the repeated focus on an ever-widening circle of others. Yet knowing that positive emotions and open, broad-minded thinking co-occur and mutually reinforce one another, from the perspective of the broaden-and-build theory, a "both–and" view of active ingredients may prove more viable than an "either–or" view. Positivity and openness may, by nature, coexist. Teasing them apart may not even be possible. Whichever attribute or attributes of the loving-kindness practice emerge as most critical, the larger test of the build hypothesis stands on solid ground: Experimentally induced positive emotions accounted for gains in resources, which in turn accounted for gains in flourishing mental health.

Although meditation—be it mindfulness, loving-kindness, or both—may be a skillful way to increase openness, it is not the only way. Another route may be to reduce certain habits of mind that tend to constrain and compartmentalize experience. New theory and research suggest that humans face a "pleasure para-dox" such that thinking too much about a pleasant experience actually dampens that experience and reduces the overall pleasantness that we can derive from it (Wilson, Centerbar, Kermer, & Gilbert, 2005). A series of experiments tested this pleasure paradox by giving study participants a gift of a $1 coin taped to an index card. By random assignment, one group of participants received an explanation for this gift, whereas another group did not. A third group received no card or gift. Researchers then assessed the magnitude of participants' pleasant feelings 5 minutes later. Results showed that the group without an explanation experienced the most enduring positive emotions. Subsequent experiments showed that people are unaware of this pleasure paradox: When given a choice, they overwhelmingly prefer more certainty about their upcoming positive events. What these data suggest is that explaining a pleasant event can paradoxically erase its pleasantness. One lesson in these findings is that it may be best to accept random acts of kindness as random. Be open to goodness however it arrives: Practice acceptance, not analysis.

Whereas habitually analyzing events may paradoxically squelch pleasant experiences, other habits of mind might expand and intensify our experience of them. *Savoring* appears to be one of these more helpful mental habits. Savoring represents the capacity to willfully generate, intensify, and prolong one's enjoyment of positive events. People's self-evaluations of their ability to savor pleasant experiences taps into a form of perceived control over positive emotions, just as their self-evaluations of their ability to cope taps into a form of perceived control over negative emotions. Moreover, these two types of perceived control over emotions—positive and negative—appear to be largely independent (Bryant, 2003). People's beliefs about savoring are hypothesized to predict the intensity and frequency of the pleasure gained from positive experiences. One study (Bryant, 2003), measured three aspects of people's savoring beliefs: their self-evaluations of their ability to savor (1) future pleasant events, (2) present pleasant events, and (3) past pleasant events. Participants were then contacted before, during, or after a vacation from college. Bryant's (2003) Savoring Beliefs Inventory showed predictive, convergent, and discriminant validity in that the relevant subscale best predicted behaviors and affect more strongly than did the subscales with other two temporal orientations. The research on savoring suggests that perhaps beyond merely accepting goodness, we should relish it, deeply appreciating each facet of its pleasantness.

Our lab group recently discovered another strategy for increasing openness completely serendipitously: Go outside. More precisely, go outside in good springtime weather. A former student of mine, Matt Keller, was keenly interested in the effects of weather on mood (as any Texas native transplanted to Michigan might be). He examined the extant literature and was surprised to learn that the mood-boosting quality of good weather was judged to be an old wives' tale, unsupported by empirical evidence (Watson, 2000). Keller reasoned that perhaps the persistent null finding could be attributed to people's limited exposure to the weather. A fact of modern life is that people are largely insulated from direct exposure to the weather, spending an average of 93% of their time indoors (Woodcock & Custovic, 1998). Noting this, Keller predicted an interaction between good weather and time spent outside on people's mood.

My laboratory routinely collects data on study participants' mood as well as their broadened thinking or cognitive openness. One spring Keller added to two simple questions to our standard battery: "How much time did you spend out-side so far today?" and "How physically active have you been today?" The latter question provided an important control for the known effects of activity level (which may covary with time spent outside) on mood. He later downloaded pre-cise metrics on the local weather (i.e., temperature and barometric pressure) from the National Climatic Data Center.

Regression analyses revealed two striking interaction effects—one predicted, the other not. People who spent more time outside when the weather was nice (high temperature or high pressure) showed the predicted boost in pleasant mood, whereas those who spent little time outside did not. What we did not expect to find was that those who spent more time outside when the weather was nice also scored higher on measures of broadened, open thinking. These included measures of digit span and openness to new information. The following spring we tested Keller's prediction experimentally, randomly assigning partici-pants to spend time outside or not, and then measured mood and broadened thinking. The same two interaction effects emerged. Later studies done year-round revealed that these were seasonal effects, evident in the spring and early summer only.

We queried the data to learn whether either effect mediated the other. They did not. In the time span in which we tested our participants, the increase in openness did not account for their boost in mood, nor did their boost in mood account for their increases in openness. These appeared to be two independent effects. Even so, other research documents that nature experiences are high on both *fascination*—they draw people's attention involuntarily—and *extent*—they provide sufficient scope and richness to fully occupy people's attention (Kaplan, 1995)—two qualities that might produce positive emotion and openness, respec-tively, and together with other characteristics (being in a different [novel] loca-tion, and being compatible with one's purposes and inclinations) are restorative. Simply put, when outdoors people can often see farther, and seeing farther may be all it takes to expand people's modes of thought, giving them more about which to feel good. These speculations merit empirical testing.

Do Good

So far, the strategies described to augment positivity emphasize internal changes, various ways of finding positive meaning, and becoming more open. A third very broad class of strategies worth mentioning, at least briefly, is to externalize posi-tive perspectives, instantiating them as behaviors, especially within social interac-tions. A classic stream of research in social psychology highlights one way to boost positivity: Help others. Helpful, compassionate actions not only spring from positive feelings (Isen, Clark, & Schwartz, 1976), but they also generate and reinforce positive feelings (Fredrickson, 2003). More recent studies report that the happiest people show more kindness to others relative to those who are less happy, and that subjective happiness increases when people increase their focus on their own acts of kindness (Otake, Shimai, Tananka-Matsumi, Otsui, & Fredrickson, 2006). That is, the habit of "counting one's own kindnesses" may function a bit like "counting one's blessings." Each strategy has been shown to boost positive affect. Another external way to augment and prolong positive affect is to share news of your good fortunes with supportive others. Diary studies confirm that when people do so, they multiply their good feelings significantly (Gable, Reis, Impett, & Asher, 2004). Related work demonstrates that when people celebrate or otherwise mark their successes, they extend the happiness they derive from them (Langston, 1994). Likewise, I would speculate that, to the extent that you are open, appreciative, and supportive of good news that you hear, you too can derive pleasure from it. Outside of social interaction, other ways to "do good" also augment positivity. Work by Folkman and Moskowitz (2000) suggests that actively working to solve problems can create important senses of mastery and control that, in turn, increase positive affect. For instance, even though caregivers whose partners were dying of AIDS in the 1990s experienced the disease itself as completely uncontrollable, many pursued realistic, attainable goals by focusing on and solving specific problems related to caregiving, such as helping to manage their dying partner's pain. The point to underscore here is that strategies for increasing positivity are not "all in your head." Externalizing positive perspectives, whether through kind acts, sharing good news, solving problems, or other routes, can also reliably increase positivity.

Be Social

Still another of Ed Diener's contributions was to closely examine the attributes of "very happy" people (Diener & Seligman, 2002). All very happy people, it appears, are highly social: Compared to less happy people, very happy people spend the least amount of time alone, the most amount of time with family, friends, and romantic partners, and have the strongest romantic and other social relationships. From these data, Diener and Seligman (2002) concluded that good social relations are a necessary condition for happiness, albeit not a sufficient condition (i.e., some less happy people showed comparable sociality). Not surprisingly, very happy people were also more extraverted, agreeable, and less neurotic than less happy people. This finding raises the interesting question of whether people might increase their positive affect by being more social. A recent series of studies tested this hypothesis directly, both within daily life and within a controlled laboratory setting (Fleeson, Malanos, & Achille, 2002). An experience sampling study revealed that rapid, within-person fluctuations in extraversion were strong predictors of rapid, within-person fluctuations in positive affect. Strikingly, this within-person association was evident for each person tested:

That is, each participant was happier when acting extraverted than when acting introverted. A laboratory experiment further revealed that when people are randomly assigned to "act extraverted" (versus "act introverted") during a group discussion, they experience more intense positive affect (Fleeson et al., 2002). So, beyond doing good for others, simply interacting with others appears to be a reliable strategy for increasing positivity.

Closing Words:
Reflect and Anticipate Diener's Legacy

This volume aims to detail the latest social science on subjective well-being, a field that would hardly exist without Ed Diener's major contributions and steering influence. The aim of this chapter was to describe a set of pathways for augmenting subjective well-being by increasing the ratio of people's pleasant to unpleasant experiences. Furthering the practical application of the science of subjective well-being, Ed Diener has recently advocated for a national well-being index (Diener & Seligman, 2004). Developed societies have long tracked the influence of various societal factors and social policies on economic well-being. It is time to look beyond money. As the data (and the Beatles) say, time and again, money can't buy love . . . or peace, joy, or any other lasting indicators of subjective well-being. Through the developing science of subjective well-being, scientists are beginning to understand the practices that can "buy" these positive states, and what they, in turn, can "buy" for us. We, as a field, owe Ed Diener a debt of gratitude for opening this possibility for us.

References

Aron, A., Aron, E. N., & Smollan, D. (1992). Inclusion of other in the self scale and the structure of interpersonal closeness. *Journal of Personality and Social Psychology, 63*(4), 596–612.

Baumeister, R. F., Bratslavsky, E., Finkenauer, C., & Vohs, K. D. (2001). Bad is stronger than good. *Review of General Psychology, 5*(4), 323–370.

Bishop, S. R., Lau, M., Shapiro, S., Carlson, L., Anderson, N. D., Carmody, J., et al. (2004). Mindfulness: A proposed operational definition. *Clinical Psychology: Science and Practice, 11*(3), 230–241.

Block, J., & Kremen, A. M. (1996). IQ and ego-resiliency: Conceptual and empirical connections and separateness. *Journal of Personality and Social Psychology, 70*(2), 349–361.

Bonanno, G. A., & Keltner, D. (1997). Facial expressions of emotion and the course of conjugal bereavement. *Journal of Abnormal Psychology, 106*(1), 126–137.

Brown, K. W., & Ryan, R. M. (2003). The benefits of being present: Mindfulness and its role in psychological well-being. *Journal of Personality and Social Psychology, 84*(4), 822–848.

Bryant, F. B. (2003). A scale for measuring beliefs about savoring. *Journal of Mental Health, 12,* 175–196.

Buysse, D. J., Reynolds, C. F., III, Monk, T. H., Berman, S. R., & Kupfer, D. J. (1989). The Pittsburgh Sleep Quality Index: A new instrument for psychiatric practice and research. *Psychiatry Research, 28,* 193–213.

Cacioppo, J. T., Gardner, W. L., & Berntson, G. G. (1999). The affect system has parallel and integrative processing components: Form follows function. *Journal of Personality and Social Psychology, 76*(5), 839–855.

Cialdini, R. B., Brown, S. L., Lewis, B. P., Luce, C., & Neuberg, S. L. (1997). Reinterpreting the empathy–altruism relationship: When one into one equals oneness. *Journal of Personality and Social Psychology, 73,* 481–494.

Csikszentmihalyi, M., & Larsen, R. W. (1987). Validity and reliability of the experience sampling method. *Journal of Nervous and Mental Disease, 175,* 526–536.

Danner, D. D., Snowdon, D. A., & Friesen, W. V. (2001). Positive emotions in early life and longevity: Findings from the nun study. *Journal of Personality and Social Psychology, 80*(5), 804–813.

Davidson, R. J. (2000). Affective style, psychopathology, and resilience: Brain mechanisms and plasticity. *American Psychologist, 55,* 1196–1214.

Davidson, R. J., Kabat-Zinn, J., Schumacher, J., Rosenkranz, M., Muller, D., Santorelli, S. F., et al. (2003). Alterations in brain and immune function produced by mindfulness meditation. *Psychosomatic Medicine, 65,* 564–570.

Diener, E. (2000). Subjective well-being: The science of happiness and a proposal for a national index. *American Psychologist, 55,* 34–43.

Diener, E., Napa-Scollon, C. K., Oishi, S., Dzokoto, V., & Suh, E. M. (2000). Positivity and the construction of life satisfaction judgments: Global happiness is not the sum of its parts. *Journal of Happiness Studies, 1,* 159–176.

Diener, E., Nickerson, C., Lucas, R. E., & Sandvik, E. (2002). Dispositional affect and job outcomes. *Social Indicators Research, 59,* 229–259.

Diener, E., & Seligman, M. E. P. (2002). Very happy people. *Psychological Science, 13*(1), 81–84.

Diener, E., & Seligman, M. E. P. (2004). Beyond money: Toward an economy of well-being. *Psychological Sciences in the Public Interest, 5*(1), 1–31.

Dunn, J. R., & Schweitzer, M. E. (2005). Feeling and believing: The influence of emotion on trust. *Journal of Personality and Social Psychology, 88*(5), 736–748.

Easterlin, B. L., & Cardena, E. (1998). Cognitive and emotional differences between short and long term Vipassana meditation. *Imagination, Cognition, and Personality, 18,* 69–81.

Emmons, R. A., & McCullough, M. E. (2003). Counting blessings versus burdens: An experimental investigation of gratitude and subjective well-being in daily life. *Journal of Personality and Social Psychology, 84*(2), 377–389.

Fleeson, W., Malanos, A. B., & Achille, N. M. (2002). An intraindividual process approach to the relationship between extraversion and positive affect: Is acting extraverted as "good" as being extraverted? *Journal of Personality and Social Psychology, 83*(6), 1409–1422.

Folkman, S., & Moskowitz, J. T. (2000). Positive affect and the other side of coping. *American Psychologist, 55*(6), 647.

Fredrickson, B. L. (1998). What good are positive emotions? *Review of General Psychology, 2*(3), 300–319.

Fredrickson, B. L. (2001). The role of positive emotions in positive psychology: The broaden-and-build theory of positive emotions. *American Psychologist, 56*(3), 218–226.

Fredrickson, B. L. (2003). Positive emotions and upward spirals in organizational settings. In K. Cameron, J. Dutton, & R. Quinn (Eds.), *Positive organizational scholarship* (pp. 163–175). San Francisco: Berrett-Koehler Publishers.

Fredrickson, B. L., & Branigan, C. (2005). Positive emotions broaden the scope of attention and thought–action repertoires. *Cognition and Emotion, 19*(3), 313–332.

Fredrickson, B. L., Cohn, M. A., Coffey, K. A., Pek, J., & Finkel, S. (2007). *Open hearts build lives: Positive emotions, induced through meditation, build consequential personal resources.* Manuscript under review.

Fredrickson, B. L., & Joiner, T. (2002). Positive emotions trigger upward spirals toward emotional well-being. *Psychological Science, 13*(2), 172–175.

Fredrickson, B. L., & Losada, M. F. (2005). Positive affect and the complex dynamics of human flourishing. *American Psychologist, 60*(7), 678–686.

Fredrickson, B. L., Mancuso, R. A., Branigan, C., & Tugade, M. M. (2000). The undoing effect of positive emotions. *Motivation and Emotion, 24*(4), 237–258.

Fredrickson, B. L., Tugade, M. M., Waugh, C. E., & Larkin, G. R. (2003). What good are positive emotions in crisis?: A prospective study of resilience and emotions following the terrorist attacks on the United States on September 11th 2001. *Journal of Personality and Social Psychology, 84*(2), 365–376.

Gable S., Reis, H., Impett, E., & Asher, E. (2004). What do you do when things go right?: The intrapersonal and interpersonal benefits of sharing positive events. *Journal of Personality and Social Psychology, 87*(2), 228–245.

Gottman, J. M. (1994). *What predicts divorce?: The relationship between marital processes and marital outcomes.* Mahwah, NJ: Erlbaum.

Harker, L. A., & Keltner, D. (2001). Expressions of positive emotion in women's college yearbook pictures and their relationship to personality and life outcomes across adulthood. *Journal of Personality and Social Psychology, 80*, 112–124.

Hayes, S. C., Follete, V. M., & Linehan, M. M. (2004). *Mindfulness and acceptance: Expanding the cognitive-behavioral tradition.* New York: Guilford Press.

Hejmadi, A., Waugh, C. E., Otake, K., & Fredrickson, B. L. (2007). *Cross-cultural evidence that positive emotions broaden views of self to include close others.* Manuscript in preparation.

Hong, Y. Y., Chiu, C., Dweck, C. S., Lin, D., & Wan, W. (1999). Implicit theories, attributions, and coping: A meaning system approach. *Journal of Personality and Social Psychology, 77*, 588–599.

Isen, A. M. (1970). Success, failure, attention, and reaction to others: The warm glow of success. *Journal of Personality and Social Psychology, 15*(4), 294–301.

Isen, A. M., Clark, M., & Schwartz, M. F. (1976). Effects of success and failure on children's generosity. *Journal of Personality and Social Psychology, 27*(2), 239–247.

Johnson, K. J., & Fredrickson, B. L. (2005). "We all look the same to me": Positive emotions eliminate the own-race in face recognition. *Psychological Science, 16*(11), 875–881.

Kabat-Zinn, J. (2003). Mindfulness-based interventions in context: Past, present, and future. *Clinical Psychology: Science and Practice, 10*(2), 144–156.

Kahn, B. E., & Isen, A. M. (1993). The influence of positive affect on variety seeking among safe, enjoyable products. *Journal of Consumer Research, 20*(2), 257–270.

Kaplan, S. (1995). The restorative benefits of nature: Toward an integrative framework. *Journal of Environmental Psychology, 15*(3), 169–182.

Keller, M., & Nesse, R. (2006). The evolutionary significance of depressive symptoms: Different adverse situations lead to different depressive symptom patterns. *Journal of Personality and Social Psychology, 91*, 316–330.

Keltner, D., & Haidt, J. (2003). Approaching awe: A moral, spiritual, and aesthetic emotion. *Cognition and Emotion, 17*, 297–314.

Kenny, D. A., Kashy, D. A., & Bolger, N. (1998). Data analysis in social psychology. In D. T. Gilbert, S. T. Fiske, & G. Lindzey (Eds.), *The handbook of social psychology* (Vol. 1, 4th ed., pp. 233–265). New York: McGraw-Hill.

Keyes, C. L. M. (2002). The mental health continuum: From languishing to flourishing in life. *Journal of Health and Social Behavior, 43*(2), 207–222.

Keyes, C. L. M., & Lopez, S. (2002). *Toward a science of mental health: Positive direction in diagnosis and interventions.* New York: Oxford University Press.

Langston, C. A. (1994). Capitalizing on and coping with daily-life events: Expressive responses to positive events. *Journal of Personality and Social Psychology, 67*(6), 1112–1125.

Larsen, R. J. (2002). Differential contribution of positive and negative affect to subjective well-being. In E. H. M. J. A. Da Silva & N. P. Riberio-Filho (Eds.), *Annual meeting of the International Society for Psychophysics* (Vol. 18, pp. 186–190). Rio de Janeiro, Brazil: Editora Legis Summa.

Levy, B. R., Slade, M. D., Kunkel, S. R., & Kasl, S. V. (2002). Longevity increased by positive self-perceptions of aging. *Journal of Personality and Social Psychology, 83*(2), 261–270.

Losada, M. (1999). The complex dynamics of high performance teams. *Mathematical and Computer Modeling, 30*(9–10), 179–192.

Lyubomirsky, S., King, L., & Diener, E. (2005). The benefits of frequent positive affect: Does happiness lead to success? *Psychological Bulletin, 131*(6), 803–855.

Lyubomirsky, S., Sheldon, K. M., & Schkade, D. (2005). Pursuing happiness: The architecture of sustainable change. *Review of General Psychology, 9*(2), 111–131.

McCullough, M. E., Emmons, R. A., & Tsang, J. (2002). The grateful disposition: A conceptual and empirical topography. *Journal of Personality and Social Psychology, 82*, 112–127.

Moskowitz, J. T. (2003). Positive affect predicts lower risk of AIDS mortality. *Psychosomatic Medicine, 65*, 620–626.

Nolen-Hoeksema, S. (2000). The role of rumination in depressive disorders and mixed anxiety/depressive symptoms. *Journal of Abnormal Psychology, 109*, 504–511.

Ostir, G. V., Markides, K. S., Black, S. A., & Goodwin, J. S. (2000). Emotional well-being predicts subsequent functional independence and survival. *Journal of the American Geriatrics Society, 48*(5), 473–478.

Otake, K., Shimai, S., Tanaka-Matsumi, J., Otsui, K., & Fredrickson, B. L. (2006). Happy people become happier through kindness: A counting kindnesses intervention. *Journal of Happiness Studies, 7,* 361–375.

Rowe, G., Hirsh, J. B., & Anderson, A. K. (2007). Positive affect increases the breadth of attentional selection. *Proceedings of the National Academy of Sciences of the United States of America, 104,* 383–388.

Schwartz, R. M., & Garamoni, G. L. (1989). Cognitive balance and psychopathology: Evaluation of an information processing model of positive and negative states of mind. *Clinical Psychology Review, 9,* 271–294.

Schwartz, R. M., Reynolds, C. F., III, Thase, M. E., Frank, E., Fasiczka, A. L., & Haaga, D. A. F. (2002). Optimal and normal affect balance in psychotherapy of major depression: Evaluation of the balanced states of mind model. *Behavioural and Cognitive Psychotherapy, 30*(4), 439–450.

Spanier, G. B. (1976). Measuring dyadic adjustment: New scales for assessing the quality of marriage and similar dyads. *Journal of Marriage and the Family, 38,* 15–28.

Stein, N., Folkman, S., Trabasso, T., & Richards, T. A. (1997). Appraisal and goal processes as predictors of psychological well-being in bereaved caregivers. *Journal of Personality and Social Psychology, 72*(4), 872–884.

Waugh, C. E., & Fredrickson, B. L. (2006). Nice to know you: Positive emotions, self–other overlap, and complex understanding in the formation of new relationships. *Journal of Positive Psychology, 1,* 93–106.

Watson, D. (2000). *Mood and temperament.* New York: Guilford Press.

Wilson, T. D., Centerbar, D. B., Kermer, D. A., & Gilbert, D. T. (2005). The pleasures of uncertainty: Prolonging positive moods in ways people do not anticipate. *Journal of Personality and Social Psychology, 88,* 5–21.

Woodcock, A., & Custovic, A. (1998). ABC of allergies: Avoiding exposure to indoor allergens. *British Medical Journal, 316,* 1075–1078.

23

Gratitude, Subjective Well-Being, and the Brain

ROBERT A. EMMONS

I would maintain that thanks are the highest form of thought, and that gratitude is happiness doubled by wonder.

—G. K. CHESTERTON

Much of human life, and for that matter, the lives of other species, centers on the giving and receiving of benefits. When a person receives a gift or benefit, a typical emotional response is gratitude directed toward the perceived source of that gift. Research in the psychology of emotion demonstrates that gratitude is a commonly experienced affect. For example, Chipperfield, Perry, and Weiner (2003) recently reported that feeling grateful was the third most common discrete positive affect experienced in a sample of older adults, reported by nearly 90% of their sample. Gratitude can also represent a broader attitude toward life—the tendency to see all of life as a gift. Gratitude thus has various meanings and can be conceptualized at several levels of analysis, ranging from momentary affect to long-term dispositions (McCullough, Emmons, & Tsang, 2002). After beginning with a brief overview of the scholarship on gratitude, I describe the relevance of recent research and perspectives on gratitude for the science of subjective well-being. The growing evidence suggests that gratitude is a key element for sparking positive and sustained changes in individual well-being. Mechanisms by which gratitude favorably impacts subjective well-being are discussed, and a tentative cognitive neuroscience of gratitude is constructed. I conclude with a consideration of the importance of cultivating gratitude as an intentional, personal discipline.

On the Meaning of Gratitude

What exactly is gratitude? Gratitude has been depicted as an emotion, a mood, a moral virtue, a habit, a motive, a personality trait, a coping response, and a way of life. The *Oxford English Dictionary* (1989) defines gratitude as "the quality or condition of being thankful; the appreciation of an inclination to return kindness" (p. 1135). The word *gratitude* is derived from the Latin *gratia*, meaning favor, and *gratus*, meaning pleasing. All derivatives from this Latin root "have to do with kindness, generousness, gifts, the beauty of giving and receiving, or getting something for nothing" (Pruyser, 1976, p. 69). We are all familiar with the feeling of gratitude—we receive a gift, and we are thankful to the person who has provided this kindness to us. We recognize that the person need not have made this gesture, but did so out of goodwill toward us.

In psychological parlance, gratitude is the positive recognition of benefits received. Gratitude has been defined as "an estimate of gain coupled with the judgment that someone else is responsible for that gain" (Solomon, 1977, p. 316). Gratitude has been said to represent "an attitude toward the giver, and an attitude toward the gift, a determination to use it well, to employ it imaginatively and inventively in accordance with the giver's intention" (Harned, 1997, p. 175). Gratitude is an emotion, the core of which is pleasant feelings about the benefit received. At the cornerstone of gratitude is the notion of *undeserved merit*. The grateful person recognizes that he or she did nothing to deserve the gift or benefit; it was freely bestowed. This core feature is reflected in one definition of gratitude as "the willingness to recognize the unearned increments of value in one's experience" (Bertocci & Millard, 1963, p. 389). The benefit, gift, or personal gain might be material or nonmaterial (e.g., emotional or spiritual). The object of gratitude is other-directed—persons as well as nonhuman intentional agents (God, animals, the cosmos; Solomon, 1977). Importantly, gratitude has a positive valence: It feels good. Solomon (1977) described it as "intrinsically self-esteeming" (p. 317).

Although a variety of life experiences can elicit feelings of gratitude, prototypically gratitude stems from the perception of a positive personal outcome, not necessarily deserved or earned, that is due to the actions of another person. Fitzgerald (1998) identified three components of gratitude: (1) a warm sense of appreciation for somebody or something, (2) a sense of goodwill toward that person or thing, and (3) a disposition to act that flows from appreciation and goodwill. Bertocci and Millard (1963) noted that the virtue of gratitude is the *willingness to recognize* that one has been the beneficiary of someone's kindness, whether the emotional response is present or not. They thus conceive of it as a "moral virtue-trait" (p. 388) that leads a person to seek situations in which to express this appreciation and thankfulness. Social psychologist Fritz Heider (1958) argued that people feel grateful when they have received a benefit from someone who (the beneficiary believes) *intended* to benefit them. Heider posited that the perceived intentionality of the benefit was the most important factor in determining whether someone felt grateful after receiving a benefit. Heider also predicted that situations in which a benefactor calls on the beneficiary's *duty* to be grateful would produce the opposite effect. Moreover, Heider noted that beneficiaries prefer to have their gratitude attributed to internal motivations rather than extrinsic ones (e.g., duty or social norm).

Gratitude from an Evolutionary Perspective

Like other emotions, gratitude can be analyzed at many levels. For example, from a biocultural or evolutionary perspective that emphasizes social-functional accounts of emotion (Keltner, 2003), gratitude helps individuals form and maintain relationships, and relationships are essential to the survival and well-being of individuals, groups, and societies. A biocultural approach to gratitude suggests that it, like other social emotions, evolved to solve certain recurring problems in the human social landscape.

Specifically, the emotion of gratitude has been hypothesized to have developed in order to solve problems of group governance. Sociologist Georg Simmel (1950) argued that gratitude was a cognitive–emotional supplement serving to sustain reciprocal obligations. Because formal social structures such as the law and social contracts are insufficient to regulate and ensure reciprocity in human interaction, people are socialized to have gratitude, which then serves to remind them of their need to reciprocate. Thus, during exchange of benefits, gratitude prompts one person (a beneficiary) to be bound to another (a benefactor) during exchange of benefits, thereby reminding beneficiaries of their reciprocity obligations. He referred to gratitude as "the moral memory of mankind. . . . If every grateful action . . . were suddenly eliminated, society (at least as we know it) would break apart" (1950, p. 388).

Gratitude also provides an emotional basis for reciprocal altruism. In his seminal article, Robert Trivers (1971) speculated on the evolutionary functions of gratitude. Trivers viewed gratitude as an evolutionary adaptation that regulates people's responses to altruistic acts. Gratitude for altruistic acts is a reward for adherence to the universal norm of reciprocity and is a mediating mechanism that links the receipt of a favor to the giving of a return favor. The effect of this emotion is to create a desire to reciprocate. From this perspective, gratitude serves as a mental mechanism that calibrates the extent of debt owed—the larger the debt, the larger the sense of gratitude. Recent research indicates that gratitude may be a psychological mechanism underlying reciprocal exchange in human and nonhuman primates (Bonnie & de Waal, 2004). I and my colleagues synthesized historical perspectives and recent research on gratitude in our theory of gratitude as a moral affect—that is, one with moral precursors and consequences (McCullough, Kilpatrick, Emmons, & Larsen, 2001). By experiencing gratitude, a person is motivated to carry out prosocial behavior, energized to sustain moral behaviors, and is inhibited from committing destructive interpersonal behaviors. Because of its specialized functions in the moral domain, we likened gratitude to empathy, sympathy, guilt, and shame. Whereas empathy and sympathy operate when people have the opportunity to respond to the plight of another person, and guilt and shame operate when people have failed to meet moral standards or obligations, gratitude operates typically when people acknowledge that they are the recipients of prosocial behavior. Specifically, we posited that gratitude serves as a *moral barometer*, providing individuals with an affective readout that accompanies the perception that another person has treated them kindly or prosocially. Second, we posited that gratitude serves as a *moral motive*, stimulating people to behave prosocially after they have been the beneficiaries of other people's prosocial behavior. Recent empirical evidence does indeed suggest that gratitude can shape costly prosocial behavior (Bartlett & DeSteno, 2006). Third, we posited that gratitude serves as a *moral reinforcer*, encouraging prosocial behavior by reinforcing people for their previous prosocial behavior.

We (McCullough et al., 2001) argued that gratitude is a human strength in that it enhances one's personal and relational well-being and is quite possibly beneficial for society as a whole. Results on the correlates of dispositional gratitude appear to bear out this viewpoint. As a disposition, gratitude is a generalized tendency to recognize and respond with positive emotions (appreciation, thankfulness) to the role of other persons' (moral agents') kindliness and benevolence in the positive experiences and outcomes that one obtains. Recent research measuring both individual differences in gratitude and the experimental cultivation of gratitude through interventions suggests that gratitude is a typically pleasant experience that is linked to emotional, physical, and relational well-being.

Gratitude as an Affective Trait

Researchers have recently begun to investigate the disposition to experience gratitude. Invoking Rosenberg's (1998) multilevel analysis of affect, we (McCullough et al., 2002) defined the disposition to experience gratitude as "a generalized tendency to recognize and respond with grateful emotion to the roles of other people's benevolence in the positive experiences and outcomes that one obtains" (p. 112). We also derived four different facets or qualities of emotional experiences that could distinguish dispositionally grateful people from less dispositionally grateful people. Compared to less grateful individuals, highly grateful individuals may feel gratitude more *intensely* for a positive event, more *frequently* or more easily throughout the day; they may have a wider *span* of benefits or life circumstances for which they are grateful at any given time (e.g., for their families, their jobs, friends, health), and they may experience gratitude with greater *density* for any given benefit (i.e., toward a more people).

In four studies, we (McCullough et al., 2002) broadly examined the correlates of the disposition toward gratitude. We developed the GQ-6 (a six-item self-report measure of the grateful disposition), showed that the GQ-6 converged with observer ratings, and found that the grateful disposition was positively associated with positive affect, well-being, prosocial behaviors/traits, and religiousness/spirituality. We also found that the grateful disposition was negatively associated with envy and materialistic attitudes. We replicated these findings in a large nonstudent sample and showed that these associations persisted even after controlling for social desirability (Paulhus, 1998). Among the Big Five dimensions of personality (John, Donahue, & Kentle, 1991), the disposition to experience gratitude was correlated with Extraversion/positive affectivity, Neuroticism/negative affectivity, and Agreeableness. Moreover, the same associations were obtained using both self-report and peer-report methods.

Specifically, we (McCullough et al., 2002) found that highly grateful people, compared to their less grateful counterparts, tend to experience positive emotions more often, enjoy greater satisfaction with life and more hope (rs ranged from .30 to .49, $ps < .01$), and also tend to experience less depression, anxiety, and envy (with most rs ranging from .18 to .39, $ps < .01$). Highly grateful individuals also tend to score higher than do their less grateful counterparts on measures of prosociality. They tend to be more empathic, forgiving, helpful, and supportive as well as less focused on materialistic pursuits, than are their less grateful counterparts (with most rs ranging from .17 to .36, $ps < .01$). Finally, people who are more strongly disposed to experience gratitude tend to be more religiously and spiritually oriented than people lower in gratitude. That is, they tend to score higher on measures of traditional religiousness (e.g., church attendance, prayer) and nonsectarian measures that assess spiritual experiences/sensibilities (e.g., sense of contact with a divine power, belief that all living things are interconnected).

More recently, researchers seeking to develop another measure of dispositional gratitude have drawn similar conclusions. Watkins, Woodward, Stone, and Kolts (2003) devised the Gratitude, Resentment, and Appreciation Test (GRAT), a self-report measure that conceptualizes dispositional gratitude as a combination of four characteristics: acknowledgment of the importance of expressing and experiencing gratitude, lack of resentment with respect to benefits received (i.e., feeling a sense of abundance rather than deprivation), appreciation for the contributions of others toward benefits received, and appreciation for "simple pleasures" (e.g., sunsets and seasons, which happen frequently) rather than extravagant pleasures (e.g., vacations and cars, which are likely to happen infrequently). They found evidence of construct validity for their dispositional measure of gratitude and various correlations that help illuminate its relationship to positive and negative affective states. Across three different undergraduate student samples, scores on the GRAT were positively related to satisfaction with life (as measured by the Satisfaction with Life Scale; Diener, Emmons, Larson, & Griffin, 1985; rs ranged from .49 to .62, $ps < .0001$) and negatively related to depression (as measured by the Beck Depression Inventory; Beck, 1972; rs ranged from −.34 to −.56, $ps < .01$).

Interventions to Promote Gratitude

Researchers have suspected for some time that the ability to notice and appreciate the good elements in one's life can improve well-being (Bryant, 1989; Janoff-Bulman & Berger, 2000; Langston, 1994), and many religious and self-help groups have adopted activities wherein its members reflect on the gifts for which they are grateful in their lives (e.g., the retreats of various church groups and Alcoholics Anonymous). The belief implicit in these self-help efforts is that the regular practice of grateful thinking should lead to enhanced psychological and social functioning. However, the only way to evaluate unambiguously whether such activity actually causes increases in well-being is to conduct experiments in which gratitude is manipulated and its effects are observed.

I and my colleague recently conducted three experiments investigating the effects of gratitude interventions on psychological and physical well-being (Emmons & McCullough, 2003). In Study 1, students were randomly assigned to one of three conditions. Participants either briefly described (e.g., in a single sentence) five things for which they were grateful in the past week (gratitude condition), five daily hassles from the previous week (hassles condition), or five events or circumstances that affected them in the last week (events condition). Participants completed these exercises along with a variety of other measures once per week for 10 consecutive weeks. A wide range of experiences sparked gratitude: cherished interactions, awareness of physical health, overcoming obstacles, and simply being alive, to name a few. Participants in the gratitude condition reported being more grateful than those in the hassles condition; thus the induction successfully impacted grateful affect. More importantly, participants in the grateful condition felt better about their lives as a whole and were more optimistic about the future than participants in either of the other comparison conditions. In addition, those in the grateful condition reported fewer health complaints and even said that they spent more time exercising than control participants did. Thus, a simple weekly intervention showed significant emotional and health benefits.

In Study 2 we (Emmons & McCullough, 2003) increased the gratitude intervention to a daily practice over a 2-week period. As in Study 1, participants were randomly assigned to one of three conditions. The gratitude and hassles conditions were identical to Study 1, but the events condition was changed to a downward social comparison manipulation. In this condition, participants were encouraged to think about ways in which they were better off than others. They added this condition to control for possible demand characteristics. This comparison condition may have inadvertently produced some grateful affect, but even so, the gratitude condition showed an impressive array of benefits. Although the health benefits from Study 1 were not evident in this study (perhaps because of the short duration of the intervention), participants in the grateful condition felt more joyful, enthusiastic, interested, attentive, energetic, excited, determined, and strong than those in the hassles condition. They also reported having offered others more emotional support or help with a personal problem, indicating that the gratitude induction increased prosocial motivation—and more directly supporting the notion of gratitude as a moral motivator (McCullough et al., 2001). Again, the gratitude manipulation showed a significant effect on positive affect as compared to the hassles condition, but no reliable impact on negative affectivity. In addition, there was some evidence that this daily intervention led to greater increases in gratitude than did the weekly practice that we examined in their first study.

In a third study we (Emmons & McCullough, 2003) replicated these effects in adults with neuromuscular diseases. Participants were randomly assigned to a gratitude condition or to a "true control condition" in which they simply completed "daily experience rating forms." Similar to the previous studies, participants in the gratitude group showed significantly more positive affect and satisfaction with life, but in addition they also showed less negative affect than the control group. Not only did the self-reports of participants in the gratitude condition indicate increased positive affect and life satisfaction, but so did the reports of significant others: Spouses of participants in the gratitude condition reported that the participants had appeared to have higher subjective well-being than did the spouses of participants in the control condition. These studies support the contention that gratitude has a causative influence on subjective well-being, opening the door for intervention possibilities with a variety of populations.

To investigate which methods of *expressing* gratitude could enhance positive affect, Watkins et al. (2003) conducted an experiment in which gratitude was manipulated in different ways (i.e., participants were instructed to think about someone to whom they were grateful, write an essay about someone to whom they were grateful, or write a letter to someone to whom they were grateful, which would allegedly be sent to that person). They had participants in the control condition write descriptively about their living rooms. They also measured positive and negative affect before and after the manipulation (using the Positive and Negative Affect Schedule; Watson, Clark, & Tellegen, 1988).

The gratitude conditions led to increases in positive affect, whereas the control condition did not. The grateful thinking condition, in particular, showed the strongest effect, perhaps because the act itself of writing an essay or a letter of gratitude on demand may have disrupted the experience of positive affect or caused some anxiety. These findings imply that in developing gratitude interventions, researchers and clinicians should consider their targets, the amount of time available for the intervention, and the kind of intervention that is most appropriate, given the circumstances. Watkins and his colleagues also found that gratitude was negatively related to depression in clinical samples (Watkins et al., 2004).

Gratitude and Sustainable Happiness

From the results of our experiments we know that gratitude has at least a temporary power to improve emotional health, relationship satisfaction, and in some regards, physical well-being. But do any of these improvements survive the test of time? Strikingly, many of our participants with neuromuscular disease continued to keep gratitude journals long after the study ended, and when we contacted them, months later, they commented on the long-term benefits of being in the study. One individual told us that "being forced, consciously, to reflect, contemplate and sum up my life on a daily basis was curiously therapeutic and enlightening. I was reminded of facets of myself that I very much like and others that could use improvement. . . . I have tried to become more aware of my level of gratitude." Another wrote: "I don't believe participating in the study changed my level of gratitude, but it made me more aware of it—I have always tried to live my life in a positive, upbeat manner. I believe my faith has helped me accomplish this."

When the well-being of participants in the gratitude group was compared to the control group, a strong and consistent pattern appeared: The gratitude group was still enjoying benefits *6 months later*. They were experiencing more positive emotions, were more satisfied with their lives, felt better about their lives as whole, and continued to feel more connected to others. The evidence contradicts the widely held view that all people have a "setpoint" of happiness that cannot be reset by any known means: in some cases, people have reported that gratitude led to transformative life changes.

In a 6-week intervention, University of California, Riverside students were instructed to contemplate "the things for which they are grateful" either once a week or three times a week (Sheldon & Lyubomirsky, 2006). They were told to make an effort to

> think about the many things in your life, both large and small, that you have to be grateful about. These might include particular supportive relationships, sacrifices or contributions that others have made for you, facts about your life such as your advantages and opportunities, or even gratitude for life itself, and the world that we live in. . . . You may not have thought about yourself in this way before, but research suggests that doing so can have a strong positive effect on your mood and life satisfaction. So, we'd like to ask you to continue thinking in this way over the next few weeks.

Examples of "blessings" listed by students included "a healthy body," "my mom," and "AOL instant messenger." Control participants only completed the happiness assessments. The results again suggested that short-term increases in happiness are possible but that optimal timing is important. Students who regularly expressed gratitude showed increases in well-being over the course of the study, relative to controls, but those increases were observed only for those students who performed the activity only once a week. Perhaps counting one's blessings several times a week led people to become bored with the practice, finding it less fresh and meaningful over time.

The benefits of gratitude were further confirmed in a recent study that compared the efficacy of five different interventions that were hypothesized to increase personal happiness and decrease personal depression (Seligman, Steen, Park, & Peterson, 2005). In a random assignment, placebo-controlled Internet study, a gratitude intervention (writing and delivering a letter of thankfulness to someone who had been especially helpful but had never been properly thanked) was found to significantly increase happiness and decrease depression for up to 1 month following the visit. Results indicated that "participants in the gratitude visitation condition showed the largest positive changes in the whole study" (Seligman et al., p. 417). Thus, the benefits of gratitude do not appear to be limited to the self-guided journal keeping methodology utilized by me and my colleague (Emmons & McCullough, 2003).

Gratitude Interventions with Children

We have conducted our gratitude research with people across the lifespan, from college age to late adulthood. Are there any groups that might be especially "gratitude challenged"? Consider children. Children are notoriously ungrateful. "Ingratitude! thou marble-hearted fiend, more hideous when thou show'st thee in a child than the sea-monster!," opined Shakespeare's *King Lear*. Envy and entitlement seem much easier developmental achievements than do gratitude and thankfulness. Research has shown that because of the perspective taking that gratitude requires, children younger than the age of 7 do not reliably understand that gratitude requires giving credit to others for positive outcomes that happen to the self.

Yet much like gratitude's happiness-instilling qualities, these assumptions regarding children's presumed inability to feel gratitude have never been put to the experimental test. One recent study (Gordon, Mushner-Eizenman, Holub, & Dalrymple, 2004) examined archival (newspaper) accounts of what school-age children said they were thankful for in the aftermath of 9/11. The most common themes mentioned were family, friends, police, firefighters, other helpers, and freedom. Girls were generally more thankful than boys, and were more thankful for family and friends, whereas boys were more grateful for material objects. One girl, age 9, wrote:

> I am thankful for my mom and dad because they help me with my homework. I am thankful for myself because my hamster got his eye scratched by my cat and I took a damp rag and washed his eye that was bleeding. I am thankful for my grandma and grandpa because they give me money to get me a Christmas gift. I am thankful for my clothes because I would around tan naked [sic]. I am thankful for my cat because my cat eats mice from the field. I am thankful for miss long [sic] because she helps kids on math and other stuff. I am thankful for my hamster because he helps me know when I have homework.

The study did not examine the link between gratitude and outcomes such as happiness, well-being, or coping, however. It remains to be seen whether counting blessings impacts on children's well-being in a manner similar to adults.

With this focus in mind, I and my colleague (Froh, Sefick, & Emmons, in press) conducted a gratitude intervention with 221 students in grades 6 and 7. A quasi-experimental design was followed in which 11 classes were randomly assigned to one of three conditions (i.e., gratitude, hassles, and control). Students in the gratitude condition were asked to list up to five things for which they were grateful since yesterday, and the hassles group was asked to do the same, though focusing on irritants. The control group just completed the measures. Aside from the counting of blessings or burdens, all students completed the same measures. Data were collected daily for 2 weeks during class instruction time, with a 3-week follow-up.

Caring/supportive relationships were the most common theme for the gratitude group. Moreover, it was also very common for kids to report being grateful for their education, health, and activities (e.g., primarily sports). Participants in both the gratitude and control condition experienced significantly less negative affect compared to those in the hassles condition at both post and follow-up. Moreover, those in the gratitude condition were significantly more optimistic about their upcoming week at follow-up compared to those in the hassles group. Within the school experience domain, the gratitude condition elicited greater satisfaction from participants than from those in the hassles and control conditions at post. Concerning residency and life overall, participants in the gratitude and control conditions were significantly more satisfied when compared to those in the hassles group at follow-up. A significant main effect for conditions related to physical symptoms approached statistical significance, with those in the gratitude group reporting being less bothered by physical problems. Lastly, the gratitude and control groups felt more grateful toward others from whom they received assistance compared to the hassles group at follow-up. This finding suggests that gratitude makes us more sensitive to perceiving kindnesses from others. Gratitude thus seemed to have a gradual yet significant effect on both the experiences of optimism and grateful feelings toward receiving aid. Even more encouraging is that the results of this study suggest that there may be better and longer-lasting ways of instilling gratitude in children than requiring the obligatory thank-you note to relatives.

Why Is Gratitude Good?: Exploring Mechanisms

The research literature to date indicates that gratitude, measured either dispositionally or activated by specific tasks, is linked to improved well-being and general positive functioning. How does one account for the psychological, emotional, and physical benefits of gratitude? A number of mechanisms has been suggested to account for the psychological benefits of grateful thinking (Watkins, 2004). Expressing gratitude for life's blessings—that is, a sense of wonder, thankfulness, and appreciation—is likely to elevate felt happiness for a number of reasons. Grateful thinking fosters the savoring of positive life experiences and situations, whereby people extract the maximum possible satisfaction and enjoyment from their circumstances. Counting one's blessings may directly counteract the effects of hedonic adaptation—the process by which our happiness level returns, again and again, to its set range—by preventing people from taking the good things in their lives for granted. If we consciously remind ourselves of our blessings, it should become harder to take them for granted and adapt to them. And the very act of viewing good things as gifts itself is likely to be beneficial for mood. Three mechanisms seem especially likely to account for the beneficial effects of grateful thinking: (1) gratitude strengthens social relationships; (2) gratitude counters negative states, especially depressive affect, and (3) gratitude is a resiliency factor in times of stress.

Gratitude Strengthens Social Ties

An unexpected benefit from gratitude journaling—one that I did not predict in advance—was that people who kept gratitude journals reported feeling closer and more connected to others, were more likely to help others, and were actually seen as more helpful by significant others in their social networks. The family, friends, partners, and others that surround them consistently reported that those who practiced gratitude seemed measurably happier and were more pleasant to be around. We also have evidence that people who are high on dispositional gratitude—the chronic tendency to be aware of blessings in life—have better relationships, are more likely to protect and preserve these relationships, are more securely attached, and are less lonely. According to the broaden-and-build model of positive emotions (Fredrickson, 2001; see also Chapter 23, this volume), gratitude is effective in increasing well-being because it builds psychological, social, and spiritual resources. Gratitude inspires prosocial reciprocity and, indeed, is one of the primary psychological mechanisms thought to underly reciprocal altruism (Trivers, 1971). Moreover, encouraging people to focus on the benefits they have received from others leads them to feel loved and cared for by others. So gratitude appears to build friendships and other social bonds. These are social resources because, in times of need, these social bonds are wellsprings to be tapped for the provision of social support.

Gratitude Counters Depressive Affect

In several studies depression has been shown to be strongly inversely related to gratitude (see Watkins, 2004, for a review). In one study that employed a structured clinical interview to assess depression, clinically depressed individuals showed significantly lower gratitude (nearly 50% less gratitude) than did non-depressed controls (Watkins, Grimm, & Kolts, 2004). How might gratitude prevent depression? If gratitude provides more focus on, and enjoyment of, benefits, then such a perspective would seem to expel depression. Gratitude should decrease the likelihood of depression to the extent individuals feeling it direct their attention to the blessings they *have* and away from things they *lack*. In providing for increased access to positive memories, gratitude could help build more positive cognitions. Although depression treatment approaches have historically emphasized correcting negative thoughts, recently some have encouraged more emphasis on building positive thoughts. A practice of gratitude could help develop a more positive way of thinking about life events and so assist in the prevention of depression. Various depression researchers have proposed that the lack of social rewards (and/or increased social punishment) is important in the etiology and maintenance of depression. If a grateful disposition actually provides for a more enjoyable social life, then it should also help to contravene depression. In one of our studies, participants were asked to recall positive and negative events from their past for 3 minutes each. A positive memory bias measure was calculated by subtracting the number of negative events from the number of positive events recalled. This number constituted the intentional recall variable. As expected, grateful individuals were more likely to have a positive memory bias. After controlling for depression, the GRAT still reliably predicted positive memory bias (Watkins, 2004). Gratitude enhances the retrievability of positive experiences by increasing the elaboration of positive information. Elaborating the event at encoding increases the retrievability of the event in our memory store. So, grateful individuals should be more likely to recall past benefits from their life and experience gratitude in response to these blessings. In other words, grateful individuals should be more likely to "count their blessings" spontaneously, not just when they are instructed to do so in a psychological experiment. People who are grateful do tend to show a *positive recall bias* (conjuring up many more pleasant memories than unpleasant ones) when asked about past life events, just as depressed individuals show a *negative recall bias* when asked to recall past events (recalling many more unpleasant than pleasant events).

Gratitude as Resiliency

In addition to the positive benefits that can accrue from the conscious practice of gratitude, additional studies have shown that gratitude can buffer a person from debilitating emotions and pathological psychological conditions. Fredrickson, Tugade, Waugh, and Larkin (2003) examined the frequency of positive and negative emotions before and after the tragic events of 9/11. Out of 20 emotions, gratitude was the second most commonly experienced (only compassion was rated more highly). They found that positive emotions were critical characteristics that actively helped resilient people to cope with the 9/11 disaster, suggesting another potential role that gratitude can play in interventions. Indeed, a whole line of research shows that benefit finding can help people cope with disasters, deadly diseases, and bereavement (Nolen-Hoeksema & Davis, 2002; Tennen & Affleck, 2002). McAdams's et al. (McAdams, Reynold, Lewis, Patten, & Bowman, 2001) analyses of redemption sequences revealed that even painful experiences could become something for which people are grateful ultimately.

Gratitude may also offer protection against psychiatric disorders. A factor-analytically derived measure of thankfulness (which included items explicitly related to gratitude, along with others that seemed to have more in common with love and acceptance) was associated with reduced risk for both internalizing (e.g., depression, anxiety) and externalizing (e.g., substance abuse) disorders in a study involving 2,616 male and female twins (Kendler, Liu, Gardner, McCullough, Larson, & Prescott, 2003).

Gratitude, Positive Emotions, and the Brain

Given the centrality of gratitude to subjective well-being and to prosocial and moral behavior, it is worth attempting to construct a tentative cognitive–affective neuroscience of gratitude. Affective neuroscience is far broader than the field of emotion because it examines the behavioral, social, and neural components of emotional processes (Schmidt, 2003).

Why bother with neural processes involved in gratitude? Well, for one reason, modeling and examining the brain correlates of a complex emotion such as gratitude, though fraught with difficulties, may help us to decide between competing accounts of the nature and functions of gratitude. In addition, it may provide clues as to how gratitude and other positive emotions can influence health, thus enhancing clinical attempts to elicit the emotion.

If, for example, investigation led us to assign gratitude to neural networks handling motivational states rather than to networks supporting consummatory pleasure or reward states, then it would be reasonable to conclude that the neurological data are more consistent with functional treatments of gratitude as promoting "reciprocity" for favors received and "moral behavior" for social debts incurred, than with nonfunctional accounts of gratitude as simply a read-out mechanism informing us that we have received an unmerited benefit. Obviously our neurological investigations could lead us to believe that gratitude involves both a pleasurable emotion and a motivational state. In this case the neurological data help us to place the psychological accounts of gratitude into a process framework, thus allowing the investigator to place further constraints on the object of his or her investigation. Measurement instruments would then need to address both the state–emotion aspects of gratitude as well as its motivational effects.

It seems likely that a process account of gratitude would involve an initial experience of relatively intense positive affect, such as joy, appreciation, or happiness, for some significant benefit received, with the intensity of this positive emotion and its concomitant motivational effects likely decreasing over time. After the initial benefit is received from a benefactor, the recipient would experience a sense of appreciation or even joy depending on the size of the gift. Arriving at a given level of intensity of gratitude (and presumably a related motivational state) would require the calculation of degree of benefit received along with anticipated costs of reciprocating. In addition, both the felt emotion and the accompanying motivational state would require a certain amount of memory of the favor received and the benefactor. In short, a process account of gratitude would involve a recipient of a benefit (1) recognizing that a gift has been received, (2) calculating costs–benefits associated with the gift, (3) experiencing an emotion that begins in appreciation and emerges into gratitude, (4) with memory of the benefit and benefactor as well as the emotion of gratitude initiating and sustaining a motivational state to reciprocate the benefit received. All four of these steps can be handled by limbic–frontal interactions (Damasio, 2003), which have been shown to support (1) assigning significance levels to events and stimuli in the individuals' environment/experience (Rolls, 2004; Schultz et al., 1995); (2) assessing probabilities and costs of current decisions and events (Adolphs, Tranel, & Denburg, 2000; Barkley, 1997); (3) supporting positive emotionality as well as motivational and approach tendencies (Berridge, 1999; Davidson, Lewis, Alloy, Amoral, Bush, & Cohen, 2002); and (4) supporting autobiographical memory retrieval as well as memory of recent social interactions (Craik, Naveh-Benjamin, Ishaik, & Anderson, 2000; Wheeler et al., 2000). The neurological data therefore support the process approach to the emergence of gratitude, and the process approach, in turn, is consistent with standard direct and indirect reciprocity accounts of the functions of gratitude. As discussed above, in the standard reciprocity account of gratitude, its function is to support human cooperation by facilitating "giving back" to a benefactor.

From the above analysis it follows that the human brain likely contains neural networks that are efficient at both detecting and displaying telltale signs of gratitude. The cues are likely to include facial expressions and vocal and behavioral displays. Thus, from the point of view of costly signaling theory, the neurology of gratitude would need to include (1) the fusiform face-processing areas near the temporal–occipital junctions, (2) the amygdala and limbic emotional processing systems that support emotional states, and (3) interactions between these two subcortical centers with the prefrontal regions that control executive and evaluative processes. Like the other social emotions, gratitude likely relies on limbic–prefrontal networks to mediate its positive effects on the individual (Blakemore, Winston, & Frith, 2004).

To test the general conclusion that gratitude differentially relies on limbic–prefrontal networks, I and a colleague (Emmons & McNamara, 2006) conducted a pilot investigation with individuals who evidence clinically significant prefrontal dysfunction—namely, individuals with midstage Parkinson disease (PD; Starkstein & Merello, 2002). If the emotion of gratitude depends on prefrontal networks then measures of gratitude should correlate with measures of prefrontal function. In addition, individuals with prefrontal dysfunction should not display the normal benefit in mood that occurs when an individual conjures up a memory of an experience that induced gratitude (Emmons & McCullough, 2003). Normally if you ask people to remember a time when they felt grateful for something that someone did for them, or for something that happened to them, their mood slightly changes into a more positive, happy one. If, however, gratitude and its beneficial effects depend critically on prefrontal networks, then we would expect no such mood improvement in persons with prefrontal dysfunction when they are asked to recall an experience involving gratitude. That is indeed what we found when testing patients with PD. We compared a group of midstage patients with PD ($n = 22$) to age-matched healthy controls ($n = 18$) on the mood induction procedure (described in Emmons & McCullough, 2003). In this procedure the subject is asked to use both an explicit self-report and an implicit unconscious report of his or her mood before and after recalling either a gratitude memory or a "control" positive memory. Whereas neither group reported a mood change when recalling a positive memory, there was a slight improvement in mood in the healthy controls after recalling a gratitude memory, but no such improvement in mood for the patients with PD. The postinduction mood scores for healthy controls, furthermore, were correlated with several measures of prefrontal function, whereas no such correlations were obtained (between postinduction mood scores and prefrontal performance) for patients with PD. In addition, though the overall score on the GQ-6 questionnaire showed no difference between the PD versus control groups (mean gratitude level out of 42 total = 36.0 [4.40] for controls and 34.8 [4.2] for patients with PD; $t < 1$, $p = .35$), it was nonetheless significantly correlated with several measures of prefrontal performance in the healthy controls but not in the patients with PD. Finally, we also found significant group differences in the latency to retrieval of a gratitude memory as well as the mean length (in number of words) of gratitude memories, with patients who had PD taking longer to retrieve memories (16.16 sec. vs. 23.45 sec.) that were also significantly wordier or more verbose than those of control subjects (100.13 words vs. 65.94 words). The latter finding was to be expected, given that a classic symptom of PD is a deficit in speech monitoring. These data merely scratch the surface of what might be accomplished by examining neurological correlates of a moral emotion such as gratitude. Further neurobiological research can lead to greater understanding of gratitude's role in promoting subjective well-being.

Cultivating Gratitude

The extant research has demonstrated that gratitude is positively related to such critical outcomes as life satisfaction, vitality, happiness, self-esteem, optimism, hope, empathy, and the willingness to provide emotional and tangible support for other people, while being negatively related to anxiety, depression, envy, materialism, and loneliness. Collectively, such studies present credible evidence that feeling grateful generates a ripple effect through every area of our lives, potentially satisfying some of our deepest yearnings—our desire for happiness, our pursuit of better relationships, and our ceaseless quest for inner peace, wholeness, and contentment.

Just because gratitude is good doesn't mean that it comes easy or naturally to most people. As a short-term fleeting emotion, the feeling of gratitude cannot be achieved through willpower alone. You can't *try* to feel grateful through sheer will any more than you can try to feel happy and successful. Although gratitude is pleasant, it is not easy. We have to work at it. It must be consciously cultivated. Albert Einstein admitted that he needed to remind himself a hundred times a day that his inner and outer life depend on the labors of other men, living and dead, and that "I must exert myself in order to give in the measure as I have received and I am still receiving." A number of personal burdens and external obstacles block grateful thoughts. A number of attitudes are incompatible with a grateful outlook on life, including perceptions of victimhood, an inability to admit one's shortcomings, a sense of entitlement, and an inability to admit that one is not self-sufficient. In a culture that celebrates self-aggrandizement and perceptions of deservingness, gratitude can be crowded out.

The benefits of gratitude come from the long-term cultivation of the disposition of gratefulness through dedicated practice. The disposition to experience gratitude, or gratefulness, is the tendency to feel gratitude frequently, in appropriate ways, in appropriate circumstances. A person with the disposition to feel grateful has established a worldview that says, in effect, that all of life is a gift, gratuitously given. Although we cannot, in any direct way, be grateful, we can cultivate gratefulness by structuring our lives, our minds, and our words in such a way as to facilitate awareness of gratitude-inducing experiences and labeling them as such. Some concrete practices include keeping a gratitude journal, using visual cues to remind oneself of one's blessings or gifts in life, and making a conscious vow to practice gratitude.

There is some research showing that swearing a vow to perform a behavior actually does increase the likelihood that the action will be executed. In one such study, members of a local YMCA who decided to participate in the 12-week "Personal Fitness Program" agreed to "exercise three days per week for 12 weeks and beyond at the Y." Once making the decision to participate, the experimental group was sworn to perform the promised behavior. A second group signed a written commitment to perform the promised behavior, and a third, control group, did not make any form of commitment. The impact of the manipulation was examined for its effect on adherence to the program. Subjects in the vow condition did demonstrate greater adherence than the other conditions, as measured by consecutive weeks of three exercise sessions without relapse (Dean, 2002). What might a vow to practice gratitude look like? It need not be elaborate. It could be something as simple as

> "I vow to not take so many things in my life for granted. I vow to pause and count my blessings at least once each day. I vow to express gratitude to someone that has been influential in my life whom I've never properly thanked."

If your vow is formalized, post it somewhere conspicuous where you will be reminded of it frequently.

German theologian Dietrich Bonhoeffer wrote that "In ordinary life we hardly realize that we receive a great deal more than we give, and that it is only with gratitude that life becomes rich" (Bonhoeffer, 1967, p. 370). Psychologists who have aligned themselves with positive psychology are quite interested in those psychological propensities that lead to a rich life, and modern research is ratifying the ancient wisdom that counting blessings is a royal road leading to the riches of happiness.

Acknowledgment

Preparation of this chapter was supported by a generous grant from the John Templeton Foundation.

References

Adolphs, R., Tranel, D., & Denburg, N. (2000). Impaired emotional declarative memory following unilateral amygdala damage. *Learning and Memory, 7*, 180–186.

Barkley, R. A. (1997). Behavioral inhibition, sustained attention, and executive functions: Constructing a unifying theory of ADHD. *Psychological Bulletin, 121*(1), 65–94.

Bartlett, M. Y., & DeSteno, D. (2006). Gratitude and prosocial behavior: Helping when it costs you. *Psychological Science, 17*, 319–325.

Beck, A. T. (1972). *Depression: Causes and treatment.* Philadelphia: University of Pennsylvania Press.

Berridge, K. C. (1999). Pleasure, pain, desire, and dread: Hidden core processes of emotion. In D. Kahneman, E. Diener, & N. Schwarz (Eds.), *Well-being: The foundations of hedonic psychology* (pp. 525–557). New York: Sage.

Bertocci, P. A., & Millard, R. M. (1963). *Personality and the good: Psychological and ethical perspectives.* New York: McKay.

Blakemore, S. J., Winston, J., & Frith, U. (2004). Social cognitive neuroscience: Where are we heading? *Trends in the Cognitive Sciences, 8*(5), 216–222.

Bonhoeffer, D. (1967). *Letters and papers from prison* (E. Bethge, Ed.). New York: Macmillan.

Bonnie, K., & de Waal, F. (2004). Primate social reciprocity and the origin of gratitude. In R. A. Emmons & M. E. McCullough (Eds.), *The psychology of gratitude* (pp. 213–229). New York: Oxford University Press.

Bryant, F. B. (1989). A four-factor model of perceived control: Avoiding, coping, obtaining, and savoring. *Journal of Personality, 57*, 773–797.

Chipperfield, J. G., Perry, R. P., & Weiner, B. (2003). Discrete emotions in later life. *Journal of Gerontology: Psychological Sciences, 58B*, 23–34.

Craik, F. I., Naveh-Benjamin, M., Ishaik, G., & Anderson, N. D. (2000). Divided attention during encoding and retrieval: Differential control effects? *Journal of Experimental Psychology, 26*, 1744–1749.

Damasio, A. (2003). The frontal lobes. In K. Heilman et al. (Eds.), *Clinical neuropsychology* (pp. 404–443). New York: Oxford University Press.

Davidson, R. J., Lewis, D. A., Alloy, L. B., Amoral, D. G., Bush, G., & Cohen, J. D. (2002). Neural and behavioral substrates of mood and mood regulation. *Biological Psychiatry, 52,* 478–502.

Dean, M. L. (2002). Effects of vow-making on adherence to a 12-week personal fitness program, self-efficacy, and theory of planned behavior constructs. *Dissertation Abstracts International: Section B: Sciences and Engineering, 62*(12-B), 5959.

Diener, E., Emmons, R. A., Larsen, R. J., & Griffin, S. (1985). The Satisfaction with Life Scale. *Journal of Personality Assessment, 49,* 71–75.

Emmons, R. A., & McCullough, M. E. (2003). Counting blessings versus burdens: Experimental studies of gratitude and subjective well-being in daily life. *Journal of Personality and Social Psychology, 84,* 377–389.

Emmons, R. A., & McNamara, P. (2006). Sacred emotions and affective neuroscience: Gratitude, costly signaling, and the brain. In P. McNamara (Ed.), *Where God and man meet: How the brain and evolutionary sciences are revolutionizing our understanding of religion and spirituality* (pp. 11–30). Westport, CT: Praeger.

Fitzgerald, P. (1998). Gratitude and justice. *Ethics, 109,* 119–153.

Fredrickson, B. L. (2001). The role of positive emotions in positive psychology: The broaden-and-build theory of positive emotions. *American Psychologist, 56,* 218–226.

Fredrickson, B. L., Tugade, M. M., Waugh, C. E., & Larkin, G. R. (2003). What good are positive emotions in crises?: A prospective study of resilience and emotions following the terrorist attacks on the United States on September 11th, 2001. *Journal of Personality and Social Psychology, 84,* 365–376,

Froh, J., Sefick, W., & Emmons, R. A. (in press). An experimental study of gratitude and well-being in school-aged children. *Journal of School Psychology.*

Gordon, A. K., Mushner-Eizenman, D. R., Holub, S. C., & Dalrymple, J. (2004). What are children thankful for?: An archival analysis of gratitude before and after the attacks of September 11. *Applied Developmental Psychology, 25,* 541–553.

Harned, D. B. (1997). *Patience: How we wait upon the world.* Cambridge, MA: Cowley.

Heider, F. (1958). *The psychology of interpersonal relations.* New York: Wiley.

Janoff-Bulman, R., & Berger, A. R. (2000). The other side of trauma: Towards a psychology of appreciation. In J. H. Harvey & E. D. Miller (Eds.), *Loss and trauma: General and close relationship perspectives* (pp. 29–44). Philadelphia: Brunner-Routledge.

John, O. P., Donahue, E. M., & Kentle, R. L. (1991). *The Big Five Inventory—Versions 4a and 54.* University of California, Berkeley, Institute of Personality and Social Research, Berkeley, CA.

Keltner, D. (2003). Expression and the course of life: Studies of emotion, personality, and psychopathology from a social–functional perspective. *Annals of the New York Academy of Sciences, 1000,* 222–243.

Kendler, K. S., Liu, X., Gardner, C. O., McCullough, M. E., Larson, D., & Prescott, C. A. (2003). Dimensions of religiosity and their relationship to lifetime psychiatric and substance use disorders. *American Journal of Psychiatry, 60,* 496–503.

Langston, C. A. (1994). Capitalizing on and coping with daily-life events: Expressive responses to positive events. *Journal of Personality and Social Psychology*, *67*, 1112–1125.

Lyubomirsky, S., Sheldon, K., & Schkade, D. (2005). Pursuing happiness: The architecture of sustainable change. *Review of General Psychology. Special Issue: Positive Psychology*, *9*, 111–131.

McAdams, D. P., Reynold, J., Lewis, M., Patten, A. H., & Bowman, P. J (2001). When bad things turn good and good things turn bad: Sequences of redemption and contamination in life narrative and their relation to psychosocial adaptation in midlife adults and in students. *Personality and Social Psychology Bulletin*, *27*, 474–485.

McCullough, M. E., Emmons, R. A., & Tsang, J. (2002). The grateful disposition: A conceptual and empirical topography. *Journal of Personality and Social Psychology*, *82*, 112–127.

McCullough, M. E., Kilpatrick, S., Emmons, R. A., & Larson, D. (2001). Gratitude as moral affect. *Psychological Bulletin*, *127*, 249–266.

Nolen-Hoeksema, S., & Davis, C. G. (2002). Positive responses to loss: Perceiving benefits and growth. In C. R. Snyder & S. J. Lopez (Eds.), *Handbook of positive psychology* (pp. 598–606). London: Oxford University Press.

Oxford English Dictionary. (1989). New York: Oxford University Press.

Paulhus, D. L. (1998). Interpersonal and intrapsychic adaptiveness of trait self-enhancement: A mixed blessing? *Journal of Personality and Social Psychology*, *74*, 1197–1208.

Pruyser, P. W. (1976). *The minister as diagnostician: Personal problems in pastoral perspective*. Philadelphia: Westminster Press.

Rolls, E. T. (2004). The functions of the orbitofrontal cortex. *Brain and Cognition*, *55*, 11–29.

Rosenberg, E. L. (1998). Levels of analysis and the organization of affect. *Review of General Psychology*, *2*, 247–270.

Schmidt, L. A. (2003). Special issue on affective neuroscience: Introductory remarks. *Brain and Cognition*, *52*, 3.

Schultz, W., Romo, R., Ljungberg, T., et al. (1995). Reward-related signals carried by dopamine neurons. In J. Houk, J. Davis, & D. Beiser (Eds.), *Models of information processing in the basal ganglia* (pp. 233–248). Cambridge, MA: MIT Press.

Seligman, M. E. P., Steen, T. A., Park, N., & Peterson, C. (2005). Positive psychology progress: Empirical validation of interventions. *American Psychologist*, *60*, 410–421.

Sheldon, K. M., & Lyubomirsky, S. (2006). How to increase and sustain positive emotion: The effects of expressing gratitude and visualizing best possible selves. *Journal of Positive Psychology*, *1*, 73–82.

Simmel, G. (1950). *The sociology of Georg Simmel*. Glencoe, IL: Free Press.

Solomon, R. C. (1977). *The passions*. Garden City, NY: Anchor Books.

Starkstein, S. E., & Merello, M. (2002). *Psychiatric and cognitive disorders in Parkinson's disease*. Cambridge, UK: Cambridge University Press.

Tennen, H., & Affleck, G. (2002). Benefit-finding and benefit-reminding. In C. R. Snyder & S. J. Lopez (Eds.), *Handbook of positive psychology* (pp. 584–597). New York: Oxford University Press.

Trivers, R. L. (1971). The evolution of reciprocal altruism. *Quarterly Review of Biology*, *46*, 35–57.

Watkins, P. C. (2004). Gratitude and subjective well-being. In R. A. Emmons & M. E. McCullough (Eds.), *The psychology of gratitude* (pp. 167–192). New York: Oxford University Press.

Watkins, P. C., Grimm, D. L., & Kolts, R. (2004). Counting your blessings: Positive memories among grateful persons. *Current Psychology: Developmental, Learning, Personality, Social, 23,* 52–67.

Watkins, P. C. Woodward, K., Stone, T., & Kolts, R. L. (2003). Gratitude and happiness: Development of a measure of gratitude and relationships with subjective well-being. *Social Behavior and Personality, 31,* 431–452.

Watson, D., Clark, L. A., & Tellegen, A. (1988). Development and validation of brief measures of positive and negative affect: The PANAS scales. *Journal of Personality and Social Psychology, 54,* 1063–1070.

Wheeler, M. A., Stuss, D. T., & Tulving, E. (1997). Toward a theory of episodic *memory*: The frontal lobes and autonoetic consciousness. *Psychological Bulletin, 121,* 331–354.

VI

CONCLUSIONS AND FUTURE DIRECTIONS

24

Myths in the Science of Happiness, and Directions for Future Research

ED DIENER

Since I began studying subjective well-being in 1981, the field has grown dramatically. Figure 25.1 presents the number of studies published per 5-year period, from 1961 to 2005, for "life satisfaction" and "happiness." As can be seen, the number of publications has increased from a handful to about 300 per year for each topic. Furthermore, there is an accelerating trend in the number of articles published on these topics. There are now about 2,000 publications per year on topics generally related to the subject of subjective well-being, and many more when ill-being is included. This trend is gratifying because our understanding of well-being has rapidly grown over these years. Despite the progress, in every field certain popular myths develop, and subjective well-being is no exception. These myths arose in part because nobody can master all of the studies in the field, in part because of our ideological beliefs and our desire to simplify findings for public consumption, and in part because rapid changes in our understanding of certain processes that influence well-being have recently refined earlier conclusions.

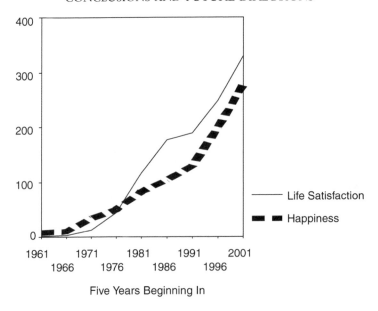

FIGURE 24.1. Growth in research on subjective well-being.

Common Myths

In this chapter I review several myths that I believe are widespread. As the science of well-being has become more popular with journalists, these myths have been promulgated to the public, and they are often readily accepted because they provide a simplified view of reality that is in accord with people's preconceptions and values. In some cases, the misunderstandings are based on early research and only recently has better evidence shown them to be myths. My purpose in reviewing these misunderstandings is not to point fingers or to blame—I have communicated these ideas too. Instead, my purpose is to describe the oversimplifications so that the field continues to develop in sophisticated and accurate directions.

Myth 1: Happiness Has an Unchanging Individual "Setpoint"

In their classic article, Brickman and Campbell (1971) suggested that we live on a hedonic treadmill in which we all strive to be happier but are doomed by adaptation to come back to hedonic neutrality. In a follow-up classic, Brickman, Coates, and Janoff-Bulman (1978) suggested that lottery winners were not happier than others and that individuals with spinal-cord injuries were not unhappier than others. Since the time of those articles, several groups have updated the original theory. The important work by the Minnesota twins research group (Tellegen et al., 1988) led to a revision in the early theory of adaptation, suggesting that people do not return to hedonic neutrality but instead return to a level of happiness set by their individual temperaments, which are largely determined by genetics (Lykken 1999). This idea, which asserted that people have individual levels of happiness determined by their temperaments and only temporarily move away from these levels after bad and good events, has been labeled the "setpoint" hypothesis, and was advanced by Headey and Wearing (1992) as well as the Minnesota twin study group. Headey and Wearing attributed the stability in people's happiness to the repetitive nature of the events they experienced because of their personalities.

Both the idea of adaptation to life circumstances and the important influence of genetically based predispositions on happiness reflect major milestones of understanding in the field. Adaptation is a force that, over time, can dampen the effects of both good and bad events and circumstances, and genetic differences between people represent some of the strongest influences leading to the individual differences in happiness. However, these findings have sometimes led to a belief in an extreme form of genetic determinism in which all long-term differences in well-being are thought to be caused by inborn temperament. This myth frequently has been reported by journalists and the media. Although people do vary in their predispositions to experience positive and negative emotions and moods, there are a number of problems with a setpoint theory that maintains that genes are all that matter for long-term subjective well-being.

Substantial evidence now indicates that the extreme setpoint theory, in which circumstances do not matter in the long run, is untenable. For example, there are significant differences between nations in happiness ratings (Diener & Suh, 2000), which closely map onto the objective conditions in nations (e.g., Diener, Diener, & Diener, 1995; Economist Intelligence Unit, 2006). Furthermore, many of these differences in subjective well-being have persisted for decades, belying the idea that people invariably adapt to all conditions over time (Inglehart & Klingemann, 2000). We also now know that people with serious health conditions that interfere with the activities of everyday life, such as quadraplegia, on average report lower levels of well-being than others (e.g., Lucas, 2007; Dijkers, 1997). Even in the classic Brickman et al. (1978) study that is cited to support the hedonic treadmill, individuals with spinal-cord injuries were substantially less happy than others. Contrary to a widespread misconception, the spinal-cord-injured sample did report significantly lower current happiness than the lottery winners. Although the Brickman et al. study found that lottery winners were not significantly happier than a comparison group, this finding might be due in part to the fact that the sample size was small. In another larger study of lottery winners, Smith and Razzell (1975) found that the winners were significantly happier and healthier than the comparison group, which was matched on other demographic factors besides income.

Although genetically influenced temperament affects happiness in important ways, and while people are likely to adapt to most conditions to some degree, my colleagues and I (Diener, Lucas, & Scollon, 2006) point to another important shortcoming in the setpoint account—people's long-term levels of happiness *can* and *do* change. Fujita and I (2005) found that over a period of many years, about one-quarter of a large sample changed significantly in baseline levels of life satisfaction. Similarly, Scollon and I (2006) found that there were significant long-term changes in life satisfaction, positive affect, and negative affect for some individuals, both at group and individual levels. Thus, "setpoint" is not destiny.

What might cause long-term changes in subjective well-being? Again, my colleagues and I (Lucas, Clark, Georgellis, & Diener, 2003) found that widowhood can decrease life satisfaction and that this effect can last for many years. Similarly, unemployment (Lucas, Clark, Georgellis, & Diener, 2004) and divorce (Lucas, 2005) can also alter people's levels of life satisfaction. In a large German sample Lucas, Clark, Georgellis, and Diener (2003) discovered that marriage did not produce a long-term change in life satisfaction. They found, however, that some individuals were more satisfied after marriage and some individuals were less satisfied after marriage, and that these conditions sometimes persisted over time. Thus, average levels of well-being following specific events may conceal individual variability in reaction and adaptation to those events. Finally, my colleagues and I (Diener, Lucas, & Scollon, 2006) reviewed evidence showing that different types of subjective well-being may move in different directions at the same time. For example, positive and negative affects might simultaneously increase or decrease, or life satisfaction might increase while positive affect decreases. These findings indicate that there cannot be a single setpoint because different aspects of people's subjective well-being move in different directions. Thus, it is clear that there are limits to the setpoint idea. Now we need to describe the factors that can alter people's long-term baseline levels of various types of well-being versus those circumstances that only temporarily change people's subjective well-being.

Myth 2: Causes of Well-Being Can Be Understood as a Pie Chart of Influences

In Figure 25.2, I present a pie chart that indicates the percentage of variance in an individual's happiness that is due to various causal factors. Please do not spend time studying this figure because such percentages are misleading for a number of reasons.

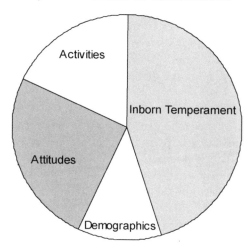

FIGURE 24.2. Misleading pie chart of causes of happiness.

One misunderstanding of percent of variance figures applied to the causes of human happiness is that the numbers are presented as though they apply to individuals. In other words, 45% an individual's happiness is said to come from inborn temperament, 12% from demographics, and so forth. The percent figures are derived, however, from the amount of variance between individuals that is "explained" or predicted by specific variables. These numbers tell us little about the absolute importance of the variables, because people in a sample may or may not differ to the same degree on each of them, and they do not tell us how individuals would change in well-being if they were to change on these variables. It is inappropriate to interpret the figures as applying to how much an *individual's* subjective well-being is derived from the various causes because the numbers are derived from *variation between people in specific samples*. The percents might be interpreted to mean that if one were to improve one's demographics from terrible to great, one's happiness might increase by 12%, but this is a misunderstanding of what the figures mean. It is important to recognize that the percent of variance between individuals, due to various causes of happiness, depends on the range and variation between people on this factor, and has no necessary connection to what might be important to altering a person's happiness.

Let me offer analogies to show why the between-subject variance figures do not apply within individuals. If we were to examine income, we might find that people's salaries predict 70% of the variance in household income, because a few people make significant amounts of money from investments. But this does not mean that 70% of an individual's income will come from his or her salary. Percentages applied to aggregates of people may have little to do with how any specific individuals earn money. For many people, virtually all income may come from their salaries, whereas for a few wealthy individuals, virtually none of their income may come from salaries. And if an individual is concerned with how to earn a lot more money, he or she should not think that 70% of income will necessarily come from salary.

Or consider an example of longevity and its causes. People might die of cancer, heart attack, stroke, aortic aneurysm, infant mortality, cirrhosis, accident, suicide, murder, animal attack, parasites, or infection—and we can assign numbers to the causes indicating the percentages of people in the world who die from each. Only a small percentage of people dies due to the parasite causing malaria; nevertheless over a million deaths per year are caused by this parasite. A person living in an area where malaria is particularly devastating would be foolish to ignore precautions against contracting malaria just because the worldwide percentage of deaths due to malaria is very small. Even if the percent figures came from malarial areas, they do not necessarily apply directly to a particular individual, or to how controllable this disease is relative to other causes of death. Thus, the percentage figures do not necessarily tell the individual what he or she should worry about the most or what he or she should do in order to live longer. For example, a person with sickle-cell anemia and good mosquito netting might need to worry little about malaria, even if many locals are dying of it. Similarly, influences on happiness may not tell the individual much about what will make him or her happy; it only tells us about the differences between people in what makes them happy.

Notice, too, that deaths due to some causes are not independent of each other, in that outcomes such as heart attack, stroke, and aortic aneurisms have several of the same underlying causes. Furthermore, "demographic variables" and "unhealthy lifestyles" are not listed as sources of death, although both of them can have a profound influence on the likelihood of contracting certain diseases. How do we divide the variance between deaths due to cirrhosis of the liver versus those due to alcoholism? These variables represent a different level of analysis wherein one cause leads to the other cause. In the same way, in presenting the causes of happiness, it does not make sense to present demographics, activities, and attitudes as separate causes of happiness or as independent of each other. They are variables that represent different levels of analysis and influence each other in complex ways. If variables from different levels of analysis are included, the pie-chart numbers should sum to more than 100! Finally, it can be seen that there are causes of death at the aggregate level that simply do not apply to individuals who are considering how to live a long and healthy life—for instance "infant mortality." In the same way, group statistics about happiness may not apply to an individual.

Happiness is sometimes said to be about one-half heritable, but this statement can easily be misunderstood. It is a descriptive statistic based on particular samples in particular life circumstances and might not apply to other samples—for example, ones in which life circumstances are more variable across people. That is, the "heritability" of happiness is not constant across samples. This point surprises some people because they do not realize that heritability is not the same as genetic effects.

Pie-chart numbers sometimes lead researchers to view some variables as being more important than other variables, and this is often mistaken. Furthermore, these figures are sometimes offered to the public as a guide to what might be most worthwhile to change in order to achieve greater happiness. However, the causes for change in an individual's happiness might diverge from what causes differences in happiness between individuals. For instance, one person might gain an enormous boost in happiness from becoming religious, even if the amount of individual differences in happiness due to religion in a population is modest. The pie-chart way of thinking is seductive, because it is clear and simple, but it can easily lead us to think about the causes of subjective well-being in misguided ways.

Imagine for a moment that income accounts for 4% of the variance in happiness in the United States. Even if only 4% of subjective well-being could be predicted by income, this prediction would encompass all individuals and all levels of income—which would not tell us how the richest and poorest might differ. If an individual were to apply the figures, erroneously, to him- or herself, he or she might think that his or her happiness would increase by 4% if he or she won a large lottery, but this is not what the findings indicate. If the person is poor, his or her well-being might increase much more than 4%. On the other hand, if the person enjoys a simple life and has few material aspirations, his or her happiness might not increase at all. The percent of variance figures derived from sample statistics do not apply to individuals.

We have adopted pie charts because they simplify things for the public, but the simplification is too great; we should not communicate numbers that can so easily mislead.

Myth 3: Money Does Not Correlate with Happiness

Although it has sometimes been said that happiness researchers have discovered that money is not important to subjective well-being, the connection between money and happiness is more intricate than that statement implies. People in rich nations are, in fact, higher in average subjective well-being than those in very poor nations. In addition, the richest of individuals is, on average, substantially higher in life satisfaction than the poorest individual, even in wealthy nations. Small correlations result from the large variability in happiness between individuals but do not indicate trivial mean-level differences between rich and poor. Another oversimplified belief is that there is little or no effect of income beyond a certain point, such as $10,000 per year (the most often-quoted figure). In fact, the place that the well-being line starts to rise less steeply depends on the sample used and on the particular dependent variable that is examined, so that the inflection point of the slope varies across studies.

In Figure 25.3 I show the life satisfaction levels of adults around age 37 who entered college in 1976 (see Diener, Nickerson, Lucas, & Sandvik, 2002). The lines show the percent of individuals by income who are dissatisfied (*very dissatisfied* and *somewhat dissatisfied* combined) and those respondents who reported being *very satisfied*. As can be seen, the relation between income and life satisfaction is not trivial. Further, as is often the case, the relation between income and life satisfaction is stronger as one rises out of poverty than at high levels of income. However, one obtains a somewhat different picture in examining dissatisfaction versus high satisfaction. For dissatisfaction, there is a sharp decline and then a relatively flat line. Levels of dissatisfaction are much higher in the lowest income group compared to the highest income groups. The line for high life satisfaction continues upward across the income groups, thus suggesting the possibility that different subjective well-being variables would show different patterns with income. As shown in the figure, high life satisfaction occurs twice as frequently in the high-income group compared to the low-income group. Thus,

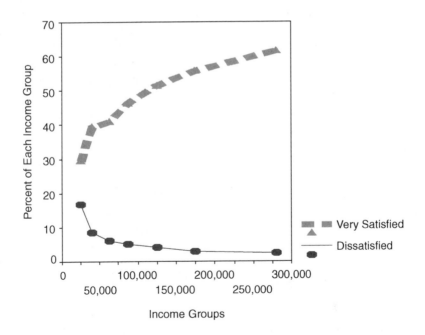

FIGURE 24.3. Income and life satisfaction.

although mean differences might not always seem large, income and well-being can show a substantial relation when examined in certain ways.

The percent of dissatisfied individuals in the poorest group is about 17, whereas only about 2% of the richest individuals are dissatisfied—an eightfold decrease. In contrast, whereas 29% of the poorest individuals say they are *very satisfied*, 62% of the richest individuals do so—over twice the proportion. The correlation between income and life satisfaction in this sample is .16. Thus, the percentage figures for rich versus poor may give a different impression of the strength of the relation of income and subjective well-being than does the correlation. The findings described above are similar to those reported by myself and a colleague (Diener & Biswas-Diener, 2002), who found that several times as many poor people as affluent people had a negative affect balance score, being higher on negative affect than on positive affect. Although the correlation between income and subjective well-being in wealthy nations is often in the .15–.20 range, the ratio of unhappiness among the poor versus the rich was 3 in one sample and 8 in the other. If poor people were three times or eight times more likely to die of cancer or heart disease, a national scandal would ensue, suggesting that the differences in subjective well-being are not trivial.

Another instance in which well-being variables can be influenced differently by income is the gap between life satisfaction and daily reporting of moods (Kahneman, Krueger, Schkade, Schwarz, & Stone, 2006). Kahneman et al. found that respondents with higher income were significantly more satisfied with their lives. However, when computing happiness by multiplying individuals' ratings of happiness in various activities by the amount of time spent in those activities, they did not find individuals with higher incomes to be happier. Richer individuals spent more time working, and because lower happiness scores were reported in work compared to leisure, the respondents with higher income did not experience higher time-adjusted happiness scores for the day. We currently have little understanding of why income might influence one form of subjective well-being but not another, although Kahneman et al. suggest that it is how people direct their attention differently when various types of measures are administered.

Money is related to subjective well-being in complex ways. As incomes in societies rise over time, the effects usually have been small or even nonexistent. In contrast, the differences between wealthy and impoverished nations, as well as between rich and poor individuals, are in some cases substantial, at least when analyzed by percentages rather than by correlations. Correlations are often low because there is a lot of variability within many income groups, but an examination of aggregated mean differences often reveals substantial differences between extreme income groups.

It is likely that income is related to happiness in part because people with high subjective well-being are more likely to earn high levels of income. Thus, much of the data do not indicate the causal influence of money on well-being.

Much more research is needed on this topic. The point I am emphasizing, however, is that the relation between money and happiness is not as small as is sometimes claimed; it is intricate and may be considerable.

People with little money may be able to experience high well-being in a culture such as the traditional Maasai (Biswas-Diener, Vitterso, & Diener, 2005), but they are likely to do less well in the mainstream of a wealthy society—for example, homeless individuals in California (Biswas-Diener & Diener, 2006). Thus, the effects of income on happiness must be taken within the context of a person's life. Money may not be the royal road to happiness, in part because of rising aspirations due to the rising incomes of one's reference group (Clark, Frijters, & Shields, 2006), and in part because money cannot fulfill certain human needs. However, we cannot assume that money matters little or not at all for happiness, and we need to be keenly aware that, in some instances, the differences between rich and poor are substantial.

A brief comment on the deleterious effects of materialism is also in order. Although early research showed that materialistic people were less happy than others, the correlation was virtually assured by the items in the early materialism measures. These measures, for example, included items that were saturated with neuroticism, such as worrying about one's material goods. In later research materialism was sometimes defined as valuing material goods and money more than other things, such as love or social relationships. The difficulty with this assessment of materialism is that it confounds the importance placed on money with the importance placed on other factors and therefore is not a pure measure of materialism per se. A "materialist" might be unhappy as a result of not valuing relationships rather than because of overvaluing money. When materialism is assessed simply as the importance placed on money, our findings are more complex regarding the detrimental effects of this state. We found that at particular levels of income, materialists are less satisfied with their lives than nonmaterialists—except at the very wealthiest level of our respondents, an income of $280,000 or more per year (Nickerson, Schwarz, Diener, & Kahneman, 2003). However, this cross-sectional finding ignores the fact that people who were materialistic were likely to gain more money in life, and this effect offset the effects of materialism. Other recent researchers such as Roberts and Robins (2000) have not found an inverse relation between material aspirations and well-being. Thus, our understanding of the relations between materialism and well-being is incomplete and depends, in part, on how materialism is assessed.

Although recent research shows that the overall relation between income and life satisfaction can be quite small in wealthy nations (Diener & Biswas-Diener, 2002), this is not the whole story. Measures of wealth and consumption can add to the prediction of subjective well-being beyond the effects of income (Headey, Muffels, & Wooden, 2004), and financial resources can buffer people's life satisfaction when problems occur (Johnson & Krueger, 2006). Furthermore, recent research with lottery winners (Gardner & Oswald, 2007) replicates the Smith and Razzell (1975) finding that lotteries can increase well-being. Thus, it is true that rising aspirations can cancel the effects of rising incomes in wealthy societies, but it is a vast oversimplification to assume that rich people do not have higher subjective well-being than poor people!

Myth 4: Correlations Show Causation If There Are Enough of Them

We all learned in our first psychology course that correlation does not equal causation, but we quickly forget this rule when we examine data on subjective well-being. We know that correlation does not prove causation, but we are seduced when we see correlations involving subjective well-being, because it is easy to assume that factors such as marriage or income have a causal influence on well-being. However, we now know that well-being can predate and influence these factors. For example, my colleagues and I (Diener et al., 2002), as well as Cacioppo et al. (Chapter 10, this volume) found that happiness can lead to later higher income. In addition, there is the selection of some individuals and not others into certain roles, such as marriage, which might lead to married people being happier but marriage itself not causing happiness (Lucas et al., 2003). Thus, we must keep reminding ourselves that the correlations between happiness and other variables can often be due to the causation going from well-being to that variable, from the influence of some third factor on both happiness and that variable, or from the self-selection of people into various levels of the independent variable we are examining.

An instructive example of correlated variables and the possible effects of a third variable regards the finding that people who report having more sex also report being happier (Blanchflower & Oswald, 2004). The authors report how much more income it would take to produce as big of an effect on subjective well-being as sex produces—and it is a lot of money. This is all good fun and games, but it may lead many readers to assume that having more sex will increase their happiness; this conclusion is intuitive and might even be correct. But the conclusion is not indicated by the correlational data. Having sex may result from having a steady partner or having a good relationship with one's partner, and this social support could be the cause of both happiness and sex. *Having sex* may be a proxy for good social partnering, lack of psychopathology, or a cheerful, outgoing disposition. Happy people might be more desirable sex partners than those who are unhappy, and thus the causal direction might again be reversed. Therefore, let us tattoo this on the back of our hand: *Hundreds of correlations, even when analyzed with meta-analyses, do not prove causation.*

Myth 5: Context Can Be Ignored

Many factors that influence subjective well-being are likely to have their effects in the broader context of people's lives. For instance, a college student's income is likely to have its influence in the context of parental income. A college student who has zero income but wealthy parents is likely to be well-off materially. In contrast, a college student from a very poor home who earns $16,000 a year while in college might be materially poor. Furthermore, money might matter more in some contexts (living in Manhattan) than in other contexts (an Amish person living in Lancaster County, PA).

We presented our longitudinal findings that married people, on average, are happier than the never-married, divorced, widowed, and separated because of selection and because of the boost in life satisfaction around the time of marriage. We were attacked for saying that marriage does not make people happier. It is important to note that we were reporting *averages*. We found that some individuals were more satisfied after marriage, even after a period of years. Furthermore, we analyzed only one sample, albeit a large one. Thus, the effects we found for marriage might not generalize to other groups. However, ours was one of the very few longitudinal studies conducted in this area, out of hundreds, and therefore the influence of selection into marriage in the cross-sectional correlational studies cannot be discounted as a cause of the correlation between marriage and subjective well-being.

What is perhaps most important to note is that the effects of marriage are likely to depend on a person's life context. For people in college, an active social and romantic life is easy without being married; in some older communities, this is likely to be much less true. Thus, the effects of marriage on a person's social life and happiness are likely to vary depending on context and culture. In our longitudinal study we found that less satisfied people were most likely to be helped in the long run by marriage—perhaps their social lives were less good before marriage, and therefore they had more to gain. In a similar vein, it was found in another study that divorce had a stronger negative correlation with well-being in some cultures than in others, although the relation was generally consistent across cultures (Diener, Gohm, Suh, & Oishi, 2000).

When we examine factors such as income, marriage, education, and age, the context of life is likely to be of extreme importance in how these factors are related to subjective well-being. But what are the contextual factors? There are myriad influences—such as values, social structure, cultural patterns, and role expectations—that can influence how these variables play out in people's lives. Returning to the example of the influence of income on happiness, people's goals, values, and expectations are likely to influence how much money they need to be happy. However, the area where they live, the cost of living in that area, and the amount needed to buy goods and services can also vary greatly across cultures and regions. We are now at the point where another correlation between income and subjective well-being is not likely to be hugely helpful to our understanding. What we need now is to understand *under what circumstances money is more and less important, and how much money is needed for quality of life in various circumstances.*

We can extend the question of context to most of the factors that researchers have related to well-being. For example, age is likely to mean different things in different cultures and in different life circumstances. Economists have found that factors such as income equality in a society have an influence on well-being that is moderated by the ideologies people hold about the importance of equality (Alesina, DiTella, & MacCulloch, 2004). It appears that what people believe about the desirability of equality influences the impact that inequality has on their well-being. This finding suggests that we must move beyond a simple input—output model of happiness, in which certain external life circumstances always produce invariant effects on well-being, to a model in which people's beliefs, values, and goals are pivotal.

Myth 6: Uncovering the Happiest Nation Is a Worthwhile Goal

Lists of the best hotels, soaps, cities, and universities have become ubiquitous. It is not surprising, then, that lists of the happiest nations and places have begun to spring up—in one list it is Nigeria (surprisingly), and in other lists it is Sweden, Switzerland, or Ireland. With the shifting top-dogs, who can keep up? The happiness ratings seem to attract sports-like competition. For instance, when I delivered talks in Switzerland and Canada, I was told that each of these populaces is, on average, happier than Americans—suggesting a kind of national "Who is happiest?" competition. Again, this is all good fun and games as long as it is not taken too seriously. When taken as fact, these country rankings can mislead us about the true differences in well-being between nations. Rankings can magnify differences in ratings that are actually quite small. For instance, when ranking cardiac surgeons based on an objective criterion such as the percent of patients who survive for 1 year after surgery, the top cardiac surgeon in a nation could differ from the 100th best surgeon by only a fraction of a percentage point. The rankings of 1 and 100 might suggest a large difference when only a trivial difference, due to chance, actually exists. Error bars of some sort around rankings might help.

Rankings also imply objective differences when, in fact, the differences could be due to spurious factors. For example, small changes over time due to national events, such as an election or a national sports event, could change the rankings of nations that are clustered tightly together at the top. Switzerland might "win" one time, and Sweden the next time, merely due to factors such as how well they are doing in the World Cup competition, because their scores are otherwise so close. Furthermore, there could be small differences in response sets, such as number-use artifacts and the reporting of moods, which can change the rankings when countries are very close in the ratings.

Another serious objection to the use of rankings is that they suggest that "happiness," or subjective well-being, is unidimensional, when in fact we know that there are separable components to it. Because rankings can change depending on which component is analyzed, the question of what nation is "happiest" is oversimplified: "Happiness" can be more than one thing. It is like asking which animal is "longest," when in fact that concept might refer to mass (a blue whale), weight in its natural environment (an elephant), height (a giraffe), or length (a giant squid). An examination of the nation-level data is instructive in this regard (Kuppens, Ceulemans, Timmerman, Diener, & Kim-Prieto, 2006). Kuppens et al. found clear negative and positive emotion factors across nations. If one wanted to know the "happiest" nation, it might be Mexico (the most positive emotions) or Canada (the fewest negative emotions). The unhappiest nation might be Kuwait (the most negative affect), China (the least positive affect), or Iran (the worst affect balance). I examined nation means in the first wave of the World Value Survey because it contained measures of positive and negative affect, as well as life satisfaction. Norway scored at the top on Positive Affect but 10th (out of 43) on Life Satisfaction and 13th on Negative Affect. Switzerland scored first on Life Satisfaction and very low on Negative Affect; however, Switzerland also scored 3rd from the bottom on Positive Affect. Because the Swiss reported little of either positive or negative emotions, their life satisfaction and positive affect score rankings diverged dramatically. Also, although Norway tended toward the top on all three measures, rankings put it at only 10th and 13th on two of them. Thus, the rankings are likely to produce an oversimplified view of the well-being of societies.

I do not mean to imply that some nations are not generally happier than others, even across a number of components of subjective well-being. However, it is important to understand the societal factors that reliably predict national differences in well-being. When the life satisfaction in a broad sample of countries correlates strongly with the average income in those nations, for example, this is a meaningful and potentially important finding. However, the parlor game of trying to pinpoint the happiest nation should be left to the popular media.

Myth 7: Most People Need to Be Happier Than They Already Are

As the field of subjective well-being has gained in popularity, a number of attempts have been made to increase happiness. For individuals who are low in subjective well-being, these interventions might be very desirable. Furthermore, the goal of increasing the long-term components of subjective well-being, such as life satisfaction, are probably worthwhile—who would argue that helping people to like their lives more is not desirable? However, it is open to question whether people should experience greater levels of positive emotions than they already feel. This issue was brought home to me when some people in Scotland said that they were happy enough and did not want American psychologists trying to make them more cheerful.

According to evolutionary theory, emotions evolved for adaptive purposes. Thus, both positive and negative emotions served a useful purpose in the past, and we need to examine whether they serve a purpose now. Most people in industrialized nations claim to be happy—above neutral most of the time in their moods and emotions (Diener & Diener, 1996). Furthermore, emotion theorists maintain that feelings of anger, fear, and sadness can all serve an adaptive function under some circumstances. Thus, it is not self-evident that all people should necessarily be happier than they are. Perhaps most people feel a functional combination of positive and negative emotions and do not need more positive emotions to function well. Certainly, some individuals may already be at an optimal level for optimal functioning. Although it seems likely that there are large numbers of individuals who might profit from more positive emotions and fewer negative emotions, we have virtually no research on this question. Thus, attempts to increase happiness are proceeding in the dark to some degree, without knowledge of how many people might want to be happier or how many people might function better if they were happier. Although happy people are, on average, more successful in a number of life domains (Lyubomirsky, King, & Diener, 2005), we do not know whether being happier still will make them more successful or less so.

In a recent paper my colleagues and I (Oishi, Diener, & Lucas, 2006) explored what we called the "optimal" level of happiness—the question of whether people with different levels of subjective well-being were successful in different realms of life. We discovered that extremely happy people are very sociable and seem to be quite successful in the social realm. However, we found that moderately happy people were most successful in certain achievement domains, such as income. Our exploration is preliminary, and much more empirical work is needed on the question of optimal levels of subjective well-being. Such work is imperative in light of the increasing attempts to increase levels of happiness.

Future Directions

In the preceding sections, I suggest that researchers in the field of well-being have sometimes seized on certain answers to questions because the answers are simple and easy to understand, when, in fact, accurate answers are much more complex and context-dependent. My intent is not to criticize but to prevent a rush to premature judgment. If our future studies on well-being are designed with an understanding of the myths I described above, they should provide more sophisticated questions and answers.

Where is the field of subjective well-being research headed in the future? After two decades of rapid progress, can we maintain the pace? I believe we can, but researchers need to be ambitious and take risks. Settling into the ways already trodden and essentially replicating past research with minor extensions will doom the field to atrophy. Thinking that integrates findings from other fields, such as sociology, experimental psychology, and neurobiology, is needed. In addition, more ambitious methods are now needed, such as larger and more in-depth studies than were usually conducted in the past.

Several future directions derive directly from understanding the myths I described above. For example, exposing the myth that the setpoint is unchanging leads to the conclusion that we need theories of within-person change as well as longitudinal findings on which to base those theories. We need much more data on context and how it moderates the influence of factors such as marriage or income. There are so many promising directions for research that I hesitate to focus on only a few. Nonetheless, here are three directions that I believe are important.

More Sophisticated Methods Are a Must

Because the field of subjective well-being grew primarily out of the sociological survey research tradition, one-time surveys based on brief self-reports of well-being are the most frequent method used. As the editor of *Journal of Happiness Studies*, I was inundated with submissions relying on one-time self-report surveys, and rarely received papers using more sophisticated methodologies. These methods have served us well but have clear limitations. Similarly, the input variables to well-being that have been emphasized so far are demographic variables and income and marriage. We now need more studies that include a broader set of input and contextual variables, as well as more diverse measures of subjective well-being, including biological, experience sampling, nonverbal, behavioral, and informant report assessments. Some argue that only self-report measures can assess subjective well-being because it is a subjective phenomenon. What they do not understand is that verbal self-reports are no more inherently tied to subjective feelings than are the other types of measures. What people say or write about their experience is not a direct measure of that experience; it is only a communication about that experience. Therefore, biological or nonverbal measures can also be used to index subjective experiences. Like self-reports, they are indirect indicators of subjective experience. Nonetheless, they complement self-report measures in terms of how they capture experience and in the measurement artifacts that are likely to influence them. The convergence and divergence between the various measurement methods can reveal much about the nature of subjective well-being. Thus, although self-reports are likely to remain a primary tool of subjective well-being researchers, they need to be supplemented by other methods.

One of the major discoveries in this field that could benefit from studies with other measures is Norman Bradburn's (1969) findings that positive and negative affect are not opposites of each other, and that different variables correlate with each. We have found that life satisfaction is also separable from the two global types of affect, even though all three forms of well-being correlate across individuals. What we need now is a more thorough analysis of when the various types of well-being converge and diverge. For example, my colleague and I (Diener & Fujita, 2006) examined whether people high in daily positive mood but low in life satisfaction, or people low in daily positive affect but high in life satisfaction, thrive more. Of course, individuals who were high in both forms of well-being were doing best. We found, however, that individuals high only in life satisfaction had more energy, self-confidence, and better health compared to individuals low in life satisfaction but high in daily positive affect. This study points toward a type of research we need much more of: examining what factors differentially predict the various forms of well-being, and how the outcomes of well-being vary depending on which type is examined. There are researchers who advocate the importance of one type of subjective well-being or another. However, what is missing from this discussion are data that shed light on the differential causes and consequences of various types of subjective well-being. There is still an unfortunate tendency in many studies to include only one type of subjective well-being, such as life satisfaction, and this shortcoming should be rectified by including a full range of measures, such as positive affect, negative affect, life satisfaction, and domain satisfactions. In addition, the assessment of both online and recalled affect should prove beneficial. In many instances, one type of well-being may correlate with a factor that other types of well-being do not. Such patterns are illuminating but can only be discovered when the various forms of well-being are assessed.

Some of the most rapid advances in psychology in the next decades are likely to come through neuroscience, immunology, genetics, and other biological approaches. Therefore, it is imperative that subjective well-being researchers learn to include biological methods in their studies. However, we also need conceptual models that recognize that different measures assess different aspects of subjective well-being (e.g., Dolan & White, 2006; Kim-Prieto, Diener, Tamir, Scollon, & Diener, 2005).

Researchers in the field also need to use many more experimental and longitudinal studies. These other methods are needed because we have already plumbed the depths of simple correlations in cross-sectional surveys. We need experimental and longitudinal studies to more deeply explore causal pathways and processes. An important first step is for researchers to understand that the methods of the past will not produce the biggest advances in the future. Studies that assess the causes of well-being need to assess, more frequently, the psychological processes that are thought to lead from the inputs to well-being.

Outcomes of Subjective Well-Being and Optimal Levels

For decades, researchers have been concerned with the causes of subjective well-being, and only recently has interest been shown in the outcomes of well-being. Although there is a robust laboratory tradition on the outcomes of induced moods and emotions, very little research has been conducted on the outcomes of long-term well-being. In 2005, my colleagues and I (Lyubomirsky et al.) reviewed the extant research in this area. Similarly, Pressman and Cohen (2005) examined the outcomes of positive affect on health, and Judge, Thoresen, Bono, and Patton (2001) examined the effects of worker satisfaction on job outcomes. Nonetheless, we have barely scratched the surface of how various types of well-being influence behavior and success in life.

Understanding Adaptation and What Can Change People's "Setpoint"

In former times, we asked what might make people happier. The realization that many things might make people happier in the short run but that adaptation is likely to occur over time led to a new question: Are there variables that can lead to a change in setpoint, to long-term changes in subjective well-being? If there are such factors, what are the processes that make them long-lasting?

The flip side of questions regarding changing the setpoint of "happiness" are issues regarding what causes adaptation or habituation. How much is active coping involved and to what extent is adaptation dependent on automatic habituation processes that occur regardless of a person's intentions and choices? Recent work on attitude change, the expression of gratitude, meditation, and so forth, suggest that specific efforts to increase feelings of subjective well-being can be effective, but we need much more research on this issue. When do such efforts produce long-term change, and when are the effects temporary? In terms of society, what improvements and progress are likely to produce increases in subjective well-being, and to which are people likely to habituate?

Studying More Than Life Satisfaction or Global Happiness

In the past, we hoped that various measures of well-being would converge. To some degree, there is convergence among different measures (e.g., Sandvik, Diener, & Seidlitz, 1993), but we know that various types of measures also diverge to some extent (Kahneman et al., 2006; Kim-Prieto et al., 2005; Oishi & Sullivan, 2006; Thomas & Diener, 1990; Wirtz, Kruger, Scollon, & Diener, 2003). Rather than being a matter of concern, this divergence can be a source of information that gives us greater insight into the nuanced nature of subjective well-being. For example, at times, global subjective well-being predicts future behavior better than momentary online well-being. Thus, future research needs to use a broader array of measures with a more complete set of variables—including life satisfaction—but also momentary positive and negative moods, and satisfaction with various life domains. Furthermore, we need to focus on more than the topic of which people are happiest—we also need to study other ways of analyzing feelings of well-being, such as the activities in which people feel most positive. For example, my colleagues and I (Pavot, Diener, & Fujita, 1990) found that both extraverts and introverts experience more positive affect in social compared to nonsocial situations, and Kahneman et al. (2006) analyzed moods within specific activities. Because people's moods and satisfaction vary across domains and activities, it is not sufficient to focus only on which individuals are, on average, happiest.

Conclusions

A number of oversimplifications and misunderstandings have crept into our beliefs about subjective well-being, and some of these myths are probably driven by our values. We want friends to matter more than money, and we do not want to defend materialism. We also desire to simplify our findings for the public. The danger is that our oversimplifications will become accepted by researchers because they are repeated so frequently. As researchers we must be critical, and this includes a skeptical stance toward our own conclusions. We want to improve society by making our findings widely known, but we must take care not to be hasty in rushing to conclusions to meet the demand for media coverage.

The chapters in this volume help point the directions for future research on well-being. They present studies based on sophisticated designs and review the past research in the field of subjective well-being. The authors of this book do much to dispel the myths I describe. I am proud to be a colleague of the outstanding set of authors represented in this volume, and I am grateful for the creativity and sophistication they bring to the field. Eid and Larsen have brought together an outstanding group of authors, and I am honored to write the concluding chapter.

The field of subjective well-being research has grown at a rapid pace, and for this I am grateful. However, the field has reached a point of saturation for certain types of descriptive cross-sectional studies. We now need to use more sophisticated methods in the study of well-being, such as multimethod measurement, longitudinal designs, and measures of context and psychological processes. I have worked in this field for 25 years and have seen such rapid progress that it substantially boosts my life satisfaction. I hope for even more progress in the next 25 years!

References

Alesina, A., DiTella, R., & MacCulloch, R. (2004). Inequality and happiness: Are Europeans and Americans different? *Journal of Public Economics*, *88*, 2009–2042.

Biswas-Diener, R., & Diener, E. (2001). Making the best of a bad situation: Satisfaction in the slums of Calcutta. *Social Indicators Research*, *55*, 329–352.

Biswas-Diener, R., & Diener, E. (2006). The subjective well-being of the homeless, and lessons for happiness. *Social Indicators Research*, *76, 185–205.*

Biswas-Diener, R., Vitterso, J., & Diener, E. (2005). Most people are pretty happy, but there is cultural variation: The Inughuit, the Amish, and the Maasai. *Journal of Happiness Research*, *6*, 205–226.

Blanchflower, D. G., & Oswald, A. J. (2004). Money, sex, and happiness: An empirical study. *Scandinavian Journal of Economics*, *106*, 393–415.

Brickman, P., & Campbell, D. T. (1971). Hedonic relativism and planning the good society. In M. H. Appley (Ed.), *Adaptation-level theory: A symposium* (pp. 287–302). New York: Academic Press.

Brickman, P., Coates, D., & Janoff-Bulman, R. (1978). Lottery winners and accident victims: Is happiness relative? *Journal of Personality and Social Psychology*, *36*, 917–927.

Clark, A. E., Frijters, P., & Shields, M. A. (2006). *Relative income, happiness and utility: An explanation for the Easterlin Paradox and other puzzles.* Manuscript submitted for publication.

Diener, E., & Biswas-Diener, R. (2002). Will money increase subjective well-being? A literature review and guide to needed research. *Social Indicators Research*, *57*, 119–169.

Diener, E., & Diener, C. (1996). Most people are happy. *Psychological Science*, *7*, 181–185.

Diener, E., & Diener, M. (1995). Cross-cultural correlates of life satisfaction and self-esteem. *Journal of Personality and Social Psychology*, *68*, 653–663.

Diener, E., Diener, M., & Diener, C. (1995). Factors predicting the subjective well-being of nations. *Journal of Personality and Social Psychology*, *69*, 851–864.

Diener, E., & Fujita, F. (2006). *Hedonists versus saints: Happy days versus a satisfying life.* Unpublished paper, University of Illinois at Urbana–Champaign.

Diener, E., Gohm, C. L., Suh, E., & Oishi, S. (2000). Similarity of the relations between martial status and subjective well-being across cultures. *Journal of Cross-Cultural Psychology*, *31*, 419–436.

Diener, E., Lucas, R., & Scollon, C. N. (2006). Beyond the hedonic treadmill: Revising the adaptation theory of well-being. *American Psychologist*, *61*, 305–314.

Diener, E., Nickerson, C., Lucas, R. E., & Sandvik, E. (2002). Dispositional affect and job outcomes. *Social Indicators Research*, *59*, 229–259.

Diener, E., & Suh, E. M. (Eds.). (2000). *Culture and subjective well-being* Cambridge, MA: MIT Press.

Dijkers, M. (1997). Quality of life after spinal cord injury: A meta-analysis of the effects of disablement components. *Spinal Cord, 35*, 829–840.

Dolan, P., & White, M. (2006). Dynamic well-being: Connecting indicators of what people anticipate with indicators of what they experience. *Social Indicators Research, 75*, 303–333.

Economics of happiness: Change and decay. (2005, August 27). *Economist, 376*(8441), 58.

Fujita, F., & Diener, E. (2005). Life satisfaction setpoint: Stability and change. *Journal of Personality and Social Psychology, 88*, 158–164.

Gardner, J., & Oswald, A. J. (2007). Money and mental well-being: A longitudinal study of medium-sized lottery winners. *Journal of Health Economics, 26*, 49–60.

Headey, B., & Wearing, A. (1992). *Understanding happiness: A theory of subjective well-being.* Melbourne, Victoria, Australia: Longman Cheshire.

Inglehart, R., & Klingemann, H. D. (2000). Genes, culture, democracy, and happiness. In E. Diener & E. M. Suh (Eds.), *Culture and subjective well-being* (pp. 165–184). Cambridge: MIT Press.

Johnson, W., & Krueger, R. F. (2006). How money buys happiness: Genetic and environmental processes linking finances and life satisfaction. *Journal of Personality and Social Psychology, 90*, 680–691.

Judge, T. A., Thoresen, C. J., Bono, J. E., & Patton, G. K. (2001). The job satisfaction–job performance relationship: A qualitative and quantitative review. *Psychological Bulletin, 127*, 376–407.

Kahneman, D., Krueger, A. B., Schkade, D., Schwarz, N., & Stone, A. A. (2006). Would you be happier if you were richer?: A focusing illusion. *Science, 312*, 1908–1910.

Kim-Prieto, C., Diener, E., Tamir, M., Scollon, C., & Diener, M. (2005). Integrating the diverse definitions of happiness: A time-sequential framework of subjective well-being. *Journal of Happiness Studies, 6*, 261–300.

Kuppens, P., Ceulemans, E., Timmerman, M. E., Diener, E., & Kim-Prieto, C. (2006). Universal intracultural and intercultural dimensions of the recalled frequency of emotional experience. *Journal of Cross-Cultural Psychology, 37*, 491–515.

Lucas, R. E. (2005). Time does not heal all wounds: A longitudinal study of reaction and adaptation to divorce. *Psychological Science, 16*, 945–950.

Lucas, R. E. (2007). Long-term disability is associated with lasting changes in subjective well-being: Evidence from two nationally representative longitudinal studies. *Journal of Personality and Social Psychology, 92*, 717–730.

Lucas, R. E., Clark, A. E., Georgellis, Y., & Diener, E. (2003). Reexamining adaptation and the set point model of happiness: Reactions to changes in marital status. *Journal of Personality and Social Psychology, 84*, 527–539.

Lucas, R. E., Clark, A. E., Georgellis, Y., & Diener, E. (2004). Unemployment alters the set-point for life satisfaction. *Psychological Science, 15*, 8–13.

Lykken, D. (1999). *Happiness: What studies of twins show us about nature, nurture, and the happiness set-point.* New York: Golden Books.

Lykken, D., & Tellegen, A. (1996) Happiness is a stochastic phenomenon. *Psychological Science, 7*, 186–189.

Lyubomirsky, S., King, L., & Diener, E. (2005). The benefits of frequent positive affect: Does happiness lead to success? *Psychological Bulletin, 131*, 803–855.

Nickerson, C., Schwarz, N., & Diener, E. (2006). *Financial aspirations, financial success, and life satisfaction: Who? And How?* Manuscript submitted for publication.

Nickerson, C., Schwarz, N., Diener, E., & Kahneman, D. (2003). Zeroing in on the dark side of the American dream: A closer look at the negative consequences of the goal for financial success. *Psychological Science, 14*, 531–536.

Oishi, S., Diener, E., & Lucas, R. E. (in press). Can people be too happy? Optimal levels of subjective well-being. *Perspectives on Psychological Science.*

Oishi, S., & Sullivan, H. W. (2006). The predictive value of daily vs. retrospective well-being judgments in relationship stability. *Journal of Experimental Social Psychology, 42*, 460–470.

Oswald, A. J. (2006). *On the common claim that happiness equations demonstrate diminishing marginal utility of money.* Unpublished manuscript, Warwick University.

Pavot, W., Diener, E., & Fujita, F. (1990). Extraversion and happiness. *Personality and Individual Differences, 12*, 1299–1306.

Pressman, S. D., & Cohen, S. (2005). Does positive affect influence health? *Psychological Bulletin, 131*, 925–971.

Roberts, B. W., & Robins, R. W. (2000). Broad dispositions, broad aspirations: The intersection of personality traits and major life goals. *Personality and Social Psychology Bulletin, 26*, 1284–1296.

Sandvik, E., Diener, E., & Seidlitz, L. (1993). Subjective well-being: The convergence and stability of self-report and non-self-report measures. *Journal of Personality, 61*, 317–342.

Scollon, C. N., & Diener, E. (2006). Love, work, and changes in extraversion and neuroticism over time. *Journal of Personality and Social Psychology, 91*, 1152–1165.

Smith, S., & Razzell, P. (1975). *The pools winners.* London: Caliban Books.

Tellegen, A., Lykken, D. T., Bouchard, T. J., Wilcox, K. J., Segal, N. L., & Rich, S. (1988). Personality similarity in twins reared apart and together. *Journal of Personality and Social Psychology, 54*, 1031–1039.

Thomas, D. L., & Diener, E. (1990). Memory accuracy in the recall of emotions. *Journal of Personality and Social Psychology, 59*, 291–297.

Wirtz, D., Kruger, J., Scollon, C. N., & Diener, E. (2003). What to do on spring break?: The role of predicted, on-line, and remembered experience in future choice. *Psychological Science, 14*, 520–524.

Author Index

515

Subject Index

Abundance scenario, 313–315, 314*t*
Academic functioning, school satisfaction and, 381
Acceptance, religiosity and, 327–328
Accommodation, pursuit of happiness and, 442
Achievement, happiness and, 301–302
Activity
    determinants of subjective well-being and, 496–499, 497*f*
    overview, 19
Adaptations
    future research and, 510
    goals and, 438–440, 443
    impediments to subjective well-being and, 63–67
    myths regarding subjective well-being and, 495, 507
    to negative events, 270–278
    to positive events, 278–281
    to promote well-being, 72–74
    relative standards and, 317
Adolescents
    life satisfaction and, 383
    parent–child relationships and, 355–357
    sibling relationships and, 361–362
Affect
    appraisals of subjective well-being and, 48–49
    attachment and, 353
    gratitude and, 472–474

    job satisfaction and, 395–396
    life satisfaction and, 31
    tranquility and, 38
Affect Balance Scale, 116, 126–127
Affective cues, momentary independence and, 115
Affective well-being
    measurement of, 142–144, 142*f*
    relation of with cognitive well-being, 116–117
    structure of, 108–115
Affectometer 2, 127
Age
    determinants of subjective well-being and, 7
    happiness and, 200–201, 201*t*, 215
    priming and, 225
    religiosity and, 325
Aggregation approach, 154
Aggression, venting and, 275
Aging
    family relationships and, 366–367
    life satisfaction and, 196–197
Agreeableness
    cognitive-motivational conflict and, 229–230
    determinants of subjective well-being and, 6
    disposition of happiness and, 199–200, 199*t*
    overview, 185–186
    school satisfaction and, 381–382
    social comparison and, 252